WB
18
ZOL

...shown below.

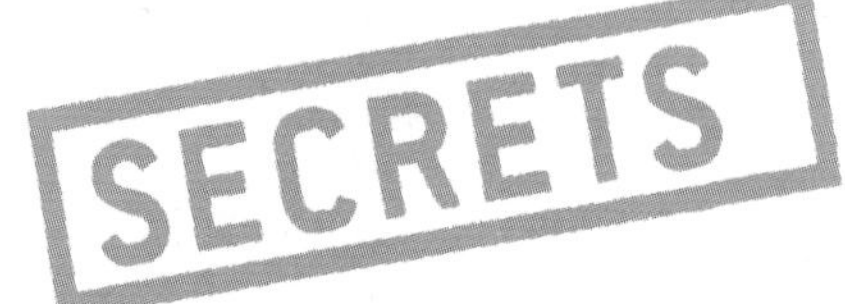

MEDICAL SECRETS

Fourth Edition

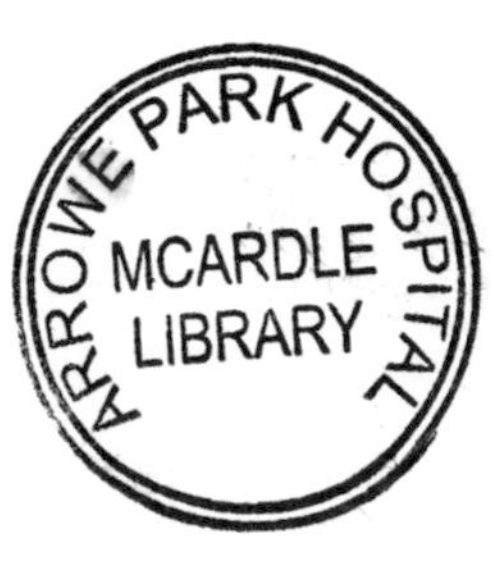

Anthony J. Zollo, Jr., M.D.
Assistant Professor
Department of Internal Medicine
Baylor College of Medicine
Houston, Texas
Chief Medical Officer
Department of Veterans Affairs Outpatient Clinic
Lufkin, Texas

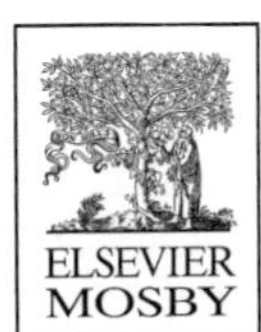

ELSEVIER
MOSBY
An Affiliate of Elsevier

The Curtis Center
170 S Independence Mall W 300E
Philadelphia, Pennsylvania 19106

Medical Secrets
Fourth Edition

ISBN: 1-56053-387-0

Copyright © 2005, 2001, 1996, 1991 by Elsevier Inc. All rights reserved.

No part of this publication may be reproduced or transmitted in any form or by any means, electronic or mechanical, including photocopying, recording, or any information storage and retrieval system, without permission in writing from the publisher. Permissions may be sought directly from Elsevier's Health Sciences Rights Department in Philadelphia, PA, USA: phone: (+1) 215 238 7869, fax: (+1) 215 238 2239, e-mail: healthpermissions@elsevier.com. You may also complete your request on-line via the Elsevier homepage (http://www.elsevier.com), by selecting "Customer Support" and then "Obtaining Permissions."

NOTICE

Medicine is an ever-changing field. Standard safety precautions must be followed, but as new research and clinical experience broaden our knowledge, changes in treatment and drug therapy may become necessary or appropriate. Readers are advised to check the most current product information provided by the manufacturer of each drug to be administered to verify the recommended dose, the method and duration of administration, and contraindications. It is the responsibility of the licensed prescriber, relying on experience and knowledge of the patient, to determine dosages and the best treatment for each individual patient. Neither the publisher nor the author assumes any liability for any injury and/or damage to persons or property arising from this publication.

Previous editions copyrighted 2001, 1996, 1991.

Library of Congress Cataloging-in-Publication Data

Medical secrets/[edited by] Anthony J. Zollo Jr.–4th ed.
p. ; cm.
Prev. ed. published by Hanley & Belfus, c2001.
Includes bibliographical references and index.
ISBN 1-56053-387-0
1. Internal medicine–Examinations, questions, etc. I. Zollo, Anthony J., 1954-[DNLM: 1. Internal Medicine–Examination Questions. WB 18.2 M4885 2005]
RC58.M43 2005
616'.0076–dc22

2004057889

Acquisitions Editor: Linda Belfus
Developmental Editor: Stan Ward
Publishing Services Manager: Joan Sinclair
Project Manager: Cecelia Bayruns

Printed in the United States of America.

Last digit is the print number: 9 8 7 6 5 4 3 2 1

CONTENTS

CONTRIBUTORS

Holly H. Birdsall, M.D., Ph.D.
Associate Professor, Departments of Otorhinolaryngology and Immunology, Baylor College of Medicine; Associate Chief of Staff for Research, Michael E. DeBakey VA Medical Center, Houston, Texas

Rhonda A. Cole, M.D.
Assistant Professor of Medicine, Gastroenterology Section, Baylor College of Medicine; Chief, Therapeutic Endoscopy, Michael E. DeBakey VA Medical Center, Houston, Texas

Charlene M. Dewey, M.D., F.A.C.P.
Associate Professor of Medicine, Baylor College of Medicine, Houston, Texas

Jane M. Geraci, M.D., M.P.H.
Assistant Professor of Medicine, Department of General Internal Medicine, University of Texas Ambulatory Treatment and Emergency Care, Division of Internal Medicine, M.D. Anderson Cancer Center, Houston, Texas

Sheila Goodnight-White, M.D.
Associate Professor of Medicine, Baylor College of Medicine; Director, Pulmonary/Critical Care Service, and Associate Chief, Medical Service, Michael E. DeBakey VA Medical Center, Houston, Texas

Gabriel B. Habib, M.D.
Associate Professor, Division of Cardiology, Department of Medicine; Associate Chief and Director of Education, Section of Cardiology, Baylor College of Medicine, Houston, Texas

Richard J. Hamill, M.D.
Professor of Medicine and Microbiology and Immunology, Department of Medicine, Baylor College of Medicine; Michael E. DeBakey VA Medical Center, Houston, Texas

Mary P. Harward, M.D.
St. Joseph Hospital, Orange, California

Teresa G. Hayes, M.D., Ph.D.
Assistant Professor of Medicine and Hematology and Oncology, Baylor College of Medicine; Attending Physician, Hematology-Oncology Section, Michael E. DeBakey VA Medical Center, Houston, Texas

Christopher J. Lahart, M.D.
Division of Infectious Diseases, Department of Internal Medicine, Baylor College of Medicine; Michael E. DeBakey VA Medical Center, Houston, Texas

Martha P. Mims, M.D., Ph.D.
Assistant Professor, Hematology-Oncology Section, Department of Medicine, Baylor College of Medicine, Houston, Texas

Sharma S. Prabhakar, M.D.
Associate Professor, Division of Nephrology, Department of Internal Medicine, Texas Tech University Health Sciences Center, Lubbock, Texas

Wayne J. Riley, M.D., M.B.A.
Vice-President & Vice Dean and Assistant Professor of Medicine, Baylor College of Medicine, Houston, Texas

Loren A. Rolak, M.D.
Director, Marshfield Clinic Multiple Sclerosis Center, Marshfield, Wisconsin; Clinical Professor of Neurology, University of Wisconsin Medical School, Madison, Wisconsin

Roger D. Rossen, M.D.
Professor, Departments of Immunology and Internal Medicine, Baylor College of Medicine; Chief, Immunology, Allergy and Rheumatology Section, Michael E. DeBakey VA Medical Center, Houston, Texas

Richard A. Rubin, M.D.
Department of Immunology, Baylor College of Medicine; Immunology, Allergy, and Rheumatology Section, The Methodist Hospital, Houston, Texas

Sarah E. Selleck, M.D.
Professor, Departments of Immunology and Internal Medicine, Baylor College of Medicine, Houston, Texas

Samuel A. Shelburne III, M.D.
Department of Medicine, Baylor College of Medicine; Michael E. DeBakey VA Medical Center, Houston, Texas

Mark M. Udden, M.D.
Associate Professor of Medicine, Hematology Oncology Section, Baylor College of Medicine; Chief, Hematology Service, Ben Taub General Hospital, Houston, Texas

Whitney W. Woodmansee, M.D.
Division of Endocrinology, Department of Medicine, University of Colorado Health Sciences Center, Denver, Colorado

Anthony J. Zollo, Jr., M.D.
Assistant Professor, Department of Internal Medicine, Baylor College of Medicine, Houston, Texas; Chief Medical Officer, Department of Veterans Affairs Outpatient Clinic, Lufkin, Texas

PREFACE

The art of Internal Medicine involves questions. It involves questions asked when taking a medical history, when forming a differential diagnosis, or when planning a diagnostic and therapeutic plan. Students of Internal Medicine, regardless of their level of training, are constantly confronted with questions posed from patients, from mentors, and from within themselves. The time-honored, question-based, Socratic approach to teaching is alive and well in the academic and clinical world of Internal Medicine. This book is intended to provide the reader with many of the questions (and answers) commonly encountered in training.

The knowledge base of Internal Medicine is substantial, probably more than any other specialty. Its acquisition is the goal of medical students, house officers, and all others who endeavor to learn and practice the discipline. Many formal textbooks of Internal Medicine provide complete coverage of all topics within the field. This work is not meant to replace the use of those texts. Rather, it is intended to focus on the lead-in questions and topics commonly encountered on teaching rounds, in clinical situations, and in examinations.

In preparing this book, we have attempted to take a middle ground between over-simplification and over-complication. We have included questions on common subjects and on "zebras," which, owing to their academic interest, are frequently discussed. We are grateful to our patients, our teachers, and our students for these questions and answers.

The editing of the each edition of this book has been an act of love. The tasks of assembling a team of contributors and editing the overall manuscript were thoroughly enjoyable, albeit very time-consuming. As editor, I am indebted to my contributors for their efforts in this enjoyable and educational undertaking. Only by utilizing the talents of experts in various subspecialties, with up-to-date knowledge of current developments, was it possible to complete this book. We are all proud of the finished product.

Anthony J. Zollo, Jr., M.D.

TOP 100 SECRETS

These secrets are 100 of the top board alerts. They summarize the most important concepts, principles, and most salient details of internal medicine. Secrets appear in the order in which the topic is covered in the main text.

1. The treatment of severe sepsis syndrome should be based on efficient resuscitation, effective antimicrobial therapy, elimination of secondary infections, euglycemia, early targeted and specific drug therapy, and establishment of therapeutic goals.

2. Acute pulmonary embolism (PE) is a difficult diagnosis to establish despite newer advances in imaging; approximately 50% of cases are diagnosed post mortem.

3. In the approach to suspected PE, keep in mind the prudent use of key diagnostic tests: (1) rapid D-dimer by ELISA is an effective screening test; (2) chest CT can help detect most PEs; and (3) a negative Doppler venous ultrasound of the legs does not exclude the diagnosis of PE.

4. The most common etiologic agent implicated in acute bacterial meningitis in the U.S. is *Streptococcus pneumoniae.*

5. In the newly diagnosed HIV patient, in addition to routine adult immunizations, immunizations against pneumococcal pneumonia, influenza, and both hepatitis A and B are indicated.

6. Metabolic syndrome is diagnosed on the basis of abdominal obesity, hypertriglyceridemia, low HDL cholesterol levels, hypertension, and fasting hyperglyceima.

7. Pituitary tumors cause problems for patients by two main mechanisms: mass effect, which applies pressure to surronding structures, and endocrine hyperfunction, which results in excessive secretion of a particular anterior pituitary hormone.

8. A key concept in evaluating patients with hyperfunctioning endocrine tumors is that biochemical diagnosis should *always* precede anatomic localization.

9. The best initial screening test for evaluation of thyroid status is the TSH, since it is the most sensitive measure of thyroid function in the majority of patients. The one exception is patients with pituitary/hypothalamic dysfunction, in whom TSH cannot reliably to assess thyroid function.

10. The most common presentation of hypogonadism is erectile dysfunction and decreased libido in men and amenorrhea and infertility in women.

11. All patients with coronary artery disease (CAD), CAD-equivalent diseases, or diabetes should be treated aggressively to reach the LDL-cholesterol target of 100 mg/dL.

12. Diabetics and patients with vascular disease should be treated with a statin lipid-lowering drug to prevent heart disease and stroke, regardless of the blood low-density lipoprotein (LDL) cholesterol level, age (from 40 to 79 years), or gender.

13. The goal blood pressure is < 130/80 mmHg in hypertensive subjects with diabetes mellitus and/or chronic kidney disease.

14. The single most life-saving treatment strategy in patients with acute ST-elevation myocardial infarction is to rapidly achieve complete reperfusion of the infarct-related artery by mechanical (balloon angioplasty or stenting) or pharmacologic means (thrombolysis).

15. Angiotensin-converting enzyme inhibitors (or angiotensin receptor blockers) and beta-adrenergic blockers are effective in reducing cardiovascular complications and improving survival in patients with systolic heart failure and are recommended in all patients with no contraindications to these drugs.

16. Noninvasive stress testing has the best predictive value for detecting CAD in patients with an intermediate (30–80%) pretest likelihood of CAD and is of limited value in patients with very low (< 30%) or very high (> 80%) likelihood of CAD.

17. In patients with *Coccidioides immitis* infections, higher titers of complement-fixing antibodies suggest more extensive disease, and rising titers suggest worsening disease.

18. Patients who present with flaccid paralysis during the summer months should be evaluated for West Nile virus infection.

19. A febrile patient with rash who presents to the emergency department during May to September in the South Atlantic and West South Central states should receive empirical doxycycline therapy for suspected Rocky Mountain spotted fever.

20. Community-acquired methicillin-resistant *Staphylococcus aureus* that is susceptible to clindamycin but resistant to erythromycin should not be treated with clindamycin because of the possibility for induction of resistance.

21. In patients with disseminated candidiasis, IV catheters should be removed and ophthalmologic examinations performed to evaluate for the presence of retinal disease.

22. Transmission of *Borrelia burgdorferi* (the causative agent of Lyme disease) from an infected *Ixodes* tick to a susceptible human requires the tick to have fed on the human for at least 40 hours.

23. Porcelain gallbladder is an incidental finding, more common in women who have gallstones. Because up to 50% of patients develop gallbladder carcinoma, prophylactic cholecystectomy is recommended.

24. Three liters of Coca-Cola administered via nasogastric lavage over a 12-hour period can dissolve gastric bezoars. It is thought that the cola acidifies the gastric contents and liberates carbon dioxide in the stomach, resulting in the disintegration of phytobezoars.

25. Regardless of what is done, GI bleeding stops spontaneously in about 80% of patients.

26. Patients with hereditary nonpolyposis colorectal cancer syndrome have a higher-than-average risk of developing colon and gastric cancer.

27. About 90% of patients with primary sclerosing cholangitis have underlying ulcerative colitis, but less than 10% of all patients with ulcerative colitis have primary sclerosing cholangitis.

28. In patients with suspected perforation, the minimum amount of free air that can be detected on an upright chest x-ray is 12 mL.

29. The three major openings in the diaphragm through which hernias may occur are the esophageal hiatus (most common), foramen of Bochdalex (3–5%, usually left-sided), and foramen of Morgagni (rare).

30. In a patient who has a malignancy involving the right hilum, look at the hand veins. If the veins in the hands are distended and do not collapse when the arms are lifted over the head, there is a high chance of superior vena cava obstruction.

31. In high-risk patients, the chance of developing breast cancer can be reduced by about 50% with the use of tamoxifen.

32. If a patient with lung cancer presents with hoarseness, look for vocal cord paralysis, a sign of mediastinal involvement (recurrent laryngeal nerve) that renders the patient inoperable.

33. Patients with head and neck cancer have a 30% chance of developing another cancer somewhere in the aerodigestive tract (head and neck, lung, or esophagus), especially if they continue to smoke and drink.

34. If a patient presents with hypercalcemia, look for a squamous cell cancer (lung, esophagus, head and neck, cervix, anus).

35. Up to 15% of breast cancers may not be detectable by mammogram. If the patient has a clinically suspicious lump, perform a biopsy.

36. The presence of bilateral small kidneys in a patient with azotemia confirms chronic renal failure.

37. In a diabetic patient with proteinuria, the presence of concomitant retinal disease suggests strongly (90% correlation) that the renal manifestations are due to diabetes.

38. Treatment of anemia of chronic renal failure by recombinant human erythropoietin is highly effective, but correction of iron deficiency and iron supplementation by oral or intravenous route is simpler, cheaper, and often by itself effective therapy.

39. In resistant hypertension, especially in younger (< 20 yr) or older (> 70 yr) patients, consider and rule out renovascular hypertension.

40. New onset of nephrotic proteinuria in an elderly patient warrants exclusion of an underlying malignancy.

41. The principal mechanism of bicarbonate reabsorption in the proximal tubule is through Na^+-H^+ exchanger (NHE3) activity.

42. D-lactic acidosis is characterized by increased serum anion gap, metabolic acidosis, and episodic encephalopathy in patients with short bowel syndrome.

43. Ethylne glycol (antifreeze) toxicity is characterized by high anion gap metabolic acidosis, neurotoxicity in the form of ataxia, seizures, and calcium oxalate crystals in the urine.

44. Bartter's syndrome is a disorder associated with normotensive hyperaldosteronism, secondary to juxtaglomerular hyperplasia, hypokalemic metabolic alkalosis, and severe renal potassium wasting.

45. Hyperkalemia is an important side effect of both ACE inhibitors and ARBs, but the problem is less frequent and smaller in magnitute with ARBs because of their less pronounced effects on aldosterone levels.

46. Hypochromic microcytic anemias are the most frequently encountered anemias in hospitalized and ambulatory patients.

47. Both iron-deficiency anemia and anemia of chronic disease have a low transferrin saturation. In iron-deficiency anemia, the TIBC is often increased, whereas anemia of chronic disease is marked by an unusually low TIBC.

48. The main clinical manifestations of sickle hemoglobinopathies are hemolytic anemia, chronic end-organ damage, periodic vaso-occlusive disease ("crises"), and hyposplenism.

49. The triad of thrombocytopenia, fragmentation hemolysis, and fluctuating neurologic signs suggests thrombotic thrombocytopenic purpura (TTP), perhaps the most spectacular of the fragmentation syndromes.

50. The cytogenetic marker of chronic myelogenous leukemia is the 9:22 translocation, in which portions of the long arms of chromosomes 9 and 22 are exchanged, resulting in a shortened 22 or Philadelphia chromosome (Ph^1). Some patients with acute lymphoblastic leukemia (ALL) also have 9:22 translocations—a poor prognostic marker in ALL.

51. The classic cell seen in the lymph nodes of patients with Hodgkin's disease is the Reed-Sternberg (RS) cell, a large cell with two nuclei, each possessing a distinct nucleolus.

52. Secondary monoclonal gammopathy must be distinguished from the monoclonal gammopathy associated with multiple myeloma, benign monoclonal gammopathy of uncertain significance, solitary plasmacytoma, amyloidosis, lymphoma, and Waldenström's macroglobulinemia.

53. Deep venous thrombosis in a young person, a family history of thrombosis, thrombosis at unusual sites (such as the mesenteric vein), or recurrent thrombosis without precipitating factors suggests a hypercoagulable state.

54. Any condition that leads to V/Q mismatching can cause hypoxemia. Most pulmonary disorders are associated with some degree of V/Q mismatching. This is the most common cause of hypoxemia and is responsive to oxygen therapy.

55. Assuming that you are at sea level and breathing room air, an easy way to calculate the A-a difference is as follows: (150–40/0.8)—PaO_2 measured by ABG.

56. Although the anterior segment of the upper lobes may be affected by TB, a lesion found only in the anterior segment suggests a diagnosis other than TB (e.g., malignancy).

57. Incidence of lung cancer now exceeds breast cancer in women. Women develop lung cancer at an earlier age and after fewer years of smoking.

58. Pleural fluid glucose < 30 mg/dL and pH < 7.30 suggest rheumatoid effusion, TB, lupus, or malignancy.

59. Mesothelioma, a pleural malignancy associated with asbestosis exposure, is not associated with tobacco use.

60. Early, aggressive intervention with disease-modifying antirheumatic drugs reduces the morbidity (deformity leading to reduced functionality and disability) and mortality associated with rheumatoid arthritis.

61. Antinuclear antibody (ANA) titers are not associated with activity of disease.

62. COX_2 NSAIDs are no more efficacious than older standard NSAIDs but are significantly less toxic.

63. A patient with low positive rheumatoid factor (RF) and arthralgia should be checked for hepatitis C, which can produce a low-grade synovitis and cryoglobulins (which in turn can produce a falsely positive RF).

64. Always check for Sjögren's antibodies (SSA/SSB) and phospholipid antibodies in a young woman with lupus before conception. Sjögren's antibodies increase the risk of neonatal lupus (rash, thrombocytopenia, heart block), and phospholipid antibodies can significantly increase the risk for miscarriage, premature labor, or intrauterine growth delay.

65. Packed red cells in freshly acquired blood may include lymphocytes that can mount a graft-versus-host reaction if the patient's own immune system is unable to rapidly kill and inactivate these transfused allogeneic leukocytes.

66. Intranasal steroids are the single most effective drug for treatment of allergic rhinitis. Decongestion with topical adrenergic agents may be needed initially to allow corticosteroids access to the deeper nasal mucosa.

67. The clinical manifestations of anaphylaxis include flushing, sense of foreboding, urticaria or angioedema, pruritus, hoarseness, stridor, bronchospasm, hypotension, tachycardia, nausea, vomiting, abdominal pain, diarrhea, headache, and syncope.

68. ACE inhibitors are often-forgotten causes of angioedema and chronic cough.

69. Chronic urticaria may require treatment with a combination of both H_1 and H_2 antihistamines, reflecting the distribution of these receptors in the skin. Work-up for an allergic etiology is rarely informative.

70. Beta blockers should be avoided whenever possible in patients with asthma because they may accentuate the severity of anaphylaxis, prolong its cardiovascular and pulmonary manifestations, and greatly decrease the effectiveness of epinephrine and albuterol in reversing the life-threatening manifestations of anaphylaxis.

71. HIV infection is preventable and treatable but never curable.

72. If you are thinking of mononucleosis as a diagnosis, think about and test for HIV.

73. Adherence to anti-HIV therapy must be > 95% for a durable response. HIV treatment guidelines change frequently—always verify your information.

74. A person under care for HIV should not develop pneumocyotic carinii pneumonia (PCP). It is entirely preventable.

75. There is a critical interaction between HIV and tuberculosis. When one infection is present, you must look for the other.

76. If you have diagnosed one sexually transmitted disease (STD), you must consider others, especially HIV.

77. Most back pain is not caused by a radiculopathy.

78. The most common cause of dizziness is benign paroxysmal positional vertigo.

79. The leading causes of death after a stroke are medical complications, not the stroke itself.

80. Heparin has no value in the acute treatment of strokes.

81. The sudden onset of a severe headache may indicate an intracranial hemorrhage.

82. Coma is usually caused by medical problems, not neurologic ones.

83. Elective surgery should be postponed for further evaluation if the patient has signs or symptoms of unstable or inadequately treated chronic disease.

84. Patients who have undergone coronary revascularization within 5 years of a proposed elective surgery and have no signs or symptoms of recurrent ischemia can usually undergo surgery without further evaluation.

85. Acute dyspnea in a patient who has had major surgery should raise the suspicion of pulmonary embolism, even if the patient has received prophylaxis.

86. All patients who take oral agents for diabetes may continue them until the day of surgery unless they have chronic liver or renal disease or are on a first-generation sulfonylurea. In these cases the oral agent should be held at least several days in advance of the surgery.

87. Pacemakers and implanted cardioverters/defibrillators should be assessed both before and after surgery, radiation therapy, or lithotripsy.

88. Surgery patients on any antiplatelet agent should be told when to stop the medication before surgery and when to resume it afterward to minimize perioperative bleeding.

89. Strict bed rest is not needed for the treatment of acute lumbosacral strain.

90. Influenza virus vaccination reduces hospitalization and death from influenza and its complications in elderly and high-risk patients.

91. Always examine the feet and pedal pulses of diabetic patients regularly, looking for ulcerations, injury, or reduced blood flow.

92. Closely monitor patients with blood pressure measurements defined as "prehypertension," and encourage lifestyle changes to prevent progression to hypertension.

93. Reduce the risk of hip fracture in elderly and high-risk patients with calcium and vitamin D supplements, exercise prescription, hip pads, and medications to treat osteoporosis, when indicated.

94. Assess a woman's risk of coronary disease, stroke, thromboembolism, and breast cancer before prescribing estrogen/progesterone therapy in menopause.

95. Older adults currently constitute the fastest-growing population in the United States—a trend that is expected to continue for the foreseeable future.

96. Commonly used instruments for a comprehensive geriatric assessment include the Mini Mental State Exam, the Geriatric Depression Scale, activities of daily living, instrumental activities of daily living, and assessment of stability and mobililty (e.g., Tinnetti or "Get Up and Go" test).

97. Dementia and short-term memory loss are not caused by aging.

98. Delirium carries tremendous mortality and morbidity rates and should be identified, worked up aggressively, and treated as any medical emergency.

99. Diastolic dysfunction, as distinct from systolic dysfunction, results from impaired relaxation in heart failure with preserved ejection fraction and may account for half of all cases of heart failure in people over 80. Although the symptoms of diastolic and systolic dysfunction may be similar, the traditional therapy for systolic dysfunction can actually worsen ventricular filling and increase the risk of orthostasis and syncope in cases of diastolic dysfunction.

100. Fifteen percent of elderly patients who fall and fracture a hip report prior falls. It is essential to ask about falls, assess for fall risk, and then act accordingly, given the significant mortality and morbidity of hip fractures.

GENERAL INTERNAL MEDICINE

Wayne J. Riley, M.D., M.B.A., Charlene M. Dewey, M.D., and Anthony J. Zollo, Jr., M.D.

1. List the principles of "diagnostic roundsmanship."

1. Common things occur commonly.
2. The race may not always be to the swift nor the battle to the strong, but it's a good idea to bet that way.
3. When you hear hoofbeats, think of horses, not zebras.
4. Place your bets on uncommon manifestations of common conditions rather than common manifestations of uncommon conditions.

Matz R: Principles of medicine. NY State J Med 77:99–101, 1977.

2. List the predominant organisms constituting the normal flora of the human body.

See Table 1-1.

TABLE 1-1. ORGANISMS CONSTITUTING NORMAL FLORA OF THE HUMAN BODY

Oropharynx	**Lower genitourinary tract**	**Skin**
Streptococcus viridans (α-hemolytic)	Staphylococci	Staphylococci (including *S. aureus*)
Staphylococci	Streptococci (including enterococci)	Corynebacteria
Streptococcus pyogenes	Lactobacilli (vaginal)	Propionibacteria
Streptococcus pneumoniae	Corynebacteria	*Candida* sp.
Moraxella catarrhalis	*Neisseria* sp.	*Malassezia furfur*
Neisseria sp.	Obligate anaerobes	Dermatophytic fungi
Lactobacilli	Aerobic gram-negative bacilli	**Large intestine and feces**
Corynebacteria	*Candida albicans*	Obligate anaerobes (including *B. fragilis*)
Haemophilus sp.	*Trichomonas vaginalis*	Aerobic gram-negative bacilli
Obligate anaerobes (not *Bacteroides fragilis*)	**Conjunctiva**	Streptococci (including enterococci)
Various protozoa	Staphylococci	*C. albicans*
Upper intestine	Corynebacteria	Various protozoa
Streptococci	*Haemophilus* sp.	
Lactobacilli	**Nasopharynx**	
Candida sp.	Staphylococci (including *S. aureus*)	
	Streptococci (including *S. pneumoniae*)	
	M. catarrhalis	
	Neisseria sp.	
	Haemophilus sp.	

Adapted from Rosebury T: Microorganisms Indigenous to Man. New York, McGraw-Hill, 1962, pp 310–384, and Mackowiak PA: The normal microbial flora. N Engl J Med 307:83–93, 1982.

3. What malignancies commonly metastasize to bone?

Metastasis to bone often comes from malignancies in the lungs, kidneys, prostate, thyroid, or breast and from soft tissue sarcomas. The "benzene ring" in Figure 1-1 is a simple way to remember the most common "metastisizers" to bone. The ring portion represents the human body. Cancers are arrayed in rough anatomic position of their site of metastasis.

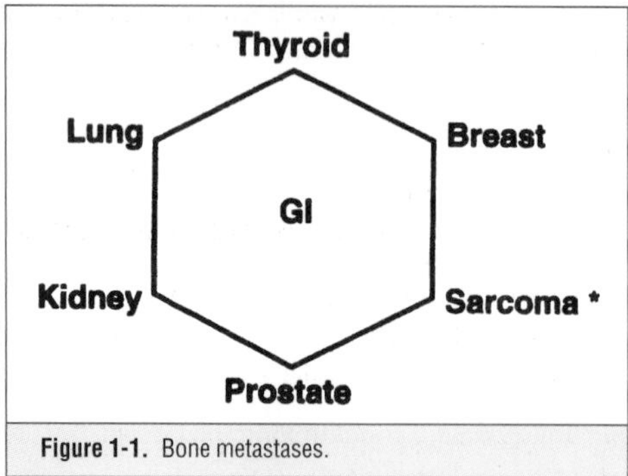

Figure 1-1. Bone metastases.

4. List the risk factors for thromboembolism.

- Age greater than 40 years
- Heart conditions: myocardial infarction (MI), atrial fibrillation, cardiomyopathy, and congestive heart failure (CHF)
- Postoperative states: especially abdominal or pelvic operations; splenectomy, orthopedic procedures of the lower extremities: total hip or knee replacements
- Neoplastic diseases, especially adenocarcinomas of lung, breast, viscera
- Fractures, especially of the pelvis, hip, and leg
- High estrogen states: pregnancy and parturition
- Prolonged immobilization or paralysis
- Previous deep venous thrombosis (DVT)/pulmonary embolism (PE)
- Nephrotic syndrome
- Inflammatory bowel disease
- Femoral vein catheters
- Varicose veins
- Drugs, especially oral contraceptives and estrogens
- Hyperviscosity syndromes and abnormal flows
- Myeloproliferative disorders with thrombocytosis, polycythemia vera
- Antithrombin III deficiency
- Protein C and protein S deficiencies
- Activated protein C resistance (factor V Leiden)
- Abnormal fibrinolysis
- Disorders of plasminogen and plasminogen activation
- Antiphospholipid antibodies and lupus anticoagulant
- Heparin-induced thrombocytopenia
- Hyperhomocystinemia
- Others: obesity, hemorrhage after strokes (CVA)

Clagett, GP et al: Prevention of venous thromboembolism. Chest 114(5)S:531S–560S, 1998.

5. **How is prothrombin time (PT) standardized for monitoring patients on anticoagulant therapy with warfarin?**
The International Normalization Ratio (INR) system standardizes PT for different thromboplastin reagents, thus providing a universal standard by which to compare any given laboratory's results with that of the World Health Organization standard. The INR is calculated as follows:

$$INR = (\text{patient PT}/\text{normal PT})^{ISI}$$

where normal PT = mean PT of the target population (in sec) and ISI = International Sensitivity Index (provided with each batch of thromboplastin reagent).

6. **List potential problems with the INR system.**
   1. Lack of reliability when used at the onset of warfarin therapy and when used to screen for a coagulopathy in patients with liver disease
   2. Relationship between precision of the INR determination and the reagent ISI
   3. Effect of instrumentation in ISI values
   4. Lack of reliability of the ISI result provided by the manufacturer
   5. Incorrect calculation of the INR resulting from the use of inappropriate control plasma
   6. Problems with citrate concentrations and interference with lupus anticoagulants with thromboplastins with low ISI values

   Hirsh J: Oral anticoagulants: Mechanism of action, clinical effectiveness, and optimal therapeutic range. Chest 114(Suppl 5):445S–469S, 1998.

7. **What is the appropriate response to an elevated INR < 5 without bleeding?**
No rapid reduction in anticoagulant medication is needed. The appropriate strategy is to decrease the dose or to skip the next dose.

8. **Give the appropriate responses to an INR of 5–9 without bleeding.**
Three approaches are recommended, depending on risk of bleeding and urgency:
   1. Omit the next 1–2 doses and monitor the INR. Restart the medication at lower dose if there is no increased risk of bleeding.
   2. Omit the next dose and monitor the INR. Administer vitamin K_1 (1–2.5 mg orally) if the risk of bleeding is increased.
   3. For urgent scenarios (e.g., dental surgery, urgent surgery), give vitamin K_1 (2–4 mg orally). After 24 hours, check the INR. If it is still high, give another 1–2 mg of vitamin K_1.

9. **What is the appropriate response to an INR > 9 without bleeding?**
Give vitamin K_1 (3–5 mg orally). Monitor the INR, and repeat the dosage of vitamin K_1, if needed, in 24–48 hours.

10. **What should be done if the patient has serious bleeding or an INR > 20?**
Give vitamin K_1, 10 mg by slow IV infusion, and supplement with fresh plasma transfusion or prothrombin complex. Concentrate may be needed, depending on urgency. This protocol may need to be repeated at 12 hours if indicated by the INR.

11. **Give the appropriate response to a life-threatening bleed or serious warfarin overdose.**
Administer prothrombin complex concentrate, supplemented with 10 mg of vitamin K_1 by slow IV infusion. This protocol can be repeated, if indicated by subsequent INR.

12. **What should be done if warfarin is to be continued after a high dose of vitamin K_1?**
Heparin can be used until the effects of vitamin K_1 are reversed and the patient becomes responsive to warfarin therapy.

Hirsh J: Oral anticoagulants: Mechanism of action, clinical effectiveness, and optimal therapeutic range. Chest 114 (Suppl 5):445S–469S, 1998.

13. Which drugs are known to alter warfarin clearance?

Warfarin clearance is altered when drugs interact or inhibit the S-isomer or R-isomer form of warfarin. The S-isomer is most important due to its strong anti–vitamin K potential. Drugs that inhibit the S-isomer can seriously potentiate its effect and prolong the PT. Drugs that inhibit the S-isomer include amiodarone, metronidazole, trimethoprim-sulfamethoxazole, phenylbutazone, sulfinpyrazole and disulfuram. Drugs that inhibit the R-isomer, resulting in less potentiation of the PT, include cimetidine and omeprazole.

14. Which drugs inhibit the effect of warfarin?

Drugs that can inhibit the effect of warfarin and may result in the need for higher doses include barbiturates, carbamazepine, cholestyramine, rifampin, sucralfate, griseofulvin, nafcillin, chlordiazepoxide, and food with large amounts of vitamin K. Other drugs such as acetaminophen, anabolic steroids, and erythromycin can potentiate the warfarin anticoagulant effect via unknown mechanisms.

Kelly WN (ed): Textbook of Internal Medicine, 3rd ed. Philadelphia, Lippincott-Raven, 1997, p 574.

Hirsh J: Oral anticoagulants: Mechanism of action, clinical effectiveness, and optimal therapeutic range. Chest 114(suppl 5):445S–469S, 1998.

15. What are the benefits and limitations of the available screening tests for DVT and thromboembolism?

See Table 1-2.

16. What is the differential diagnosis of DVT?

Blood vessel disorders

- Panniculitis
- Lipodermatosclerosis
- Chronic venous insufficiency
- Varicose veins
- Superficial thrombophlebitis
- Neoplasm
- Hematoma
- Arterial aneurysm

Orthopedic disorders

- Ruptured popliteal membrane
- Ruptured Baker's cyst
- Ruptured calf muscle or tendon
- Severe muscle cramp
- Bone fracture
- Arthritis
- Compartment syndrome

Infection

- Cellulitis
- Joint sepsis

Lymphatic disorders

- Lymphedema
- Lymphangitis

Others

- Neuropathy
- Reperfusion edema
- Paralyzed limb
- Genealized edematous state

TABLE 1-2. BENEFITS AND LIMITATIONS OF SCREENING TESTS FOR DEEP VENOUS THROMBOSIS (DVT) AND THROMBOEMOBLISM

Study	PPV/NPV	Benefits	Limitations
Contrast venography	Gold standard, 100% sensitive and specific	Highly specific, useful from IVC to calf	Invasive, painful, and expensive; therefore not first line. Contra-indicated in renal failure and chronic renal insufficiency
Venous ultrasound	Sensitivity: 80–100% Specificity: 86–100% PPV: 92–100%	Highly accurate for proximal DVT, noninvasive; allows differentiation of fresh versus old DVT; compression with venous imaging has best prediction, portable	Insensitive for DVT suspected in the calf; reader-dependent, less accurate for chronic DVT, massive obesity, severe edema, casts
Impedance plethys-mography	Sensitivity: 93% Specificity: 94%	Reliable for proximal DVT; excellent screening test when used with I^{125}-labeled fibrinogen scan; less expensive and portable; non-invasive; no radiation exposure	Insensitive for calf; sensitivity/specificity dependent on adherence to study protocol; potential false positives; cannot be used to assist with other potential diagnoses
I^{125}-labeled fibrinogen scan (symptomatic)	Sensitivity: 56% Specificity: 84%	Sensitive for calf and distal thigh DVT	Insensitive for proximal and iliac vein thrombosis; may not become positive until 72 hours; cannot be used with leg casts or bandages
D-dimer (ELISA, e.g., VIDAS DD)	Sensitivity: 94–100% NPV: 92–100%	Minimally invasive; suggests thrombus; acts as marker of activation of coagulation; newer tests are rapid, costly	Negative D-dimer (normal level) cannot rule out DVT; nonspecific; currently not endorsed for widespread use in screening; restrict to low–moderate risk patients; can be timely

(*continued*)

TABLE 1-2. BENEFITS AND LIMITATIONS OF SCREENING TESTS FOR DVT AND THROMBOEMOBLISM *(continued)*

Study	PPV/NPV	Benefits	Limitations
Latex (e.g., SimpleRed)	Sensitivity: 89–100% NPV: 95–100%	Minimally invasive; rapid, economical	Subjective; nonspecific; currently not endorsed for widespread use in screening; restrict to low–moderate risk patients
Spiral (helical) CT	Sensitivity: 64–100% Specificity: 89–97%	Rapid; noninvasive; actually identifies thrombus; identifies other disease states; can be used in face of abnormal chest films; can provide alternative causes for symptoms; possibly cost effective	Cannot detect emboli in subsegmental pulmonary arteries where up to 36% of emboli are located; use as a "rule-in" study; cannot rule out secondary to unable to detect in the subsegmental areas; expensive, reader-dependent
MRI	Sensitivity: near 100% Specificity: 90–100%	Demonstrates an actual clot in leg or lung simultaneously; noninvasive; no nephrotoxic iodine; excellent sensitivity/specificity for DVT; safe; can detect alternative diagnoses; no contrast or radiation needed	Limited studies on use; less sensitive for calf and pulmonary emboli; not as sensitive as angiography for pulmonary emboli; insufficient evidence for replacement of previous standards ($\dot{V}/\dot{Q}$ and angiogram) restricted among patients who are claustrophobic, morbidly obese, have metallic implants

IVC = inferior vena cava, PPV = positive predictive value, NPV = negative predictive value, CT = computed tomography, MRI = magnetic resonance imaging.

Kelley WN (ed): Textbook of Internal Medicine, 3rd ed. Philadelphia, Lippincott-Raven, 1997.

Van der Graaf F, et al: Exclusion of deep venous thrombosis with D-dimer testing. Thromb Haemost 83:191–198, 2000.

Gill P, Nahum A: Improving detection of venous thromboembolism. Post Grad Med 108(4):24–40, 2000.

Tapson V: The diagnostic approach to acute venous thromboembolism: Clinical practice guideline. Am J Respir Crit Care Med 160(3):1043–1066, 1999.

17. **List the differential diagnoses of PE.**
   - Pneumonia or bronchitis
   - Exacerbation of chronic obstructive pulmonary disease (COPD)
   - Asthma
   - Acute myocardial infarction (MI)
   - Dissection of the aorta
   - Pericardial tamponade
   - Pulmonary hypertension
   - Lung cancer
   - Pneumothorax
   - Costochondritis
   - Rib fracture
   - Musculoskeletal pain
   - Anxiety

KEY POINTS: DIAGNOSIS OF PULMONARY EMBOLISM 

1. Acute PE is a very difficult diagnosis to establish despite newer advances in imaging.
2. Approximately 50% of cases are diagnosed postmortem.
3. Rapid D-dimer by enzyme-linked immunosorbent assay (ELISA) is an effective screening test.
4. Chest computed tomography (CT) can be helpful in detecting most PEs.
5. A negative Doppler venous ultrasound of the legs does not exclude the diagnosis of PE.

18. **Describe the mechanism by which grapefruit juice causes a clinically significant drug-food interaction.**
Grapefruit juice is an inhibitor of the cytochrome P-450 3A4 system in the intestines. Such inhibitions can lead to elevations in the serum concentrations of many drugs and create conditions that result in lack of drug efficacy and/or supratherapeutic drug levels. The list of drugs affected by concomitant grapefruit juice consumption is long and extensive. Thus, it is prudent to advise patients to "wash down" their medications with water and limit grapefruit juice consumption.
   Kane GC, et al: Drug-grapefruit juice interactions. Mayo Clin Proc 75:933–942, 1999.

19. **What screening tests should be used in the evaluation of a patient with involuntary weight loss?**

Initial testing
Complete blood count
Electrolytes, calcium
Glucose
Urinalysis
Abdominal CT/magnetic resonance imaging (MRI)

Additional testing
HIV test
Upper and/or lower GI endoscopy
Thyroid-stimulating hormone
Chest x-ray
Chest CT scan
Recommended cancer screening

20. **Define sensitivity, specificity, and predictive value of a test. How are they calculated?**
These terms are frequently used in the assessment of a test and its ability to rule in or rule out a given condition (also called the **accuracy** of the test). To use these values, you must understand

how they are derived. Since a test can be positive or negative (if we disregard inconclusive results), and a patient either has or does not have a condition, there are four possible outcomes in any test situation: true positive, false positive, true negative, and false negative. These results are used to calculate sensitivity, specificity, and predictive value (Fig. 1-2).

Last JM: A Dictionary of Epidemiology, 2nd ed. New York, Oxford University Press, 1988.

		Disease: Present	Disease: Absent
Test result	+	a	b
	−	c	d

a = True positive

b = False positive

c = False negative

d = True negative

Sensitivity = $\frac{a}{a+c}$ = Percentage of patients who have the disease and test positive

Specificity = $\frac{d}{b+d}$ = Percentage of persons who do not have the disease and test negative (True-Negative).

Positive predictive value = $\frac{a}{a+b}$ = Percentage of patients who test positive and actually do have the disease.

Negative predictive value = $\frac{d}{c+d}$ = Percentage of patients who test negative and really do not have the disease.

Figure 1-2. Calculation of sensitivity, specificity, and predictive value.

21. Distinguish between the urinary indices of prerenal azotemia and oliguric acute renal failure.

See Table 1-3.

TABLE 1-3. URINARY INDICES OF PRERENAL AZOTEMIA AND OLIGURIC ACUTE RENAL FAILURE

Index	Prerenal Azotemia	Oliguric Acute Renal Failure
BUN/P_{cr} ratio	>20:1	10–15:1
Urine Na (mEq/L)	< 20	>40
Urine osmolality (mosmol/L)	>500	< 350
Fractional excretion of Na	<1%	> 2%
Urine/P_{cr}	> 40	< 20

BUN = blood urea nitrogen, P_{cr} = plasma creatinine, Na = sodium.

22. **List common causes of jaundice in adults.**

Biliary tract obstruction	**Hepatocellular dysfunction**
Gallstones	Hepatitis
Tumor	Viral
Pancreatic neoplasm	Alcohol-induced
CHF	Drug-induced
Hepatocellular carcinoma	Cirrhosis

23. **Outline the current recommendations by the various organizations for colorectal cancer screening in patients who are asymptomatic and not members of a high-risk group.**
See Table 1-4.

TABLE 1-4. RECOMMENDATIONS FOR COLON CANCER SCREENING IN PERSONS AT AVERAGE RISK

American Cancer Society	Starting at age > 50 with either (1) fecal occult blood test (FOBT) yearly plus flexible sigmoidoscopy every 5 years or (2) full colonoscopy every 10 years or double-contrast barium enema (DCBE) every 5–10 years
U.S. Preventive Services Task Force	Starting at age > 50 with annual FOBT or sigmoidoscopy or both.
American College of Physicians	Between 50–70 years with flexible sigmoidoscopy, colonoscopy, or DCBE. FOBT for those who refuse.

From American Cancer Society Colon and Rectum Resource Center at www3.cancer.org and Guide to Clinical Preventive Services, 2nd ed. Report of the US Preventive Services Task Force. Baltimore, Williams & Wilkins, 1996, pp 89–103.

24. **What conditions can lead to false-positive results with the HemOccult Test?**
The HemOccult Slide Test (Smith-Kline Diagnostics) detects the presence of hemoglobin in feces. **False-positive** results can be produced by the dietary intake of rare beef or fruits and vegetables that contain peroxidases. This effect is seen mainly in tests performed on rehydrated stool specimens. Oral iron preparations also have been implicated in some studies but not in others. False-positive results can occur due to blood from sources other than colorectal carcinoma, such as gastric blood loss caused by nonsteroidal antiinflammatory drugs (NSAIDs).

25. **What conditions can lead to false-negative results with the HemOccult Test?**
False-negative results are obtained in patients with colonic neoplasms that are not bleeding (lesions < 1–2 cm, nonulcerated lesions), that bleed intermittently, or that are not producing the 20 mL of blood per day required for a reliably positive result. Stool that is stored prior to testing and large doses of ascorbic acid may also lead to false-negative results.

Fleischer DE, et al: Detection and surveillance of colorectal cancer. JAMA 261:580–586, 1989.

26. **What screening programs for colorectal cancer are recommended for patients in high-risk groups, according to the American Cancer Society?**
See Table 1-5.

TABLE 1-5. AMERICAN CANCER SOCIETY GUIDELINES FOR EARLY DETECTION OF COLORECTAL POLYPS AND CANCER

Risk Category	Recommendations*	Age to Begin	Interval
Family history of familial adenomatous polyposis	Early surveillance with endoscopy, counseling to consider genetic testing and reference to a specialty center	Puberty	If genetic test (+) or polyposis confirmed, consider colectomy, once weekly endoscopy for 1–2 years
Family history of hereditary nonpolyposis colon cancer	Colonscopy and counseling to consider genetic testing	Age 12 yr	If genetic test (+) or if patient has had genetic testing, colonoscopy every 2 years until age 40, then every 1 year
Inflammatory bowel disease	Colonoscopies with biopsies for dysplasia	8 years after start of pancolitis 12–15 years after start of (L) side colitis	Every 1–2 years

*Digital rectal exam should be done at the time of each sigmoidoscopy, colonoscopy, or DCBE.
Copyright American Cancer Society (from www.cancer.org).

27. What is the erythrocyte sedimentation rate (ESR)?

The ESR is a nonspecific index of inflammation. The normal values for patients under age 50 are 0–15 mm/h in men and 0–20 mm/h in women. The normal values increase with age and may be higher in people over age 60, even in the absence of disease. Whether the ESR is normal, increased, or decreased depends on the sum of forces acting on the erythrocytes (RBCs). These forces include the downward force of gravity (dependent on the mass of the RBC), upward buoyant forces (dependent on the density [mass/volume] of the RBC), and bulk plasma flow (created by the downward-moving RBCs).

28. What conditions cause the ESR to increase?

- Inflammatory disorders
- Hyperfibrinogenemia
- Rouleaux formation
- Anemia (hypochromic, microcytic)
- Pregnancy
- Hyperglobulinemia
- Hypercholesterolemia

29. What conditions cause the ESR to decrease?

- Increased serum viscosity
- Hypofibrinogenemia

- Sickle cell disease
- Leukemoid reaction
- Polycythemia
- Spherocytosis
- Anisocytosis
- High-dose corticosteroids
- CHF
- Cachexia

30. Describe the four stages of alcohol withdrawal.

1. **Tremulousness** occurs 8–12 hours after cessation of drinking. The tremor is aggravated by intention or agitation and may be accompanied by nausea and vomiting, insomnia, headache, diaphoresis, tachycardia, and anxiety. The symptoms usually subside within 24 hours, unless the patient progresses to the next stage.
2. **Alcoholic hallucinosis** usually occurs 12–24 hours after the cessation of drinking but may take 6–8 days to develop. Auditory or visual hallucinations alternate with periods of lucidity. The symptoms of the first stage continue and worsen.
3. **Grand mal seizures** ("rum fits") occur in 90% of cases between 6–48 hours after cessation of drinking. The seizures are generalized and usually multiple. This stage occurs in 3–4% of untreated patients.
4. **Delirium tremens** usually occurs 3–4 days after the cessation of drinking but may not develop for up to 2 weeks. It manifests as confusion, hallucinations, tremors, and signs of autonomic hyperactivity (fever, tachycardia, dilated pupils, diaphoresis). It is a medical emergency and carries a mortality of 5–15% despite treatment. Death is usually due to cardiovascular collapse.

31. How quickly can a healthy person clear ethanol from his or her body?

A normal person can metabolize 150 mg of ethanol/kg body weight/h. In a normal 70-kg person, this rate leads to a decrease in blood ethanol level of approximately 20 mg/dL/h.

32. What constellation of symptoms constitutes the Wernicke-Korsakoff syndrome?

This syndrome most commonly occurs in the malnourished, alcoholic patient and includes the following symptoms:

Ocular
Horizontal/vertical nystagmus
Paralysis of conjugate gaze
External rectus muscle paralysis

Ataxia
Stance and gait affected
Cannot walk without assistance

Altered mental status
Alcohol withdrawal
Global confusion (apathetic, inattentive, lethargic, slurred speech, irrational)
Korsakoff's amnesic psychosis
Anterograde amnesia (impairment of learning new ideas)
Past memory disturbances (confabulation)

33. Which laboratory tests should be done in evaluating a person with altered mental status?

- Complete blood count
- Full chemistry panel
- Vitamin B_{12}
- Serum folate
- Urinalysis
- Urine toxicology screen
- Electrocardiogram
- CT scan (in selected patients)
- Electroencephalogram (in selected patients)
- ESR
- Serologic test for syphilis (VDRL)
- Thyroid function tests (thyroid-stimulating hormone, free thyroxine)
- Arterial blood gas
- HIV test
- Lumbar puncture (in selected patients)
- Chest x-ray
- MRI scan (in selected patients)

34. List the metabolic-toxic causes of dementia.

- Anoxia
- Pernicious anemia
- Pellagra
- Folic acid deficiency
- Hypothyroidism
- Bromide intoxication
- Hypoglycemia
- Hypercalcemia associated with hyperparathyroidism
- Organ system failure
  - Hepatic encephalopathy
  - Uremic encephalopathy
  - Respiratory encephalopathy
- Chronic drug-alcohol-nutritional abuse

35. List the structural causes of dementia.

- Alzheimer's disease
- Vascular disease
  - Multi-infarct dementia
- Binswanger's dementia
- Huntington's chorea
- Multiple sclerosis
- Pick's disease
- Cerebellar degeneration
- Wilson's disease
- Amyotrophic lateral sclerosis
- Progressive multifocal leukoencephalopathy
- Progressive supranuclear palsy
- Brain tumor
- Irradiation to frontal lobes
- Surgery
- Normal-pressure hydrocephalus
- Brain trauma
  - Chronic subdural hematoma
  - Dementia pugilistica

36. List the infectious causes of dementia.

- Neurosyphilis (general paresis)
- Tuberculous and fungal meningitis
- Viral encephalitis
- HIV-related disorders
- Gerstmann-Straussler syndrome

37. Summarize the differential diagnosis of delirium (acute confusional state).

See Table 1-6.

38. What are the indications for lumbar puncture?

A lumbar puncture (LP) is extremely useful in determining the diagnosis in a number of disorders affecting the central nervous system (CNS), such as viral, bacterial, and fungal infections; demyelinating disorders (e.g., multiple sclerosis); subarachnoid hemorrhage; malignancies; and other complex CNS disorders such as Guillain-Barré: syndrome. Examination of cerebrospinal fluid (CSF) is the sine qua non for the diagnosis of meningitis in patients presenting with altered mental status, headache, or fever.

www.UpToDate.com

TABLE 1-6. DIFFERENTIAL DIAGNOSIS OF DELIRIUM

NEUROLOGIC

Trauma
Concussion
Intracranial hematoma
Subdural hematoma

Vascular disorders
Multiple infarctions
Right hemisphere or posterior circulation infarcts
Hypertensive encephalopathy
Vasculitis (e.g., systemic lupus erythematosus [SLE] polyarteritis nodosa, giant-cell arteritis)
Air and fat embolism
Subarachnoid hemorrhage

Inflammations
Acute disseminated encephalomyelitis
Postinfectious encephalitis

Neoplasia
Multiple parenchymal metastases
Meningeal carcinomatosis
Midline brain tumors
Brain tumors causing brain stem compression, edema, or hydrocephalus
Paraneoplastic syndromes (limbic encephalitis)

Infections
Meningitis and encephalitis (viral, bacterial, fungal, protozoal)
Multiple abscesses
Progressive multifocal leukoencephalopathy

Epilepsy
Postictal state
Temporal lobe status (complex partial status)

SYSTEMIC

Substrate depletion
Hypoglycemia
Diffuse hypoxia (pulmonary, cardiac, carbon monoxide poisoning)

Metabolic encephalopathy
Diabetic ketoacidosis
Renal failure
Liver failure
Electrolyte, fluid, and acid-base imbalance (especially calcium, sodium, magnesium)
Hereditary metabolic disease (e.g., porphyria, metachromatic leukodystrophy, mitochondrial cytopathy

Vitamin deficiency
Thiamine (Wernicke's encephalopathy)
Nicotinic acid (pellagra)
Vitamin B_{12}

Endocrine, over- or underactivity
Thyroid
Parathyroid
Adrenal

Infection
Septicemia
Malaria
Subacute bacterial endocarditis
Focal infection (e.g., pneumonia)

Thermal injuries
Hypothermia
Heat stroke

Hematologic disorders
Hyperviscosity syndrome
Severe anemia

Toxic causes
Drug and alcohol intoxication (therapeutic, social, illegal)
Drug withdrawal (e.g., alcohol, barbiturates, narcotics)
Chemical toxins (e.g., heavy metals, organic toxins)

(*continued*)

TABLE 1-6. DIFFERENTIAL DIAGNOSIS OF DELIRIUM *(continued)*

PSYCHIATRIC	
Acute mania	Schizophrenia
Depression or extreme anxiety	Hysterical fugue states

From Brown MM, Hachinski VC: Acute confusional states, amnesia, and dementia. In Isselbacher KJ, et al (eds): Harrison's Principles of Internal Medicine, 13th ed. New York, McGraw-Hill, 1994, p 140, with permission.

KEY POINTS: LUMBAR PUNCTURE

1. With new imaging modalities such as CT and MRI, the absolute indications for LP have been narrowed.
2. LP is still the procedure of choice for confirming the presence of a CNS infection and subarachnoid bleed in the setting of a negative CT scan.
3. Bacterial meningitis can be rapidly fatal; thus the administration of empirical IV antibiotics should not be delayed before obtaining imaging studies and performing LP for CSF analysis and culture.

39. Which organisms are implicated in meningitis of the adult?

Streptococcus pneumoniae is the most common cause of bacterial meningitis in the adult, followed by *Neisseria meningitis. Haemophilus influenzae* has decreased in frequency by 82% due to the vaccination available against this organism. A newer epidemic is being seen with antibiotic-resistant strains of *S. pneumoniae.*

Bacterial	**Viral**
S. pneumoniae	Enterovirus (polio, coxsackie, echo)
N. meningitis	Herpes simplex types 1 and 2
H. influenzae	Varicella-zoster virus
Staphylococcus aureus	Adenoviruses
Treponema pallidum	Epstein-Barr virus
Enterobacteriaceae	Lymphocytic choriomeningitis virus
Klebsiella sp.	HIV
Pseudomonas sp.	Influenza virus types A and B
Listeria monocytogenes	**Fungal**
Borrelia burgdorferi	*Cryptococcus neoformans*
Neisseria gonorrhoeae	*Histoplasma capsulatum*
Clostridium sp.	*Coccidioides immitis*
Mycobacterium tuberculosis	*Blastomyces dermatitidis*
Proteus sp.	**Parasites**
Ehrlichia bruella	*Toxoplasma gondii*
	Taenia solium (cysticercosis)

Pruitt AA: Infections of the nervous system. Neurol Clin North Am 16(2):419–447, 1998.

40. How do the CSF findings differ among bacterial, tuberculous, fungal, and viral meningitis?

See Tables 1-7 and 1-8.

TABLE 1-7. CSF FINDINGS IN BACTERIAL AND NONBACTERIAL MENINGITIS

	Bacterial	Viral	Mycobacterial or Fungal
Total cells (per mL)	Usually > 500	Usually < 500	Usually < 500
WBCs	Predominantly PMN	Predominantly mononuclear	Predominantly mononuclear
Glucose (% of blood)	≤ 40%	> 40%	≤ 40%
Protein (mg/dL)	> 50	> 50	> 50
Gram stain	Positive (65–95%)	Negative	Negative

WBC = white blood cell, PMN = polymorphonuclear.

TABLE 1-8. DIFFERENTIAL DIAGNOSIS OF CSF PLEOCYTOSIS

Predominantly Polymorphonuclear (> 90% pmns)	Predominantly Mononuclear (< 90% pmns)
Bacterial meningitis	Viral meningitis or encephalitis
Early viral meningitis	Tuberculous or fungal meningitis
Early tuberculous or fungal meningitis	Partially treated bacterial meningitis
Brain abscess or subdural empyema with rupture into subarachnoid space	Brain abscess or subdural empyema
Chemical arachnoiditis	Listeriosis (variable)
	Neurosyphilis
	Neuroborreliosis (Lyme disease)
	Neurocysticercosis
	Neurosarcoidosis
	Primary amoebic meningoencephalitis
	Guillain-Barré syndrome
	CNS vasculitis, tumor, hemorrhage
	Multiple sclerosis
	Others

From Kelly WN (ed): Textbook of Internal Medicine, 3rd ed. Philadelphia, Lippincott-Raven, 1997, p 2373.

41. Name the five leading etiologies of cerebrovascular disease (stroke).

- Embolism
- Atherosclerotic disease
- Lacunar infarcts
- Hypertensive hemorrhage
- Ruptured aneurysms/arteriovenous (AV) malformation

42. What are the major risk factors for cerebrovascular disease?
Cerebrovascular disease is the third leading cause of adult deaths. The major risk factors include hypertension, hypercholesterolemia, smoking, and cardiovascular disease (particularly atrial fibrillation and recent MI). Other causes include advanced age, diabetes mellitus, migraine headaches, and the use of oral contraceptive agents.

43. What are the types and causes of peripheral neuropathies in adults?
See Table 1-9.

TABLE 1-9. TYPES AND CAUSES OF PERIPHERAL NEUROPATHIES IN ADULTS

Motor	Sensory	Sensorimotor	
Guillain-Barré syndrome	Alcohol	Diabetes mellitus	Alcohol
Porphyria	Diabetes mellitus	Uremia	Inherited neuropathies
Lead poisoning	Vascular disease	Chronic inflammatory polyradiculopathy	Metronidazole
Sulfonamides	Neoplasm	Clofibrate	Colchicine
Amphotericin B	Uremia	Chlorpropamide	Chlorambucil
Dapsone	Arsenic	Phenytoin	Tolbutamide
Imipramine		Nitrofurantoin	Ergotamine
Amitriptyline		Ethambutol	Streptomycin
Gold		Penicillamine	Ethionamide
		Indomethacin	Gold
			Phenylbutazone

From Farrante JA: Focusing on peripheral neuropathies. Emerg Med 22:57–62, 1990.

44. Which cranial nerves (CNs) are commonly affected in tuberculous meningitis?
These CN palsies may be either unilateral or bilateral and most commonly occur in CN VI (abducens, usually bilateral). Palsies may also develop in CN III (oculomotor) > CN IV (trochlear) > CN II (optic).

Johnson JL, Ellner JJ: Tuberculous meningitis. In Evans RW, Baskins DS, Yatsu FM: Prognosis of Neurological Disorders. Oxford, Oxford University Press, 1992.

45. Which common viral illnesses are frequently seen in adults?

- Influenza A > influenza B
- Epstein-Barr virus
- Herpes simplex virus I and II
- Varicella-zoster virus
- Cytomegalovirus
- Respiratory viruses
- Rhinoviruses
- Coronaviruses
- Respiratory syncytial virus
- Parainfluenza virus
- Adenoviruses

46. Which groups are most susceptible to infection by the herpes zoster virus?

- Elderly people (age > 60)
- Patients with Hodgkin's and non-Hodgkin's lymphoma
- Immunocompromised patients (cancer, organ transplant, HIV infection)
- Patients on high-dose steroid therapy

47. Which organism is responsible for the cellulitis of marine workers and fishermen?

Vibrio vulnificus is a ubiquitous, invasive, gram-negative rod found in warm, salty, coastal waters. It is found in zooplankton and shellfish and has been associated with two disease syndromes: (1) sepsis in alcoholics and persons with liver disease and (2) wound infections from minor abrasions and/or lacerations. Advanced cases can result in necrotizing vasculitis and gangrene.

48. What organisms are usually involved in adult viral pneumonia?

Influenza, parainfluenza, RSV, adenovirus, and hantavirus

49. List the organisms commonly involved in community-acquired pneumonia in the following scenarios.

Smoker	*S. pneumoniae, H. influenzae, M. catarrhalis*
Postviral bronchitis	*S. pneumoniae*, rarely *S. aureus*
Alcoholic	*S. pneumoniae*, anaerobes, coliforms
IV drug abuser	*S. aureus*
Epidemics	Legionnaire's disease
Bird handlers	Psittacosis
Rabbit handlers	Tularemia
COPD patients	Anaerobes
No comorbid diseases/risks	Mycoplasma, chlamydia, viral

50. List the organisms commonly involved in hospital-acquired pneumonia in the following scenarios.

Mechanical ventilator	Coliforms, *Pseudomonas aeruginosa, S. aureus*
Steroid use	Yeast, *Pneumocystis carinii*
Airway obstruction	Anaerobes
Poststroke (CVA)	*S. pneumoniae*, anaerobes

Eilbert DN, Moellening RC Jr, Sande MA: Sanford Guide to Antimicrobial Therapy, 30th ed. Hyde Park, NY, Antimicrobial Therapy Inc., 2000, p 28.

51. What factors predispose to acquiring toxic shock syndrome (TSS)?

TSS is secondary to infection caused by *S. aureus.* It should be considered in any patient presenting with fever, rash, and hypotension. Risk factors include:

- Use of high-absorbency tampons
- Diaphragm placement for contraception
- Postoperative wounds (breast augmentation, cesarean section, indwelling catheters)
- Cutaneous infections (especially in the axillary or perianal areas): cellulites, insect bites, burns, abscesses

Cunha BA: Case studies in infectious diseases: Toxic shock syndrome. Emerg Med 21:119–126, 1989.

52. Which organisms are commonly implicated in infective endocarditis?

See Table 1-10.

53. For which dental procedures is endocarditis prophylaxis recommended in patients with moderate- and high-risk cardiac problems?

- Dental extractions
- Periodontal procedures (surgery, scaling and root planning, probing, and recall maintenance)
- Dental implant placement and reimplantation of avulsed tooth
- Endodontic instrumentation or surgery only beyond the apex

TABLE 1-10. INCIDENCE OF MICROBIAL PATHOGENS IN INFECTIVE ENDOCARDITIS

Organisms	Native Valve (%)		Prosthetic Valve (%)	
	Nonaddicts	Addicts	Early (< 2 Mo)	Late (> 2 Mo)
Streptococci	50–70	20	5–10	25–30
Enterococci	10	8	< 1	5–10
Staphylococci	25	60	45–50	30–40
(*S. aureus*)	(90)	(99)	(15–20)	(10–12)
(*S. epidermidis*)	(10)	(1)	(25–30)	(23–28)
Gram-negative bacilli	< 1	10	20	10–12
Fungi	< 1	5	10–12	5–8
Diphtheroids	<1	2	5–10	4–5
Miscellaneous	5–10	1–5	1–5	1–5
Multiple	< 1	5	8	8
Culture negative	5–10	10–20	5–10	5–10

From Gorbach, et al (eds): Infectious Diseases. Philadelphia, W.B. Saunders, 1992, p 549.

- Subgingival placement of antibiotic fibers or strips
- Initial placement of orthodontic bands but not brackets
- Intraligamentary local anesthetic injection
- Prophylactic cleaning of teeth or implants when bleeding is anticipated

54. For which dental procedures is endocarditis prophylaxis *not* recommended?

- Restoration dentistry (filling cavities, replacement of missing teeth, operative or prosthodontic with or without retraction cord)
- Local anesthetic injections
- Intracanal endodontic treatment, post placement and buildup
- Placement of rubber dams
- Postoperative suture removal
- Placement of removable prosthodontic or orthodontic appliances
- Taking of oral impressions
- Fluoride treatments
- Taking of oral radiographs
- Orthodontic appliance adjustment
- Shedding of primary teeth

www.UpToDate.com

55. What is the differential diagnosis of generalized lymphadenopathy?

See Table 1-11.

56. What is spontaneous bacterial peritonitis (SBP)? Who gets it?

SBP is an infection of preexisting ascites without an obvious cause for peritoneal contamination (such as trauma or perforation) and has an incidence of 10–25% among patients with liver disease and ascites. It occurs most frequently in patients with Laennec's cirrhosis but also has been described in patients with other types of liver disease, such as chronic active hepatitis, acute viral hepatitis, and metastatic disease. Children with ascites due to nephrosis are also at risk.

TABLE 1-11. CAUSES OF GENERALIZED LYMPHADENOPATHY*

Infections		Neoplasms	Miscellaneous
Bacterial		Lymphoma	Sarcoidosis
Scarlet fever	Tuberculosis	Acute lymphocytic leukemia	Other chronic granulomatous disorders
Syphilis	Atypical mycobacteria		
Brucellosis	(Melioidosis)	Chronic lymphocytic leukemia	
Leptospirosis	(Glanders)		Systemic lupus erythematosus
Viral		Other lymphoproliferative disorders	
HIV/AIDS	Rubella		Rheumatoid arthritis
Epstein-Barr virus	(Dengue fever)	Immunoblastic lymphadenopathy	Hyperthyroidism
Cytomegalovirus	(West Nile fever)		Lipid storage diseases
Hepatitis B	(Epidemic hemorrhagic fever)	Reticuloendothelioses	Generalized dermatitis
Measles			Serum sickness
	(Lassa fever)		Phenytoin
Parasitic			
Toxoplasmosis	(African trypanosomiasis)		
(Kala azar)			
(Chagas' disease)	(Filariasis)		
Rickettsial	**Fungal**		
(Scrub typhus)	Histoplasmosis		

*Parentheses indicate infections that are uncommon or not reported in the United States. Other infections that characteristically may produce regional lymphadenopathy (e.g., tularemia, Lyme disease, lymphogranuloma venereum) rarely cause generalized lymphadenopathy.
Adapted from Libman H: Generalized lymphadenopathy. J Gen Intern Med 2:48–58, 1987.

57. How does SBP present? How is it diagnosed?

SBP usually presents as fever, chills, and abdominal pain or tenderness, but it may be asymptomatic and should be looked for in any patient with ascites who presents with a sudden onset of hypotension or hepatic encephalopathy. It can be diagnosed by demonstrating an ascitic fluid leukocyte count $> 1000/\mu L$ or an absolute polymorphonuclear (PMN) cell concentration $> 250\ \mu L$.

58. Which organisms are most likely to cause SBP?

Greater than 60% of SBP cases are due to gram-negative enteric bacteria, with *Escherichia coli* and *Klebsiella pneumoniae* being the most frequently isolated organisms. About 25% of cases are due to gram-positive cocci, with streptococcal species topping the list. Anaerobic isolates are infrequently found.

59. How is this profile different in selective intestinal decontamination (SID)?

SID, generally accomplished with fluorinated quinolones, suppresses gram-negative bacteria but not gram-positive bacteria. Therefore, patients on SID may have an increased frequency of gram-positive organisms as the etiology for SBP episodes.

Such J, Rungon BA: Spontaneous bacterial peritonitis. Clin Infect Dis 27:669–676, 1998.

60. **Which areas of the GI tract can be involved in Crohn's disease?**
Crohn's disease had been reported to affect all areas from the mouth to the anus. The major site of involvement is the colon.

61. **What is the most common cause of infectious diarrhea?**
Enterotoxigenic *E. coli* is the most frequently documented pathogen and the most likely cause of "traveler's diarrhea." There are also a host of viral, bacterial, protozoal, and parasitic causes.

62. **Name the common causes of upper GI hemorrhage.**
The four most common causes are peptic ulcer disease, varices, esophagitis, and Mallory-Weiss tears. Other causes include erosive gastritis, carcinoma, and AV malformations.

63. **Name the common causes of lower GI hemorrhage.**
The four most common causes are hemorrhoids, angiodysplasia, diverticulosis, and carcinoma. Other causes include inflammatory bowel disease (Crohn's disease, ulcerative colitis), polyps, and ischemic colitis.

64. **What characterizes hepatic encephalopathy? Who is at risk?**
Hepatic encephalopathy is a syndrome composed of altered mentation (lethargy, obtundation), fetor hepaticus (peculiar odor of the breath in patients with liver disease), and asterixis ("wrist-flapping" tremor). It occurs in patients with underlying hepatic insufficiency.

65. **What factors cause hepatic encephalopathy?**

Factors causing increased blood ammonia

GI hemorrhage	Increased dietary protein
Constipation	Metabolic alkalosis
Onset of renal insufficiency (dehydration, diuretics, or acute tubular necrosis)	Insufficient treatment with laxatives and lactulose

Factors leading to worsened hepatic insufficiency

Sedatives and tranquilizers	Hepatorenal syndrome
Analgesics	Progressive hepatocellular dysfunction
Viral hepatitis	Ethanol use

Systemic factors

Infections	Hypercarbia
Electrolyte abnormalities	Hypokalemia
Hypoxemia	

Fraser CL: Hepatic encephalopathy. N Engl J Med 313:865–873, 1985.

66. **What are the characteristics of liver diseases associated with pregnancy?**
See Table 1-12.

67. **What are the three most common causes of acute pancreatitis?**
Alcoholism and gallstones are the most common causes, accounting for 60–80% of cases, and idiopathic acute pancreatitis is the third leading cause, representing up to 15% of cases.

68. **What are the iatrogenic causes of acute pancreatitis?**
Iatrogenic causes include the postoperative state (after abdominal or nonabdominal surgery) and endoscopic retrograde cholangiopancreatography (ERCP), especially manometric studies of blunt abdominal trauma to the sphincter of Oddi. Pancreatitis occurs in 3% of renal transplant patients and is due to many factors, including surgery, hypercalcemia, drugs (glucocorticoids, azathioprine, L-asparaginase, diuretics), and viral infections.

TABLE 1-12. CHARACTERISTICS OF LIVER DISEASES IN PREGNANCY

Disease	Symptoms	Jaundice	Trimester	Incidence in Pregnancy	Laboratory Values	Adverse Effects
Hyperemesis gravidarum	Nausea, vomiting	Mild	1st or 2nd	0.3–1.0%	Bilirubin < 4 mg/dL, ALT < 200 U/L	Low birth weight
Intrahepatic cholestasis of pregnancy	Pruritus	In 20–60%, 1–4 wk after pruritus starts	2nd or 3rd	0.1–0.2% in US	Bilirubin < 6 mg/dL, ALT < 3000 U/L increased bile acids	Stillbirth, prematurity, bleeding; fetal mortality 3.5%
Biliary tract disease	Right upper quadrant pain, nausea, vomiting, fever	With common bile duct obstruction	Any	Unknown	If CBD stone, increased bilirubin and GGT	Unknown
Drug-induced	None or nausea, vomiting, pruritus	Early (in cholestatic hepatitis)	Any	Unknown	Variable	Unknown
Acute fatty liver of pregnancy	Upper abdominal pain, nausea, vomiting, confusion late in disease	Common	3rd	0.008%	ALT < 500 U/L, low glucose; DIC in > 75%, increased bilirubin and ammonia late in disease	Increased maternal mortality (≤ 20%) and fetal mortality (13–18%)
Preeclampsia and eclampsia	Upper abdominal pain, edema, hypertension, mental status changes	Late, 5–14%	2nd or 3 rd	5–10%	ALT < 500 U/L (unless infarction), proteinuria, DIC in 7%	Increased maternal mortality (~1%)
HELLP syndrome	Upper abdominal pain, nausea, vomiting, malaise	Late, 5–14%	3rd	0.1% (4–12% of women with pre-eclampsia)	ALT < 500 U/L, platelets < 100,000/mm^3, hemolysis; increased LDH; DIC in 20–40%	Increased maternal mortality (1–3%) and fetal mortality (35%)
Viral hepatitis	Nausea, vomiting, fever	Common	Any	Same as general population	ALT greatly increased (> 500 U/L), increased bilirubin; DIC rare	Maternal mortality increased with hepatitis E

ALT = alanine aminotransferase, CBD = common bile duct, GGT = gamma glutamyl transferase (GGT), DIC = disseminated intravascular coagulation, HELLP = hemolysis, elevated liver enzymes, and low platelet count, LDH = lactate dehydrogenase.
From Knox TA, Olans LB: Liver diseases in pregnancy. N Engl J Med 335:569–576, 1996, with permission.

69. List the metabolic causes of acute pancreatitis.

- Hypertriglyceridemia
- Apolipoprotein C-II deficiency syndrome
- Hypercalcemia (e.g., hyperparathyroidism)
- Renal failure
- Acute fatty liver of pregnancy (also occurs in otherwise uncomplicated pregnancy, most often in association with cholelithiasis)

70. List the infectious causes of acute pancreatitis.

- Mumps
- Viral hepatitis
- Other viral infections (coxsackievirus, echovirus, cytomegalovirus)
- Ascariasis
- Infections with *Mycoplasma*, *Campylobacter*, *Mycobacterium avium* complex, other bacteria

71. Which drugs are associated with acute pancreatitis?

Definite association: azathioprine, 6-mercaptopurine, sulfonamides, thiazide diuretics, furosemide, estrogens (oral contraceptives), tetracycline, valproic acid, pentamidine, dideoxyinosine (ddI).

Probable association: acetaminophen, nitrofurantoin, methyldopa, erythromycin, salicylates, metronidazole, NSAIDs, angiotensin-converting enzyme (ACE) inhibitors.

72. List the vascular and connective tissue disorders associated with acute pancreatitis.

Vascular: ischemic-hypoperfusion state (after cardiac surgery), atherosclerotic emboli
Connective tissue disorders with vasculitis: systemic lupus erythematosus, necrotizing angiitis, thrombotic thrombocytopenic purpura.

73. What other conditions may be associated with acute pancreatitis?

- Hereditary pancreatitis
- Obstruction of the ampulla of Vater: regional enteritis, duodenal diverticulum
- Pancreas divisum

74. What causes should be considered in patients who have recurrent bouts of acute pancreatitis without an obvious cause?

- Occult disease of the biliary tree or pancreatic ducts, especially occult gallstones (microlithiasis, sludge)
- Drugs
- Hypertriglyceridemia
- Pancreas divisum
- Pancreatic cancer
- Sphincter of Oddi dysfunction
- Cystic fibrosis
- Truly idiopathic disease

Fauci AS, et al: Harrison's Principles of Internal Medicine, 14th ed. New York, McGraw-Hill, 1998, p 1742.

75. Define carcinoid syndrome.

Carcinoid syndrome is a symptom complex caused by carcinoid tumors, which are the most common endocrine tumors of the digestive tract. These tumors arise from enterochromaffin cells and have the ability to produce a wide variety of biologically active amines and peptides, including serotonin, bradykinin, histamine, adrenocorticotropic hormone (ACTH), prostaglandins, and others. Because the liver, via the portal circulation, receives blood from the digestive tract and clears these products from the blood prior to their entry into the systemic circulation, most patients do not manifest symptoms until hepatic metastases occur.

76. How do patients with carcinoid syndrome present?
Patients usually present with episodes of cutaneous flushing, which typically are red in the beginning and then become purple, start on the face and then spread to the trunk, and last for several minutes. These episodes are often accompanied by tachycardia and hypotension. Symptoms are paroxysmal in character and provoked by alcohol, stress, or palpation of the liver and may be triggered by the administration of catecholamines, pentagastrin, or reserpine. The tumors can also cause diarrhea, crampy abdominal pain, obstruction, GI bleeding, and malabsorption.

77. Which drugs can cause gingival hyperplasia?
Phenytoin, cyclosporine, and nifedipine.

Butler RT, et al: Drug-induced gingival hyperplasia: Phenytoin, cyclosporine and nifedipine. J Am Dent Assoc 114:56–60, 1987.

78. Which drugs are frequently abused in the U.S.? Give their common street names.

- Alcohol: booze, spirits
- Marijuana (no.1 illegal drug used): weed, joints, grass, pot, reefers, Acapulco gold, Mary Jane, blunts
- Cocaine: crack, rock
- PCP (phencyclidine): angel dust, hog, dust, bromide fluid, elephant tranquilizer, animal tranquilizer, monkey dust, killer weed, rocket fuel, supergrass
- Amphetamine: white crosses, black beauties
- Dextroamphetamine: dexies
- Methamphetamine: speed, ice, crystal, meth, Hawaiian ice, crank
- Gamma-hydroxybutyrate (GHB): easy lady, liquid X, Georgia home boy, gamma-oh, everclear, water, wolfies, vita G, poor man's heroin, goop
- Flunitrazepam (rohypnol): roophies, circles, forget pill, Mexican Valium, drop drug, roaches
- MDA (3,4 methylenedioxyamphetamine; amphetamine analog): love drug, love pulls
- MMDA (3,4-methylenedioxymethamphetamine; amphetamine analog): ecstasy, XTC, Adam, California sunrise, E, hug drug, love drug, M&M, ice
- MDEA (3,4-methylenedioxymethamphetamine; amphetamine analog): Eve
- Alphamethyl fentanyl: white china
- LSD (lysergic acid diethylamide; hallucinogen): acid, dots, microdots, cubes, window panes, blotters, acid, doses, trips
- Psilocybin (psychedelic mushrooms): shrooms
- Volatile substances: glue, cement, gasoline, airplane glue (toluene), amyl nitrate; fluorinated hydrocarbons (freon), typewriter fluid (trichloroethylene). *Sniffing, huffing,* and *bagging* are terms identifying how they are inhaled.
- Prescription drugs: benzodiazepines (diazepam [Valium] and alprazolam [Xanax]), narcotic analgesics (e.g., codeine, morphine, fentanyl, meperidine, hydrocodone).

Schulz JE: Illicit drugs of abuse. Substance abuse. Prim Care 20(1):221–230, 1993.

Drug Enforcement Administration, U.S. Department of Justice, at www.usdoj.gov/dea/index.htm

Ropero-Miller JD, Goldberger BA: Recreational drugs: Current trends in the 90's. Toxicol Clin Lab Med 18(4):727–746, 1998.

Finen J: Prescription drug abuse. Substance abuse. Prim Care 20:231–239, 1993.

79. What are the three major stages of cocaine use and cessation?

- **The high:** euphoria, increased self-confidence, increased energy, increased ability to do work.
- **Levels drop:** feeling depressed, irritable, restless, and generally uncomfortable.
- **Abstinence syndrome:** crash, cravings, withdrawal, and extinction.

A major side effect with continued abuse is paranoia, also called "armed paranoia." Combined with their increased energy levels, abusers often exhibit erratic and aggressive or violent behaviors.

80. Characterize the four elements of the abstinence stage.

- Crash: depression, anxiety, and agitation.
- Craving: prolonged sleeping followed by intense food cravings.
- Withdrawal: decreased energy, anhedonia, dysphoria, and reduced normal activities; lasts 6–18 weeks after last use (a common time for relapse).
- Extinction phase: return to usual state of activities, energy, and interests.

81. What antidotes are available for common drug and chemical overdoses?
See Table 1-13.

TABLE 1-13. ANTIDOTES FOR COMMON DRUG AND CHEMICAL OVERDOSES

Drug	Antidote and Dosage
Acetaminophen	N-acetylcysteine (Mucomyst, Mucosil-10): 140 mg/kg initially, followed by 70 mg/kg every 8 h for 17 doses.
Narcotics	Naloxone (Narcan): 0.4–2.0 mg IV. Can be repeated at 2- to 3-minute intervals.
Benzodiazepines	Flumazenil (Romazicon): 0.3 mg IV. Additional doses of 0.5 mg over 30 sec at 1-min intervals to a cumulative dose of 3 mg.
Anticholinergic agents	Physostigmine: 2 mg by slow IV. Repeat in 20 min if no improvement; follow with 1–2 mg IV for recurrent symptoms
Methanol, ethylene glycol	Ethanol (absolute): 1 mL/kg in D_5W IV over 15 min. Maintenance dose: 125 mg/kg/h IV in D_5W.
Digoxin	Digoxin immune FAB (ovine; Digibind): dose varies with serum concentration of digoxin, but on average, 10 vials can be given to start. For large, unknown amounts of digoxin, give 20 vials (760 mg) IV reconstituted with sterile water for injection, preferably through a micron membrane.
Phenothiazines, haloperidol, Loxitane	Diphenhydramine: 25–50 mg; or benztropine: 1–2 mg (may be given IV or IM).
Cyanide	Sodium nitrite: 300 mg IV, or sodium thiosulfate: 12.5 gm.
Organophosphates (insecticides)	Atropine sulfate: 2–5 mg IV. Repeat every 10–30 min to maintain a decrease in bronchial secretions. After atropine, pralidoxime: 1 mg IV for 2 doses. Repeat every 8–12 h for 3 doses if muscle weakness is not relieved.

FAB = fragment antigen binding.
From Guzzardi LJ: Role of the emergency physician in poisoning. Med Clin North Am 2:10–11, 1982, and Physician's Desk Reference, 54th ed. Montvale, NJ, Medical Economics Company, Inc., 2000.

82. A 19-year-old woman is admitted with salicylate poisoning. What acid-base disturbances are seen in this condition on serial blood gas monitoring?

Acute salicylate intoxication is characterized by profound effects on acid-base balance. Early in the course of intoxication, primary **respiratory alkalosis** results from direct stimulation of the respiratory center in the medulla by salicylates. This causes an increase in pH and a fall in $PaCO_2$. A **compensatory metabolic acidosis** due to renal excretion of bicarbonate may be seen, which tends to bring the pH back toward normal. In young adults and children (especially with toxic doses), a **primary metabolic acidosis** ensues. It is normochloremic and associated with a high anion gap. The continuation of primary respiratory alkalosis and metabolic acidosis should give a clue to the diagnosis of acute salicylate intoxication. In more severe cases, primary respiratory acidosis occurs due to the depression of the respiratory center at very high salicylate levels.

83. What causes the primary metabolic acidosis in salicylate poisoning?

1. Impaired hepatic carbohydrate metabolism, leading to accumulation of ketones and lactate in plasma.
2. Accumulated salicylic acid itself, which displaces several mEq of bicarbonate.
3. Dehydration and hypotension impair renal excretion of inorganic acids and cause further metabolic acidosis.

84. List the initial steps in the assessment and treatment of a patient with a suspected drug overdose.

1. Control airway
2. Check vital signs (blood pressure, respiration, pulse, temperature)
3. Stabilize any abnormalities in vital signs
4. Check mental status/level of consciousness
5. Obtain blood for laboratory studies (chemistries, arterial blood gases, toxicology screen)
6. IV fluid: D_5W with thiaminenaloxone
7. Quick physical exam (heart, lungs, abdomen, neurologic)

Goldfrank LJR, et al: Management of overdose with psychoactive medications. Med Clin North Am 2:65, 1982.

85. Which organs are frequently damaged by intravenous drug abuse (IVDA)?

In descending order of frequency: the lung, heart, and kidneys.

86. Which infectious diseases are commonly observed among IV drug abusers?

Persons who engage in IVDA run a high risk of acquiring serious infections from all classes of pathogens, and any organ system may be affected (Table 1-14).

87. Which valves are most frequently affected in rheumatic heart disease?

In order of frequency: the mitral valve is the most commonly involved. The aortic valve is often involved, and the tricuspid, although rare, is more frequently involved than the pulmonic valve.

88. What are the causes of the common cardiac arrhythmias in adults?

See Table 1-15.

89. How do you differentiate the common tachyarrhythmias?

See Table 1-16.

90. What are the causes of prolonged QT intervals?

The QT interval can be prolonged due to congenital causes (Romano-Ward syndrome and Jervell-Lange-Nielson syndrome) or acquired causes (usually secondary to medications). Hypomagnesemia, hypokalemia, and bradycardia can contribute to the risk.

TABLE 1-14. COMMON INFECTIONS IN IV DRUG ABUSERS

Central nervous system	**Lungs**	**Heart**
Meningitis	Septic pulmonary emboli	Endocarditis
Mycotic aneurysm	Pneumonia	*S. aureus* (> 50% of cases)
Focal neurologic infections:	*S. pneumoniae*	Strep. groups A, B & G (2nd most common)
1. Abscess	*S. aureus*	Polymicrobial
2. Subdural empyema	Aspiration (anaerobes)	Noncandidal sp. (5%)
Eye	*P. aeruginosa*	Enterococcus (+ frequency)
Endophthalmitis	Abscess	Gram-negative bacilli (infrequent)
Fungal *(Candida)*	Empyema	
Bacterial *(S. aureus)*	Tuberculosis	
Abdomen	**Muscle**	**Noncardiac vascular infections**
Hepatitis A, B, C, D, G	Necrotizing fascitis ± myositis	Septic thrombophlebitis
Splenic abscess	Pyomyositis	Mycotic aneurysms (both due to *S. aureus*)
Skin	**Joints**	**HIV infection** (most common infection in IVDAs)
Cellulitis	Osteomyelitis (esp. lumbar spine)	AIDS and AIDS-related
S. aureus	Septic arthritis (mostly knee)	*Pneumocystis carinii* pneumonia
Streptococci	Genitourinary	Cytomegalovirus
Gram negative bacilli	Sexually transmitted diseases (gonorrhea and syphilis)	Toxoplasmosis
Suppurative phlebitis	Renal abscesses	Cryptococcal meningitis
Skin ulcers		*Mycobacterium avium* complex
		H. influenzae pneumonia

From Levine DP, Brown PD: Infections in injection drug users. In Mandell GL, Bennett JE, Dolin R (eds): Principles and Practice of Infectious Disease, 5th ed. New York, Churchill Livingstone, 2000, pp 3112–3126.

91. **What special management does a non–Q-wave MI require?**
A non–Q-wave MI has a better short-term prognosis, but patients are at higher risk of reinfarction or extension of the infarct area, early onset of postinfarction pain, and an overall higher late mortality rate. Fig. 1-3 summarizes the approach to treatment.

92. **When is corrective surgery indicated in patients with aortic stenosis?**
Once symptoms of AS develop, patients should be considered for valve replacement. The typical symptoms include heart failure, angina, and syncope. Any of these symptoms depict severe AS (estimated valve area < 0.8 cm^2) and has an estimated 3-year mortality of 50%.

93. **When do ventricular premature depolarizations (VPDs) warrant medical therapy?**
VPDs, or premature ventricular contractions (PVCs), occur in asymptomatic people without cardiac problems, in acute situations such as post-MIs, and in patients with cardiac diseases. Each is treated differently. When VPDs occur in asymptomatic people, therapy is usually not

TABLE 1-15. COMMON CARDIAC ARRHYTHMIAS IN ADULTS

Arrhythmia	Rate (bpm)	Etiologies
Sinus tachycardia	100–200	Fever, pain, drugs, hyperthyroidism, hypertension
Paroxysmal supraventricular	130–220 (usually 160)	Pre-excitation syndrome (Wolff-tachycardia [PSVT] Parkinson-White syndrome), AV nodal reentry, congenital abnormalities, atrial septal defect, concealed accessory bypass tracts
Atrial flutter Ventricular	Atrial, 250–350 150–220	Mitral valve disease, COPD, pulmonary embolus, alcohol abuse, organic heart disease, MI, cardiac surgery
Atrial fibrillation Ventricular	Atrial, 350–500 100–160	Myocardial ischemia, MI, organic heart disease, rheumatic heart disease, alcohol abuse, CHF, elderly patients, febrile illness, hyperthyroidism, chest surgery
Ventricular tachycardia	100–230	Ischemic heart disease, MI, mitral valve prolapse, cardiomyopathy, hypercalcemia, hypokalemia, hypomagnesemia, hypoxemia

TABLE 1-16. DIFFERENTATION OF COMMON TACHYARRHYTHMIAS

	Sinus Tachycardia	Paroxysmal Atrial Tachycardia	Atrial Fibrillation	Atrial Flutter	Ventricular Tachycardia
Rate	100–200	169–190	160–190	140–160	100–230
Rhythm	Regular	Regular	Irregular	Regular	Slightly irregular
QRS shape	Normal*	Normal*	Normal*	Normal*	Abnormal
Atrial activity	Sinus P wave†	Absent or nonsinus P wave†	Absent	Flutter waves	Sinus P waves†
P-QRS relation	Yes	May be masked by rapid ventricular rate	No	May be masked by rapid ventricular rate	No
Carotid massage	Slows	No response, or converts to sinus rhythm	No response	Increased block	No response

* Unless intraventricular conduction disturbance.
† Sinus P waves are upright in lead II and occur at least 0.12 sec before the QRS complex begins.
From Gottlieb AJ, et al: The Whole Internist Catalog. Philadelphia, W.B. Saunders, 1980, p 158.

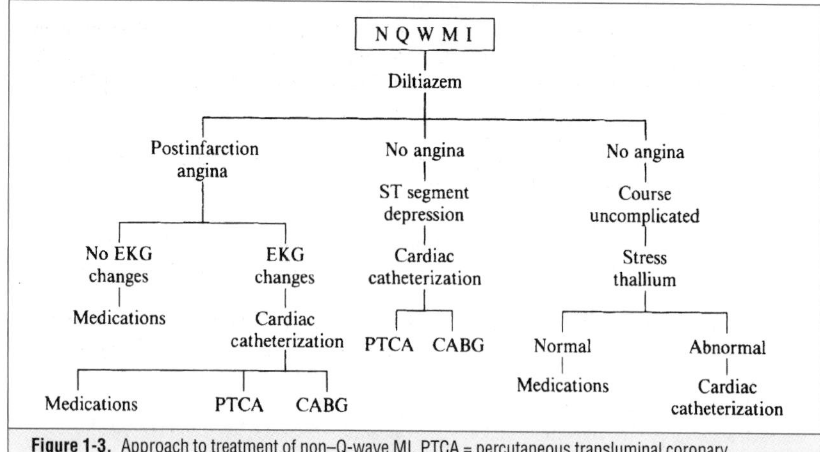

Figure 1-3. Approach to treatment of non–Q-wave MI. PTCA = percutaneous transluminal coronary angioplasty, CABG = coronary artery bypass grafting.

warranted, and patients should be counseled to avoid aggravating factors (e.g., caffeinated products, tobacco, stimulants) and given reinforcement. VPDs after an MI are usually accepted as a "warning arrhythmia" and treated with IV lidocaine as the drug of choice. In cardiac conditions, patients face a higher risk of sudden death, and PVCs are usually suppressed with beta blockers. Newest data conclude that asymptomatic middle-aged men with PVCs during exertion may have an increased long-term risk of death from cardiovascular diseases.

Myerburg RJ, Kessler KM, Castellanos A: Recognition, clinical assessment, and management of arrhythmias and conduction disturbances. In Alexander RW, et al (eds): Hurst's The Heart, 9th ed. New York, McGraw-Hill, 1998, pp 905–909.

Jouven X, et al: Long-term outcome in asymptomatic men with exercise-induced premature ventricular depolarizations. N Engl J Med 343(12):826–833, 2000.

94. What is torsades de pointes?

Torsades de pointes, or "twisting of the points," is a polymorphic ventricular tachycardia characterized by QRS complexes that change in amplitude and electrical polarity, appearing to "twist" around the isoelectric line. A prolonged QT interval must be present (Fig. 1-4). There may also be U waves.

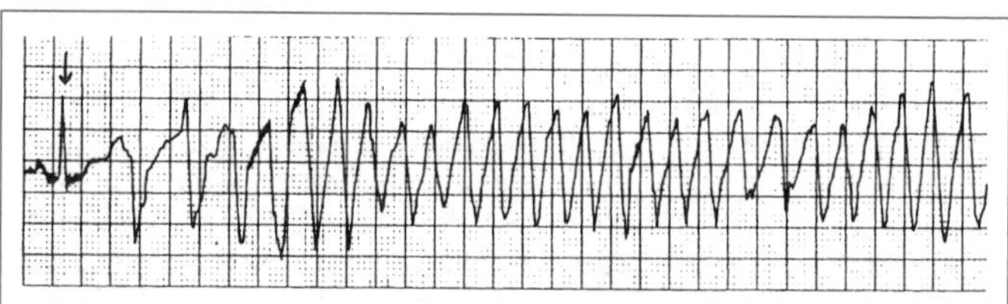

Figure 1-4. Torsades de pointes. A single sinus beat (arrow) is followed by ventricular tachycardia with an oscillating or swinging pattern of QRS complexes. (From Selig CB: Simplified EKG Analysis. Philadelphia, Hanley & Belfus, 1992, p 75.)

95. List the causes of torsades de pointes.

- Quinidine
- Psychotropics
- Phenothiazines
- Lithium
- TCAs
- Hypokalemia
- Myocardial ischemia
- Tumors
- Severe bradycardia
- Disopyramide
- Hypomangesemia
- Procainamide
- Subarachnoid hemorrhage
- Third-degree heart block
- Amiodarone
- Myocarditis
- Trauma
- CNS lesions

Saffer J, et al: Polymorphous ventricular tachycardia associated with normal and long Q-T intervals. Am J Cardiol 49:2021–2029, 1982.

96. List the major risk factors for development of coronary artery disease (CAD).

- Age (males: 45 yr; females: 55 yr or premature menopause without estrogen replacement therapy)
- Family history of premature CAD (definite MI or sudden death before age 55 in father or other male first-degree relative, or before age 65 in mother or other female first-degree relative)
- Current cigarette smoking
- Hypertension (BP 140/90 mmHg confirmed by several measurements or taking anti-hypertensive medication)
- Elevated low-density lipoprotein (LDL) cholesterol
- Low high-density lipoprotein (HDL) cholesterol (< 35 mg/dL or 0.9 mmol/L confirmed by several measurements)
- Diabetes mellitus

97. What major negative risk factor decreases the risk of CAD?

High HDL cholesterol (> 60 mg/dL or 1.6 mmol/L)

Summary of the second report of the National Cholesterol Education Program (NCEP) expert panel on detection, evaluation, and treatment of high blood cholesterol in adults (Adult Treatment Panel II). JAMA 269:3015–3023, 1993.

98. A 35-year-old male with a past history of nephrotic syndrome is admitted for elective knee surgery. He has been taking ibuprofen for 3 weeks. On admission, serum creatinine is 3 mg/dL. What points help you to differentiate acute renal failure (ARF) from chronic renal failure (CRF)?

The patient has a previous history of nephrotic illness, has been taking an NSAID and has a moderate degree of renal insufficiency. This insufficiency could be ARF induced by the NSAID or unrecognized progressive CRF. Urinary sediment can be useful in this situation. Acute interstitial nephritis is associated with RBC and white blood cell (WBC) casts, whereas CRF is associated with broad casts (usually 2–3 times the diameter of a WBC). The presence of significant anemia, hyperphosphatemia, and hypocalcemia and changes of renal osteodystrophy are suggestive of advanced CRF. The most important confirmation of chronicity is demonstration of shrunken or small kidneys by ultrasound or CT scanning.

99. How do NSAIDs cause acute renal failure?

The NSAIDs inhibit cyclooxygenase, an enzyme responsible for synthesizing prostaglandins from arachidonic acid. The intrarenal production of prostaglandins, especially PGE_2, contributes significantly to the maintenance of renal blood flow (RBF) and glomerular filtration rate (GFR) in states of diminished effective arterial blood volume. In any of the prerenal states, angiotensin II and norepinephrine production is increased, which in turn increases renal vasodilator prostaglandin synthesis and thus leads to improvement of renal ischemia. The NSAIDs have the potential to significantly lower RBF and GFR in certain disease states (such as hypovolemia, CHF, nephrotic syndrome, and lupus nephritis) and to produce ARF. An acute interstitial nephritis associated with nephrotic syndrome may also occur, particularly after the use of fenoprofen.

100. Who is at highest risk for NSAID-induced renal failure?

- Elderly patients
- Patients taking ACE inhibitors and/or beta blockers
- Patients receiving > 1 NSAID (e.g., aspirin and indomethacin)
- Diabetics
- Patients on diuretics or who are dehydrated
- Patients with underlying CHF

101. Which conditions related to pregnancy predispose to ARF?

Although its incidence has declined markedly with control of septic abortions and antenatal care, ARF is not uncommon in pregnancy. Toxemia of pregnancy, antepartum hemorrhage, and postpartum hemorrhage are associated with an increased risk of ARF. Other predisposing factors include postpartum sepsis, abortion, postpartum hemolytic uremia syndrome, and amniotic fluid embolism. In addition, acute fatty liver and urinary tract obstruction are occasionally associated with ARF during pregnancy.

102. Describe the physiologic changes in the kidney during pregnancy.

Pregnancy is associated with an increase in GFR of about 50% and a mild decrease in plasma creatinine and blood urea nitrogen (BUN). There is a slight increase in kidney size (about 1 cm) and dilation and tortuosity of the ureters. These changes were believed secondary to pressure by the gravid uterus, but it is now known that these changes can be related to increased progesterone levels. Other physiologic changes include increased uric acid clearance, resulting in slight hypouricemia.

103. List the most common causes of ARF in hospitalized patients.

- Hypoperfusion (approximately 50%)
- Dehydration
- CHF
- Postoperative renal failure
- Obstruction
- Drugs (especially aminoglycosides)
- Sepsis
- Arrhythmia
- IV contrast dye
- Hepatorenal syndrome

104. Which class of antihypertensive agents is contraindicated in patients with bilateral renal artery stenosis?

ACE inhibitors. In bilateral renal artery stenosis or stenosis to a solitary kidney, the renal perfusion pressure (and thus GFR) depends on the local renin-angiotensin system. When the system is blocked by an ACE inhibitor, a marked decrease in the efferent arterial pressure with subsequent decrease in renal perfusion pressure results, causing a diminished GFR.

105. What does the presence of eosinophils in urine denote?

Normal urine does not contain eosinophils; their presence in a urine sample points to renal disease. The contribution of eosinophils to the immune response is not clearly known, but they are activated by antigens and antigen-induced hypersensitivity reactions. Eosinophils in the urine are characteristic of tubulointerstitial disease (i.e., interstitial nephritis), especially if they comprise > 5% of the total number of WBCs in the sample. Eosinophils in the urine are seen in interstitial nephritis, acute tubular necrosis, urinary tract infections, hepatorenal syndrome, and kidney transplant rejection

Carwin HL, et al: Clinical correlates of eosinophiluria. Arch Intern Med 145:1097–1099, 1985.

106. What three findings comprise the hyporeninemic-hypoaldosteronism syndrome?

1. Low serum aldosterone levels (due to impaired secretion)
2. Low serum renin levels
3. Hyperkalemia (which is more severe than expected by the degree of renal insufficiency)

107. List the clinical characteristics of patients with hyporeninemic hypoaldosteronism.

- Mean age: 65 years
- Asymptomatic hyperkalemia (75%)
- Chronic renal insufficiency (70%)
- Diabetes mellitus (50%)
- Cardiac arrhythmias (25%)
- Normal aldosterone response to ACTH (25%)

108. In chronic renal failure, what is the importance of the calcium-phosphate product ($Ca^{2+} \times PO_4^-$–product)?

When the product of the serum concentrations of calcium and phosphate exceeds 70, metastatic calcifications are more likely to occur. Calcium phosphate ($CaPO_4$) may precipitate out of the plasma and deposit in arteries, soft tissues, periarticular areas, and viscera.

109. List the common causes of diffuse bilateral interstitial lung infiltrates.

- Pulmonary edema
- Miliary tuberculosis
- *Pneumocystis carinii* pneumonia
- Lymphangitic spread of carcinoma (breast, gastric)
- Sarcoidosis
- Lymphoma
- Chlorambucil
- Idiopathic
- Drugs/toxins
- Nitrofurantoin
- Amiodarone
- Sulfonamides
- Zidovudine
- Bleomycin
- Methotrexate
- Cyclophosphamide

Crystal RG, et al: Interstitial lung disease of unknown cause. N Engl J Med 310:154–166, 235–244, 1984.

110. Where do you find Hampton's hump?

Hampton's hump, named after Aubrey Otis Hampton (1900–1955), a U.S. radiologist, is a radiographic finding that is highly suggestive of a pulmonary infarction. It is a dense, homogeneous, wedge-shaped consolidation in the middle and lower lobes. The base is contiguous with the pleura, but the apex points, in a convex fashion, toward the hilum. This pattern gives the appearance of a hump.

111. How are lung cancers classified? What are the most common types?

Lung cancers are classified into small cell lung cancer (SCLC) and non–small cell lung cancer (NSCLC). NSCLC accounts for over 80% of all lung cancers. There are several types of non–small cell cancers; adenocarcinoma makes up the majority of the NSCLCs (32%). Others include squamous cell, large cell, epidermoid, bronchioloalveolar carcinoma, and mixed versions of all of these.

112. Which skin cancer is most common in adults?

Nonmelanoma skin cancers are the most common and include basal cell carcinoma (the most common skin neoplasm worldwide) and squamous cell carcinoma. Basal cell carcinoma occurs 4–10 times as frequently as squamous cell carcinoma. The primary risk factor is excessive sun exposure, especially in fair-skinned individuals, and 90% of tumors occur in sun-exposed areas of the skin. Basal cell carcinomas are divided into six types: nodular, pigmented, cystic, sclerosing, superficial, and nevoid. Metastasis is rare, and the prognosis is usually excellent, although deaths from local extension do occur. Therapy is based on location and extent of the tumor. Removal of the tumor, by a variety of means, is curative in 90% of the cases.

Jerant AF, et al: Early detection and treatment of skin cancer. Am Fam Physician 62(2):357–368, 2000.

113. What criteria should be remembered in evaluating a lesion suspicious for a melanoma?

The **ABCD** rule lists the key criteria for evaluating these lesions:

A = **A**symmetry
B = **B**order irregularity
C = **C**olor variation (usually purple/black)
D = **D**iameter > 6 mm

Jerant AF, et al: Early detection and treatment of skin cancer. Am Fam Physician 62(2):357–368, 2000.

114. Are tinea versicolor and vitiligo manifestations of the same disease?

No. The differences are shown in Table 1-17.

TABLE 1-17. VITILIGO VERSUS TINEA VERSICOLOR

	Vitiligo	Tinea
Etiology	? Autoimmune	Fungal infection
Pathology	Destruction of melanocytes	Decreased melanosomes in the stratum corneum
Incidence	1%	Common
Age of onset	Young adults	Young adults
Description	Macular depigmented areas Absence of melanin	Small hypopigmented-to-tan macules with a bran-like scale
Associated conditions	Graves' disease, pernicious anemia, diabetes mellitus, Addison's disease	Seborrhea
Diagnosis	Chalk-white under Wood's lamp Absence of melanocytes on skin biopsy	Gold fluorescence on Wood's lamp Spores/hyphae on skin biopsy KOH = positive, "spaghetti and meatballs" appearance
Therapy	Trioxsalen with sun exposure at least two times a week	Selenium sulfide, sulfur ointments, ketoconazole, salicylic acid

115. How do a chancre and a chancroid ulcer differ?

See Table 1-18.

116. List the cutaneous manifestations of hyperthyroidism.

- Warm, moist, "velvety" texture of skin
- Increased palmar/dorsal sweating
- Facial flushing
- Palmar erythema
- Vitiligo
- Altered hair texture
- Alopecia
- Pretibial myxedema

117. How common is asymptomatic bacteriuria in patients over age 65? Is treatment necessary?

Asymptomatic bacteriuria is present in at least 20% of women and 10% of men over age 65. Treatment is not necessary unless it is associated with an obstructive uropathy.

Boscia JA, et al: Asymptomatic bacteriuria in the elderly. Infect Dis Clin North Am 1:893–905, 1987.

TABLE 1-18. CHANCRE VERSUS CHANCROID ULCER

	Chancre	Chancroid Ulcer
Disease	Syphilis	Chancroid (a disease in itself)
Organism	*Treponema pallidum*	*Haemophilus ducreyi*
Description	Painless papule that rapidly erodes. Edge feels cartilaginous. Indurated.	Painful, superficial ulcer with ragged edges. Base is covered by necrotic exudate. More often multiple.
Location	Penis, cervix/labia, and anus/rectum/mouth in homosexuals	Males: Preputial orifice, prepuce, frenulum Females: labia, clitoris, vestibule
Treatment	Penicillin G, tetracycline	Trimethoprim/sulfamethoxazole, erythromycin

118. Headaches in an elderly patient should always alert one to the possibility of which rheumatologic disease?
Temporal (giant cell) arteritis should be considered in any patient over age 50 with a headache, especially if it is continuous, throbbing, and unilateral. Untreated temporal arteritis can result in irreversible monocular blindness.

119. What other symptoms suggest temporal arteritis?
- Claudication of jaw when chewing and/or talking
- Transient loss of vision (amaurosis fugax), visual-field deficits, diplopia, sudden visual loss
- Symptoms of polymyalgia rheumatica (girdle-hip pain) seen in 50% of patients
- Tender, swollen, red, nodular temporal artery with decreased pulsation on palpation (two thirds of patients)
- Fever
- Weight loss

120. What are the leading causes of blindness in the elderly?
Cataracts, glaucoma, retinopathies, temporal arteritis, and diabetes mellitus (DM).

121. What are the common presentations of type 1 DM versus type 2 DM?
See Table 1-19.

TABLE 1-19. TYPE 1 VERSUS TYPE 2 DIABETES MELLITUS

	Type 1	Type 2
Age	< 40 years	> 40 years, elderly
Onset	Short period	Insidious, found incidentally on lab tests
Complications	Diabetic ketoacidosis	Hyperosmolar coma
Body habitus	Normal, thin	Obese (generally)
Pathology	Islet cells destroyed	Insulin resistance, low insulin secretion, islet cells intact
Ketosis prone	Yes	Yes, but much less common than type 1
Therapy	Insulin	Weight loss, balanced diet, oral hypoglycemic agents, perhaps insulin

122. What are the predisposing factors for the development of diabetic foot ulcers?

- Friction from poorly fitting and/or new shoes
- Untreated calluses and corns
- Self-treated calluses and corns
- Foot trauma (often unnoticed)
- Walking barefoot
- Burns
- Paronychia
- Self-inflicted foot lesions (rare)
- Heel friction in bed-bound patients
- Foot deformities (bunions, hammer toes, edema)

Adapted from Watkins PJ: The diabetic foot. BMJ 326:977–979, 2003.

123. Summarize the effects of chronically elevated blood glucose on the skin, eyes, and peripheral nerves.

Skin: dermopathy, diabetic foot/leg ulcers, greater susceptibility to skin infections, necrobiosis lipoidica diabeticorum.

Eyes: cataracts, retinopathy.

Peripheral nerves: peripheral neuropathy, mononeuropathy (median nerve).

124. What are the effects of chronically elevated blood glucose on the genitourinary system and kidneys?

Genitourinary system: impotence, retrograde ejaculation, neurogenic bladder, diabetic amyotropy, neuropathic cachexia.

Kidneys: renal insufficiency, end-stage renal disease, nephritic syndrome, repeated urinary tract infections.

125. List the gastrointestinal effects of chronically elevated blood glucose.

- Gastroparesis
- Diabetic diarrhea
- Constipation
- Esophageal dysfunction
- Gastroesophageal reflux disease

126. Summarize the effects of chronically elevated blood glucose on the CNS.

- Coma (due to diabetic ketoacidosis or hyperosmolar coma)
- Personality changes
- Autonomic insufficiency

127. List the cardiovascular effects of chronically elevated blood glucose.

- Increased risk of CAD, CVA, DVT
- Silent MI
- Cardiomyopathy
- Hypertriglyceridmia
- Elevated total cholesterol
- Lowered HDL cholesterol
- Hypertension
- Peripheral vascular disease
- Impaired cardiovascular reflexes

128. **What are the clinical stages of hypoglycemia? How are they characterized?**
Mild: symptoms related to stimulation of the adrenergic or CNS in response to a low blood sugar.
Moderate: symptoms related to CNS effects of hypoglycemia are more pronounced, but the patient is still capable of assisting him- or herself. Symptoms include impaired motor function, confusion, and inappropriate behaviors.
Severe: symptoms of hypoglycemia result in coma, seizure, or altered mental status, impairing the patient's ability to seek help or get a sugar source.

KEY POINTS: DIABETES MELLITUS

1. The diagnosis of diabetes can be made only with a fasting blood glucose > 126 mg/dL, a random glucose level > 200 mg/dL, or a 2-h glucose > 200 mg/dL after a 75-gm glucose load. It is not acceptable to use HbA1c to confirm the diagnosis.
2. Diabetes ketoacidosis (DKA) can occur quickly in type 1 diabetic patients when insulin is withheld; thus they need a continuous supply of insulin to prevent DKA relapse.
3. Insulin therapy is frequently needed in type 2 diabetics when oral agents fail to control blood sugar. This is caused by an inability of pancreatic beta cells to produce insulin.
4. Control of blood sugar is not the only goal in treating diabetics; control of blood pressure and lipids is also important in preventing both the microvascular and macrovascular complications.

129. **Define hypoglycemia unawareness.**
Hypoglycemia unawareness is an iatrogenic syndrome, usually occurring in type 1 DM, in which patients become resistant to or unaware of early defense signs such as tachycardia and sweats. Patients may progress to coma and/or seizures without warning signs.
Lebovitz HE, et al: Therapy for Diabetes Mellitus and Related Disorders, 3rd ed. Alexandria, VA, American Diabetes Association, 1998, pp 241–251.

130. **What are consistent laboratory findings in adrenal insufficiency?**
- Hyponatremia (rarely < 120 mEq/L)
- Hyperkalemia (rarely > 7 mEq/L)
- Hypocarbia (HCO_3 ~15–20 mEq/L)
- Hypoglycemia
- Elevated BUN
- Elevated eosinophils
- Elevated lymphocytes

131. **Benign neutropenia is most commonly observed in which peoples?**
Africans, West Indian blacks, and African Americans. This is not a genetic trait but rather an acquired one. The neutropenia probably results from an abnormal release of neutrophils by the bone marrow. The WBC count ranges from 3000 to 4000 in African Americans. This is a normal response to infections, steroids, and pregnancy.

132. **What complaints in elderly hypothyroid patients most commonly bring them to medical attention?**
- Constipation
- Difficulty in thinking
- Lethargy, easy fatigability
- Cold intolerance

Bartuska DG: Thyroid disease in the news. Contemp Intern Med (Jun):23–32, 1989.

133. What protection is afforded to patients with the heterozygous sickle cell gene?
The high frequency of the sickle cell gene in areas endemic for malaria is an example of balanced polymorphism. The sickle cell gene protects the host from lethal *Plasmadium falciparum* malaria. The actual mechanism is not fully understood, but it is postulated that the entry of the parasite into the host cell lowers RBC oxygen saturation. This desaturation leads to sickling and arrests the maturation of the parasite. The sickled cells are cleared by the phagocytic system.

Luzzatto L: Genetics of red cells susceptibility to malaria. Blood 54:961–976, 1979.

134. Name the five types of crises in sickle cell disease.
1. Vaso-occlusive (painful): The typical "sickle crisis" whose symptoms depend on the location of occlusion.
2. Aplastic: Bone marrow suppression due to infection.
3. Sequestration: Seen in younger patients (aged 1–5 yr) while the spleen is still intact.
4. Hemolytic: Look for G6PD deficiency or malaria.
5. Megaloblastic: Seen in conditions of increased folate requirements (as in pregnancy).

135. Describe the acute chest syndrome.
Acute chest syndrome is a medical emergency frequently seen in patients with sickle cell disease. It is characterized by acute chest pain, arterial hypoxemia, and pulmonary infiltrates. This life-threatening complication is most often treated with exchange transfusion and aggressive critical care monitoring.

136. Which drugs are most commonly implicated in drug-induced (immune) thrombocytopenia?
Antibacterials: sulfonamides, rifampin, trimethoprim, ampicillin, cephalosporins, p-aminosalicylate, nitrofurantoin, isoniazid.

Anticonvulsants: carbamazepine, phenytoin, sodium valproate, diphenylhydantoin, phthalazinol.

Antihypertensives: methyldopa, chlorothiazide, hydrochlorothiazide, diazoxide, furosemide.

Cinchona alkaloids: quinine, quinidine.

NSAIDs: aspirin, indomethacin, phenylbutazone, sulindac.

Others: heroin, chlorpropamide, bleomycin, desipramine, gold, heparin, cimetidine, digitoxin, acetaminophen.

137. List the differential diagnoses of macrocytic anemias.
- Liver disease
- Vitamin B_{12} deficiency
- Folate deficiency
- Myelodysplastic syndrome
- Drugs that impair DNA synthesis: 6-mercaptopurine, zidovudine, 5-fluorouracil, hydroxyurea

138. What are the differential diagnoses of microcytic anemias?
- Iron deficiency (most common type of anemia worldwide)
- Hemoglobinopathies: thalassemia, sickle cell anemia, sickle cell disease
- Sideroblastic anemias
- Anemia of chronic disease

139. What are the American College of Rheumatology criteria for the diagnosis of gout?
The American College of Rheumatology states that the confirmation of the diagnosis of gout can be established by the presence of at least 6 of 12 specific criteria:
- Maximum joint inflammation within 1 day
- More than one attack over time

- Monoarticular arthritis (although gout can affect many joints)
- Redness of the joint
- Great toe pain or swelling
- Unilateral great toe involvement
- Unilateral tarsal involvement
- Suspected presence of a tophus
- Hyperuricemia
- Asymetrical swelling within the joint on plain x-rays
- Subcortical cysts without erosion on x-ray
- Negative joint fluid culture for infectious causes during an attack

Adapted from Gout, Teal, G.P. & Fuchs, H.A. PIER, Clinical Guidance from American College of Physicians, http://pier.acponline.org

140. Which enzyme is usually elevated in lymphoma?

Lactate dehydrogenase (LDH) is elevated in many lymphomas and other lymphoproliferative disorders. The source is believed to be tumor cells, and LDH is used as a measurement of disease activity.

WEB SITES

1. www.UpToDate.com
2. www.MDConsult.com
3. www.pier.acponline.org

BIBLIOGRAPHY

1. Alexander RW, et al (eds): Hurst's The Heart, 9th ed. New York, McGraw-Hill, 1998.
2. Beers MH, Berkow R: The Merck Manual of Diagnosis and Therapy, 17th ed. Whitehouse Station, NJ, Merck Research Laboratories, 1999.
3. Fauci AS, et al (eds): Harrison's Principles of Internal Medicine, 14th ed. New York, McGraw-Hill, 1998.
4. Guide to Clinical Preventive Services, 2nd ed. Report of the US Preventive Services Task Force. Baltimore, Williams & Wilkins, 1996.
5. Kelley WN (ed): Textbook of Internal Medicine, 3rd ed. Philadelphia, Lippincott-Raven, 1997.
6. Klippel JH (ed): Primer on the Rheumatic diseases, 11th ed. Atlanta, GA, The Arthritis Foundation, 1997.
7. Lebovitz HE, et al: Therapy for Diabetes Mellitus and Related Disorders, 3rd ed. Alexandria, VA, American Diabetes Association, 1998.
8. Mandell GL, Douglas GD, Bennett JE (eds): Principles and Practice of Infectious Disease, 5th ed. New York, Churchill Livingstone, 2000.
9. Physician's Desk Reference, 54th ed. Montvale, NJ, Medical Economics Company, Inc., 2000.
10. Sanford Guide to Antimicrobial Therapy, 13th ed. Hyde Park, NY, Antimicrobial Therapy, Inc., 2000.
11. Tapson VP (Committee chair): The Diagnostic Approach to Acute Venous Thromboembolism: Clinical Practice Guidelines. Am J Respir Crit Care Med 160(3):1043–1066, 1999.
12. Tierney LM, McPhee SJ, Papdakis MA: Current Medical Diagnosis and Treatment, 38th ed. Norwalk, CT, Appleton & Lange, 1999.

ENDOCRINOLOGY

Whitney W. Woodmansee, M.D.

CHAPTER 2

DIABETES MELLITUS AND GLYCEMIC DISORDERS

1. **List the three main categories of diabetes mellitus (DM).**
   - Type 1 (previously called insulin-dependent DM or juvenile-onset DM)
   - Type 2 (previously called non–insulin-dependent DM or adult-onset DM)
   - Gestational diabetes (diabetes diagnosed in pregnancy)

2. **Describe type 1 DM.**
   Type 1 DM accounts for approximately 5–10% of patients and is generally due to autoimmune destruction of the pancreatic beta-cells, leading to absolute insulin deficiency. Although typically diagnosed in patients before age 30, it can present at any age due to variability in the rate of beta-cell destruction.

3. **What are the major characteristics of type 2 DM?**
   The majority of patients have type 2 DM, which is associated with insulin resistance and relative insulin deficiency. Most patients are obese (predominantly abdominal accumulation). Type 2 DM is diagnosed in adulthood, and patients are not prone to develop ketoacidosis except in association with the stress from another illness.

4. **Compare and contrast the general features of type 1 and type 2 DM.**
   See Table 2-1.

TABLE 2-1. CHARACTERISTICS OF DIABETES MELLITUS

Type 1 Diabetes Mellitus	Type 2 Diabetes Mellitus
Usually presents at a younger age	Typically presents age > 40
Normal weight or thin	Obese
Usually no family history	Strong family history
Autoimmune markers may be positive (anti-GAD and anti-islet cell antibodies)	Not autoimmune in nature
Insulin sensitive	Insulin resistant
Requires insulin for treatment	Often managed with diet or oral agents
	Usually eventually require insulin

GAD = glutamic acid decarboxylase.

5. **What is gestational DM?**
Gestational DM, which is diagnosed during pregnancy, occurs in approximately 4% of pregnant women and usually presents in the second or third trimester when insulin resistance normally occurs. It is associated with increased fetal morbidity and mortality. Glucose tolerance usually returns to normal after delivery, but 30–40% of women with gestational DM develop type 2 DM within 10 years.

6. **Summarize other specific types of DM.**
Other specific types of DM include genetic defects in beta-cell function, also known as maturity-onset diabetes of the young, genetic defects in insulin action (i.e., mutations in the insulin receptor), diseases of the exocrine pancreas (e.g., hemochromatosis, neoplasm, cystic fibrosis), endocrinopathies (e.g., Cushing's syndrome, acromegaly, somatostatinoma, glucagonoma), drug-induced DM (e.g., pentamidine, glucocorticoids, alpha interferon), infections, and other rare genetic disorders.

7. **Summarize the two sets of criteria in routine clinical use for the diagnosis of DM.**
   - Symptoms of diabetes plus casual plasma glucose (PG) concentration ≥ 200 mg/dL (11.1 mmol/L). *Casual* is defined as any time of day without regard to last meal. The classic symptoms of diabetes include polyuria, polydipsia, and unexplained weight loss.

     or
   - Fasting PG ≥ 126 mg/dL (7.0 mmol/L). *Fasting* is defined as no caloric intake for at least 8 hours.

8. **What caveat applies to both sets of criteria?**
In the absence of unequivocal hyperglycemia with acute metabolic decompensation, these criteria should be confirmed by repeat testing on a different day.

9. **What is the oral glucose tolerance test (OGTT)?**
The OGTT is a specialized test for the diagnosis of DM. The test should be performed as described by the World Health Organization, using a glucose load containing the equivalent of 75 gm of anhydrous glucose dissolved in water. A positive test is defined as 2-hour PG ≥ 200 mg/dL (11.1 mmol/L). The OGTT is an accepted method for diagnosing DM; it is just not used routinely because it is more cumbersome than the other criteria described in question 7.

10. **What is the role of hemoglobin A_{1c} in the diagnosis of DM?**
Hemoglobin A_{1c} is not used to diagnose DM.

11. **What is "pre-diabetes"?**
Pre-diabetes refers to an intermediate group of people who have glucose values too high to be considered normal but do not fit the criteria for the diagnosis of DM. They are at high risk of developing DM. This group includes patients with impaired glucose tolerance (IGT) and impaired fasting glucose (IFG).

12. **Define IGT and IFG.**
IGT is defined as a 2-hour postload glucose of 140–199 mg/dL (7.8–11.1 mmol/L), using the OGTT. **IFG** is defined as fasting PG of 100–125 mg/dL (5.6–6.9 mmol/L). IGT and IFG are not truly disease entities but are associated with the metabolic syndrome and a high risk of developing DM and cardiovascular disease.

13. **List the characteristics of the metabolic syndrome.**
The metabolic syndrome refers to a constellation of signs and symptoms that are associated with an increased risk of cardiovascular disease and include:
   - Pre-diabetes or diabetes (hyperinsulinemia)

- Abdominal (central) obesity
- Hypertension
- Atherosclerosis
- Polycystic ovarian syndrome
- Atherogenic dyslipidemia (elevated triglycerides, apolipoprotein B, small dense LDL and low HDL)
- Altered coagulant state (impaired fibrinolysis, increased plasminogen activator inhibitor–1)
- Proinflammatory state (elevated C-reactive peptide)

KEY POINTS: DIAGNOSTIC FEATURES OF METABOLIC SYNDROME (THREE OR MORE OF THE FOLLOWING)

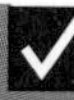

1. Abdominal obesity (waist circumference: men > 40 inches (102 cm), women > 35 inches (88 cm)
2. Hypertriglyceridemia (≥ 150 mg/dL)
3. Low HDL cholesterol (men < 40 mg/dL, women < 50 mg/dL)
4. Hypertension (≥ 130/85 mmHg)
5. Fasting hyperglycemia (≥ 110 mg/dL)

14. Describe the pathophysiology of diabetic ketoacidosis (DKA).

The pathogenesis of DKA involves an increase in counter-regulatory hormones (catecholamines, cortisol, glucagon, and growth hormone), accompanied by insulin deficiency. All of these hormonal factors contribute to increased hepatic and renal glucose production and decreased peripheral glucose utilization. These hormonal changes also serve to enhance lipolysis and ketogenesis as well as glycogenolysis and gluconeogenesis and serve to worsen hyperglycemia and acidosis. Lipolysis leads to increased free fatty acid synthesis for ultimate conversion by the liver to ketones. This state is associated with increased production and decreased utilization of glucose and ketones. Glucosuria leads to osmotic diuresis and dehydration that is associated with reduced renal function and worsening acidosis.

15. List the clinical features of DKA.

Clinical features vary with the severity of DKA: polydipsia, polyphagia, polyuria, severe dehydration, altered mental status (ranges from normal to coma), gastrointestinal distress (nausea, vomiting, abdominal pain), weight loss, and weakness.

16. What physical exam findings are associated with DKA?

Physical exam findings also vary with the severity of DKA: dehydration, poor skin turgor, Kussmaul breathing (deep, sighing respiration) mental status changes (wide range), hypotension, tachycardia, musty (fruity) breath, hyporeflexia, and hypothermia. Untreated DKA can progress to coma, shock, and death.

17. Summarize the lab data associated with DKA.

Lab data, which vary with the severity of DKA, include PG > 250 mg/dL, arterial pH < 7.3, serum bicarbonate < 18 mEq/L, positive serum and urine ketones, and elevated anion gap (> 10–12). Although the above lab results are diagnostic for DKA, one may see other abnormalities, including: elevated blood urea nitrogen and creatinine with dehydration, leukocytosis, low serum sodium, and elevated serum potassium due to extracellular shifting caused by insulin deficiency.

18. How is DKA managed?

In general, successful treatment of DKA includes fluid resuscitation, insulin therapy, and careful monitoring and correction of electrolyte imbalances. It is extremely important to identify precipitating factor(s) when possible. The most common precipitating factor is infection. The hospitalized patient should have appropriate bacterial cultures (e.g., blood, urine) and antibiotic therapy if infection is suspected.

19. What factors other than infection may precipitate DKA?

Other precipitating factors include myocardial infarction, stroke, pancreatitis, trauma, alcohol abuse, or medications (particularly inadequate insulin therapy).

20. Should patients with DKA be hospitalized?

Hospitalization depends on the severity of DKA, and very mild DKA in experienced patients with type 1 DM can be managed in the outpatient setting. Most patients, however, require hospitalization for IV fluid management, insulin (IV insulin infusion is the treatment of choice), and correction of electrolytes (sodium, potassium, phosphate, bicarbonate).

21. What principle should be kept in mind when patients are transitioned from IV to subcutaneous (SC) insulin?

The SC insulin must be given prior to discontinuing IV insulin (usually 1–2 hours to allow for adequate plasma insulin levels) to avoid return of hyperglycemia and/or DKA.

22. What is hyperglycemic hyperosmolar nonketotic syndrome (HHNS)?

Patients with HHNS present with severe hyperglycemia, profound dehydration, and some degree of alteration in mental status (50%). Typically patients have type 2 DM and mild renal impairment. The plasma glucose is frequently very elevated (> 600 mg/dL). Ketosis is usually only very mild or absent. Patients typically have severe dehydration, and plasma hyperosmolarity (> 340 mOsm/L) is one hallmark of this condition.

23. How is HHNS treated?

Treatment consists of aggressive fluid replacement, insulin, and correction of electrolyte disturbances. As with DKA, a search for the precipitating factor is warranted.

24. What is hemoglobin A_{1c}?

Hemoglobin A_{1c} (glycohemoglobin) is glycosylated hemoglobin and is used as a measure of average serum glucose concentrations over the prior 2–3 months.

25. How is hemoglobin A_{1c} used clinically?

Hemoglobin A_{1c} is an overall indicator of glycemic control. It should be measured biannually in patients who meet treatment goals (typically $A_{1c} < 7\%$) or quarterly in patients whose therapy is actively changing. Although an ideal goal for A_{1c} is < 7%, this goal must be individualized. Less intensive goals may be indicated in patients with frequent hypoglycemia, and more intensive goals may be desired in some patients to further reduce diabetes complications.

26. What are the currently recommended goals for glycemic control in patients with DM?

- Hemoglobin $A_{1c} < 7\%$
- Preprandial glucose 90–130 mg/dL
- Postprandial glucose < 180 mg/dL

27. Summarize the management of cardiovascular risk factors and screening guidelines for coronary disease in patients with diabetes mellitus.

- Blood pressure control. The goal is < 130/80 mmHg. Therapy should be individualized for each patient. First-line agents include angiotensin-converting enzyme (ACE) inhibitors and angiotensin receptor blockers. Second-line agents include diuretics, beta blockers, and dihydropyridine calcium channel blockers.
- Smoking cessation.
- Lipid management. Test annually or more frequently if patient has not met the following goals: LDL < 100 mg/dL, triglycerides < 50 mg/dL, and HDL > 40 mg/dL.
- Consider aspirin therapy for primary or secondary prevention.
- Consider screening for coronary artery disease.

28. What guidelines are recommended for screening of diabetic nephropathy?
Screen for microalbuminuria annually with spot albumin-to-creatinine ratio, and treat if detected. Microalbuminuria is defined as 30–299 μg albumin/mg creatinine and must be confirmed on repeated exams. Clinical albuminuria is defined as ≥ 300 μg albumin/mg creatinine. Start screening patients with type 1 DM when they have had DM for > 5 years and patients with type 2 DM at the time of diagnosis.

29. Summarize the screening recommendations for diabetic retinopathy.
Patients with type 1 DM should receive a comprehensive dilated eye exam within 3–5 years of diagnosis and annually thereafter. Patients with type 2 DM should receive a comprehensive dilated exam at the time of diagnosis and annually. The eye care specialist may determine altered timing of follow-up exams.

30. How are patients screened for diabetic neuropathy?
Patients should be assessed with monofilament sensory testing. Perform a good foot exam, and educate patients about foot care.

31. What other educational elements are important in the management of DM?
All diabetic patients should be educated about nutrition and lifestyle modifications.

32. Summarize the immunization guidelines for diabetic patients.
Annual influenza vaccine should be given to all patients with DM greater than age 6 months. Pneumococcal vaccine is recommended for all diabetic adults at least once.

33. Identify the oral agents available for the treatment of type 2 DM.
Type 2 DM can be treated with diet, exercise, oral agents, and insulin alone or in combinations. Table 2-2 lists oral medications available for treatment.

34. Describe the different types of insulin.
See Table 2-3.

35. Where is insulin cleared?
Approximately 50% of insulin is cleared via first pass through the liver. Once insulin is in the periphery, 30% is cleared by the kidney. Intravenous insulin has an extremely short half-life regardless of the type of insulin used (e.g., regular or Lispro). As soon as the insulin IV infusion is discontinued, it is generally cleared quickly from the circulation.

36. What are the indications for an insulin pump?
Although both continuous subcutaneous insulin infusion (CSII) and multiple daily insulin injections can effectively control blood glucose values, some patient and physician preferences may lead to the

TABLE 2-2. AVAILABLE ORAL AGENTS FOR THE TREATMENT OF TYPE 2 DM

Class	Generic Name (Brand Name)	Common Side Effects
Augment insulin release		
Sulfonylureas	Glyburide (Micronase, DiaBeta, Glynase)	Hypoglycemia, dizziness, GI upset
	Glipizide (Glucotrol, Glucotrol XL)	
	Glimepiride (Amaryl)	
Meglitinides	Repaglinide (Prandin)	Hypoglycemia, GI upset
	Nateglinide (Starlix)	
Insulin sensitizer		
Biguanides	Metformin (Glucophage)	Anorexia, diarrhea, GI upset, lactic acidosis (rare). Do not use in renal disease (Cr > 1.4 women, 1.5 men) or CHF.
	Metformin XL (Glucophage XL)	
Thiazolidinediones	Rosiglitazone (Avandia)	Weight gain, fluid retention (do not use in CHF), hepatotoxicity, hypoglycemia when used with insulin
	Pioglitazone (Actos)	
Alpha-glucosidase inhibitor	Acarbose (Precose)	Flatulence, diarrhea, GI distress
	Miglitol (Glyset)	
Mixtures	Glyburide/metformin (Glucovance)	Same as single agents
	Glypizide/metformin (Metaglip)	
	Metformin/rosiglitazone (Avandamet)	

Cr = creatinine, CHF = congestive heart failure, GI = gastrointestinal.

use of an insulin pump (CSII). This method of insulin delivery frequently affords the patient greater flexibility in insulin dosing and meal timing. CSIIP works very well for highly motivated patients with variable meal schedules but requires significant patient education, meticulous monitoring, and supervision by a health care provider who is comfortable with this mode of insulin delivery.

37. List the chronic complications of DM.

Microvascular

- Neuropathy (painfulparesthesias, autonomic neuropathy)
- Retinopathy (nonproliferative and proliferative retinopathy, blindness)
- Nephropathy (spectrum of disease from microalbuminuria to end-stage renal disease)

TABLE 2-3. TYPES OF INSULIN

Insulin Type	Time of Onset	Peak	Duration of Onset
Rapid-acting			
Lispro (Humalog)	< 30 min	30–90 min	3–5 h
Aspart (Novolog)	< 0.25 h	1–3 h	3–5 h
Short-acting			
Regular	0.5–1 h	2–4 h	6–12 h
Intermediate-acting			
NPH	1–2 h	4–14 h	10–24 h
Lente	1–3 h	6–16 h	12–24 h
Long-acting			
Glargine (Lantus)	1 h	No real peak	24 h
Ultralente	4–8 h	10–30 h	18–36 h
Mixtures			
70% NPH/30% Regular	30 min	4–8 h	16–24 h
50% NPH/50% Regular	30 min	7–12 h	16–24 h
75% NPL/25% Lispro	< 30 min	Lispro 30–90 min	
		Protamine 2–4 h	6–12 h
70% NPA/25% Aspart	< 0.25 h	1–4 h	12–24 h

NPH = neutral protamine Hagedorn, NPL = neutral protamine lispro, NPA = neutral protamine aspart. These values are highly variable among individual patients. Even in a given person, these values vary depending on the site and depth of injection, skin temperature, and exercise. *Note:* Insulin glargine cannot be mixed with other insulins due to the low pH of its diluent. Rapid-acting insulins can be mixed with NPH, Lente, and Ultralente.

Macrovascular (cardiovascular and peripheral vascular disease)

- Nonhealing ulcers, amputations
- Hypertension
- Dyslipidemia

38. **What are the symptoms of hypoglycemia?**
Symptoms can be divided into two categories: **adrenergic** (due to excess secretion of epinephrine) and **neuroglycopenic** (due to cerebral dysfunction). Patients with DM typically develop symptoms of hypoglycemia when blood glucose values fall below 50–60 mg/dL but severity of symptoms can vary with the individual. Additionally, some fasting individuals (particularly women) without DM can be completely asymptomatic with glucose values around 50 ng/dL. See Table 2-4.

39. **Describe hypoglycemia-associated autonomic failure.**
Hypoglycemia-associated autonomic failure refers to a syndrome of inappropriate response to hypoglycemia that occurs in patients with DM. Under normal physiologic conditions, hypoglycemia induces a reduction in insulin levels and an enhancement of glucagon and epinephrine

TABLE 2-4. SYMPTOMS OF HYPOGLYCEMIA

Adrenergic	Neuroglycopenic
Sweating	Dizziness
Tachycardia	Headache
Tremor	Decreased cognition, confusion
Anxiety	Clouded vision
Hunger	Seizures
	Coma

secretion, both of which serve to defend against continued hypoglycemia. Patients with type 1 DM and many patients with type 2 DM have defective glucose counter-regulation. Since they cannot reduce exogenous insulin levels and have impaired glucagon and epinephrine responses to hypoglycemia, they become prone to severe iatrogenic hypoglycemia. Additionally, they frequently have attenuated sympathoadrenal responses to hypoglycemia. Hypoglycemia-associated autonomic failure is induced by hypoglycemia and reversed by avoidance of hypoglycemia.

40. What is hypoglycemic unawareness?
Hypoglycemic unawareness refers to hypoglycemia that occurs unnoticed by the patient because it is not associated with any adrenergic symptoms. It is not uncommon for such patients to have exceedingly low glucose levels without cognitive impairment or other symptoms. They may go into an altered mental state without warning due to the lack of associated adrenergic symptoms.

41. What is the diagnostic approach to hypoglycemia in patients without diabetes?
First, hypoglycemia should be established using Whipple's triad: presence of symptoms consistent with hypoglycemia (such as sweating, hunger, palpitations, and weakness), documented low plasma glucose at the time of symptoms, and relief of symptoms when the plasma glucose concentration is raised to normal levels. Hypoglycemia in the fasting state is typically more clinically concerning than reactive (postprandial) hypoglycemia. Although the exact criteria are debated, glucose levels of < 50 mg/dL in men and < 40 mg/dL in women are generally accepted as indicative of hypoglycemia.

42. Summarize the differential diagnosis of adult hypoglycemia not related to diabetes.

- Drug-induced or factitious hypoglycemia. It is important to rule out exposure to exogenous insulin and oral antidiabetic agents, particularly sulfonylureas. Other drugs associated with hypoglycemia include ethanol (inhibits gluconeogenesis), salicylates, sulfonamides, pentamidine, monoamine oxidase (MAO) inhibitors, and quinine.
- Critical illness, including liver and renal failure.
- Adrenal insufficiency (lack of the counter-regulatory hormone cortisol).
- Insulinoma: tumor of the pancreatic beta cell that produces too much insulin.
- Non–beta-cell tumors, including mesenchymal tumors such as fibrosarcoma, mesothelioma, and leiomyosarcoma, that produce insulin-like growth factor I (IGF-I) or IGF-II.
- Insulin or insulin receptor autoantibodies (rare).

43. How do you distinguish between endogenous and exogenous hyperinsulinemia?
Insulin and C-peptide levels are helpful to distinguish between endogenous and exogenous hyperinsulinemia since insulin and its cleavage product C-peptide are secreted by the pancreatic beta cell in equimolar amounts. If a patient is getting exogenous insulin, insulin levels will be high and C-peptide levels low. Both values are elevated in patients with surreptitious sulfonylurea use since these drugs stimulate release of endogenous insulin and C-peptide. Sulfonylurea blood levels can also help rule out drug-induced hypoglycemia in this setting.

44. List the most common pancreatic endocrine tumors.
These tumors are derived from the islet cells of the pancreas and are named for the hormones that they secrete. They are listed below along with their clinical presentations:

- **Insulinoma** (secretes insulin): hypoglycemia.
- **Gastrinoma** (secretes gastrin): Zollinger-Ellison syndrome, associated with excess gastric acid secretion and peptic ulcer disease.
- **Glucagonoma** (secretes glucagon): DM, weight loss, anemia, necrolytic migratory erythema.
- **Somatostatinoma** (secretes somatostatin): somatostatin inhibits secretion of insulin gastric acid and pancreatic enzymes, leading to diabetes, weight loss, hypochlohydria, steatorrhea, and gallstones.
- **VIPoma** (secretes vasoactive intestinal peptide): watery diarrhea, hypokalemia, achlorhydria.
- **PPoma** (secretes pancreatic polypeptide alone or in combination with other pancreatic peptides): watery diarrhea.

45. Identify the hereditary syndrome associated with pancreatic tumors.
Multiple endocrine neoplasia syndromes (MEN) are characterized by neoplastic transformation in multiple endocrine glands. MEN type 1 (MEN1) is associated with pancreatic tumors. MEN1 is now known to be caused by a mutation in the tumor suppressor MEN1 gene, whose product is named *menin.*

46. What are the components of MEN1?
Components of MEN1 include the 3 Ps:

- Pituitary tumors (most commonly prolactinoma)
- Primary hyperparathyroidism (typically due to parathyroid hyperplasia)
- Pancreatic tumors (most commonly gastrinoma, followed by insulinoma)

47. What are MEN2A and MEN2B?
MEN2A and MEN2B are due to activating mutations of the *RET* proto-oncogene. MEN2A includes neoplasms of the thyroid (medullary thyroid carcinoma), parathyroid (primary hyperparathyroidism), and adrenal gland (pheochromocytoma). MEN2B includes medullary thyroid carcinoma, pheochromocytoma, and mucosal neuromas.

OBESITY

48. How is obesity currently defined?
Obesity is the level of overweightness associated with significant mortality and morbidity. Obesity is determined by body mass index (BMI). The BMI is calculated by dividing weight in kilograms by height in meters squared (weight in kg)/(height in meters)^2. Individuals are currently considered overweight if the BMI is greater than 25. Levels of obesity are defined as follows:

- BMI < 25: Normal
- BMI 25–29.9: Overweight

- BMI 30–34.9: Mild obesity
- BMI 35–39.9: Moderate obesity
- BMI > 40: Severe obesity

49. How significant is waist circumference in diagnosing obesity?
Waist circumference can also be used to diagnose obesity. Health risks of obesity are correlated with visceral (abdominal) adiposity. People with larger waist sizes have increased risks of obesity-related disorders such as hypertension, cardiovascular disease, and diabetes. Waist circumference is determined by placing a tape measure horizontally around the abdomen at the level of the iliac crest. Measurements should be taken at the end of a normal expiration. The tape measure should be snug but not compress the skin. Increased risk of obesity-related disease occurs in men with a waist circumference ≥ 40 inches (102 cm) and women with a waist conference ≥ 35 inches (88 cm).

50. List the health risks associated with obesity.
- Diabetes
- Hypertension
- Hyperlipidemia
- Coronary artery disease
- Cerebral vascular disease
- Degenerative arthritis
- Obstuctive sleep apnea
- Gallbladder disease
- Cancers of endometrium, breast, colon, and prostate
- Psychological complications (depression, poor self-esteem, discrimination)
  Stein CJ, Colditz GA: The epidemic of obesity. JCEM 89(6):2522–2525, 2004.

51. How common is obesity?
Obesity is now thought to be one of the leading health disorders in the United States. Its prevalence has increased dramatically and it is now estimated that approximately one third of the U.S. population is obese (BMI > 30). The prevalence is higher in ethnic minorities and is rapidly increasing in children and adolescents.

52. What causes people to gain weight?
Weight gain occurs when a person is not in energy balance. Weight maintenance occurs when people consume as many calories as they expend per day. Obesity occurs in the setting of increased caloric intake or decreased energy expenditure relative to caloric intake.

53. List the three components of total daily energy expenditure (EE).
- Basal metabolic rate (approximately 65% of total daily EE)
- Energy of physical activity (30% of average person's daily EE)
- Thermic effect of food (energy cost of digesting food, which accounts for 5% of daily EE)

54. What factors control energy homeostasis?
Energy homeostasis is achieved by complex interactions between the brain and neural factors that control appetite and satiety, nutrient metabolism, and hormonal systems. Much research is currently being conducted in the neural mechanisms that regulate feeding and energy balance. Most evidence suggests that obese people do not have major alterations in their basal metabolic rates. In fact, since total energy expenditure is linearly related to BMI, obese people actually require more calories for weight maintenance than lean people. It is much more likely that obesity develops as a multifactorial process involving genetic predisposition as well as environmental and behavioral factors.

55. **Who should be treated for obesity?**
Obese people should be instructed about proper diet and exercise to prevent obesity-related complications. People with more severe obesity or those who already have obesity-related complications should be treated more aggressively.

56. **Describe the general approach to treatment of obesity.**
Treatment must be individualized, and the patient's goals must be discussed. Frequently, patients want a rapid, substantial weight loss. Unfortunately, this goal is usually not healthy or attainable in the patient's desired time frame. Since 1 lb of fat stores approximately 3500 kcal, in order to lose 1 lb of weight per week, the person must decrease caloric intake by roughly 500 kcal/day. This regimen is often extremely difficult to follow. Consequently, a more moderate approach is to restrict caloric intake (250–500 kcal reduction from basal intake) and increase energy expenditure (30 minutes of moderate physical activity most days of the week).

57. **When should pharmacotherapy be considered for the treatment of obesity?**
Typically, the first approach is diet and exercise with behavioral modifications followed by the addition of pharmacotherapy. Pharmacotherapy should be considered in patients with a BMI over 30, a BMI over 27 with comorbidities, or minimal response after 6 months of lifestyle modifications.

58. **What medications are used for the treatment of obesity?**
- Phentermine, a norepinephrine agonist (15–30 mg/day)
- Sibutramine, a combination norepinephrine/serotonin reuptake blocker (5, 10, and 15 mg; start with 10 mg and titrate)
- Orlistat, a pancreatic lipase inhibitor (120 mg 3 times/day before meals)

59. **How effective are medications in treating obesity?**
In general, medications require chronic use for effectiveness and can be expected to produce a 5–10% weight loss in most people.

60. **Summarize the role of surgery in the treatment of obesity.**
Surgery is generally reserved for people with severe obesity (BMI > 40) who have failed other forms of therapy. The most frequently performed procedures are the vertical banded gastroplasty and gastric bypass.

PITUITARY GLAND

61. **Summarize the general functions of the pituitary gland.**
The pituitary gland is the "master gland" of the endocrine system. It is involved in many body functions, including growth and development, metabolism, and reproduction. These functions are regulated by the secretion of hormones that interact at specific target organ sites.

62. **Describe the anterior pituitary gland.**
The anterior pituitary or adenopypophysis, which composes 80% of the entire gland, is derived embryologically from Rathke's pouch and is oral ectoderm in origin. Anterior pituitary hormones are synthesized in the pituitary by specific cell types and are regulated by hypothalamic and target organ factors.

63. **List the six major hormones secreted by the anterior pituitary.**
- Somatotropin (growth hormone [GH])
- Prolactin

- Corticotropin (ACTH)
- Thyrotropin (thyroid-stimulating hormone [TSH])
- Luteinizing hormone (LH)
- Follicle-stimulating hormone (FSH)

64. **How is secretion of these hormones regulated?**

All of these hormones are regulated by positive and negative feedback mechanisms. Most hormones are stimulated by a hypothalamic hormone and inhibited by a target organ hormone. The one exception is prolactin, which is is under tonic inhibitory control by hypothalamic dopamine neurons. A schematic diagram is represented in Fig. 2-1.

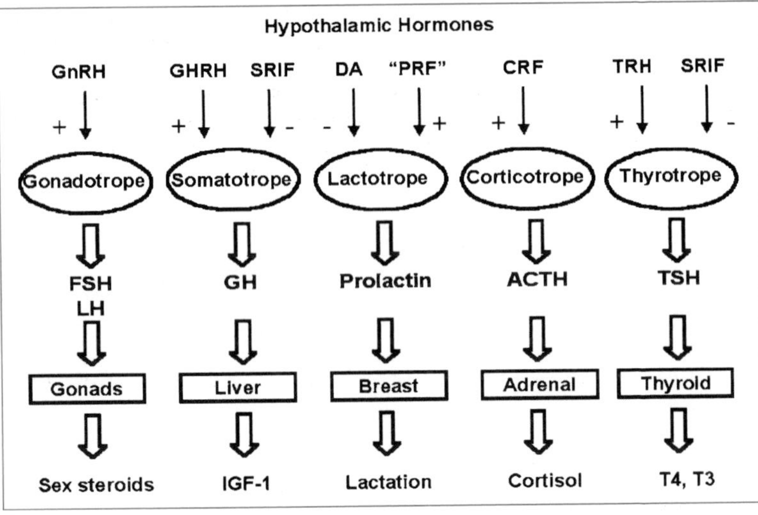

Pituitary Cell Type	Hormone	Hypothalamic Factor
Corticotrope	Corticotropin (ACTH)	CRH stimulates
Thyrotrope	Thyrotropin (TSH)	TRH stimulates and SRIF inhibits
Gonadotrope	Luteinizing hormone (LH) Follicle-stimulating hormone (FSH)	GnRH
Somatotrope	Growth hormone (GH)	GHRH stimulates and SRIF inhibits.
Lactotrope	Prolactin	Dopamine inhibits prolactin-releasing factors (e.g., TRH, suckling)

Figure 2-2. Hormones of the anterior pituitary gland. CRH = corticotropin-releasing hormone, TRH = thyrotropin-releasing hormone, SRIF = somatostatin, GnRH = gonadotropin-releasing hormone, GHRH = growth hormone–releasing hormone, PRF = prolactin releasing factors.

65. **Describe the posterior pituitary. What hormones does it secrete?**
The posterior pituitary or neurohypophysis is an extension of the floor of the third ventricle and originates from cells of the central nervous system. Posterior pituitary hormones included arginine vasopressin (AVP, antidiuretic hormone) and oxytocin. These hormones are synthesized in the cell bodies of hypothalmic neurons and stored in the axons that terminate in the posterior pituitary.

66. **Describe the general approach to evaluating a patient with pituitary disease.**
It is important to take a good history and ask specific questions related to hormonal hyper- or hypofunction. Think specifically about assessing anterior and posterior pituitary function.

67. **In particular, what should be evaluated in patients with pituitary tumors?**
Questions should identify clinical problems associated with pituitary tumors, which include hormonal abnormalities and mass effects. Mass effects can include neurologic symptoms and impaired anterior pituitary function. It is rare to have posterior pituitary dysfunction as a consequence of a pituitary tumor, but it can be seen in patients with pituitary trauma or disorders of the pituitary stalk. Headache and disruption of cranial nerve function (cranial nerves II, III, IV, and VI) are the most common neurologic symptoms. Pituitary tumors that compress the optic nerves or optic chiasm are typically associated with visual field deficits (bitemporal hemianopsia) or visual loss.

KEY POINTS: MECHANISMS BY WHICH PITUITARY TUMORS CAUSE PROBLEMS 

1. Mass effect: tumors apply pressure to surrounding structures causing functional disruption that may lead to:
   - Headaches
   - Visual disturbance/visual field defects
   - Cranial nerve dysfunction
   - Anterior pituitary hormone deficiencies
2. Endocrine hyperfunction: due to excessive secretion of a particular anterior pituitary hormone by the tumor.

68. **What factors should be the focus of the physical exam?**
On physical exam it is important to perform a full neurologic exam with visual field testing by confrontation and to look for clinical evidence of hormonal hyperfunction (e.g., enlarged hands and feet, skin tags, and facial features of acromegaly) or hypofunction (e.g., loss of body hair in hypogonadal men or delayed deep tendon reflexes as a sign of hypothyroidism).

69. **What causes acromegaly?**
Acromegaly is caused by a tumor of the GH-secreting cell.

70. **How does acromegaly present clinically?**
If the tumor occurs in childhood before the closure of the epiphyses, the effect is known as gigantism. Patients frequently present late in the disease with large tumors (macroadenomas in 85%) due to the very slow development of the clinical features. It often goes unrecognized by the patient, his or her family, and the primary care provider because the physical changes occur

so slowly. Such patients can present with soft tissue hypertrophy; headache; arthritis/carpal tunnel syndrome; increased size of hands, head, and feet; organomegaly, including cardiomegaly with congestive heart failure; and obstructive sleep apnea.

71. What physical exam findings are suggestive of acromegaly?
Physical exam findings include soft tissue characteristics (large doughy hands), frontal bossing, widening spaces in teeth, skin tags, organomegaly, large body size, signs of hyperprolactinemia, hypogonadism, and visual field deficits.

72. How is acromegaly diagnosed?
Diagnosis is based on clinical features, laboratory evaluation, and magnetic resonance imaging (MRI) of the pituitary. Diagnostic lab abnormalities include elevated GH with failure to suppress with oral glucose administration and an elevated IGF-1 (somatomedin-C). Patients may also have insulin resistance/DM, hyperprolactinemia due to stalk compression, hypogonadism, and hypercalciuria/nephrolithiasis. They are at higher risk of colon polyps/cancer and have increased mortality rates.

73. Explain the goal for treatment of acromegaly.
The goal of treatment is to normalize anterior pituitary function and GH secretion. Mortality rates return to baseline levels if the GH is normalized (normal GH, normal IGF-1, and normal GH suppression [$< 1\ \mu g/L$] following oral glucose).

74. How can this goal be achieved?
Transsphenoidal surgical resection is typically the treatment of choice. Medical treatment is often required because many tumors are too large at presentation to be completely excised by surgery. In such cases, somatostatin analogs are indicated for medical therapy to control GH secretion. GH cells have somatostatin receptors and treatment with somatostatin analogs (octreotide), have been shown to decrease GH levels and induce tumor shrinkage. A new GH receptor antagonist, pegvisomant, has also been approved for medical therapy. Although less effective, dopamine agonists such as bromocriptine or cabergoline can also be tried to control GH levels. Finally, radiation therapy can be offered to patients who fail surgical and medical interventions.

Melmed S, et al: Consensus guidelines for acromegaly management. JCEM 87(9):4054–4058, 2002.

75. Prolactinomas are the most common type of pituitary tumor. In general, how do they present?
The clinical picture of hyperprolactinemia is variable, depending on age, sex, duration of hyperprolactinemia, and tumor size. Hypogonadism is common and due to prolactin inhibition of gonadotropin-releasing hormone neurons and leads to suppression of the hypothalamic-pituitary-gonadal axis. Women of reproductive age present earlier with amenorrhea and galactorrhea. Men and postmenopausal women usually present later in the disease course with mass effect such as headache and visual deficits.

76. List the clinical features of hyperprolactinemia.

- Galactorrhea
- Amenorrhea/menstrual irregularities
- Infertility
- Hirsutism
- Gynecomastia and erectile dysfunction in men
- Growth arrest/delayed puberty
- Mass lesions/visual field defects (primarily in men and postmenopausal women)
- Osteopenia (due to hypogonadism)

77. **What is the differential diagnosis of hyperprolactinemia?**
- Pregnancy (normal physiologic cause of hyperprolactinemia)
- Neurogenic disorder (chest wall lesion, suckling; do not measure prolactin after a breast exam.)
- Drugs: dopamine depletion or antagonists (usually psychoactive medications)
- Cirrhosis
- Primary hypothyroidism (thyrotropin-releasing hormone [TRH] also stimulates prolactin secretion)
- Ectopic production (ovarian tumors)
- Pituitary tumors/prolactinomas
- Idiopathic disease

78. **What are the treatment options for hyperprolactinemia?**
Treatment obviously depends on the etiology. When due to a medication, it is obviously best to stop the offending agent if possible. Medical therapy with dopamine agonists is the treatment of choice for prolactinomas. Oral contraceptives can be used to restore normal menstrual cycles and protect against bone loss in female patients who have mild elevations in prolactin in the absence of a visible pituitary tumor. Surgery is not typically the treatment of choice for prolactinomas due to a high recurrence rate (especially for macroadenomas) but can be considered in invasive tumors or tumors resistant to medication. Radiation can always be considered in patients who fail other modalities.

79. **How do dopamine agonists work?**
Dopamine agonists have been shown to inhibit prolactin secretion and cause tumor shrinkage. Examples include bromocriptine, pergolide, and the newer, more potent agent, cabergoline. All must be started at low doses and titrated upward very slowly to avoid side effects. The most common side effects include nausea, vomiting, and orthostatic hypotension. Cabergoline appears to be the best tolerated but most expensive option.

80. **What is the "stalk effect"?**
Large non–prolactin-secreting tumors compress the pituitary stalk, thus interrupting the tonic inhibitory effect of dopamine (or prolactin-inhibiting factor) on the pituitary. The result is elevation of prolactin levels up to 200 ng/mL.

81. **What is pituitary apoplexy?**
Pituitary apoplexy is defined as sudden headache, visual change, ophthalmoplegia, and altered mental status caused by the acute hemorrhage or infarction of the pituitary gland. Most cases are due to pituitary hemorrhage of a previously undiagnosed pituitary adenoma (65%). Patient presentation may range from asymptomatic to symptoms of severe retro-orbital headache, visual defects, meningeal signs, altered sensorium, seizure, or coma depending on the extent of the lesion. Clinical symptoms and signs plus CT scan or MRI of the pituitary aid in the diagnosis. This condition can be life-threatening if unrecognized.

82. **How is pituitary apoplexy treated?**
Treatment consists of stress doses of steroids (for cerebral edema and presumed adrenal insufficiency) and/or neurosurgical decompression. Hormonal deficiencies following apoplexy are the rule, and panhypopituitarism is common. Hypogonadism occurs in nearly 100%, GH deficiency in 88%, hyperprolactinemia in 67%, adrenal insufficiency in 66%, hypothyroidism in 42%, and diabetes insipidus in 3%.

83. **What is a thyrotropinoma?**
As the name suggests, it is a tumor of the TSH-producing cell. This rare tumor occurs in approximately one in a million people. It produces a clinical syndrome of hyperthyroidism that is indistinguishable from other more common causes (e.g., Graves' disease, toxic nodular goiter).

It is differentiated from primary hyperthyroidism by an inappropriately normal or elevated TSH in the setting of elevated thyroid hormone levels. Since TSH is secreted as a dimer peptide comprised of the TSH beta and alpha subunits, alpha subunit levels are typically elevated. Patients have an elevated molar ratio of alpha-SU/TSH > 1.

84. **How is a thyrotropinoma diagnosed?**
Pituitary MRI typically demonstrates a tumor. If not, since these tumors display somatostatin receptors, octreotide scanning may be helpful for tumor localization.

85. **What causes hypopituitarism?**
It is possible to have an isolated hormonal deficiency or complete anterior pituitary hormonal dysfunction (panhypopituitarism). Causes of hypopituitarism include:

- Mass lesions from tumors (pituitary adenoma, craniopharyngiomas, metastatic lesions)
- Iatrogenic causes (pituitary surgery, radiation)
- Infiltrative disease (hemochromatosis, lymphoma, sarcoid, histiocytosis X)
- Pituitary infarction (Sheehan syndrome, after coronary artery bypass grafting, trauma)
- Pituitary apoplexy
- Genetic disease (transcription factor mutations)
- Empty sella syndrome (typically secondary)
- Hypothalamic dysfunction (mass lesions, infiltrative diseases, radiation, trauma, infection)
- Autoimmune lymphocytic hypophysitis
- Miscellaneous (abscess/infection; aneurysm)

86. **How do patients with hypopituitarism present?**
Patients present with signs and symptoms of hormonal deficiency. Evaluation is aimed at documenting deficiency and may include stimulation testing (i.e., adrenal insufficiency, GH deficiency).

87. **How is hypopituitarism treated?**
Treatment consists of correcting the hormonal deficiency. Patients with adrenal insufficiency need to be educated about stress-dose steroids for acute illness, and all patients should wear medical alert jewelry.

88. **What is diabetes insipidus (DI)? How is it treated?**
DI is characterized by an inability to concentrate urine due to insufficient arginine vasopressin (AVP, antidiuretic hormone) release or activity. Large amounts of dilute urine are excreted in the setting of hyperosmolality and hypernatremia.

89. **What are the two types of DI?**
Central (neurogenic) DI, which is due to impaired or inadequate secretion of AVP from the posterior pituitary, and nephrogenic DI, which is due to resistance to AVP. Central DI can be partial or complete and is typically an acquired condition related to trauma or infiltrative disease of the hypothalamus/posterior pituitary. Nephrogenic DI can be acquired due to hypercalcemia, hypokalemia, drug-induced (lithium), or congenital.

90. **How do patients with DI present?**
Patients present with polyuria (typically large volumes with osmolality < 200 mOsm/kg), polydipsia, and hypernatremia if the patients do not have an intact thirst mechanism or do not drink water. Diagnosis is confirmed by performing a water deprivation test.

91. **How is DI treated?**
Treatment depends on diagnosis. Central DI is typically treated with AVP replacement in the form of dDAVP (desmopressin), a synthetic AVP agonist. There are no good therapies for

nephrogenic DI, but treatment is usually aimed at volume contraction using thiazide diuretics, salt depletion or prostaglandin synthesis inhibitors. These agents decrease renal blood flow by volume contraction and decrease urine output by reducing glomerular filtration rates.

ADRENAL GLANDS

92. List the hormones secreted by the adrenal gland.
See Table 2-5.

TABLE 2-5. ADRENAL HORMONES

Hormone	Synthesis	Syndromes
Cortisol	Synthesized from cholesterol in the adrenal cortex (zona fasciculata, zona reticularis)	Hyperfunction: Cushing's syndrome Hypofunction: Adrenal insufficiency
Aldosterone	Synthesized from cholesterol in the adrenal cortex (zona glomerulosa)	Hyperfunction: Hyperaldosteronism Hypofunction: Adrenal insufficiency
Androgens/sex steroids	Synthesized from cholesterol in the adrenal cortex (zona fasciculata, zona reticularis)	Hyperfunction: Hirsutism/virilization Hypofunction: No clear syndrome
Catecholamines (norepinephrine, epinephrine)	Synthesized in the adrenal medulla	Hyperfunction: Pheochromocytoma Hypofunction: Hypotension

93. Differentiate Cushing's syndrome from Cushing's disease.
Cushing's syndrome refers to hypercortisolemia and its associated signs and symptoms due to any cause. *Cushing's disease* refers specifically to hypercortisolemia due to ACTH overproduction by a pituitary adenoma. The most common cause of Cushing's syndrome is iatrogenic due to exogenous steroid treatment for a variety of conditions (rheumatologic, organ transplant, reactive airway disease). If one excludes iatrogenic hypercortisolemia, the most common cause of Cushing's syndrome is Cushing's disease, which accounts for approximately two thirds of all cases.

94. What are the signs and symptoms of Cushing's disease?
- Atrophic, thin skin, easy bruising, purple striae (abdomen, axilla, hips, thighs)
- Weight gain or central obesity
- Dorsocervical (buffalo hump) and supraclavicular fat accumulation
- Moon facies
- Menstrual irregularities
- Hirsutism
- Diabetes or insulin resistance
- Muscle weakness

- Hypertension
- Increased susceptibility to infection
- Osteoporosis (or osteopenia)
- Psychiatric symptom (depression, mood changes, even psychosis)
- Hypercoagulable state

95. List the four steps involved in evaluating a patient for Cushing's syndrome.

- Step 1: Screen for and document Cushing's syndrome (hypercortisolemia).
- Step 2: Differentiate between ACTH-dependent and ACTH-independent causes.
- Step 3: Distinguish pituitary Cushing's disease from ectopic ACTH secretion.
- Step 4: Anatomic imaging and surgical resection of the tumor once identified.

96. Who should be considered for Cushing's syndrome screening?

This is a difficult question because many people have symptoms that could be associated with Cushing's syndrome, such as weight gain, hypertension, diabetes, and depression. Consider screening adults with weight gain and an abnormal fat distribution, proximal muscle weakness, large (> 1 cm wide) purple striae, and new cognitive/depression complaints; children with linear growth failure and continued weight gain; and young people with nontraumatic bone fractures, cutaneous atrophy, or hypertension. Patients with multiple clinical features should be screened particularly if the symptoms become more severe over time.

97. How should one screen for Cushing's syndrome?

First-line screening tests include the low-dose (1 mg) overnight dexamethasone test and 24-hour urine free cortisol levels.

Arnaldi G, Angeli A, Atkinson AB, et al: Diagnosis and complications of Cushing's syndrome: A consensus statement. J Clin Endocrinol Metab 88(12):5593–5602, 2003.

98. How is the low-dose dexamethasone suppression test performed?

Give 1 mg of dexamethasone at 11 PM the night before. This dose should suppress 8 AM cortisol to < 1.8 μg/dL if a sensitive assay is used (the old cutoff value was < 5 μg/dL).

99. How is the 24-hour urine free cortisol test done?

This test should be normal in patients without Cushing's syndrome (most assays define normal as = < 100 mg/24 h). This test may be repeated up to three times if the first test is normal and there is a high index of suspicion. It must always be performed with a creatinine level to ensure adequacy of the urine collection.

100. What is the late evening salivary cortisol test?

Some clinicians advocate this test because it is easy to perform and salivary and plasma cortisol levels are highly correlated. Patients are instructed to obtain late night (11 PM) salivary samples. Cortisol levels should be low and confirm normal diurnal variation. Cushing's patients have abnormally high late-night levels. This test can be considered as a screening test, particularly in patients with episodic hypercortisolemia, but it has not replaced the other two tests as first-line modalities. Normal ranges are assay-dependent and must be validated for each laboratory.

101. Once hypercortisolemia has been documented, what is the next step in evaluating a patient with Cushing's syndrome?

After ruling out ingestion of exogenous steroids, the next step is to differentiate between ACTH-dependent (80%) and ACTH-independent (20%) disease. ACTH-dependent disease is associated with pituitary adenoma (80%), ectopic ACTH (20%), and corticotropin-releasing hormone (CRH) hypersecretion (rare). ACTH-independent disease is associated with adrenal adenoma (40–50%), adrenal carcinoma (40–50%), nodular dysplasia (rare), and McCune-Albright syndrome (rare).

102. What is the best way to make this distinction?
The best method is simultaneous measurement of ACTH and cortisol. If the ACTH is >10 pg/mL, the patient most likely has an ACTH-dependent cause of Cushing's syndrome. Additionally, an ACTH value > 10 pg/mL following peripheral CRH administration suggests ACTH dependency.

103. Once ACTH-dependent Cushing's syndrome has been confirmed, what is the final step in making the biochemical diagnosis?
The final step involves differentiating between a corticotrope adenoma and an ectopic ACTH-secreting tumor. A high-dose (8-mg) dexamethasone test can be performed. Patients with a pituitary source of ACTH retain suppressibility of cortisol to high-dose dexamethasone, whereas patients with ectopic ACTH tumors do not.

104. How is the dexamethasone test confirmed?
Many clinicians confirm the diagnosis with inferior petrosal sinus sampling (IPSS). This test takes advantage of the concentration gradient between pituitary venous drainage via the inferior petrosal sinus (IPS—central) and peripheral venous values of ACTH to further determine whether an ACTH-producing corticotroph adenoma is present in the pituitary; the inclusion of CRH stimulation adds greater sensitivity to the test.

105. Explain how the IPSS is done.
Samples of ACTH and cortisol are obtained simultaneously from the IPS (central) and from a peripheral site (e.g., inferior vena cava [IVC]). In patients with Cushing's disease, the central/peripheral ratio (C/P = IPS/IVC ratio) of ACTH is > 2. In patients with ectopic ACTH, the ratio is < 2 and selective venous sampling (e.g., of the pulmonary, pancreatic, or intestinal beds) may localize the ectopic tumor.

106. How does the inclusion of CRH increase diagnostic accuracy?
Administration of CRH during bilateral IPS sampling has increased the diagnostic accuracy of the test by eliciting an ACTH response in the few patients with pituitary tumor who did not have a diagnostic C/P gradient in the basal samples. All patients with Cushing's disease have had a C/P ratio > 3 after CRH, whereas patients with ectopic ACTH or adrenal disease have had C/P ratios < 3 after CRH.

107. What is the most significant limitation of IPSS with or without CRH?
It is important to note that IPSS with or without CRH has not been extensively performed in normal subjects. Thus correct interpretation of the results requires that the patient be hypercortisolemic at the time of the study so that the response of normal corticotropes to CRH is suppressed. One approach is represented in Fig. 2-2. If results indicate an ectopic source, a CT or MRI of the chest is usually performed first since most are due to small cell carcinoma or bronchial or thymic carcinoid tumors.

108. What is pseudo-Cushing's syndrome?
This is a clinical state characterized by mild overactivity of the hypothalamic-pituitary-adrenal axis that is not associated with true Cushing's syndrome (hypercortisolemia). It is typically seen in a variety of psychiatric states (depression, anxiety), alcoholism, uncontrolled diabetes, and severe obesity. The dexamethasone-CRH stimulation test can be used to help distinguish this disorder from true Cushing's syndrome. Alternatively, an elevated midnight plasma cortisol level rules out pseudo-Cushing's because, unlike patients with true Cushing's syndrome, patients with pseudo-Cushing's retain the diurnal rhythym of cortisol secretion.

109. Explain how the dexamethasone-CRH stimulation test is done.
Patients take 0.5 mg of dexamethasone every 6 hours for 8 doses starting at noon. At 8 AM (after the 8 doses of dexamethasone), CRH (human recombinant CRH [Acthrel]) is given

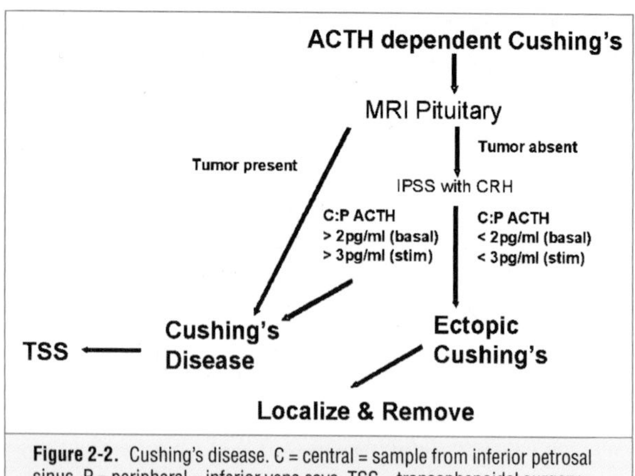

Figure 2-2. Cushing's disease. C = central = sample from inferior petrosal sinus, P = peripheral = inferior vena cava, TSS = transsphenoidal surgery.

intravenously at a dose of 1 μg/kg, and cortisol is measured 15 minutes later. A cortisol value > 1.4 mg/dL indicates Cushing's syndrome.

110. **What is Nelson's syndrome?**
Nelson's syndrome occurs in up to 30% of patients following bilateral adrenalectomy and is due to corticotrope hyperplasia/adenoma. Patients often present with mass effects associated with the adenoma and hyperpigmentation due to high levels of ACTH (with resultant high levels of melanocyte-stimulating hormone).

111. **Define adrenal insufficiency.**
As the name suggests, this disorder is caused by insufficient release of adrenal hormones (typically hormones of the adrenal cortex: cortisol and aldosterone).

112. **What causes adrenal insufficiency?**
The causes can be divided into two categories: primary and central. Primary adrenal insufficiency (Addison's disease) is due to adrenal gland dysfunction. Central adrenal insufficiency includes both secondary (pituitary) and tertiary (hypothalamic) causes.

113. **List the causes of primary adrenal sufficiency.**
Autoimmune destruction (70–80%), tuberculosis (20%), adrenal destruction by bilateral hemorrhage or infarction, tumor, infections (other than tuberculosis), surgery, radiation, drugs, amyloidosis, sarcoidosis, hyporesponsiveness to ACTH, and congenital abnormalities.

114. **List the cause of central adrenal insufficiency.**
Withdrawal of exogenous steroids (common), following cure of Cushing's syndrome, pituitary adenoma/infarction, and hypothalamic abnormalities (rare).

115. **What are the major symptoms and signs of Addison's disease?**
See Table 2-6.

116. **How do Addison's disease and central adrenal insufficiency differ in their presentation?**
Primary adrenal insufficiency (Addison's disease) is caused by failure or destruction of the adrenal glands, leading to underproduction of glucocorticoids and mineralocorticoids. This

TABLE 2-6. CLINICAL PRESENTATION OF PRIMARY ADRENAL INSUFFICIENCY (ADDISON'S DISEASE)

Symptoms	Signs
Weakness, fatigue	Hyperkalemia (mild)
Anorexia, weight loss	Hyponatremia
Dizziness	Orthostatic hypotension
GI upset: nausea, vomiting, diarrhea, abdominal pain	Hyperpigmentation (buccal mucosa, skinfolds, extensor surfaces, new scars)
Salt craving	Vitiligo
	Adrenal calcifications

results in an increase in ACTH production by the pituitary. Its signs and symptoms are described above. **Central** adrenal insufficiency is caused by deficient production of ACTH, leading to underproduction of glucocorticoids. The manifestations are the same as those of Addison's disease with the following exceptions:

- Hyperpigmentation is not seen in central disease. Patients do not have hypersecretion of melanocyte-stimulating hormone (a product of the propiomelanocortin gene, like ACTH) that is responsible for the hyperpigmentation.
- Electrolyte abnormalities (hyponatremia, hyperkalemia) are not typically present in central disease because the aldosterone system is largely intact.
- Central disease may involve other manifestations of hypopituitarism.
- Hypoglycemia is more commonly seen with central disease due to the presence of combined ACTH and GH deficiency.

117. Summarize the differences in treatment of primary and central adrenal insufficiency.

In terms of treatment, patients with Addison's disease typically require replacement of both glucocorticoids (prednisone or hydrocortisone) and mineralocorticoids (Florinef), whereas patients with central adrenal insufficiency typically need only glucocorticoids. Patients with central disease do not usually require mineralocorticoids because aldosterone secretion is largely unaffected. All patients should be instructed to increase steroid replacement during times of illness and should wear medical alert jewelry. The goal of treatment is to ameliorate the signs and symptoms of adrenal insufficiency without causing Cushing's syndrome due to exogenous glucocorticoid replacement. Always use the lowest possible doses that control symptoms to avoid side effects.

118. What is the gold standard test to assess adequacy of the hypothalamic-pituitary-adrenal axis?

Although a number of tests are available to assess function of the hypothalamic-pituitary-adrenal axis, the insulin tolerance test (ITT) is the gold standard. The principle of the test is to induce hypoglycemia (plasma glucose < 40 mg/dL) with IV insulin, which acts as a major stressor to stimulate production of ACTH, cortisol, and GH.

119. What test do most clinicians use to assess adrenal insufficiency?

Because the ITT is cumbersome and requires close monitoring, most clinicians perform an ACTH stimulation test. In the classic test, a baseline cortisol is drawn and 250 μg of IV synthetic ACTH (Cortrosyn) is given. Blood samples for cortisol are collected at 30 and 60 minutes. A normal response is a stimulated cortisol value of > 20 μg/dL. A normal response rules out adrenal insufficiency in the majority of cases. A rare exception is the patient with acute central adrenal insufficiency (i.e., pituitary apoplexy or head trauma); since the adrenal glands have not had sufficient time to become atrophic and unresponsive to ACTH. Lack of a normal response indicates decreased adrenal reserve but does not differentiate between primary and central adrenal insufficiency.

120. How do you distinguish between primary and central adrenal insufficiency?
An ACTH level is used to determine whether the adrenal insufficiency is primary (high ACTH) or central (low or normal ACTH). More recently, clinicians have considered the 250-μg ACTH test less accurate in detecting patients with mild adrenal insufficiency (since it is a supraphysiologic dose) and have recommended a 1-μg ACTH stimulation test. The test is performed the same way as the higher dose test but requires dilution of the ACTH. ACTH (Cortrosyn) is available only in a 250-μg vial and must be diluted for this low-dose test. Therefore, careful attention must be given to ensure proper administration of the drug to avoid a high false-positive rate.

121. Why is it important to rule out adrenal insufficiency in pituitary patients with central hypothyroidism?
Pituitary patients with central hypothyroidism metabolize cortisol more slowly than euthyroid patients. Thyroid hormone replacement increases cortisol metabolism and can precipitate adrenal crisis in a patient with undiagnosed central adrenal insufficiency. It is important to detect and treat adrenal insufficiency before starting thyroid hormone replacement to avoid this complication.

122. Describe the clinical presentation of pheochromocytoma. What is the "classic triad" of symptoms?
Patients with pheochromocytomas present with signs and symptoms attributable to catecholamine excess. These symptoms include the classic triad (episodic headache, diaphoresis, and tachycardia) with or without hypertension (may be paroxysmal hypertension). Other symptoms may include anxiety/psychiatric disturbances, tremor, pallor, visual changes (papilledema, blurred vision), weight loss, polyuria, polydipsia, hyperglycemia, dilated cardiomyopathy, and arrhythmias. Most patients have two of the three symptoms of the classic triad. If the patient is hypertensive and has the classic triad of symptoms, the sensitivity and specificity for pheochromocytoma are both > 90%.

123. What other diagnoses should be considered?
It is important to consider other potential diagnoses, including anxiety/panic attacks, alcoholism (or alcohol withdrawal), sympathomimetic drugs (cocaine, amphetamines, phencyclidine, epinephrine, phenylephrine, terbutaline, phenylpropanolamine [a popular over-the-counter decongestant]), combined ingestion of MAO inhibitor and tyramine-containing food, hyperthyroidism, menopause, hypoglycemia, and abrupt discontinuation of short-acting sympathetic antagonists (e.g., clonidine).

124. What is the "rule of 10" for pheochromocytomas?
- 10% are extra-adrenal
- 10% are bilateral
- 10% are familial
- 10% are malignant

125. How do you evaluate a patient with suspected pheochromocytoma?
The most important strategy is to make a biochemical diagnosis before embarking on radiographic imaging. This step is crucial because people can have incidental adrenal tumors that do not hypersecrete catecholamines.

126. **Describe the two main screening tests for pheochromocytoma.**
Some clinicians recommend plasma-free normetanephrine and metanephrine levels as the initial biochemical test. If these values are more than four-fold higher than the upper limit of the normal reference range, proceed to radiographic imaging (CT of abdomen initially) to localize the tumor. Unfortunately, these tests are not always widely available. In such cases, obtain measurements of 24-hour urine normetanephrine and metanephrine.

127. **What other tests may be helpful?**
Other helpful tests include 24-hour urine fractionated catecholamines and catecholamine metabolites homovanillic acid and vanillylmandelic acid as well as plasma catecholamines. A clonidine suppression test may also be used to confirm the diagnosis. In borderline cases, multiple tests need to be performed or repeated.

128. **How is the 24-hour urine test performed?**
Since catecholamine hypersecretion may be episodic, it is best to collect the urine samples when the patient is symptomatic. If possible, testing should be performed after discontinuing medications. Caffeine, alcohol, and tobacco should be avoided during testing.

129. **Describe the clonidine suppression test.**
Plasma catecholamines are measured before and 3 hours after oral administration of 0.3 mg of clonidine. Failure to suppress plasma catecholamines suggests the diagnosis of pheochromocytoma. This test must not be performed in hypovolemic patients or patients taking diuretics, beta blockers, or tricyclic antidepressants.

130. **After the biochemical diagnosis is made, how is the tumor localized?**
The tumor is localized by using CT or MRI (first of the adrenals, then of the chest, abdomen, and pelvis). If the tumor cannot be localized with standard imaging, peform an ^{123}I metaiodobenzylguanidine (MIBG) scan to localize functional catecholamine-rich tissue.

Pacek K, et al: Recent advances in genetics, diagnosis, localization, and treatment of pheochromocytoma. Ann Intern Med 134:315–329, 2001.

131. **What is the treatment of choice for patients with pheochromocytomas?**
After tumor localization, the treatment of choice is surgery. All patients must be preoperatively treated with alpha-adrenergic (phenoxybenzamine) and beta-adrenergic (atenolol) blockade to avoid stress-induced catecholamine excess and hypertensive crisis during surgery. It is critical to avoid beta-adrenergic blockade in the presence of unopposed alpha agonists because it may lead to peripheral vasoconstriction and an exacerbation of the patient's hypertension.

132. **What is an adrenal incidentaloma?**
Approximately 1% of all abdominal CT scans reveal a previously unsuspected adrenal mass, termed *adrenal incidentaloma*. These tumors fall into three categories: nonfunctioning mass, hyperfunctioning mass, and pseudoadrenal mass. Since approximately 10% are hormonally active and < 3% are adrenocortical carcinomas, it is important to assess hormonal hyperfunction and malignant potential.

133. **How do you evaluate an adrenal incidentaloma?**
Although there are numerous approaches, evaluations should be individualized. It is important to perform a careful history and physical exam, looking for signs and symptoms of hormone excess. It is usually recommended that patients be screened for Cushing's syndrome (24-hour urine free cortisol and/or 1-mg overnight dexamethasone suppression test) and pheochromocytoma (24-hour urine metanephrines/catecholamines or plasma metanephrines). One can consider screening for hyperaldosteronism, particularly if the patient is hypertensive and has a

serum potassium < 3.9. Plasma aldosterone concentration (PAC) and plasma renin activity (PRA) may be used to test for an aldosterone-secreting tumor, looking for an PAC:PRA ratio > 20–25. Nonfunctioning tumors < 4 cm are typically observed for growth. Functional tumors or tumors > 4 cm (or growing) are typically removed by surgery.

Aron DC (ed): Endocrine incidentalomas. Endocrinol Metab Clin North Am 29:69–186, 2000.

134. **What is primary hyperaldosteronism?**
Primary hyperaldosteronism is excessive production of aldosterone independent of the renin-angiotensin system. It is observed in approximately 0.5–2% of the population, and the differential diagnosis includes solitary aldosterone-producing adenoma (65%), bilateral or unilateral adrenal hyperplasia, adrenal carcinoma, and glucocorticoid remediable aldosteronism.

135. **How do patients with primary hyperaldosteronism present?**
Patients present with hypertension, hypokalemia (weakness, muscle cramping, paresthesias, headaches), low magnesium levels, and metabolic alkalosis.

136. **How should patients with primary hyperaldosteronism be evaluated?**
The first step is assess upright plasma aldosterone concentration and PRA in the absence of drugs that alter the renin-aldosterone axis (such as most antihypertensives: spironolactone, ACE inhibitors, and diuretics). A ratio of plasma aldosterone concentration (ng/dL) to PRA (ng/mL/h) of > 20–25 makes the diagnosis likely.

137. **How is the diagnosis of primary hyperaldosteronism confirmed?**
Confirmation requires a high 24-hour urine aldosterone level in the presence of normokalemia and adequate volume status or inadequate suppression of aldosterone levels using the saline suppression or salt-loading test. As always, biochemical diagnosis should precede diagnostic imaging. Treatment depends on the etiology but usually includes surgery except in cases of adrenal hyperplasia or glucocorticoid-remediable hyperaldosteronism.

THYROID GLAND

138. **Diagram the hypothalamic-pituitary-thyroid axis.**
See Figure 2-3.

139. **Describe the lab findings in hyperthyroidism and hypothyroidism.**
See Table 2-7.

140. **Distinguish between subclinical and overt thyroid disease.**
Thyroid disease occurs along a continuum. At either end is hyperthyroidism or hypothyroidism. Milder forms of thyroid dysfunction are often referred to as **subclinical** disease, meaning below the limit of detection by clinical evaluation. **Overt** disease refers to hyperthyroidism or hypothyroidism with classic clinical signs and symptoms, abnormal TSH, and abnormal hormone levels.

141. **Discuss the significance of subclinical thyroid disease.**
Subclinical disease was originally thought to be a laboratory diagnosis in which patients had an abnormal TSH and normal thyroid hormone levels and were "asymptomatic." We now know that subclinical disease is often associated with subtle clinical signs and symptoms and that it represents an early, mild form of thyroid disease. Although these milder forms of thyroid dysfunction have been shown to be associated with abnormal physiology (particularly subclinical hypothyroidism), treatment is currently quite controversial. Many thyroidologists believe that treatment should be initiated in patients with mild forms of the disease. However, a recent con-

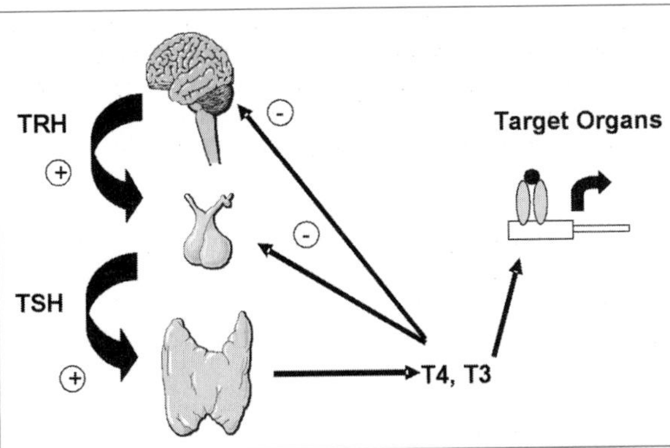

Figure 2-3. Hypothalamic-pituitary-thyroid axis. Thyrotropin-releasing hormone (TRH) is made in the hypothalamus and stimulates the pituitary thyrotropes to release thyroid-stimulating hormone (TSH, thyrotropin), which acts at the level of the thyroid gland and directs release of two hormones, T_4 (L-thyroxine) and T_3 (L-triiodothyronine). These two hormones circulate in the blood bound to protein, primarily thyroid-binding globulin. It has been thought that most of the actions of thyroid hormone are mediated by the binding of T_3 to nuclear hormone receptors and the altering of gene transcription (either positively or negatively) of the thyroid hormone–responsive gene in target tissues. The axis is regulated as a classic negative feedback system as shown above.

TABLE 2-7. LABORATORY TESTING IN THYROID DISEASE

Laboratory Test	Hyperthyroidism	Hypothyroidism
TSH	Low or undetectable	High
Free T_4	High	Low
Total T_4	High	Low
Free T_3 (not often accurate)	High	Low
Total T_3	High	Low
T_3 resin uptake Inverse measure of thyroid hormone binding sites on TBG	Usually high if no TBG abnormality	Usually low if no TBG abnormality

TSH = thyroid-stimulating hormone, T_3 = triiodothyronine, T_4 = thyroxine, TBG = thyroid-binding globulin.

sensus panel concluded that the data regarding benefits of detection and treatment of subclinical cases were not well established. Therefore, clinical judgement should prevail.

Col NF, et al: Subclinical thyroid disease: Clinical applications. JAMA 291: 239–243, 2004.

Sirks MI, et al: Subclinical thyroid disease: Scientific review and guidelines for diagnosis and management. JAMA 291:228–238, 2004.

Helfand M: Screening for subclinical thyroid dysfunction in nonpregnant adults: A summary of the evidence for the U.S. Preventive Services Task Force. Ann Intern Med 140:128–141, 2004.

142. How common is thyroid disease?

Thyroid disease is relatively common. It affects more women than men, and subclinical thyroid disease is more common than overt disease. The prevalence of hypothyroidism increases with age in both men and women. In fact, more than 20% of women over the age of 60 have hypothyroidism. General overall prevalence rates are as follows.

- Hyperthyroidism: 1.3% (0.5% overt and 0.7% subclinical).
- Hypothyroidism: 4.6% (0.3% overt and 4.3% subclinical).

Hollowell JG, et al: Serum TSH, T(4), and thyroid antibodies in the United States population (1988 to 1994): National Health and Nutrition Examination Survey (NHANES III). J Clin Endocrinol Metab 87:489–499, 2002.

Canaris GJ, et al: The Colorado thyroid disease prevalence study. Arch Intern Med 160:526–534, 2000.

KEY POINTS: THYROID GLAND

1. The best initial screening test for evaluation of thyroid status is the TSH level.
2. TSH is the most sensitive measure of thyroid function in the majority of patients.
3. The one exception is patients with pituitary/hypothalamic dysfunction, in whom TSH cannot be used to reliably to assess thyroid function.

143. How do you evaluate a patient with hyperthyroidism?

Hyperthyroidism is diagnosed by history, physical exam, and thyroid function tests: low or undetectable TSH, high or normal T_4, and high or normal T_3. Normal hormone levels in the presence of low or undetectable TSH typically suggest subclinical hyperthyroidism. The one major exception is the pituitary patient with low or normal hormone levels in the setting of a suppressed TSH. TSH as a measure thyroid status is not a reliable indicator of hyperthyroidism in patients with pituitary dysfunction. The etiology of hyperthyroidism can be confirmed by performing a thyroid I^{123} scan.

144. Describe the presentation of patients with hyperthyroidism.

See Table 2-8.

145. What is the differential diagnosis of hyperthyroidism?

Hyperthyroidism results from tissue exposure to excess thyroid hormone. The excess thyroid hormone can come from thyroid gland hyperfunction (Graves' disease, autonomously functioning nodule), from inflammation and destruction of all or part of the gland with resultant release of stored hormone (thyroiditis), or from an exogenous source outside the thyroid.

146. How does the thyroid I^{123} scan help differentiate among the different causes of hyperthyroidism?

A thyroid I^{123} scan can help differentiate among the causes based on the pattern and degree of I^{123} uptake by the thyroid gland (Table 2-9). Graves' disease is the most common cause of endogenous hyperthyroidism. It is an autoimmune disease in which patients develop antibodies that mimic TSH by binding to its receptor on thyroid cells to stimulate thyroid hormone production.

147. What is thyroid storm?

Thyroid storm is a dramatic, life-threatening exacerbation of hyperthyroidism (thyrotoxicosis). It is the extreme of a continuum of severity of hyperthyroidism that is associated with a 20% mortality rate if untreated. It is a clinical diagnosis based on the severity of hyperthyroidism.

TABLE 2-8. CLINICAL PRESENTATION OF HYPERTHYROIDISM

Symptoms	Signs
Lethargy, fatigue	Tremor
Anxiety/palpitations	Tachycardia/atrial arrhythmias/hypertension
	Rarely congestive heart failure; often hyperdynamic precordium
Hyperactivity	Agitation (mental status alterations if severe or in elderly patients)
Increased defecation	Goiter
Weight loss	Increased deep tendon reflexes
Sleep disturbance/insomnia	Warm, moist, soft skin
Heat intolerance	Proximal muscle weakness
Menstrual irregularities in women	Ophthalmopathy: lid lag, stare (Graves' disease:
Erectile dysfunction in men	proptosis, diplopia, color vision changes, optic
Infertility	neuropathy, chemosis, eye irritation, extra-ocular muscle dysfunction)
Increased appetite	Brittle nails
Poor exercise capacity, dyspnea	Edema (Graves'disease: pretibial myxedema)

148. Describe the presentation of thyroid storm.
Patients present with severe signs and symptoms of hyperthyroidism that can also include severe tachycardia and arrhythmias, heart failure, fever, gastrointestinal disturbances (hepatitis, jaundice), and mental status changes.

149. How is thyroid storm treated?
In addition to general supportive care (often in the intensive care unit), treatment involves initiation of the following medications:

- Antithyroid medication (propylthiouracil [PTU]) to block thyroid hormone synthesis and peripheral conversion of T_4 to T_3.
- Beta blockers to inhibit the adrenergic system (propranolol or esmolol IV).
- Saturated solution of potassium iodide or other iodine-rich compounds (Gastrograffin, ipodate) to block the release of preformed thyroid hormones.
- Glucocorticoids may also be part of the initial management because thyroid hormones increase metabolism of endogenous cortisol and steroids can inhibit conversion of T_4 to T_3.

150. Summarize the treatment approach to hyperthyroidism.
Treatment is based on the etiology of the hyperthyroidism. The most common causes are overly zealous replacement of thyroid hormone, Graves' disease, hyperfunctioning nodular disease, and thyroiditis. Over-replacement is easily treated by titrating down the thyroid hormone dose. All hyperthyroid patients benefit from beta blockers to treat the hyperadrenergic state.

151. How is Graves' disease treated?
Graves' disease is treated with I^{131} radioiodine ablation or antithyroid drugs (ATDs). Surgery can be performed to remove the Graves' gland, but most patients prefer the nonsurgical options.

TABLE 2-9. CAUSES OF HYPERTHYROIDISM

Etiology	I^{123} Scan Pattern	RAIU (%)	Pathogenesis
Common causes			
Graves' disease	Homogenous	High uptake (can be high normal)	Stimulating TSH receptor antibody
Multinodular goiter	Patchy	Moderate uptake	Autonomous thyroid function
Solitary toxic nodule	Suppressed gland with one area of high uptake	Normal gland with suppressed uptake, high nodule uptake	Autonomous thyroid function
Thyroiditis Silent Subacute Drug-induced Radiation-induced	Homogeneous	Low uptake	Release of preformed hormone
Exogenous thyroid hormone ingestion	Homogeneous	Low uptake	Excess thyroid hormone in drug or food
Less common causes			
Hashitoxicosis	Patchy	Moderate uptake	Release of preformed hormone
Iodine (jod-basedow)	Homogeneous	Low uptake	Iodine excess
Hyperemesis gravidarum	Do not scan due to pregnant state	Would expect high uptake	Circulating hCG
Lithium	Variable	High uptake	Variable
Rare causes			
TSH-producing pituitary adenoma	Homogeneous	High uptake (can be normal)	Excess TSH production from tumor
Pituitary resistance to thyroid hormone	Homogeneous	High uptake (can be normal)	Excess TSH production from impaired feedback
Choriocarcinoma Trophoblastic disease	Homogeneous	High uptake	Circulating hCG cross-reacts with TSH receptor
Struma ovarii (teratoma)	Homogeneous	Low uptake	Ovarian teratoma
Metastatic thyroid cancer	Homogeneous	Low uptake	Foci of functional autonomous tissue
Thyroid adenoma infarction	Homogeneous	Low uptake	Release of preformed hormone

TSH = thyroid-stimulating hormone, RAIU = radioactive iodine uptake, hCG = human choriogonadotropin.

152. **How is nodular disease treated?**
Hyperthyroid patients with nodular goiter (solitary or multinodular) are typically treated with I^{131} ablation or surgery (particularly if the gland is large and the patient has compressive symptoms). ATDs can be used in this setting to render patients euthyroid, but they are typically not recommended for the long term because they do not address the underlying pathophysiology of the disease. The hyperthyroidism invariably returns if the ATD is discontinued.

153. **Describe the treatment of thyroiditis.**
Thyroiditis, due to inflammation and release of preformed hormone, is typically treated with beta blockers and time. Some patients with painful or subacute thyroiditis can be treated with steroids if the pain is particularly severe.

154. **How are ATDs used in Graves' patients?**
ATDs can be used as primary treatment for Graves' disease or for short-term management in preparation for I^{131} radioablation. If the second approach is chosen, the ATD must be discontinued 7–10 days prior to the I^{131} ablation so that it will not inhibit iodine uptake into the gland. ATDs should be titrated to normalize the TSH and T_4 (total or free T_4). Because normalization of TSH lags behind normalization of the T_4 level (by approximately 4–6 weeks), both lab tests must be monitored initially to avoid induction of hypothyroidism. Patients are typically treated with an ATD for 12–18 months, then tapered off to determine whether they have remained in remission. Relapse rates are high (50–60%) within the first year and are highest in patients with large goiters and more severe hyperthyroidism.

155. **Compare the two available ATDs.**
Both ATDs, PTU and methimazole (Tapazole), inhibit T_4 and T_3 synthesis by the thyroid gland and are effective for treating hyperthyroidism. PTU has a shorter plasma half-life (60 min) and is approximately 75% protein-bound. For this reason, it is the preferred drug for treating pregnant patients. Additionally, PTU blocks the peripheral conversion of T_4 to T_3 and is thus preferred for treatment of thyroid storm. Methimazole is more convenient than PTU due to its once-daily dosing (half-life = 4–6 h). It is generally avoided during pregnancy due to the association with a rare congenital scalp defect known as aplasia cutis.

156. **Summarize the side effects of ATDs.**
ATDs are generally well tolerated. Side effects include rash (most common), abnormal taste agranulocytosis (0.2–0.5%), mild elevated transaminases, fulminant hepatitis (rare), and vasculitis. Side effects typically occur within the first 3 months of therapy at generally higher doses of methimazole. There is no dose relationship of side effects with PTU.

157. **What is T_3 toxicosis?**
This term refers to patients with hyperthyroidism that is due primarily to high T_3 levels. Such patients have a low or undetectable TSH, normal T_4, and elevated T_3. It is important to check the T_3 level in patients whom you suspect of having subclinical hyperthyroidism to rule out T_3 toxicosis. The differential diagnosis, evaluation, and treatment are otherwise the same as for patients with hyperthyroidism due to any cause.

158. **How do you evaluate a patient with hypothyroidism?**
Hypothyroidism is diagnosed by history, physical exam, and thyroid function tests: elevated TSH, low or normal T_4, and low or normal T_3. Normal hormone levels in the presence of an elevated TSH suggest subclinical hypothyroidism. The concept is that the TSH is a much more sensitive marker of thyroid disease than circulating hormone levels and that even if the T_4 or T_3 is normal with regard to the laboratory reference range, it may not be "normal" for that particular patient. Thyroid I^{123} scans are not usually performed in patients with hypothyroidism. Sometimes antithyroid antibodies (antithyroid peroxidase or antithyroglobulin) are checked

because they are frequently positive in patients with the most common cause of primary hypothyroidism, autoimmune thyroiditis (Hashimoto's thyroiditis).

159. How do hypothyroid patients present clinically?
Patients can present with the signs and symptoms listed in Table 2-10. Note that symptoms associated with hypothyroidism can be vague and nonspecific. Hypothyroid patients generally have more symptoms than euthyroid patients, but in a given patient it can be difficult to detect hypothyroidism based on symptoms alone. For example, fatigue and weight gain are very common complaints that lead a clinician to check thyroid status. Unfortunately, these complaints are also common in the general population; therefore, laboratory testing is required to determine whether these symptoms are related to abnormal thyroid status.

TABLE 2-10. CLINICAL PRESENTATION OF HYPOTHYROIDISM

Symptoms	Signs
Lethargy, fatigue	Goiter
Dry skin	Dry skin (common in dry climates)
Hair loss, brittle hair, brittle nails	Coarse hair, alopecia, brittle nails
Decreased energy	Delayed relaxation phase of deep tendon reflexes
Constipation	Periorbital edema, edema
Weight gain (not usually > 50 lb)	Deepened voice
Hoarseness	Hypothermia
Cold intolerance	Lipid abnormalities (elevated cholesterol, LDL)
Menstrual irregularities in women	Elevated transaminases, creatinine phosphokinase
Erectile dysfunction in men	Reduced respiratory effort
Infertility	Proximal muscle weakness
Children: precocious or delayed puberty, abnormal growth/cognition	Bradycardia, hypertension, cardiomegaly
Depression, cognitive dysfunction	Neuropathy
Poor exercise capacity, dyspnea	
Muscle pain, joint stiffness	
Chest pain/angina	
Paresthesias	

160. What causes hypothyroidism?
Hypothyroidism is a clinical syndrome caused by the cellular responses to a deficiency of thyroid hormone. It can be divided into four categories based on mechanism: primary, secondary, tertiary, and peripheral (generalized) resistance to thyroid horomone.

161. Explain the mechanisms of primary hypothyroidism.
Primary hypothyroidism is due to a pathologic process intrinsic to the thyroid gland, leading to defective production of thyroid hormone or destruction of the gland. The most common cause is destruction due to autoimmune thyroiditis (Hashimoto's thyroiditis). Other causes of primary hypothyroidism include other forms of thyroiditis (silent, painful/subacute, postpartum,

drug-induced), "burnt-out" Graves' disease, thyroid ablation from any cause (radiation, radioactive iodine, surgical resection, metastatic tumor/neoplasia), thyroid hormone biosynthetic defects, iodine deficiency, and thyroid agenesis or dysgenesis.

162. How does secondary hypothyroidism develop?

Secondary hypothyroidism is due to a deficiency of TSH from the pituitary (central hypothyroidism). It is observed most frequently in patients with pituitary tumors or damage to the pituitary (e.g., radiation, surgery).

163. Name the major cause of tertiary hypothyroidism.

A deficiency of TRH from the hypothalamus (central hypothyroidism).

164. What is peripheral (generalized) resistance to thyroid hormone?

This is a rare genetic cause of hypothyroidism in which patients have generalized tissue resistance to thyroid hormone. This disorder is due to mutations in the thyroid hormone beta-receptor gene. There is also a form that seems to cause primarily pituitary resistance to thyroid hormone. Unlike patients with generalized resistance, these patients present with symptoms of tissue hyperthyroidism and high T_4 and T_3 levels accompanied by an elevated or "inappropriately" normal TSH.

165. How should hypothyroidism be treated?

The treatment of choice is levothyroxine (T_4) for most patients. The goal is to reverse the clinical syndrome by restoring the TSH and hormone levels to the normal range. A typical replacement dose is 1.6 μg/kg/day in young healthy patients. Elderly patients often require lower doses. The best approach is to "start low, go slow." Measure the TSH every 4–6 weeks (because the half-life of the drug is 7 days and you need to wait until the patient is in equilibrium) until a goal TSH between 1 and 2 is attained. Avoid over- or under-replacement. Once the patient is on a stable dose, the TSH can be monitored annually unless there are changes in the patient's clinical status.

166. How does iodide affect thyroid gland function?

Iodide has multiple inhibitory effects on thyroid function, including decreased iodide transport, decreased iodide organification, and decreased thyroid hormone secretion.

167. Describe the Wolff-Chaikoff effect.

The Wolff-Chaikoff effect refers to the normal transient inhibitory effect of an iodide load on thyroid function. Most patients "escape" from these inhibitory effects within 2–4 weeks after iodide exposure.

168. What is the jodbasedow phenomenon?

The jodbasedow phenomenon refers to iodide-induced thyrotoxicosis. This phenomenon typically occurs in elderly patients with underlying nodular thyroid disease after they receive an iodide load (radiographic contrast). In iodide-deficient countries, the jodbasedow phenomenon can occur following reintroduction of iodide in patients with goiter.

169. Describe postpartum thyroiditis.

Postpartum thyroiditis is an inflammation of the thyroid that can cause both hyperthyroidism and hypothyroidism. It occurs in approximately 5–9% of women following pregnancy, with a higher frequency (25%) in women with type 1 diabetes. Pathology reveals an inflammatory process that is indistinguishable from lymphocytic thyroiditis (Hashimoto's disease). In fact, women with positive antithyroid antibodies are at much higher risk of developing postpartum thyroiditis and permanent thyroid dysfunction.

170. How is postpartum thyroiditis treated?

Patients are treated according to their phase of presentation. One third of women go through the classic three phases: hyperthyroid phase (1–3 months), hypothyroid phase (4–8 months), and return to a euthyroid state. Since only 25–30% of women develop permanent hypothyroidism, it is important to assess whether a woman has moved into the euthyroid phase to avoid unnecessary lifelong therapy with thyroid hormone.

171. List the risk factors for malignancy in a thyroid nodule.

Risk factors include positive family history of thyroid cancer; extremes of age (< 20 yr or > 60 yr); rapid growth of a preexisting nodule; large, painful, or firm nodule; invasive and compressive symptoms; presence of lymphadenopathy; fixation of nodule to adjacent structures; vocal cord paresis; and history of head and neck irradiation. Any nodule ≥ 1–1.5 cm should be evaluated in a clinically euthryoid patient.

172. What is the most cost-effective method for evaluating a thyroid nodule?

Fine-needle aspiration biopsy (FNAB). Most clinicians confirm the euthyroid state by checking a TSH. It is no longer recommended that all nodules be evaluated with a thyroid I^{123} scan to determine their functionality. FNAB is recommended for cold nodules (do not concentrate iodine) because the risk of malignancy is approximately 5–10%, and most nodules (> 95%) are cold. Therefore, the thyroid I^{123} scan can be avoided in many patients. Hyperfunctioning or "hot" nodules on thyroid scan are not typically biopsied since they carry an extremely low risk of malignancy (< 1%).

173. What is the 5–10% rule for thyroid nodules?

- 5–10% of people have palpable nodules (more common in women).
- 5–10% of nodules are cancerous (overall lifetime risk of thyroid cancer = 1%).
- 5–10% of thyroid cancer is associated with high morbidity and mortality rates.

174. List the types of thyroid cancer.

- Thyroid epithelial cell cancers: papillary (75%), follicular (10%), Hurthle cell, anaplastic. Papillary and follicular thyroid cancer are considered "differentiated" thyroid cancer.
- Thyroidal C-cell cancer (calcitonin-secreting): medullary thyroid cancer.
- Primary thyroid lymphoma.

175. Summarize the staging systems for thyroid cancer.

Multiple staging systems are used for thyroid cancer. The most widely accepted is the American Joint Committee on Cancer TNM staging system. There are separate staging systems for papillary and follicular cancer, anaplastic cancer and medullary thyroid cancer. The stage typically increases (worsening prognosis) with age (> 45 yr), size of tumor, invasiveness, presence of cancer-containing lymph nodes, and metastatic spread. National Collaborative Cancer Network (guidelines may be accessed at *www.nccn.org.*)

176. How should differentiated thyroid cancer be treated?

Overall, differentiated thyroid cancer has an excellent prognosis if treated appropriately. Most patients receive a thyroidectomy followed by radioiodine (I^{131}) remnant ablation. Patients are treated with thyroid hormone to keep the TSH suppressed. The level of TSH suppression is determined by the aggressiveness of the disease (initial stage), risk of recurrence, and time elapsed from initial diagnosis. This therapy has been shown to decrease cancer recurrence and mortality and to facilitate monitoring for residual/recurrent cancer.

177. Describe the typical follow-up for patients with differentiated thyroid cancer.

Standard monitoring of patients with differentiated thyroid cancer includes serial physical exams, thyroglobulin (tumor marker) measurements both on thyroid hormone suppression therapy and after TSH stimulation, diagnostic whole-body I^{131} scans (WBS), and thyroid ultrasound. Previously, TSH stimulation was achieved by induction of hypothyroidism following withdrawal of thyroid hormone. Since an elevated TSH is required to stimulate I^{131} uptake into thyroid cells, patients typically discontinue thyroid hormone replacement a number of weeks prior to the WBS and thyroglobulin test. As expected, hypothyroidism is uncomfortable for most patients, and some patients experience very severe symptoms and refuse or delay these cancer-monitoring procedures.

National Collaborative Cancer Network (guidelines may be accessed at *www.nccn.org*) and Schlumberger MJ: Papillary and follicular thyroid carcinoma. N Engl J Med 338:297–306, 1998.

178. What other option for monitoring is available?

Fortunately, the development of recombinant human TSH (rhTSH) provides a tool whereby TSH levels can be elevated without the need for the patient to become hypothyroid. This discovery has revolutionized care of patients with thyroid cancer. Although rhTSH is currently approved by the U.S. Food and Drug Administration (FDA) for diagnostic monitoring of differentiated thyroid cancer, many other potential uses for rhTSH are under investigation. The overall goal is to have no evidence of disease based on negative imaging studies and undetectable thyroglobulin levels.

Woodmansee WW, Haugen BR: A review of the potential uses for recombinant human TSH in patients with thyroid cancer and nodular goiter. Clin Endocrinol 61:163–173, 2004.

REPRODUCTIVE ENDOCRINOLOGY

179. Define erectile dysfunction (ED).

ED is the inability to obtain and maintain an erection sufficient for sexual intercourse. ED is usually multifactorial in etiology, and most men have at least some psychogenic factors that contribute to the disorder (i.e., performance anxiety can exacerbate underlying organic etiology).

180. List the six main categories of ED.

- **Hormonal:** hypogonadism (primary or secondary), hyperprolactinemia (with resultant hypogonadism), hyperthyroidism or hypothyroidism, and diabetes. Less common: adrenal insufficiency and Cushing's syndrome.
- **Pharmacologic:** long list of implicated medications: antihypertensives (clonidine, beta blockers, vasodilators, thiazide diuretics, spironolactone); antidepressants (selective serotonin reuptake inhibitors [SSRIs], tetracyclic antidepressants), antipsychotics, anxiolytics, cimetidine, phenytoin, carbamazepine, ketoconazole, metoclopramide, digoxin. Alcohol is a major culprit. Illicit drugs include marijuana, cocaine, and heroin.
- **Systemic disease:** any severe illness can cause ED and hypogonadotrophic hypogonadism.
- **Vascular:** diabetes, peripheral vascular disease.
- **Neurologic:** diabetes, spinal cord injury, neuropathy.
- **Psychogenic:** uncommon in isolation, but contributes to most cases due to other etiologies. It is a diagnosis of exclusion.

181. Describe the typical evaluation of a patient with ED.

A typical initial evaluation includes history (with particular attention to medications), physical exam, and laboratory testing to rule out endocrine abnormalities. Start by checking TSH, prolactin, and testosterone and ruling out systemic disease with urinalysis, complete chemistry panel and blood count, and HbA1c level in patients with diabetes. Carefully review the patient's medication list and ascertain alcohol consumption to assess possible etiologies for ED. Nocturnal penile tumescence testing is available to assess erectile function.

182. What is the most important step in the management of ED?

The most important step is to reverse the underlying organic etiologies and discontinue any offending medications, if possible.

183. What are the potential treatment options for men with ED?

- Correction of any hormonal abnormality (testosterone replacement for hypogonadism after carefully determining etiology, correction of thyroid dysfunction, maximal glycemic control in diabetes, treatment of hyperprolactinemia with dopamine agonist)
- Treatment of any underlying systemic disorders, including depression (SSRIs can cause ED but may help to prevent premature ejaculation)
- Medical therapy (see question 184)
- Mechanical devices (rings, vacuum pump device): cumbersome to some patients, but side effects are minimal
- Surgical interventions: typically used as a last resort; options include revascularization, removal of venous shunts, and penile implants
- Supportive counseling

184. What medical therapies are available for ED?

- $Alpha_2$-adrenergic receptor blocker: yohimbine (oral).
- Phosphodiesterase 5 inhibitors: sildenafil (Viagra), vardenafil (Levitra), tadalafil (Cialis). All three are administered orally, but none should be used in combination with nitrates.
- Intracavernosal injections of vasodilating medications: alprostadil (Caverject), prostaglandin E_1, papaverine, phentolamine.
- Transurethral alprostadil suppositories (MUSE)

185. List the three etiologic categories of gynecomastia.

Idiopathic, physiologic, and pathologic.

186. List the physiologic causes of gynecomastia.

- Newborn (due to maternal estrogens during pregnancy)
- During puberty (due to increased estrogen-to-androgen ratio)
- Older ages (mechanism not entirely clear but possibly due to combined effect of decreasing testosterone with age and increased estrogen due to peripheral aromatization of androgens to estrogens in adipose tissue)

187. What causes pathologic gynecomastia?

Pathologic gynecomastia is typically due to estrogen excess from either overproduction or peripheral aromatization. Categories include:

- Drugs: any drug that increases estrogen activity or production or reduces testosterone activity or production. Main mechanisms: estrogen-like properties, stimulation of estrogen production, increase in estrogen precursor molecules, reduction of testosterone levels.
- Tumors: examples of tumors with increased human chorionic gonadotropin (hCG) or estrogen production include testicular tumors (Leydig cell, Sertoli cell, germ cell, granulosa cell), choriocarcinoma, or adrenal tumors. Male breast cancer is an uncommon cause.
- Decreased androgens or androgen resistance (hypogonadism due to any cause, Klinefelter's syndrome, Kallmann's syndrome).
- Increased aromatase activity (obesity, hyperthyroidism, genetic mutations).
- Displacement of estrogens from sex hormone–binding globulin.
- Others: end-stage liver disease, renal disease, HIV infection, familial syndrome, starvation refeeding.

188. What are the causes of amenorrhea?

It is important to determine whether amenorrhea is primary (the patient has never had menses) or secondary (cessation of menses after she has started). It is also important to rule out pregnancy as a cause of amenorrhea. After pregnancy is ruled out, consider the following three broad categories: anatomic/outflow tract defect, ovarian failure, and chronic anovulation.

KEY POINTS: REPRODUCTIVE ENDOCRINOLOGY

1. The most common presentation of hypogonadism in men is erectile dysfunction and decreased libido.
2. The most common presentation of hypogonadism in women is amenorrhea and infertility.

189. Give examples of anatomic/outflow tract defects.

- Imperforate hymen
- Asherman's syndrome
- Müllerian agenesis
- Sexual differentiation disorders

190. What are the causes of primary ovarian failure?

In primary ovarian failure **(hypergonadotrophic hypogonadism)** levels of LH and FSH are generally high. Congenital causes include genetic alterations (Turner's syndrome [XO], enzyme deficiencies, LH or FSH receptor or postreceptor defects). Acquired causes include autoimmune destruction and physical insults (e.g., radiation, chemotherapy, viral infection, surgery).

191. Summarize the causes of secondary ovarian failure.

Secondary ovarian failure **(hypogonadotropic hypogonadism)** is associated with low level of FSH and LH and induces chronic anovulation. Most causes in this category are acquired and include hypothalamic dysfunction (induced by exercise or eating disorders), pituitary dysfunction (tumors, hypopituitarism), and androgen excess (adrenal tumors, polycystic ovarian syndrome, tumors with high human choriogonadotropin, congenital adrenal hyperplasia). Other causes include hyperthyroidism and hypothyroidism, liver disease, renal disease, obesity, and adrenal dysfunction.

192. Describe the polycystic ovary syndrome (PCOS).

PCOS (Stein-Leventhal syndrome) is a disorder characterized by (1) oligo- or anovulation, (2) hyperandrogenism, and (3) polycystic ovaries. Patients can be diagnosed with PCOS if they have at least two of the features and other etiologies have been excluded.

193. How do women with PCOS typically present?

Women typically present with menstrual dysfunction, hirsutism, and insulin resistance. Long-term consequences of PCOS include increased risk of developing type 2 diabetes, hyperlipidemia, and endometrial cancer.

194. Describe the management of PCOS.

Management is aimed at correcting the underlying metabolic disorder and addressing cosmetic concerns related to hirsutism. Weight loss and treatment of insulin resistance (thiozolidenediones, metformin) are recommended. Oral contraceptives are used to regulate menstrual cycles and suppress hyperandrogenism. Since most patients have impaired ovulation, fertility must also be addressed. Most women can be treated with the ovulation induction drug, clomiphene citrate, either alone or in combination with insulin-sensitizing medication. Hirsutism is treated by suppressing androgen production (oral contraceptives, androgen receptor blockers, or 5-alpha-reductase inhibitors) and appropriate cosmetic treatments.

195. Summarize the traditional rationale behind hormonal treatment of menopausal women.

Menopause represents the time in a woman's life that cyclic ovarian function ceases. Hormone replacement therapy (HRT), which consists of combined estrogen and progesterone in women with an intact uterus and estrogen only for women without a uterus, has become extremely controversial over the past few years. HRT was frequently given to women at the time of menopause and continued indefinitely. It was initially thought that HRT offered a number of clinical benefits to women, including amelioration of vasomoter symptoms (hot flashes), improved lipids, and decreased risk of cardiovascular disease, osteoporosis, and dementia.

196. How have the recommendations HRT changed in current practice?
The Women's Health Initiative study and subgroup studies have now altered our practices regarding HRT. HRT was associated with an increased risk of breast cancer, thromboembolic diseases, and cardiovascular disease (coronary artery disease and stroke) and a reduced risk of colon cancer and osteoporosis. Although the absolute risk of these disorders is small, HRT is no longer recommended for disease prevention. HRT is now mainly indicated for the short-term treatment of menopausal vasomotor symptoms, using the lowest effective dose.

U.S. Preventative Task Force: Postmenopausal hormone replacement therapy for primary prevention of chronic conditions: Recommendations and rationale. Ann Intern Med 137:834–839, 2002.

National Institutes of Health Web Site: www.nih.gov.

PARATHYROID HORMONE, CALCIUM, AND BONE DISORDERS

197. Identify the principal organs responsible for maintaining serum calcium in the normal range.
Overall, calcium homeostasis is tightly regulated in three regions of the body.

- Bone: storage of calcium
- Kidney: excretion of calcium
- Intestine: absorption of calcium

Marx SJ: Medical progress: Hyperparathyroid and hypoparathyroid disorders. N Engl J Med 343:1863–1875, 2000.

198. List the three main hormones involved in calcium regulation.
Parathyroid hormone (PTH), vitamin D, which increase serum levels of calcium, and calcitonin, which decreases serum levels of calcium.

199. Describe how PTH works to increase serum calcium levels.
PTH is synthesized and secreted by the parathyroid glands in response to low serum levels of calcium. Its mechanisms of action include:

- Increases bone resorption
- Increases 1,25 (OH)2 vitamin D production
- Increases renal calcium retention
- Increases renal phosphate excretion

200. Describe how vitamin D works to increase serum calcium levels.
The most active form is 1,25 (OH) 2 vitamin D, which is synthesized in the kidney by conversion of 25 (OH) vitamin D by 1-alpha hydroxylase. Its mechanisms of action include:

- Increases bone resorption
- Increases renal calcium and phosphate retention
- Enhances intestinal calcium absorption

201. How does calcitonin work to decrease serum calcium levels?
Calcitonin is synthesized by thyroidal C cells. Its mechanisms of action include:

- Promotes calcium deposition in bone
- Inhibits osteoclastic bone resorption

KEY POINTS: CALCIUM HOMEOSTASIS

1. Calcium homeostasis is tightly regulated to keep calcium in a very narrow physiologic range.
2. The three organs involved in calcium homeostasis are the bone (storage), kidney (excretion), and intestine (absorption).
3. The three hormones involved in calcium homeostasis are parathyroid hormone, vitamin D, and calcitonin.
4. Parathyroid hormone and vitamin D work to increase calcium levels.
5. Calcitonin works to decrease calcium levels.

202. List the signs and symptoms of hyper- and hypocalcemia.
See Table 2-11.

TABLE 2-11. CLINICAL PRESENTATION OF CALCIUM DISORDERS*

Hypercalcemia		Hypocalcemia	
Symptoms	**Signs**	**Symptoms**	**Signs**
CNS: cognitive impairment (variable), weakness GI symptoms (N/V), reflux, constipation Renal – impaired function, polyuria, polydipsia, nephrocalcinosis Osteopenia Pancreatitis	Dehydration (patient may have hypotension if severe) Hypertension Arrhythmias (shortened QT interval)	Perioral and peripheral paresthesias (initially) Carpal-pedal spasm Irritability Tetany Seizures Congestive heart failure (rare)	Chvostek's sign Trousseau's sign Bradycardia/ arrhythmias, prolonged QT interval Hypotension Laryngospasm Bronchospasm

* All signs and symptoms are a function of severity of calcium abnormality, acuteness of onset, and centralpatient's underlying medical status (often more severe in elderly patients).
CNS = central nervous system, GI = gastrointestinal.

203. Identify the two most common causes of hypercalcemia.
Primary hyperparathyroidism (55%) and hypercalcemia of malignancy (35%) account for the majority of cases of hypercalcemia.

204. Describe how you would distinguish between the two.
Hypercalcemia diagnosed on an outpatient basis is usually due to primary hyperparathyroidism, whereas malignancy is the most common cause in hospitalized patients. The PTH level distinguishes between hypercalcemia of malignancy (undectetable PTH with high levels of PTH-related peptide) and primary hyperparathyroidism (high PTH level).

205. What are the uncommon causes of hypercalcemia?
Thyrotoxicosis, granulomatous disease (sarcoidosis, tuberculosis, histoplasmosis, coccidiomycosis), drug-induced (thiazides, lithium vitamins A and D intoxication, aluminum toxicity in renal failure, immobilization, renal insufficiency, tertiary hyperparathyroidism), and total parenteral nutrition. Another possibility is total parenteral nutrition.

206. List the rare causes of hypercalcemia.
Adrenal insufficiency, pheochromocytosis, pancreatic islet-cell tumors, familial hypocalciuric hypercalcemia (FHH), and milk alkali syndrome.

207. Describe the diagnosis of primary hyperparathyroidism.
Primary hyperparathyroidism is usually due to a single parathyroid adenoma. Diagnosis rests on elevated levels of calcium and PTH level and hypercalciuria.

208. How is primary hyperparathyroidism treated?
Surgery is recommended for patients with any of the severe complications (e.g., bone lesions, nephrolithiasis, nephrocalcinosis, or overt muscle disease). However, some patients do not present with classic signs and symptoms and are believed to have a mild form of the disease that has been termed **asymptomatic hyperparathyroidism**. Many of these patients have mild elevations in calcium and complain of mild cognitive symptoms or symptoms of depression that are not always clearly related to the disease. Since a large number of patients are "asymptomatic" and may be observed, a list of indications for surgery has been developed. Table 2-12 lists the guidelines as revised in 2002.

Bilezikian JP, et al: Summary statement from a workshop on asymptomatic primary hyperparathyroidism: a perspective from the 21st century. JCEM 87:5353–5361, 2002.

TABLE 2-12. INDICATIONS FOR SURGERY IN PRIMARY HYPERPARATHYROIDISM

Measurement	Indication for Surgery
Serum calcium (amount above normal)	1 mg/dL
24-hr urine calcium	> 400 mg/day
Creatinine clearance	Reduced 30%
Bone mineral density	T score: 2.5 at any site (spine, hip, forearm)
Age	< 50 years

209. Differentiate between osteoporosis and osteopenia.
Osteoporosis is a systemic skeletal disease characterized by low bone mass and deterioration of bone microarchitecture that result in an increase in bone fragility and susceptibility to fracture. The World Health Organization defines it as bone density greater than 2.5 standard deviations below the mean for young adults (T score > –2.5).

Osteopenia is a radiologic diagnosis of reduced bone mass. Some use the term to refer to patients with low bone mass who have not experienced fractures. The World Health Organization defines it as a bone density between 1 and 2.5 standard deviations below the mean for young adults (T score: –1 to –2.5).

210. Identify the risk factors for low bone density and fractures.
See Table 2-13.

TABLE 2-13. RISK FACTORS FOR FRACTURES: FALLS AND LOW BONE DENSITY

	Low Bone Density	
Falls	**Modifiable**	**Nonmodifiable**
Low bone mineral density Previous fractures Frequent falls	Nutrition: calcium/vitamin D intake Physical activity Habits: smoking, caffeine, alcohol Medications Secondary causes	Age Race/genetics Body habitus (slender) Family history Early menopause

211. How is osteoporosis classified?
Osteoporosis is classified as primary or secondary.

212. What are the three categories of primary osteoporosis?
Juvenile, idiopathic, and involutional. Involutional osteoporosis is further divided into type 1 (associated with menopause) and type 2 (associated with aging).

213. List the causes of secondary osteoporosis.
- **Endocrine:** DM, hyperthyroidism, hypogonadism, Cushing's syndrome, hyperparathyroidism, osteomalacia.
- **Gastrointestinal:** gastrectomy /malabsorption syndromes (patients may develop calcium and vitamin D deficiencies), malnutrition (also seen in anorexia nervosa), liver disease (patients may develop vitamin D deficiency).
- **Malignancy:** multiple myeloma, metastatic carcinoma.
- **Renal disease**
- **Connective tissue disorders**
- **Medications:** steroids (most common), thyroid hormone (chronic overreplacement), anticonvulsants, heparin, isoniazid, loop diuretics, cyclosporin A, transplant antirejection medications.
- **Miscellaneous:** lifestyle factors such as poor nutrition, use of alcohol and/or tobacco, immobilization.

214. How should patients be screened for secondary causes of osteoporosis?
It is important to perform a careful history and physical exam to assess fracture risk factors and symptoms suggestive of a secondary cause of osteoporosis. Approximately one third of osteoporotic women have an undiagnosed disorder of bone or mineral metabolism (usually calcium disorder). An initial laboratory evaluation with serum calcium, PTH, and TSH as well as 24-hour urine calcium has been shown to identify the majority of secondary causes.

Tannenbaum C, et al: Yield of laboratory testing to identify secondary contributors to osteoporosis in otherwise healthy women. J Clin Endocrinol Metab 87:4431–4437, 2002.

215. List the treatment options for patients with osteoporosis. Which agents have been shown both to increase bone mineral density and to reduce fractures?
See Table 2-14.

TABLE 2-14. MEDICATIONS CURRENTLY AVAILABLE FOR THE TREATMENT OF OSTEOPOROSIS

Drug	Mechanism of Action	Increases BMD Data Available	Reduces Fractures Data Available
Calcitonin	Antiresorptive	Yes	Hip: not significant Spine: yes
Estrogen/HRT	Antiresorptive	Yes	Hip: uncertain Spine: yes
Raloxifene	Antiresorptive	Yes	Hip: not significant Spine: yes
Bisphosphonates			
Alendronate	Antiresorptive	Yes	Hip: yes Spine: yes
Risedronate	Antiresorptive	Yes	Hip: yes Spine: yes
Pamidronate (off-label use)	Antiresorptive	Yes	Hip: no data Spine: uncertain
Zoledronate (off-label use)	Antiresorptive	Yes	Hip: no data Spine: no data
Teriparatide (human recombinant PTH aa 1–34)	Anabolic	Yes	Hip: uncertain (reduced nonvertebral fractures) Spine: yes

Not significant: indicates effect on hip has been examined but no significant differences found. Trial may have been underpowered to detect differences. Hip data may have been combined in all nonvertebral fractures.
Uncertain: results variable or data insufficient to determine.
No data: has not been examined yet, or trial is under way.
FDA-approved drugs for prevention and treatment of osteoporosis: alendronate, risedronate, and raloxifene are approved for treatment and prevention. HRT is approved for prevention. Calcitonin and teriparatide are approved for treatment.
Off-label use: drug has been used in this setting but is not FDA-approved for osteoporosis treatment.
BMD = bone mineral density.

216. What is the current role of HRT in the treatment of postmenopausal osteoporosis?

Hormone replacement has been used for decades for treatment of postmenopausal osteoporosis. It has been shown to increase bone mineral density and reduce vertebral fractures. However, since the Women's Health Initiative Study demonstrated increased risk of other disorders, it is no longer first-line therapy (see question 196). All patients should receive adequate calcium (1500 mg combined as food and supplement) and vitamin D (400–800 U/day).

217. What is FHH?

FHH is a very rare autosomal dominant genetic disorder that has a high penetrance (nearly 100%). It is due to an inactivating germ-line mutation in the calcium-sensing receptor, resulting in insensitivity of the parathyroid cells to inhibition by calcium. Renal tubule cells are also insensitive to calcium.

218. Summarize the clinical characteristics of FHH.
FHH is generally a benign disorder that results in alteration of the calcium "set point." Patients have lifelong moderately elevated calcium, normal to slightly elevated intact PTH, and normal to low calcium excretion. The fractional excretion of calcium (which normalizes calcium excretion for glomerular filtration rate) is usually low. Most patients have a ratio of calcium clearance (C_{Ca}) to creatinine clearance (C_{Cr}) of < 0.01. This ratio is calculated by the following equation:

$$C_{Ca}:C_{Cr} = [Ca_u \times Cr_s]/[Ca_s \times Cr_u]$$

where Ca_u = urinary calcium, Cr_u = urinary creatinine, Ca_s = serum calcium, and Cr_u = urinary creatinine. Due to the abnormal calcium sensor, patients have "relative hypocalciuria" (unusually normal for the degree of hypercalcemia).

219. Why is it necessary to distinguish FHH from primary hyperparathyroidism?
It is important to distinguish FHH (using the 24-hour urine calcium and creatinine levels) from primary hyperparathyroidism to avoid unnecessary parathyroid surgery.

220. What is Paget's disease?
Paget's disease is characterized by abnormal bone remodeling. It can affect one or more skeletal sites and begins with abnormal bone resorption followed by compensatory bone formation. This process results in disorganized bone remodeling that predisposes the affected region to deformity and fracture. The exact etiology is unknown. Patients may be asymptomatic and present only with elevated serum alkaline phosphatase levels, or they may present with bone pain and deformity.

221. Summarize the management of Paget's disease.
Indications for medical therapy with bisphosphonates include progressive bone pain, planned surgery at an active bone site, and prevention of disease progression at sites that are at high risk for future complications.

222. What causes hypocalcemia?
Hypocalcemia can be divided into two broad categories: hypoparathyroidism or nonhypoparathyroidism. Hypoparathyroidism causes can be divided into PTH deficiency (e.g., surgical, autoimmune, congenital aplasia, radiation-induced, infiltrative diseases) or PTH resistance (PTH antibodies, pseudohypoparathyroidism). Nonhypoparathyroid causes include vitamin D deficiency or resistance (dietary deficiency, lack of sunlight, liver and renal disease), accelerated bone mineralization (hungry bone syndrome following parathyroidectomy), drugs (anticalcemic, antineoplastic), and acute complexing/sequestration of calcium (rhabdomyolysis, tumor lysis syndrome, pancreatitis, phosphate infusions, blood transfusions).

223. How should hypocalcemia be treated?
Treatment depends on the severity and duration of symptoms. Patients with acute hypocalcemia should be hospitalized with telemetry monitoring and given intravenous calcium supplementation. Patients with chronic hypocalcemic disorders are managed with oral calcium and vitamin D supplementation. *Note:* Never give calcium with phosphate.

LIPID DISORDERS

224. What are the major classes of lipoprotein particles?
Lipoproteins are named based on their density and are composed of nonpolar (and therefore water-insoluble) cholesterol esters and triglycerides surrounded by a layer of polar (and therefore water-soluble) proteins and lipids (unesterified cholesterol and phospholipids). This structure allows the entire particle to remain miscible in serum. The major lipoproteins are listed in Table 2-15.

TABLE 2-15. LIPOPROTEIN PARTICLES

Lipoprotein Particle	Location of Origin	Composition	Apoproteins	Associated Disorders
Chylomicron	Intestine	80–95% TG 3–7% chol	Apo B48	Chylomicronemia
VLDL	Liver	50–65% TG 20–30% chol	Apo B100	Familial hypertriglyceridemia Familial combined hyperlipidemia
Remnants and IDL	Catabolism of VLDL & chylomicrons	30–40% TG 30–50% chol	Depends on particle of origin	Familial dysbetalipoproteinemia (Broad beta disease)
LDL	IDL, VLDL remnants	4–10% TG 45–55% chol	B-100	Familial hypercholesterolemia, Familial combined hyperlipidemia
HDL	Liver, intestine	3–7% TG 25% chol	Apo A	Tangier's disease

VLDL = very low density particle, LDL = low-density particle, ID = intermediate density particle, HDL = high-density particle, TG = triglycerides, chol = cholesterol.

225. How can you estimate a patient's LDL cholesterol using measurements of total cholesterol, HDL, and triglycerides?

$$\text{LDL} = \text{total cholesterol} - \text{HDL} - \text{triglycerides}/5$$

226. What is familial hypercholesterolemia (FH)?
FH is an autosomal dominant disorder due to a mutation in the LDL receptor (causing a deficient or defective receptor) that leads to altered LDL catabolism and increased cholesterol synthesis. Approximately 1/500 people are heterozygous carriers of a mutation and 1/1,000,000 are homozygous for the disorder. Such people have much higher rates of

premature atherosclerosis and can have myocardial infarctions at a very young age. Physical exam often reveals tendinous xanthomas (cholesterol deposition in the extensor tendons) and corneal arcus. Management is aimed at aggressive LDL-lowering to reduce cardiovascular risk.

227. What is the chylomicronemia syndrome?

The chylomicronemia syndrome typically occurs when triglyceride levels are > 1000 mg/DL. Patients develop severe triglyceride elevations when the enzyme lipoprotein lipase (LPL), which is responsible for triglyceride hydrolysis of chylomicrons and very low density lipoprotein (VLDL), becomes saturated and is no longer able to clear chylomicrons from the circulation. When the LPL enzyme becomes saturated, chylomicrons accumulate, and the patient's serum becomes lipemic. Severe chylomicronemia typically develops in patients with a combined genetic and acquired cause of hypertriglyceridemia.

228. Describe the physical manifestations of chylomicronemia syndrome.

Physical manifestations of this syndrome include lipemia retinalis, eruptive xanthomas, and hepatomegaly. Patients are at increased risk of developing pancreatitis.

229. How is chylomicronemia syndrome treated?

Treatment is aimed at reducing triglyceride levels and may require fasting to lower the triglyceride levels into a safer range.

230. How should you screen for lipid disorders?

Current recommendations for screening and treatment are based on the National Cholesterol Education Program guidelines that were last revised in 2001. It is recommended that adults 20 years or older have a screening fasting lipid profile obtained every 5 years (more often if they are at high risk). Treatment is based on determining the patient's LDL cholesterol (LDL-c) goal. This goal is modified by cardiovascular risk factors (independent of LDL levels).

231. List the important risk factors for cardiovascular disease.

- Age: male ≥ 45 years, female ≥ 55 years
- Family history: coronary heart disease (CHD) in a male first-degree relative < 55 years or female first-degree relative < 65 years
- Current cigarette smoking
- Hypertension (≥ 140/90 mmHg or on antihypertensive medications)
- Low HDL cholesterol: < 40 mg/dL (*Note:* High HDL-c is a negative risk factor; if the patient has a level > 60 mg/dL, subtract one risk factor.)

232. How do you determine a patient's goal for LDL cholesterol?

Goal LDL-c is determined by patient evaluation and summation of risk factors. Patients at highest risk (known CHD, other forms of atherosclerotic disease, or diabetes) are treated to a goal LDL-c of < 100mg/dl. For patients with two or more risk factors, the 10-year risk for coronary disease must be calculated to determine whether they should be treated as a CHD-equivalent (10 year risk ≥ 20%). A point-scoring system for calculation of this risk was derived from the Framingham cohort data. This calculation can be done by adding the points for all the risk factors (from the original article) or using a handheld PDA (a free program for calculating risk can be downloaded from the National Institutes of Health at http://hin.nhlbi.nih.gov/atpiii/atp3palm.htm).

Executive Summary of the Third Report of the National Cholesterol Education Program (NCEP) Expert Panel on Detection, Evaluation, and Treatment of High Blood Cholesterol in Adults (Adult Treatment Panel III). JAMA 285:2486–2497, 2001.

233. Once you have obtained a lipid profile and evaluated a patient's CHD risk factors, what are the treatment recommendations?
See Table 2-16.

TABLE 2-16. LDL CHOLESTEROL GOALS

Risk Category	LDL-C goal	Start TLC	Consider Medication
CHD or CHD risk equivalent (10-yr risk of ≥ 20%)	100 mg/dL	≥ 100 mg/dL	≥ 130 mg/dL
≥ 2 risk factors (10-yr risk is < 20%)	130 mg/dLl	≥ 130 mg/dL	10-yr risk 10–20%: ≥ 130 mg/dL 10-yr risk <10%: ≥ 160 mg/dL
0–1 risk factor	160 mg/dL	≥ 160 mg/dL	≥ 190 mg/dL

CHD equivalent: other atherosclerotic disease (peripheral artery disease, abdominal aortic aneurysm, symptomatic carotid artery disease, diabetes or patients with multiple risk factors that confer a 10-year CHD risk of > 20%).
CHD = coronary heart disease, TLC = therapeutic lifestyle change (diet, weight reduction, exercise).

A recent update to the NCEP ATPIII Guidelines indicated that an *optional* LDL goal for *very high risk* patients could be < 70 mg/dL. A *very high risk* person was defined as a patient with known cardiovascular disease and multiple and/or uncontrolled risk factors, multiple risk factors of the metabolic syndrome or an acute coronary syndrome.

Executive summary of the third report of the National Cholesterol Educational Program (NCEP) expert panel on detection, evaluation, and treatment of high blood cholesterol in adults (Adult Treatment Panel III). JAMA 285:2486–2497, 2001.

Grundy SM et al. Implications of recent clinical trials for the National Cholesterol Education Program Adult Treatment Panel III Guidelines. Circulation 110:227–239, 2004.

234. List the currently available lipid-lowering agents.
See Table 2-17.

TABLE 2-17. LIPID-LOWERING AGENTS

Class	Drugs	Mechanism	TG	LDL	HDL	Side Effects
HMG CoA reductase inhibitors or "statins" (drugs of choice for lowering LDL)	Fluvastatin Pravastatin Lovastatin Simvastatin Atorvastatin Rosuvastatin (in order of ↑ potency)	Inhibits HMG CoA reductase (rate-limiting enzyme in cholesterol synthesis) ↑LDL receptor activity	↓,↓↓ (dose-related)	↓↓↓	↑	Overall well-tolerated ↑ LFTs Rhabdomyolysis Myositis Drug interactions
Cholesterol absorption inhibitor	Ezetamibe	Inhibits cholesterol absorption from gut	↔	↓↓	↔	↑ LFTs (w/ statins) GI upset/bloating
Bile acid resins	Colestipol Cholestyramine Colesevelam	Bind bile acids ↑Hepatic LDL receptor activity	↔, ↑	↓↓	↑	Constipation Steatorrhea Bloating Bind other drugs
Fibrates (drugs of choice for lowering TG)	Clofibrate Gemfibrozil Fenofibrate	↓VLDL synthesis ↑VLDL clearance	↓↓↓	↔, ↓*	↑	Overall well-tolerated Gallstones Myopathy Drug interactions
Bile acid resins	Colestipol Cholestyramine Colesevelam	Bind bile acids ↑Hepatic LDL receptor activity	↔, ↑	↓↓	↑	Constipation Steatorrhea Bloating Bind other drugs

(continued)

TABLE 2-17. LIPID-LOWERING AGENTS *(continued)*

Class	Drugs	Mechanism	TG	LDL	HDL	Side Effects
Nicotinic acid (drug of choice for raising HDL)	Crystalline niacin Niaspan (long-acting niacin)	↓VLDL secretion ↓Adipose lipolysis	↓↓	↓	↑↑	Flushing with short-acting form. ↑ LFTs Glucose intolerance Hyperuricemia Rash
Omega 3 fatty acids	Fish oils	↓VLDL synthesis and secretion	↓↓	?	?	Glucose intolerance Smell like fish

TG = triglycerides, LDL = low-density lipoprotein, HDL = high-density lipoprotein, LFT = liver function tests, VLDL = very low density lipoprotein, GI = gastrointestinal.
* Fenofibrate has more LDL-lowering effect than gemfibrozil.

235. List the genetic causes of lipid abnormalities.
See Table 2-18.

TABLE 2-18. GENETIC DISORDERS OF LIPID METABOLISM

Disorder	Mechanism	Lipid Profile
Familial hypercholesterolemia (increased CHD risk)	Autosomal dominant mutation in LDL receptor	Elevated LDL
Familial defective Apo B-100 (increased CHD risk)	Autosomal dominant Impaired binding of LDL to receptor. Mutant Apo B-100 ligand	Elevated LDL
Familial combined hyperlipidemia (increased CHD risk)	Overproduction of VLDL Specific gene defect unknown High Apo B	Elevated LDL and TG
Polygenic hypercholesterolemia (increased CHD risk)	Genetics poorly understood Abnormal LDL metabolism Apo E4 phenotype	Elevated LDL
Familial hypertriglyceridemia	Autosomal dominant Overproduction and secretion of VLDL	Elevated TG
Familial dysbetalipoproteinemia (broad beta disease) (increased CHD risk)	Altered IDL and remnant metabolism Apo E2 phenotype	Elevated LDL and TG
Lipoprotein lipase deficiency	Mutation in LPL gene Decreased TG metabolism	Elevated TG, low HDL
Familial hypoalphalipoproteinemia (increased CHD risk)	Autosomal dominant. Mutation in *Apo A-1* gene	Low HDL
Apo C-II deficiency (cofactor for LPL)	Decreased TG metabolism	Elevated TG
Tangier's disease: cholesterol esters accumulate in tissues: tonsils (orange), peripheral nerves, liver, spleen lymph nodes, cornea Unclear CHD risk	Autosomal recessive Mutation in the *ABC-A1* gene that allow cellular cholesterol efflux; abnormal intracellular cholesterol transport	Low HDL

(*continued*)

TABLE 2-18. GENETIC DISORDERS OF LIPID METABOLISM *(continued)*

Disorder	Mechanism	Lipid Profile
Familial HDL deficiency like Tangier disease but no systemic finding		
LCAT deficiency (corneal opacities)	Mutation in the LCAT gene Abnormal cholesterol esterification	Low HDL
CETP excess	High CETP activity (allows cholesterol ester transfer from HDL to TG-rich lipoproteins); gene variants with altered activity	Low HDL

CHD = coronary artery disease, VLDL = very low density lipoprotein, TG = triglycerides, LDL = low-density lipoprotein, HDL = high-density lipoprotein, IDL = intermediate-density lipoprotein, LCAT = lecithin-cholesterol acyltransferase, CETP = cholesterol ester transfer protein, Apo = apolipoprotein.

236. Identify some secondary/acquired causes of hyperlipidemia.
See Table 2-19.

TABLE 2-19. SECONDARY AND ACQUIRED CAUSES OF HYPERLIPIDEMIA

Increased LDL, Cholesterol	Increased TG	Decreased HDL
Hypothyroidism Poorly controlled diabetes Obesity/Metabolic syndrome Drugs: anabolic steroids Nephrotic syndrome Primary biliary cirrhosis Diet high in saturated fat	Hypothyroidism Poorly controlled diabetes Obesity/metabolic syndrome Drugs: oral estrogens, alcohol, beta blockers, protease inhibitors, thiazides, glucocorticoids, retinoids Nephrotic syndrome	Tobacco use Poorly controlled diabetes Obesity/metabolic syndrome Drugs: androgens, progesterone, beta blockers Sedentary lifestyle Diet restricted in fat

USEFUL ENDOCRINE-RELATED WEB SITES

1. The Endocrine Society: www.endo-society.org
2. Uptodate Reference: www.uptodate.com
3. Endotxt.org (Web-based source of information about endocrine diseases directed to physicians)
4. American Association of Clinical Endocrinologists: www.aace.com
5. Pituitary Society: www.pituitarysociety.org
6. American Thyroid Association: www.thyroid.org
7. American Diabetes Association: www.diabetes.org
8. American Society for Bone and Mineral Research: www.ASBMR.org
9. National Osteoporosis Foundation: www.nof.org
10. American Heart Association: www.americanheart.org

BIBLIOGRAPHY

1. American Diabetes Association: Clinical Practice Recommendations 2004. Diabetes Care 27(Suppl 1): S1–S150, 2004.
2. Basa ALP, Afsharkharaghan H (Zollo A, ed): Endocrinology in Medical Secrets, 3rd ed. 2001.
3. Braverman LE, Utiger RD (eds): Werner and Ingbars' Thyroid. A Fundamental and Clinical Text. Philadelphia, Lippincott Williams & Wilkins, 2000.
4. Favus MJ (ed): Primer on the Metabolic Bone Diseases and Disorders of Mineral Metabolism, 5th ed. Washington, DC, American Society of Bone and Mineral Research, 2003.
5. Larson PR, et al: Williams Textbook of Endocrinology, 10th ed. Philadelphia, W.B. Saunders, 2003.
6. Pickett CA: Diagnosis and management of pituitary tumors: Recent advances. Prim Care Clin Office Pract 30:765–789, 2003.
7. Wierman ME (ed): Diseases of the Pituitary: Diagnosis and Treatment. Totowa, NJ, Humana Press, 1997.

CARDIOLOGY

Gabriel B. Habib, Sr., M.D., and Anthony J. Zollo, Jr., M.D.

CHAPTER 3

Of all the ailments which may blow out life's little candle, heart disease is the chief.

William Boyd
Pathology for the Surgeon

Art is long and Time is fleeting
And our hearts, though stout and brave,
Still, like muffled drums are beating
Funeral marches to the grave.

Henry Wadsworth Longfellow
A Psalm of Life

PHYSICAL EXAMINATION

1. **What is cardiac tamponade?**
When the clinical triad of cardiac tamponade was first described by Beck in 1935, it consisted of hypotension, elevated systemic venous pressure, and a small, quiet heart. The condition was commonly due to penetrating cardiac injuries, aortic dissection, or intrapericardial rupture of an aortic or cardiac aneurysm. Today the most common causes are neoplastic disease, idiopathic pericarditis, acute myocardial infarction (MI), and uremia.

2. **Summarize the physical examination findings in cardiac tamponade.**
   - **Jugular venous distention:** almost universally present except in patients with severe hypovolemia.
   - **Pulsus paradoxus:** defined as a decrease in systolic blood pressure (BP) in excess of 10 mmHg during quiet inspiration. Pulsus paradoxus is difficult to elicit in volume-depleted patients.
   - **Tachycardia**, with a thready peripheral pulse: sometimes severe cardiac tamponade may restrict left ventricle (LV) and right ventricle (RV) filling enough to cause hypotension, but a thready and rapid pulse is almost invariably present.

3. **What is Kussmaul's sign?**
Kussmaul's sign, an inspiratory increase in systemic venous pressure, is commonly present in chronic constrictive pericarditis but is rarely detected in acute cardiac tamponade.

4. **What is the third heart sound (S_3)? What is a physiologic S_3?**
An S_3 (or ventricular gallop) is a low-frequency sound that is heard just after the second heart sound (S_2). When found in normal young patients, it is called a physiologic S_3.

5. **What is a pathologic S_3?**
An S_3 is also found in a variety of pathologic conditions (pathologic S_3), including congestive heart failure (CHF), mitral valve prolapse, thyrotoxicosis, coronary artery disease (CAD), cardiomyopathies, pericardial constriction, mitral or aortic insufficiency, and left-to-right shunts.

6. **Describe the mechanism behind an S_3.**
The mechanism behind an S_3 is controversial. It may be due to an increase in the velocity of blood entering the ventricles (rapid ventricular filling). It usually represents myocardial decompensation when associated with heart disease.

7. **What is an S_4?**
An S_4, or atrial gallop, occurs just before S_1 and reflects decreased ventricular compliance (a stiff ventricle). It is associated with CAD, pulmonic or aortic valvular stenosis, hypertension, and ventricular hypertrophy from any cause.

8. **How are heart murmurs graded?**

Grade	Physical Examination Findings
1	Barely audible intensity (only a cardiologist can hear it!)
2	Low-intensity murmur (the upper-level resident can hear it)
3	Loud murmur (everyone can hear it)
4	Loud murmur with palpable thrill
5	Loudest murmur audible (still requires a stethoscope placed on the chest)
6	Murmur loud enough to be heard with the stethoscope off the chest

9. **Explain the normal splitting of S_2.**
S_2 is normally split into aortic (A_2) and pulmonic components (P_2) caused by the closing of the two respective valves. The degree of splitting varies with the respiratory cycle (physiologic splitting). With inspiration, the negative intrathoracic pressure leads to increased venous return to the right side of the heart and a decrease to the left side; this causes P_2 to occur slightly later and A_2 to occur slightly earlier, which leads to a widening of the splitting of S_2. With expiration, the negative intrathoracic pressure is eliminated and A_2 and P_2 occur almost **simultaneously.**

10. **What is paradoxical splitting of S_2? What causes it?**
Paradoxical splitting of S_2 refers to the situation in which the split of A_2 and P_2 seems to widen with expiration and shorten with inspiration (the opposite of normal). This paradox is caused by P_2 preceding A_2 during expiration and is usually due to conditions that delay A_2 by delaying ejection of blood from the LV and therefore closure of the aortic valve. Causes include aortic insufficiency, aortic stenosis, hypertrophic obstructive cardiomyopathy, MI, left bundle branch block, or an RV pacemaker.

11. **What causes fixed splitting of S_2?**
In fixed splitting of S_2, the interval between A_2 and P_2 does not change with the respiratory cycle. It is typically associated with atrial septal defects or RV dysfunction.

12. **How do you measure the jugular venous pulse at the bedside?**
The patient's chest should be elevated to the point that the pulsations are maximally visualized (usually 30–45° of elevation). The height of this oscillating venous column above the sternal angle (angle of Louis) can then be measured (Fig. 3-1). Since the sternal angle is about 5 cm from the right atrium (RA) (regardless of elevation angle), central venous pressure can be estimated by adding 5 cm to the measurement. Normal central venous pressure is 5–9 cmH_2O.

13. **Name the three waves composing the jugular venous pulse.**
    1. **a-wave**, produced by right atrial contraction, occurs just before S_1.
    2. **c wave** is caused by bulging upward of the closed tricuspid valve during RV contraction (often difficult to see).
    3. **v wave** is caused by right atrial filling just before opening of the tricuspid valve.

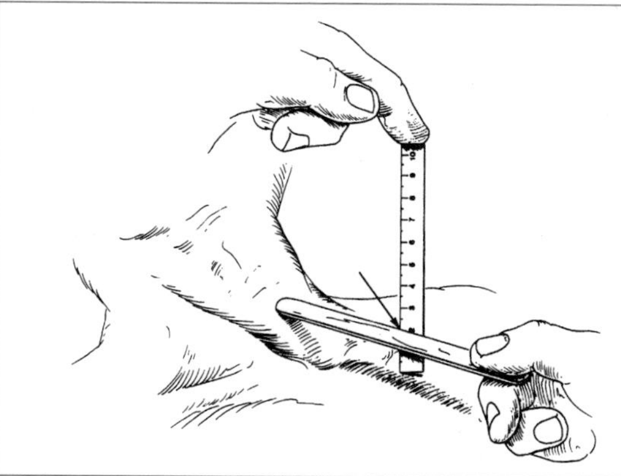

Figure 3-1. Measurement of venous jugular pressure at the bedside. (From Adair OV, Havranek EP: Cardiology Secrets. Philadelphia, Hanley & Belfus, 1995, p 6, with permission.)

14. **What are "cannon" a-waves?**
These very large and prominent a-waves occur when the atria contract against a closed tricuspid valve. Irregular "cannon" a-waves are seen in atrioventricular (AV) dissociation or ectopic atrial beats. Regular "cannon" a-waves are seen in a junctional or ventricular rhythm in which the atria are depolarized by retrograde conduction.

15. **What is the likely cause of a systolic ejection murmur, best heard at the second right intercostal space, in an 82-year-old asymptomatic man?**
By far, the most common cause in this setting is aortic sclerosis. This valvular abnormality is characterized by thickening and/or calcification of the aortic valve, and unlike valvular aortic stenosis, it is typically *not* associated with any significant transvalvular systolic pressure gradient.

16. **How can aortic stenosis be differentiated from aortic sclerosis?**
The following findings are present with aortic stenosis but absent with aortic sclerosis:
   - Diminished carotid upstroke
   - Diminished peripheral pulses
   - Late peaking of systolic murmur
   - Loud S_4
   - Syncope, angina, or heart failure
   - Loud systolic murmur and thrill

17. **How do standing, squatting, and leg-raising affect the intensity and duration of the systolic murmur heard on dynamic auscultation in a patient with idiopathic hypertrophic subaortic stenosis (IHSS)?**
In IHSS, a decrease in the size of the LV increases the dynamic LV outflow obstruction, leading to an increased intensity of the murmur. A decrease in LV volume occurs on standing. In contrast, leg-raising and squatting increase venous return and thereby increase LV volume, decreasing the dynamic LV obstruction and the murmur intensity.

18. **Define pulsus paradoxus. What medical diseases can present with pulsus paradoxus?**
Pulsus paradoxus was first described by Kussmaul in 1873 as the apparent disappearance of the pulse during inspiration despite persistence of the heartbeat. In fact, pulsus paradoxus is an exaggeration of the normal decline in systolic BP and LV stroke volume on inspiration.

19. Describe the mechanism behind pulsus paradoxus.
The fall in intrathoracic pressure is rapidly transmitted through the pericardial effusion and results in an exaggerated increase in venous return to the right side of the heart. This, in turn, causes bulging of the interventricular septum toward the LV, thereby resulting in a smaller LV volume and LV stroke volume during inspiration.

20. What medical diseases can present with pulsus paradoxus?
Pulsus paradoxus is **not** a sine qua non of cardiac tamponade. It may also occur in patients with severe chronic obstructive pulmonary disease complicated by the need for large negative intrathoracic pressures on inspiration. Interestingly, pulsus paradoxus is usually absent in chronic constrictive pericarditis.

ELECTROCARDIOGRAPHY

21. Describe the three phases of the evolution of an acute MI on electrocardiography (ECG).

1. **Abnormal T wave**, which is tall, prolonged, inverted, or upright. Hyperacute tall T waves are typically seen in the first hour or two of MI evolution. The T wave usually becomes inverted after ST-segment elevation has occurred and may remain inverted for days, weeks, or years.
2. **ST-segment elevations** in leads facing the infarcted myocardial wall and reciprocal ST depressions in opposite leads. ST-segment changes are the most common ECG signs of acute MI. ST-segment elevations rarely persist > 2 weeks except in patients with a ventricular aneurysm.
3. **Appearance of new Q waves**, often several hours or days after the onset of MI symptoms. Alternatively, the amplitude of the QRS complex is decreased. Q waves may develop earlier when thrombolytic therapy is administered (Fig. 3-2).

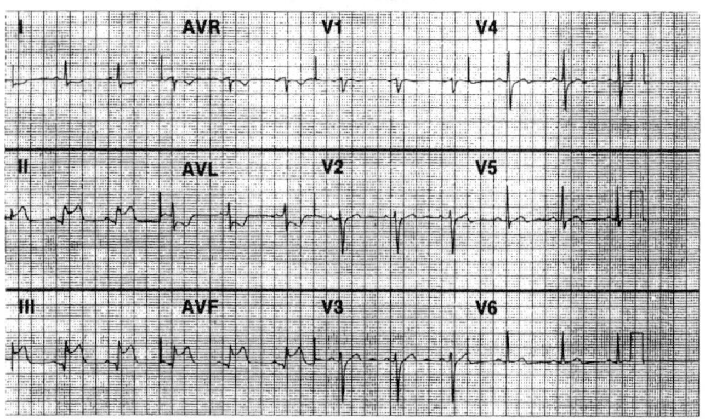

Figure 3-2. Acute MI localized to inferior leads (II, III, and aVF). The ECG shows ST elevation with hyperacute peaked T waves and the early development of significant Q waves. Reciprocal ST depression is also seen (leads I and aVL). (From Seelig CB: Simplified ECG Analysis. Philadelphia, Hanley & Belfus, 1997, p 13.)

22. What are the ECG manifestations of atrial infarction?

1. Depressed or elevated PR segment
2. Atrial arrhythmias
   - Atrial flutter
   - Atrial fibrillation
   - AV nodal rhythms

23. **Where does the venous a-wave appear in the cardiac cycle?**
During the course of one cardiac cycle, the electrical events (ECG) initiate and therefore precede the mechanical (pressure) events, and the latter precede the auscultatory events (heart sounds) that they produce. Shortly after the P wave, the atria contract to produce the a-wave; S_4 may succeed the latter.

24. **Where does an S_3 occur in relation to the QRS complex?**
The QRS complex initiates ventricular systole, followed shortly by LV contraction and the rapid buildup of LV pressure. Almost immediately, LV pressure exceeds left atrial (LA) pressure to close the mitral valve and produces S_1. When LV pressure exceeds aortic pressure, the aortic valve opens, and when aortic pressure is once again greater than LV pressure, the aortic valve closes to produce S_2 and terminate ventricular ejection. The decreasing LV pressure drops below LA pressure to open the mitral valve, and a period of rapid ventricular filling commences. During this time, an S_3 may be heard (Fig. 3-3). (For simplification, right-sided heart pressures have been omitted.)

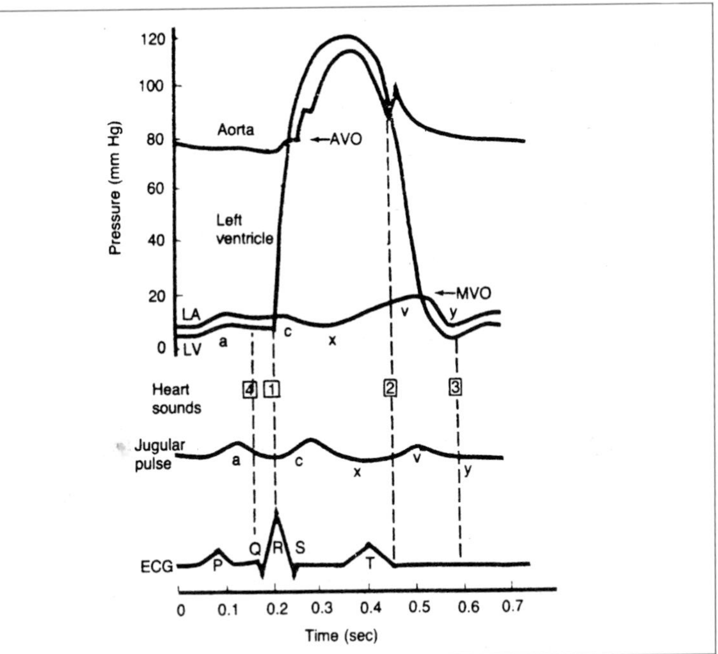

Figure 3-3. Production of S_1, S_2, S_3, and S_4 in the cardiac cycle. AVO = aortic valve opens, MVO = mitral valve opens. (From Andreoli TE, et al [eds]: Cecil Essentials of Medicine, 2nd ed. Philadelphia, W.B. Saunders, 1990, p 8.)

25. **Which arrhythmias can be detected in young patients without apparent heart disease?**
In a study of 24-hour continuous ECG monitoring performed on 50 male medical students, severe sinus bradycardia (40 bpm or fewer), sinus pauses of up to 2 sec, and nocturnal AV nodal block were frequently found. Frequent premature atrial or ventricular beats were not commonly found.

Brodsky M, et al: Arrhythmias documented by 24-hour continuous electrocardiographic monitoring in 50 male medical students without apparent heart disease. Am J Cardiol 39:390–395, 1977.

26. How do you differentiate atrial fibrillation (AF) from the other types of supraventricular tachycardias (SVTs)?
AF differs from all other SVTs by having totally disorganized atrial depolarizations without effective atrial contraction. An ECG may occasionally show small, irregular waves of variable amplitude and morphology, occurring at a rate of 350–600/min, but these are often difficult to recognize on a routine 12-lead ECG.

27. How do you differentiate atrial tachycardia and atrial flutter?
Unlike AF, atrial tachycardia (or paroxysmal atrial tachycardia) and atrial flutter demonstrate a regular ventricular rhythm and are characterized by regular and slower atrial rhythms (Table 3-1). The flutter rate (i.e., the atrial rate) in atrial flutter ranges between 250 and 350 bpm. The most common flutter rate is 300 bpm, and the most common ventricular rates are 150 and 75 bpm, respectively. Atrial tachycardias have slower atrial rates, ranging from 150 to 250 bpm. The most common cause of atrial tachycardia with block is digitalis toxicity.

TABLE 3-1. COMPARISON OF SUPRAVENTRICULAR TACHYCARDIAS

	Atrial Fibrillation	Atrial Flutter	Atrial Tachycardia
Atrial rate	> 400	240–350	100–240
Atrial rhythm	Irregular	Regular	Regular
AV block	Variable	2:1, 4:1, 3:1, or variable	2:1, 4:1, 3:1, or variable
Ventricular rate	Variable	150, 75, 100, or variable	Variable

28. What is the significance of capture and fusion beats on ECG in differentiating between ventricular tachycardia (VT) and SVT with aberrancy?
Three ECG findings are virtually pathognomonic of VT: AV dissociation, capture beats, and fusion beats (Table 3-2). A capture beat is a normally conducted sinus beat interrupting a wide-complex tachycardia. A fusion beat has a QRS morphology intermediate between a normally

TABLE 3-2. DISTINGUISHING FEATURES OF WIDE-COMPLEX VT AND SVT

	VT	SVT
History of MI	Yes	No
Ventricular aneurysm	Yes	No
Fusion beats	Yes	No
Capture beats	Yes	No
Complete AV dissociation	Yes	No
Similar QRS when in sinus rhythm	No	Yes
RBBB + QRS > 0.14 sec	Yes	No
LBBB + QRS > 0.16 sec	Yes	No
Positive concordance in V_1–V_6	Yes	No
LBBB + right QRS axis	Yes	No
Intermittent cannon waves	Yes	No

LBBB = left bundle branch block, RBBB = right bundle branch block.

conducted narrow beat and a wide-complex ventricular beat. The clinical hallmark of AV dissociation is the presence of intermittent cannon waves in the jugular neck veins.

29. Summarize the role of exercise stress testing.

Exercise stress testing is widely used to detect and assess the functional significance of CAD. It also has been shown to predict survival in patients recovering from an acute MI. Because exercise stress testing is commonly requested, its contraindications should be widely known and clearly understood so that use of this test is appropriate and safe.

30. What are the medical contraindications to exercise ECG testing?

1. MI acute or pending
2. Unstable angina
3. Acute myocarditis or pericarditis
4. Left main CAD
5. Severe aortic stenosis
6. Uncontrolled hypertension
7. Uncontrolled cardiac arrhythmias
8. Second- or third-degree AV block
9. Acute noncardiac illness

31. What are the types of AV block?

1. **First-degree AV block:** Prolongation of the PR interval due to a conduction delay at the AV node.
2. **Second-degree AV block:** Manifested by dropped beats in which a P wave is not followed by a QRS complex (no ventricular depolarization and therefore no ventricular contraction). It is divided into two types:
   - **Type I:** (Wenckebach phenomenon): The PR interval lengthens with each successive beat until a beat is dropped and the cycle repeats itself.
   - **Type II:** The PR intervals are prolonged but do not gradually lengthen until a beat is suddenly dropped. The dropped beat may occur regularly, with a fixed number (X) of beats for each dropped beat (called an X:1 block). Type II is much less common than type I and is commonly associated with bundle branch blocks.
3. **Third-degree AV block** (complete heart block): The atria and ventricles are controlled by separate pacemakers. It is associated with widening of the QRS complex and a ventricular rate of 35–50 bpm.

32. What ECG changes are seen in hyperkalemia?

A tall, peaked, symmetrical T wave with a narrow base (so-called tented T wave) is the earliest ECG abnormality and is usually present in leads II, III, V_2, V_3, and V_4. Shortening of the QT interval, widening of the QRS interval, ST-segment depression, flattening of the P wave, and PR-interval prolongation follows this. Eventually, the P waves disappear and the QRS complexes assume a configuration similar to a sine wave, eventually degenerating into ventricular fibrillation (VF). Widening of the QRS complex can assume a configuration consistent with atypical right bundle branch block (RBBB) or left bundle branch block (LBBB) making the recognition of hyperkalemia more difficult. Unlike typical RBBB, hyperkalemia often causes prolongation of the entire QRS complex.

33. Summarize the sequence of ECG changes in experimental hyperkalemia.

Tall, symmetrical T waves	$K^+ > 5.7$ mEq/L
Reduced P wave amplitude	$K^+ > 7.0$ mEq/L
Prolongation of PR interval	$K^+ > 7.0$ mEq/L
Disappearance of P waves	$K^+ > 8.4$ mEq/L
Widening of QRS interval	$K^+ = 9–11$ mEq/L
VF	$K^+ > 12$ mEq/L

34. What ECG signs suggest hypercalcemia? Are similar changes seen in other conditions?

Hypercalcemia shortens the QT interval, particularly the interval between the beginning of the QRS complex and the peak of the T wave. The abrupt slope to the peak of the T wave is most characteristic of hypercalcemia. Another cause of shortened QT interval is digitalis toxicity.

35. What is the normal range for PR and QT intervals on a 12-lead ECG? Do these intervals vary with heart rate, sex, or age?

The normal range for the **PR interval** is 0.12–0.20 sec. It is not significantly related to age, sex, or heart rate.

The normal range for the **QT interval** also is unrelated to age, but it does vary with heart rate. As the heart rate increases, the QT interval shortens. To help evaluate a QT interval independent of heart rate, the corrected QT interval (QTc) can be calculated:

QTc (in msec) = measured QT (in msec)/square root of the R-R interval (in sec)

The normal range for the **QTc** is 0.36–0.44 sec. A prolonged QTc is defined as QTc > 0.44 sec.

36. In the frontal plane, is a QRS axis of +120° compatible with a diagnosis of left anterior hemiblock?

This diagnosis requires the presence of a QRS of –60° to –90° in the frontal plane. A frontal plane QRS axis of +120° is consistent with right axis deviation and is therefore not compatible with a diagnosis of left anterior hemiblock (left anterior fascicular block).

37. List the diagnostic criteria for left anterior fascicular block.

- QRS axis –60° to –90°
- Small q-wave in lead I
- Small r-wave in lead III

38. Describe the ECG manifestations of RV hypertrophy.

- R-wave > S-wave in V_1 or V_2
- R-wave > 5 mm in V_1 or V_2
- Right axis deviation
- Persistent rS pattern (V_1–V_6)
- Normal QRS duration

39. What are the congenital causes of a prolonged QT interval?

- With deafness: Jervell syndrome
- Without deafness: Romano-Ward syndrome

40. List the acquired causes of a prolonged QT interval.

- Drugs: class IA/IC antiarrhythmics, tricyclic antidepressants, and phenothiazines
- Electrolyte abnormalities: low K^+, Ca^{2+}, Mg^{2+}
- Hypothermia
- Central nervous system injury (least common cause)
- Liquid diets
- CAD
- Cardiomyopathy
- Mitral valve prolapse

41. What is the clinical significance of a prolonged QT interval?

Prolongation of the QT interval is associated in certain patients with a definite increase in risk of VF and death.

DIAGNOSIS

42. How are cardiac and noncardiac causes of chest pain differentiated?

See Tables 3-3 and 3-4.

TABLE 3-3. CARDIAC CAUSES OF CHEST PAIN

Condition	Location	Quality	Duration	Aggravating/ Relieving Factors	Associated Signs and Symptoms
Angina	Retrosternal, radiates to neck, left arm	Pressure, burning, squeezing	< 10 min	Aggravated by exercise, cold, emotional stress, after meals Relieved by rest, nitroglycerin	S_4, paradoxically split S_2, murmur of papillary muscle
Rest or crescendo angina	Same as angina	Same as angina	> 10 min	Same as angina with gradually decreasing tolerance for exertion	Same as angina
Myocardial infarction	Substernal; may radiate like angina	Heaviness, pressure, burning, constriction	30 min or longer, variable	Unrelieved	Shortness of breath, diaphoresis, nausea, vomiting, weakness, anxiety
Pericarditis	Substernal or cardiac apex; may radiate to left arm	Sharp, stabbing, knifelike	Hours to days	Aggravated by deep breathing, rotating chest, or supine Relieved by sitting up and leaning forward.	Pericardial friction rub, cardiac tamponade, pulsus position, paradoxsus
Dissecting aortic aneurysm	Anterior chest, back, abdomina	Excruciating, tearing, knifelike	Sudden onset, lasts for hours	Unrelated to anything	Lower BP in one arm, absent pulses, murmur of aortic insufficiency, paralysis, pulsus paradoxsus

TABLE 3-4. NONCARDIAC CAUSES OF CHEST PAIN

Condition	Location	Quality	Duration	Aggravating/ Relieving Factors	Associated Signs and Symptoms
Pulmonary embolism	Substernal or over area of pulmonary infarction	Pleuritic or like angina	Sudden onset, min to > 1 h	May be aggravated by breathing	Dyspnea, tachypnea, tachycardia, hypotension, signs of right-sided (CHF), rales, pleural rub, hemoptysis (with infarction)
Pulmonary hyper-tension	Substernal	Pressure	—	Aggravated by effort	Dyspnea, signs of pulmonary HT
Pneumonia with pleuritis	Over area of consolidation	Pleuritic, well-localized	—	Aggravated by breathing	Dyspnea, cough, fever, dull to percussion, bronchial breath sounds, pleural rub
Spontaneous pneumothorax	Unilateral	Sharp, well-localized	Sudden onset, hours	Painful breathing	Dyspnea, hyperresonance, and decreased breath and voice sounds
Musculoskeletal	Variable	Aching	Short or long	Aggravated by movement, history of muscle exertion	Tender to pressure or movement
Herpes zoster	Dermatomal distribution	—	Prolonged	None	Rash appears in area of discomfort
GI disorders (esophageal reflux, ulcer)	Lower substernal, epigastric	Burning, colicky, aching	—	Precipitated by recumbency or meals, partial relief with antacids	Nausea, vomiting, food intolerance, melena, hematemesis, jaundice
Anxiety	Often localized to a point, moves	Sharp, burning, variable	Variable	Situational anger, usually brief	Sighing respirations, often chest wall tenderness

HT = hypertension.
From Andreoli TE, et al (eds): Cecil Essentials of Medicine, 2nd ed. Philadelphia, W.B. Saunders, 1990, pp 12–13.

43. A 31-year-old man complains of a sudden onset of sharp left chest pain, increased by deep inspiration and coughing. Physical findings, chest x-ray, and ECG are normal. What is your differential diagnosis?

- Acute pleuritis (coxsackievirus A, B)
- Acute pericarditis (coxsackievirus B)
- Pneumonia (viral, bacterial)
- Pulmonary embolus or infarction
- Pneumothorax

In this patient, the most likely clinical diagnosis causing pleuritic chest pain in the presence of a normal physical, chest x-ray, and ECG findings is acute viral pleuritis or pericarditis.

44. A 56-year-old man presents to the emergency center with acute onset of squeezing and diffuse, anterior chest pain associated with diaphoresis and dyspnea. What is your differential diagnosis?

1. Acute MI
2. Angina pectoris
3. Acute aortic dissection
4. Acute pericarditis
5. Acute pulmonary embolus
6. Acute pneumothorax

45. Which tests will help confirm your clinical suspicions?

Among these diagnoses, the first three are most common and should be carefully considered in the diagnostic work-up of this patient. A **12-lead ECG** is performed to look for ST-segment elevations (evidence of acute myocardial injury due to infarction or pericarditis), ST-segment depressions (evidence of subendocardial ischemia), or T-wave changes. Determination of **serial cardiac enzymes** (creatine kinase and MB isoenzyme) over the first 24–48 hours of hospitalization will help to confirm a diagnosis of acute MI. The absence of any ECG changes of acute MI or ischemia in a patient with severe anterior chest pain radiating to the back should suggest the clinical diagnosis of acute aortic dissection. Finally, a **chest x-ray** is helpful in the work-up of patients with acute chest pain to look for evidence of pneumothorax, cardiac enlargement suggestive of cardiac failure, or wedge-shaped pulmonary consolidation suggestive of acute pulmonary embolus.

46. Identify the types of shock and their causes.

See Table 3-5.

47. What is a pseudoinfarction? What is its differential diagnosis?

Some patients exhibit ECG changes similar to those of MI but do not have any other definitive evidence of an MI. Such patients are said to have ECG evidence of "pseudoinfarction." Causes include:

1. LV or RV hypertrophy
2. LBBB
3. Wolff-Parkinson-White syndrome
4. Hypertrophic cardiomyopathy
5. Hyperkalemia
6. Early repolarization
7. Cardiac sarcoid or amyloid
8. Intracranial hemorrhage

48. A patient presents to the cardiac care unit with clinical signs and symptoms suggestive of acute RV MI. How would an ECG help to confirm this clinical diagnosis?

About one third of patients with acute inferior wall MI develop a RV infarction. The clinical syndrome of RV MI should be suspected when the following clinical triad is present in a patient suffering from an inferior wall MI:

- Hypotension
- Elevated jugular veins
- Clear lungs

TABLE 3-5. CLASSIFICATION OF SHOCK STATES

Type	Primary Mechanism	Clinical Causes
Hypovolemic	Volume loss	Exogenous Blood loss due to hemorrhage Plasma loss due to burn, inflammation Fluid/electrolyte loss due to vomiting, diarrhea, dehydration, osmotic diuresis (diabetes) Endogenous Extravasation due to inflammation, trauma, tourniquet, anaphylaxis, snake venom, and adrenergic stimulation (pheochromocytoma)
Cardiogenic	Pump failure	MI, CHF, cardiac arrhythmias, intracardiac obstruction (incl valvular stenosis)
Distributive (vasomotor dysfunction)		
1. High or normal resistance	Expanded venous capacitance	Hypodynamic septic shock due to gram-negative enteric bacillemia; autonomic blockade; spinal shock; tranquilizer, sedative, or narcotic overdose
2. Low resistance	AV shunting	Pneumonia, peritonitis, abscess, reactive hyperemia
Obstructive	Extracardiac obstruction of main blood flow channels	Vena caval obstruction (supine hypotensive syndrome), pericarditis (tamponade), pulmonary embolism, dissecting aortic aneurysm, aortic compression

(From Weil MH, et al: Acute circulatory failure [shock]. In Braunwald E [ed]: Heart Disease: A Textbook of Cardiovascular Medicine, 3rd ed. Philadelphia, W.B. Saunders, 1988, p 569, with permission.)

The clinical recognition of RV infarction is important. The clinical suspicion can be confirmed by performing a right-sided ECG. The presence of at least 1 mm of ST-segment elevation in lead V_3R or V_4R is characteristically present in RV MI. Further confirmation can be derived from non-invasive assessment of RV systolic function using radionuclide techniques or two-dimensional echocardiography.

49. **Name the three types of cardiomyopathies. How are they distinguished?**
See Table 3-6.

50. **An 89-year-old woman was found unconscious in her backyard. She "woke up" a few minutes after arrival at the emergency department. Physical, neurologic, ECG, and chest x-ray findings are all normal. She feels fine and demands to be released. Would you admit her to the hospital?**
Syncope, defined as a transient loss or impairment of consciousness, can be due to a wide variety of etiologies, both cardiovascular and noncardiovascular. Patients most likely to have cardiovascular syncope are older and may or may not have a prior history of documented cardiac disease (manifested by angina pectoris, MI, or sudden cardiac death). It is desirable to hospitalize patients

TABLE 3-6. CLASSIFICATION OF CARDIOMYOPATHY

Type	Characteristics	Symptoms/Signs	Laboratory Diagnosis
Dilated (congestive)	Cardiac dilation, generalized hypocontractility	LV and RV failure	X-ray: cardiomegaly with pulmonary congestion ECG: sinus tachycardia, nonspecific ST-T changes, arrhythmias,conduction disturbances, Q waves Echo: dilated LV, generalized decreased wall motion, mitral valve motion consistent with low flow Catheterization: dilated hypocontractile ventricle, mitral regurgitation
Hypertrophic	Ventricular hypertrophy, esp. of the septum, with or without outflow tract obstruction Typically good systolic but poor diastolic (compliance) ventricular function	Dyspnea, angina, pre-syncope, syncope, palpitations Large jugular a-wave,bifid carotid pulse, palpable S_4 gallop, prominent apical impulse, "dynamic" systolic murmur and thrill, mitral regurgitation murmur	X-ray: LV predominance, dilated left atrium ECG: LV hypertrophy, Q waves, nonspecific ST-T waves; ventricular arrhythmias Echo: hypertrophy, usually asymmetric (septum > free wall); systolic anterior motion of mitral valve; midsystolic closure of aortic valve Catheterization: provokable outflow tract gradient; hypertrophy with vigorous systolic function and cavity obliteration; mitral regurgitation
Restrictive	Reduced diastolic compliance impeding ventricular filling; normal systolic function	Dyspnea, exercise intolerance, weakness Elevated jugular venous pressure, edema, hepatomegaly, ascites, S_4 and S_3 gallops, Kussmaul's sign	X-ray: mild cardiomegaly, pulmonary congestion ECG: low voltage, conduction disturbances, Q waves Echo: characteristic myocardial texture in amyloidosis with thickening of all cardiac structures Catheterization: square root sign, M-shaped atrial waveform, elevated left and right filling pressures

From Andreoli TE, et al (eds): Cecil Essentials of Medicine, 2nd ed. Philadelphia, W.B. Saunders, 1990, p 106.

who are at high risk for cardiovascular syncope, since they have a much worse prognosis and may have potentially life-threatening complications of their underlying cardiovascular disease. This elderly woman should be hospitalized since she is at high risk for cardiovascular syncope.

51. List the common cardiovascular causes of syncope.

- **Tachyarrhythmias**, such as VT or SVT (AF, atrial flutter, or paroxysmal SVT).
- **Bradyarrhythmias**, such as second- or third-degree AV block, AF with a slow ventricular response rate, or sinus bradycardia due to sick sinus syndrome.
- **LV outflow obstruction** due to fixed lesions (valvular, subvalvular, or supravalvular aortic stenosis) or dynamic obstruction such as hypertrophic cardiomyopathy. Characteristically, these patients present with syncope during or immediately after exercise.
- **LV inflow obstruction** due to severe mitral stenosis or a large LA myxoma.
- **Primary pulmonary hypertension**

52. Should a thorough work-up be done on all patients with syncope?

No. The routine use of expensive or invasive studies into the cause of syncope is not warranted. The etiology of syncope will be undetermined in 30–50% of cases even after a thorough (and expensive) work-up. In up to 85% of cases in which an etiology is identifiable, it will be identified or at least suggested by the initial history, physical exam, and ECG. Further studies should be ordered on the basis of the results of this initial evaluation.

53. A 68-year-old man with hypertension presents with a 2-week history of progressive exertional dyspnea, orthopnea, and paroxysmal nocturnal dyspnea. What is the differential diagnosis of congestive heart failure in hypertensive patients?

- CAD
- Diastolic dysfunction associated with hypertension
- Dilated cardiomyopathy (idiopathic or alcoholic)
- Valvular heart disease (mitral regurgitation, aortic stenosis, aortic insufficiency)
- Restrictive heart disease (amyloidosis)
- Hypertrophic cardiomyopathy (idiopathic hypertrophic subaortic stenosis)

54. What is a hyperdynamic precordial impulse?

It is a thrust of exaggerated height that falls away immediately from the palpating fingers. It is typically found in patients with a large stroke volume. The clinical conditions include thyrotoxicosis, anemia, beriberi, AV shunts or grafts, exercise, or mitral regurgitation. A hyperdynamic precordial impulse should be differentiated from the sustained apical impulse, a graphic equivalent of a heave, detected in the presence of LV hypertrophy due to hypertension or aortic stenosis.

55. What is the differential diagnosis of an abnormal early diastolic sound heard at the apex and lower left sternal border?

- Loud P_2
- S_3 gallop
- Opening snap
- Pericardial knock
- Tumor plop (atrial myxoma)

An early diastolic sound may be due to wide splitting of S_2, with or without a loud pulmonic closure sound. An atrial septal defect (ASD) causes wide and fixed splitting of S_2.

56. Explain the significance of a loud P_2.

A loud P_2 usually indicates the presence of pulmonary hypertension, whether primary or secondary to chronic pulmonary disease.

57. **How is S_3 best heard?**
Unlike other causes of an early diastolic sound, a third heart sound (S_3) can best be heard using the bell of the stethoscope. Unlike a physiologically split A_2–P_2, the A_2–S_3 interval does not change during respiration. Associated physical findings of CHF, such as pulmonary rales, distended neck veins, or edema are usually present along with an S_3.

58. **What is an opening snap?**
An opening snap may be the only finding in a patient with a mild noncalcified and pliable mitral valve. In such a patient, a loud S_1 is also commonly present. A diastolic rumble at the apex confirms the physical diagnosis of mitral stenosis.

59. **What causes a pericardial knock?**
In patients with chronic constrictive pericarditis, the sudden slowing of LV filling in early diastole associated with the restriction of a rigid pericardium acting as "a rigid shell" causes the pericardial knock.

60. **What is a tumor plop?**
In some patients with large atrial myxomas protruding through the mitral valve during diastole, the sudden cessation of LV filling, caused by the tumor's obstruction to the flow of blood, creates an audible tumor plop. Cardiac auscultation in various positions helps to detect a tumor plop. Likewise, cardiac symptoms in these patients are often related to body position.

61. **Summarize the pathophysiology and significance of an opening snap in patients with mitral stenosis. Does its presence imply a more severe degree of stenosis?**
An opening snap is typically present only when the mitral valve leaflets are pliable, and it is therefore usually accompanied by an accentuated S_1. Diffuse calcification of the mitral valve can be expected when an opening snap is absent. If calcification is confined to the tip of the mitral valve, an opening snap is still commonly present. The interval between the aortic closure sound and opening snap (A_2–OS) is inversely related to the mean LA pressure. A short A_2–OS interval is a reliable indicator of severe mitral stenosis; however, the converse is not necessarily true.

62. **What is the "figure 3" sign? What congenital cardiac disease does it most likely suggest?**
A routine chest x-ray may reveal a characteristic "3" sign, which results from post-stenotic dilatation of the descending aorta and the dilated left subclavian artery. A barium swallow may reveal a reverse "3" sign. Along with rib notching, the presence of the "3" sign is almost pathognomonic for **aortic coarctation**.

63. **What are the major and minor Jones criteria for diagnosing acute rheumatic fever?**

Major Jones Criteria	Minor Jones Criteria
Carditis	Fever
Polyarthritis	Arthralgia
Chorea	Prolonged PR internal
Erythema marginatum	Elevated erythrocyte sedimentation rate or positive C-reactive protein
Subcutaneous nodules	Previous rheumatic fever or rheumatic heart disease

The clinical diagnosis of acute rheumatic fever is made if two major criteria or one major and two minor criteria are present in a patient with a preceding streptococcal infection (as evidenced by recent scarlet fever, positive throat culture for group A streptococci, or increased antistreptococcal antibody or other streptococcal antibody titer).

CORONARY ARTERY DISEASE

64. Is aspirin effective in the treatment of unstable angina pectoris?

Unequivocal evidence from two clinical trials, the VA and Canadian Cooperative Trials, indicates that aspirin reduces subsequent MI and mortality in unstable angina patients. Both mortality and MI are reduced by about 50% in aspirin-treated patients. On the other hand, there is less evidence to suggest a beneficial effect of aspirin in chronic stable angina pectoris.

Lewis HD, et al: Protective effects of aspirin against acute myocardial infarction and death in men with unstable angina: Results of a Veterans Administration Cooperative Study. N Engl J Med 309:396–403, 1983.

Cairns JA, et al: Aspirin, sulfinpyrazone, or both in unstable angina: Results of a Canadian multicenter trial. N Engl J Med 313:1369–1375, 1985.

65. Define acute coronary syndrome.

Acute coronary syndrome is a clinical syndrome characterized by ischemic cardiac chest pains associated with ST or T-wave changes, but, unlike classic acute MI, there is no acute ST segment elevation. Thus, it is called the non-ST elevation acute coronary syndrome. This includes two diseases: unstable angina and non–Q-wave MI, which are differentiated based on the presence or absence of an elevation of the creatinine kinase MB fraction (MB CK) or troponin I or T levels.

66. Describe the pathophysiologic mechanism of acute coronary syndromes.

The pathophysiologic mechanism of acute non-ST elevation coronary syndrome is intermittent and/or incomplete coronary occlusion by platelet-rich "white" recent thrombus resulting from platelet aggregation at the site of a damaged inner surface of a coronary artery. The trigger for this platelet aggregation is usually rupture of an atherosclerotic plaque. This type of thrombus is in sharp contrast to the mature red blood cell and fibrin-rich "red" or "mature" thrombus, which is the hallmark pathologic finding in patients with acute ST elevation MI. Unlike the platelet-rich "white" thrombus, a mature "red" thrombus results in a complete and/or persistent coronary artery occlusion resulting in severe transmural ischemia characterized by acute ST segment elevation. An intermittent or incomplete occlusion of a coronary artery usually causes acute subendocardial ischemia, which presents with ST segment depression or T wave changes that are transient or dynamic in nature.

67. Compare and contrast acute coronary syndromes to acute ST-elevation MI.

Interestingly, the clinical presentations of these pathophysiologically distinct clinical syndromes are quite different. Patients with acute ST elevation MI present with a persistent relentless chest pain lasting for over 30 min (and up to several hours). In contrast, patients with non-ST segment elevation acute coronary syndromes usually present with a waxing and waning of intermittent and recurrent episodes of ischemic cardiac chest pains.

68. Is clopidogrel recommended in patients admitted with unstable angina or acute non-ST elevation coronary syndromes already treated with aspirin?

The American Heart Association/American College of Cardiology (AHA/ACC) guidelines recommend clopidogrel in patients admitted with acute coronary syndromes with no ST segment elevation in addition to aspirin therapy. This class I recommendation is based on the CURE trial which showed a significant reduction in recurrent cardiac events with the addition of clopidogrel to standard therapy including aspirin, beta blockers, and statins.

Braunwald E, Antman EM, Beasley JW, et al, for the American College of Cardiology/American Heart Association Committee on the Management of Patients with Unstable Angina: ACC/AHA guideline update for the management of patients with unstable angina and non–ST-segment elevation myocardial infarction: A report of the ACC/AHA Task Force on Practice Guidelines. Circulation 106:1893–1900, 2002.

The Clopidogrel in Unstable Angina to Prevent Recurrent Events Trial investigators: Effects of clopidogrel in addition to aspirin in patients with acute coronary syndrome without ST segment elevation. N Engl J Med 345:494–502, 2001.

69. How successful is the combination of thrombolysis and 2b/3a inhibitors?

Three clinical trials have evaluated the angiographic results of thrombolytics in combination with an inhibitor of the platelet glycoprotein 2b/3a receptor: the TIMI 14, SPEED GUSTO, and INTRO-AMI trials. All three specifically evaluated angiographic outcome at 60 and 90 min after thrombolytics when combined with a platelet glycoprotein 2b/3a receptor. The TIMI 14 and GUSTO SPEED trials revealed that the proportion of patients who completely reperfuse (as evidenced by a TIMI flow grade 3) is significantly higher with the combination of half-dose t-PA or r-PA with the platelet glycoprotein 2b/3a receptor inhibitor abciximab (Reopro). The INTRO-AMI trial confirmed these results using the platelet glycoprotein 2b/3a receptor inhibitor eptifibatide (Integrelin) and showed a similar increase in rate and extent of thrombolysis at 90 min after thrombolysis is initiated. However, despite these promising angiographic results, none of the mortality trials showed any survival advantages for the combination of lysis + 26/3a inhibitors. This combination is *not* routinely recommended.

Antman EM, Giugliano RP, Gibson CM, et al, for the TIMI 14 Investigators: Abciximab facilitates the rate and extent of thrombolysis: Results of the Thrombolysis in Myocardial Infarction (TIMI) 14 trial. Circulation 99:2720–2732, 1999.

Trial of abciximab with and without low-dose reteplase for acute myocardial infarction: Strategies for Patency Enhancement in the Emergency Department (SPEED) Group. Circulation 101:2788–2794, 2000.

KEY POINTS: PLATELET AGGREGATION

1. Platelet aggregation is the key pathophysiologic mechanism causing non-ST elevation acute coronary syndrome.
2. Strategies specifically targeting the inhibition of platelet aggregation, such as aspirin, low-molecular-weight or unfractionated heparin, and clopidogrel, are routinely recommended.
3. The use of more potent platelet aggregation inhibitors (the glycoprotein IIB/IIIA inhibitors such as tirofiban, eptifibatide or abciximab) are reserved for patients with acute coronary syndromes at substantially high risk for major cardiovascular complications because of greater bleeding risk.

70. Is primary angioplasty (a mechanical reperfusion therapy) using a balloon-tipped catheter as effective as pharmacologic reperfusion therapy with a thrombolytic drug?

The primary angioplasty in myocardial infarction (PAMI) trial is the first published clinical trial designed specifically to compare balloon angioplasty with t-PA as the primary reperfusion therapy in patients with acute ST-elevation MI. Survival rates (at 30 days and at 2 years) after primary angioplasty were similar to those with t-PA in acute MI, but angioplasty conferred greater freedom from recurrent ischemia, reinfarction, and need for readmission to the hospital. Another important advantage of balloon angioplasty over thrombolytic drug therapy is freedom from intracranial hemorrhage, a dreadful complication of thrombolysis, particularly in elderly patients.

Nunn CM, O'Neill WW, Rothbaum D, et al: Long-term outcome after primary angioplasty: Report from the primary angioplasty in myocardial infarction (PAMI-I) trial. J Am Coll Cardiol 33:640–646, 1999.

71. **Do nitrates differ in efficacy when used in the management of vasospastic angina compared with classic effort angina?**
Patients with both forms of angina respond promptly to nitrates.

72. **Do beta blockers differ in efficacy and safety when used in the management of vasospastic angina compared with classic effort angina?**
Although the response of patients with effort angina to beta blockers is uniformly good, the response of patients with Prinzmetal's angina is variable. In some patients, the duration of episodes of angina pectoris may be prolonged during therapy with propranolol, a noncardioselective beta blocker. In others, especially those with associated fixed atherosclerotic lesions, beta blockers may reduce the frequency of anginal episodes. Noncardioselective beta blockers may, in some patients with variant angina, leave a receptor-mediated coronary arterial vasoconstriction unopposed and thereby worsen anginal symptoms.

73. **Do calcium blockers differ in efficacy and safety when used in the management of vasospastic angina compared with classic effort angina?**
In contrast to beta blockers, calcium blockers are quite effective in reducing the frequency and duration of episodes of variant angina. Along with nitrates, calcium blockers are the mainstay of treatment of Prinzmetal's angina because of their proven efficacy and safety.

74. **Is treadmill exercise ECG testing helpful in confirming the diagnosis of exertional angina?**
Exercise testing is the most common provocative test used by clinicians to confirm the clinical diagnosis of exertional angina pectoris. An exercise ECG test is considered positive for CAD if it shows at least a 1-mm horizontal or downsloping ST-segment depression during exercise. Myocardial ischemia is induced in these patients by an increase in myocardial O_2 demand, primarily due to the increase in heart rate with exercise.

75. **Is treadmill exercise ECG testing helpful in confirming the diagnosis of variant angina?**
In patients with variant angina, myocardial ischemia is primarily due to a decrease in O_2 supply rather than to an increase in O_2 demand. Exercise testing is thus of limited diagnostic value in these patients. It may show ST-segment elevation, ST-segment depression, or no change in ST segments during exercise.

76. **A 78-year-old asthmatic man has stable exertional angina of 3 years' duration. His past medical history reveals intermittent claudication after walking 50 yards. What is your approach to medical management of his anginal symptoms?**
This elderly man has three medical problems: asthma, intermittent claudication, and chronic stable angina. Of the available antianginal drugs, beta blockers are contraindicated because of the presence of asthma. Cardioselective beta blockers, such as metoprolol (Lopressor) or atenolol (Tenormin), may be used cautiously in low doses in asthma, but noncardioselective beta blockers are not safe in this patient. However, the presence of peripheral vascular disease, as manifested by intermittent claudication, also is a contraindication for the use of any beta blocker. Calcium antagonists or nitrates are thus the antianginal drugs of choice in this patient.

77. **How common are acute coronary syndromes, including unstable angina?**
Acute coronary syndrome (unstable angina or non-ST elevation myocardial infarction) is a common potentially life-threatening medical condition. In 2003, it accounted for over 750,000 hospital admissions in the United States.

78. **Based on clinical history, physical examination, and initial admission ECG, which patients with acute coronary syndromes (unstable angina or non-ST elevation myocardial infarction) are at highest risk for death or recurrent MI?**
The risk of death or recurrent non-fatal MI is highest in patients with acute coronary syndrome complicated by any of the following features:
- Ongoing prolonged chest pain > 20 min in duration
- Acute pulmonary edema (by physical exam or chest x-ray)
- New or worsening mitral regurgitation murmur
- Rest angina with dynamic ST-segment changes ≥ 1 mm
- S_3 gallop or lung rales
- Hypotension
- Positive enzymatic markers of MI such as MBCK or troponin I or T.

Patients with one or more of these high-risk indicators should generally be admitted to the coronary care unit for ECG monitoring and intensive medical therapy with IV nitrates, heparin, aspirin, and beta blockers.

Braunwald E, et al: Diagnosing and managing unstable angina. Circulation 90:613–622, 1994.

79. **Which patients with unstable angina should undergo cardiac catheterization?**
Cardiac catheterization should be entertained in patients with unstable angina and any of the following features:
- Unstable angina refractory to medical management
- Prior revascularization, including percutaneous angioplasty, coronary stenting, or bypass surgery
- Depressed LV function (LV ejection fraction < 50%)
- Life-threatening "malignant" ventricular arrhythmias
- Persistent or recurrent angina/ischemia
- Inducible myocardial ischemia (provoked by exercise, dobutamine, adenosine, or dipyridamole) at a low exercise level

Braunwald E, et al: Diagnosing and managing unstable angina. Circulation 90:613–622, 1994.

80. **A 48-year-old man presents with acute severe epigastric pain, anorexia, nausea, vomiting, and diaphoresis. Which myocardial wall is likely affected? Explain the rationale for such an unusual clinical presentation.**
Patients with an **acute inferior wall MI** sometimes present with epigastric pain associated with gastrointestinal symptoms, as in this case. Less commonly, they present with hiccupping, which may at times be intractable. These unique clinical manifestations are thought to be related to increased vagal tone and irritation of the diaphragm by the adjacent infarcted inferior wall.

81. **Does early administration of thrombolytic therapy after MI decrease mortality?**
The effect of IV thrombolytic therapy on MI mortality is well established. In the GISSI trial published in 1986, 11,806 patients with acute MI presenting within 12 hours of symptom onset were randomly assigned to receive IV streptokinase or placebo. The hospital mortality was significantly reduced in patients treated with streptokinase within the first 6 hours. Most importantly, there was a remarkable 50% reduction in hospital mortality in patients treated within 1 hour of symptom onset. Subsequent clinical trials of various thrombolytic drugs including streptokinase (SK), t-PA (Activase), r-PA (Retavase), and the most recent FDA-approved thrombolytic TNK–t-PA (Tenectaplase) confirmed the consistent improvement in survival with thrombolytic therapy in patients with acute ST elevation MI.

82. Summarize the benefits of thrombolytic therapy.

Thrombolysis is the most effective life-saving pharmacologic therapy in acute MI. It saves about 40 lives for every 1000 treated patients and reduces 30-day and 1-year mortality by about 25%. Patients presenting up to 12 hours after symptom onset may benefit from thrombolysis.

83. Outline the standard of care for patients with acute ST-elevation MI.

The current standard of care for patients with acute ST-elevation (or transmural) MI includes administration of IV thrombolytic therapy in all patients admitted within 12 hours of symptom onset (in the absence of contraindications). Contraindications include bleeding disorders, severe uncontrolled hypertension (blood pressure > 180/120 mmHg), recent history of thromboembolic cerebrovascular accident (within 2 months), any prior history of a hemorrhagic cerebrovascular accident, prolonged cardiopulmonary resuscitation (over 10 min), or active bleeding from a peptic ulcer or other noncompressible source, or known brain metastasis or cerebrovascular AVM or aneurysm.

GISSI Trial: Effect of time to treatment on reduction in hospital mortality observed in streptokinase-treated patients. Lancet 1:397–401, 1986.

AHA/ACC Task Force: Guidelines for management of acute myocardial infarction. Circulation July 2004, accessed via ACC or NIH Web sites.

84. Which drug is more effective in achieving successful reperfusion of a thrombosed coronary artery: SK, t-PA, r-PA, or TNK–t-PA?

In the TIMI trial, t-PA resulted in about twice as many successful reperfusions (due to clot lysis) as SK. In the GUSTO trial, t-PA was more effective than SK in opening coronary arteries and preventing death in the first 30 days after acute MI. In the RAPID I and RAPID II trials, about 60% of r-PA-treated patients experienced complete reperfusion at 90 min compared with about 50–55% of patients treated with t-PA. In the large-scale GUSTO III trial, however, despite the higher TIMI flow grade 3 in patients treated with r-PA, survival was similar in patients who received t-PA or r-PA. Angiographic trials of TNK–t-PA showed similar coronary angiographic success compared with t-PA, and the ASSENT-2 trial confirmed the equivalent efficacy of both agents in improving survival. Recent mortality trials of TNK–t-PA showed no survival benefit over t-PA. In summary, t-PA is clearly angiographically superior to SK in opening arteries and saving lives, whereas the newer r-PA and TNK-t-PA thrombolytics are not clearly superior to t-PA in overall efficacy, but are more convenient to administer as a bolus (single bolus for TNK–t-PA and double boluses, 30 min apart for t-PA).

GUSTO Angiographic Investigators: The effects of tissue plasminogen activator, streptokinase, or both on coronary-artery patency, ventricular function and survival after acute myocardial infarction. N Engl J Med 329:1615–1622, 1993.

85. Should oral nitrates be administered routinely to all patients with uncomplicated MI?

IV, transdermal, and/or oral nitrates have traditionally been used routinely in all patients admitted with suspected acute MI. However, despite the encouraging results of early small clinical studies, two large multi-center clinical trials, ISIS-4 and GISSI-3, consisting of about 78,000 patients, showed no significant benefit of early oral nitrates on survival, infarct size, or ventricular function. Their routine administration should thus be limited to patients with well-established indications for nitrates, such as postinfarction angina ischemia or CHF.

Gruppo Italiano per lo Studio della Sopravivenza nell' Infarto Miocardio (GISSI-3): Effects of lisinopril and transdermal glyceryltrinitrate singly and together on 6-week mortality and ventricular function after acute myocardial infarction. Lancet 343:1115–1122, 1994.

ISIS-4: A randomized factorial trial assessing early oral captopril, oral mononitrate, and intravenous magnesium sulphate in 58,050 patients with suspected acute myocardial infarction. Lancet 345:669–685, 1995.

Morris JL, et al: Nitrates in myocardial infarction: Influence on infarct size, reperfusion, and ventricular remodeling. Br Heart J 73:319, 1995.

86. What is the most common cause of death in the first 48 hours after an acute MI?
Ventricular fibrillation. Other causes of death include cardiac rupture, pump failure due to massive infarction, acute mechanical complication such as ventricular septal rupture or acute mitral regurgitation, and cardiogenic shock.

87. What is the official recommendation for use of statins in patients with CAD?
The National Cholesterol Education Program Adult Treament Panel III recommends that all patients with CAD be treated with statins if the LDL cholesterol level is > 130 mg/dL with a goal LDL of < 100 mg/dL. Recent recommendations extend the benefit of statins in patients with CAD (with metabolic syndrome, diabetes, multiple risk factors, or poorly controlled or uncontrolled risk factors) to new target LDL levels < 70 mg/dL.

Third Report of the Expert Panel on Detection, Evaluation, and Treatment of High Blood Cholesterol in Adults (Adult Treatment Panel III) Executive Summary. JAMA May 16, 2001.

Grundy, Scott, et al. July 12, 2004. Circulation 2004. NCEP report.

88. Do statins help prevent MI and stroke in patients with CAD (or other vascular disease) and/or diabetes mellitus, regardless of the LDL cholestrol level?
The Heart Protection Study investigated the effect of simvastatin (40 mg/day) on fatal or nonfatal coronary heart disease events in about 20,000 patients, aged 40–79 years, with vascular disease and/or diabetes mellitus and a mildly elevated low-density cholesterol level of about 130 mg/dL. This trial showed the same overall 24% reduction in cardiovascular mortality and 30–35% reduction in coronary heart disease events and stroke in the 3800 patients with a baseline LDL cholesterol of < 100 mg/dL as in patients with higher LDL cholesterol levels (100–130 or >130 mg/dL). These results indicate that patients aged 40–79 years with known vascular disease and/or diabetes mellitus should receive statin therapy, regardless of the LDL cholesterol level. A recent study of atorvastatin (10 mg/day) in diabetics 40–79 years reported similar results. As a result, the American Diabetes Association has recommended statin therapy in all diabetics 40 years or older regardless of LDL unless total cholesterol is < 135 mg/dL.

Heart Protection Study Investigators: The Heart Protection Study. Lancet 360:7–22, 2002.

Collaborative Atorvastatin Diabetes Study (CARDS).

89. Cardiac rupture is almost always a fatal complication of acute MI. List the three risk factors for its development.
- Female sex
- Hypertension
- First MI

90. List the clinical features of cardiac rupture.
- LV to RV infarction ratio of 7:1
- Seen in anterior or lateral wall MI
- Usually with large MI (> 20%)
- Usually 3–6 days after MI
- Rare with LV hypertrophy or good collateral vessels

91. What complication of acute inferior wall MI typically presents with hypotension, elevated neck veins, clear lungs, and a normal cardiac silhouette on chest x-ray?
This is the classic triad of RV MI. The diagnosis can be confirmed by demonstrating at least 1-mm ST elevation in right-sided chest leads V_3R or V_4R. Clinical management consists of volume expansion in combination with IV dopamine. In these patients, we should avoid diuretics or preload reducing drugs such as nitrates, as they further worsen the low cardiac output state and hypotension. It is recommended to perform a right-sided ECG in all patients presenting with acute inferior wall (MI).

92. Which lipid-lowering drug has been proved in a prospective placebo-controlled clinical trial to reduce cardiovascular mortality in acute MI survivors with "average" blood cholesterol levels?

Pravastatin, a potent 3-hydroxy-3-methylglutaryl coenzyme A (HmG Co-A) reductase inhibitor, has been evaluated in MI patients in the CARE (Cholesterol and Recurrent Events) Trial. In this double-blind trial, 3583 men and 576 women who had survived a recent MI and had plasma total cholesterol levels below 240 mg/dL and LDL levels of 115–174 mg/dL received pravastatin (40 mg/day) or placebo for 5 years. The primary endpoint was a fatal coronary event or a nonfatal MI. The frequency of the primary endpoint was 10.2% in the pravastatin group and 13.2% in the placebo group (24% reduction in risk). Subgroup analysis revealed that most of the benefit occurred in patients with baseline serum LDL cholesterol levels > 125 mg/dL. In practical terms, patients with LDL cholesterol > 125 mg/dL and prior MI should receive an HmG CoA reductase inhibitor for at least 5 years.

Sacks FM, Pfeffer MA, Moye LA, et al, for the Cholesterol and Recurrent Events Trial investigators: The effect of pravastatin on coronary events after myocardial infarction in patients with average cholesterol levels. N Engl J Med 335:1001–1009, 1996.

93. Do angiotensin-converting enzyme (ACE) inhibitors improve survival in patients recovering from acute MI?

Long-term oral ACE inhibitors started 3–16 days after acute MI and maintained for about 3 years reduce mortality by about 19% in patients with asymptomatic LV systolic dysfunction (LVEF < 40%), as demonstrated in the Survival and Ventricular Enlargement (SAVE) Trial. Subsequent trials (ISIS-4 and GISSI-3) specifically showed that even a short 6-week course of an ACE inhibitor started within 24 hours of infarct onset decreases 6-week mortality by 7–12%, corresponding to 5 deaths prevented for every 1000 treated patients.

Pfeffer MA, Braunwald E, Moye LA, et al, on behalf of the SAVE Investigators: Effect of captopril on mortality and morbidity in patients with left ventricular dysfunction after myocardial infarction. Results of the Survival and Ventricular Enlargement Trial. N Engl J Med 327:669–677, 1992.

ISIS-4: A randomized factorial trial assessing early oral captopril, oral mononitrate, and intravenous magnesium sulphate in 58,050 patients with suspected acute myocardial infarction. Lancet 345:669–685, 1995.

Gruppo Italiano per lo Studio della Sopravvivenza nell' Infarto Miocardio (GISSI-3): Effects of lisinopril and transdermal glyceryltrinitrate singly and together on 6-week mortality and ventricular function after acute myocardial infarction. Lancet 343:1115–1122, 1994.

94. Why should IV ACE inhibitors be avoided in the first 24 hours after acute MI?

IV ACE inhibitors should be avoided in the first 24 hours of acute MI evolution since they may cause a potentially harmful acute decrease in BP with a resultant reduction in coronary blood flow, as demonstrated in the CONSENSUS-II trial.

Swedberg K, et al: Effects of the early administration of enalapril on mortality in patients with acute myocardial infarction: Results of the cooperative New Scandinavian Enalapril Survival Study II (CONSENSUS-II). N Engl J Med 327:678–684, 1992.

95. Summarize the current guidelines for use of an ACE inhibitor in patients with acute MI.

The current guidelines for the management of patients with acute MI specifically recommend the routine use of an ACE inhibitor in the first 6 weeks after onset of an MI. This regimen is followed in patients with an impaired LV systolic function (as defined by an LVEF < 40%) by lifelong use of an ACE inhibitor.

96. What is the differential diagnosis of a new systolic murmur and acute pulmonary edema appearing 3 days after an acute anterior wall MI?

(1) Acute mitral regurgitation due to papillary muscle rupture and (2) interventricular septal rupture. Both are potentially fatal complications and are most common 3–6 days after infarction. Rupture of

the posteromedial papillary muscle, associated with inferior wall MI, is more common than rupture of the anterolateral papillary muscle. Unlike rupture of the interventricular septum, which occurs with large infarcts, papillary muscle rupture occurs with a small infarction in about 50% of cases.

97. **How do you differentiate between acute mitral regurgiation and ventricular septal rupture?**
Differentiation between acute mitral regurgitation and ventricular septal rupture is difficult at the bedside. Two-dimensional and Doppler echocardiography at the bedside can demonstrate the presence and severity of mitral regurgitation and localize the site of a ventricular septal defect (VSD). Further confirmation of the presence of a left-to-right shunt across a VSD can be obtained by a step-up in blood oxygen saturation from the RA to the pulmonary artery, documented by blood sampling using a Swan-Ganz catheter.

98. **What is the most likely cause of a persistent ST-segment elevation several weeks after recovery from a large transmural anterolateral wall MI?**
Persistent ST-segment elevation is not an uncommon complication of a large anterolateral transmural MI. It may be a manifestation of dyskinesis of the thinned-out infarcted myocardium. However, persistent ST-segment elevations should suggest the presence of an **LV aneurysm**, and noninvasive confirmation of this diagnosis by two-dimensional echocardiography or radionuclide ventriculography should be sought.

99. **Which myocardial infarctions are most commonly complicated by LV aneurysms?**
A ventricular aneurysm develops in 12–15% of survivors of an **acute transmural MI**. Aneurysms range from 1–8 cm in diameter. They are four times more common at the apex and anterior wall than in the inferoposterior wall, and they are more common in patients with larger infarcts. The mortality is about six times higher in patients with an LV aneurysm than in those with comparable global LV function. Death is often sudden, suggesting an increased risk of sustained VT and VF in these patients.

100. **How common is restenosis after balloon angioplasty and bare-metal non-coated coronary stent placement?**
Restenosis has been reported in about 40–45% of patients undergoing balloon angioplasty and about 25–35%% of patients undergoing coronary stent placement.

KEY POINTS: PERCUTANEOUS CORONARY BALLOON ANGIOPLASTY 

1. Restenosis is the most common complication of percutaneous coronary balloon angioplasty.
2. The incidence of restenosis is significantly reduced with bare metal coronary artery stents.
3. The incidence is even more reduced with sirolimus or paclitaxel-coated drug-eluting coronary artery stents.

101. **Are drug-eluting coronary stents more or less likely to be complicated by restenosis compared to bare metal stents?**
Two types of drug-eluting stents, sirolimus- and paclitaxel-eluting stents, have been extensively investigated in patients with CAD. These two coated stents have been developed specifically to inhibit proliferation of vascular smooth muscle cells, the primary mechanism for restenosis over the first 6 months after stent placement. Both drug-eluting coronary stents have now been demonstrated in large randomized clinical trials to cause significantly less restenosis than the so-called bare metal stents. Overall, restenosis occurs in 2–6% of patients receiving a drug-eluting coronary stent compared to about 25–35% with bare metal stents. Coated stents are

also associated with substantially decreased need for readmission with recurrent angina and repeat coronary interventions.

Moses JW, Leon MB, Popma JJ, et al, for the SIRUS investigators: Sirolimus-eluting stents versus standard stents in patients with stenosis in a native coronary artery. N Engl J Med 349:1315–1323, 2003.

Schofer J, Schluer M, Gershlick AH, et al, for the E-SIRIUS Investigators: Sirolimus-eluting stents for Treatment of Patients with long Atherosclerotic lesions in small coronary arteries: Double-blind, randomized controlled trial (E-SIRIUS). Lancet 362:1093–1099, 2003.

Colombo A, Drzewiecki J, Banning A, et al, for the TAXUS II Study Group: Randomized study to assess the effectiveness of slow- and moderate-release polymer-based paclitaxel-eluting stents for coronary artery lesions. Circulation 108:788–794, 2003.

102. Beta blockers are effective in the treatment of stable exertional angina pectoris. Should you recommend routine administration of oral beta blockers in MI survivors who are angina-free?

Several large-scale, multicenter clinical trials conducted in the U.S. and abroad have shown a consistent reduction in total and cardiovascular mortality in survivors of acute transmural MI treated with oral beta blockers for 1–3 years. The largest published U.S. trial is the Beta-Blocker Heart Attack Trial, which randomized 3837 MI survivors to either propranolol (180 or 240 mg/day) or placebo. At 3 years of follow-up, a 26% reduction in mortality was found in patients treated with propranolol compared with placebo-treated patients. Thus, regardless of the presence or absence of angina, the routine administration of oral beta blockers—propranolol (180–240 mg), timolol (10 mg bid), or metoprolol (100 mg b.i.d.), to be started 5–21 days post-MI and continued for at least 7 years—is recommended in survivors of transmural MI.

Beta-Blocker Heart Attack Trial Research Group: A randomized trial of propranolol in patients with acute myocardial Infarction: 1. Mortality results. JAMA 247:1707–1714, 1982.

103. A 67-year-old man has stayed in bed for the past 3 days with flu-like symptoms. A 12-lead ECG reveals new Q waves in leads V_1 to V_6 and ST-segment elevation of 3 mm in leads V_2–V_5, I, and aVL. What do you suspect in this patient?

This patient has ECG changes indicative of the recent evolution of an extensive anterolateral MI, as evidenced by:

- 3-mm ST-segment elevations in anterolateral leads V_2–V_5, I, and aVL
- New Q waves in all anterolateral chest leads

The most likely clinical diagnosis is an acute, extensive anterolateral MI that occurred 3–4 days ago, when he first complained of flu-like symptoms.

104. Is plasma creatinine kinase (CK) likely to be high in this patient?

The laboratory confirmation of this clinical diagnosis is routinely done by measuring serum CK containing M and B subunits (MBCK) and CK levels at 6-hour intervals for 24–48 hours. Serum MBCK and CK levels are elevated starting at 4–8 hours after symptom onset, reach a peak at 18–24 hours, and normalize within 3–4 days. Thus, serum MBCK and CK levels in this patient are likely to be normal.

105. What other laboratory tests are helpful in establishing the diagnosis of MI?

Cardiac troponins T and I are newer, more specific enzymatic markers of MI that remain elevated up to 10–14 days after an MI. Troponins T and I are now routinely obtained in patients with chest pain syndromes and are of particular value in diagnosing MI in patients presenting late (over 12–24 h) after MI symptom onset as well as in risk-stratifying patients presenting with acute coronary syndromes.

106. What is Dressler's syndrome?

Dressler's syndrome, first described in 1854, is post-MI chest pain *not* due to coronary insufficiency. Its exact etiology is unclear, but it is characterized by inflammation of the pericardium and surrounding tissues. It occurs 2–10 weeks after MI in 3–4% of cases and can be treated with corticosteroids and NSAIDs.

107. How does Bayes' theorem help determine the value of exercise ECG testing in the detection of CAD?

Bayes' theorem allows prediction of the presence or absence of CAD in a patient, given the prevalence of CAD in the population and the sensitivity and specificity of the diagnostic test. In general, the ability of noninvasive stress tests (treadmill exercise ECG test, treadmill thallium myocardial scintigraphy, treadmill or dobutamine echocardiography, or bicycle exercise radionuclide ventriculography) to predict the presence or absence of CAD in patients with a very low or very high pretest probability of CAD is poor. Thus, at both ends of the spectrum of pretest probability, noninvasive testing does not help the clinician decide whether to perform or not perform a definitive diagnostic test, such as coronary arteriography. On the other hand, patients with an intermediate pretest probability of CAD (30–70%) are good candidates for noninvasive stress testing (Table 3-7). In the patient with typical exertional angina pectoris and ≥ 2 coronary risk factors (associated with ≥ 80% pretest probability of CAD), a negative treadmill ECG and thallium myocardial scintigram predict < 30% probability of CAD. However, a positive treadmill thallium test in the same patient predicts a 90% probability of CAD. In such patients, coronary angiography is recommended in the latter case (positive treadmill thallium test) but not in the former.

TABLE 3-7. PROBABILITY OF CORONARY ARTERY DISEASE

Pretest Probability	After Treadmill ECG		After Treadmill Thallium
80%	Positive test: 95%	→	Positive test: 99%
		→	Negative test: 85%
	Negative test: 60%	→	Positive test: 90%
		→	Negative test: 30%

HYPERTENSION

108. A 45-year-old hypertensive woman has been treated with amlodipine 10 mg/day orally, for chronic stable angina pectoris and hypertension. She complains of ankle edema that worsened after her dose of amlodipine was recently increased. Are diuretics indicated?

Ankle edema is a common side effect of dihydropyridine calcium channel blockers, occurring in 7–20% of patients treated. It is a dose-dependent side effect and readily responds to down-titration of the calcium channel blocker dose. Another novel strategy to minimize the occurrence of this ankle edema is to combine calcium channel blockade with ACE inhibition. This combination is more effective than monotherapy with either drug in lowering blood pressure and is associated with lower prevalence of any dose-related side effects, including ankle edema.

109. Define hypertension and prehypertension.

Optimal blood pressure is defined as a blood pressure of 120/80 mmHg. Hypertension (HTN) is defined as a sustained elevation of blood pressure greater than 140/90 mmHg. Prehypertension is defined as a blood pressure ranging from 120/80 to 140/90 mmHg. Patients with prehypertension are at a significantly greater risk for cardiovascular complications of HTN and should be advised of therapeutic lifestyle changes: regular exercise, reduction of dietary saturated fat consumption, and weight reduction to prevent the subsequent development of sustained HTN.

110. How do you classify or stage HTN severity? Is this classification practically useful in your approach to antihypertensive drug therapy?

HTN is now classified into two stages, depending on whether BP is > 160/100 mmHg. Patients with stage 2 HTN (BP >1 60/100 mmHg) are rarely controlled to a goal BP of < 140/90 mmHg on a single BP-lowering drug. In fact, the ALLHAT trial as well as several other trials have shown that at least two or more drugs are needed in two thirds of hypertensives; in one third of hypertensive patients, three BP-lowering drugs may be needed to get BP to goal.

111. What are current guidelines for treatment of HTN?

To maximize BP control, the current guidelines recommend routine initiation of two BP-lowering drugs in patients with stage 2 HTN. This combination can include any of the following classes of antihypertensive drugs: thiazide diuretics, beta blockers, ACE inhibitors, or calcium channel blockers. Since thiazide diuretics are readily available, inexpensive, and as effective as calcium channel blockers or beta blockers in reducing cardiovascular complications of hypertension, they are generally recommended as an important part of any antihypertensive drug regimen. However, the selection of a specific antihypertensive drug class should take into consideration comorbid conditions associated with HTN, such as diabetes mellitus, heart failure, CAD, or renal failure as well as the patient's tolerance of specific drug classes.

The Seventh Report of the Joint National Committee on Prevention, Detection, Evaluation, and Treatment of High Blood Pressure: the JNC 7 report. JAMA 2003 May 21; 289:2560–2572.

112. Describe your approach to the initial evaluation of a patient with possible secondary causes of HTN. What is the value of findings such as postural HTN, paroxysmal HTN, and hypokalemia in the diagnostic work-up of such patients?

The initial evaluation of the hypertensive patient should be focused on historical or physical clues to the various causes of secondary HTN, including:

- Alcohol consumption
- Muscle weakness
- Headache
- Nervousness
- History of renal parenchymal disease
- Documented postural hypotension
- Dietary salt intake
- Paroxysmal episodes of palpitation
- Sweating
- Nausea or vomiting
- Concomitant history of generalized atherosclerotic vascular disease

A careful history (including age at onset of HTN and family history of HTN), physical examination, laboratory panel (urinalysis, microscopy, complete blood cell count, blood electrolytes, serum creatinine), chest x-ray, and 12-lead ECG should be obtained in all patients evaluated for HTN.

113. What do paroxysmal and postural HTN suggest?

Pheochromocytoma.

114. Which findings suggest renal artery stenosis?

Generalized atherosclerosis and abdominal or flank bruits.

115. What do muscle weakness and unexplained hypokalemia suggest?

Aldosteronism.

116. Which findings suggest parenchymal renal disease?

Prior history of renal parenchymal disease and the presence of abnormal urine sediment suggest secondary HTN due to parenchymal renal disease.

117. It is generally accepted that antihypertensive therapy lowers the risk of stroke, but does it have any effect on risk of MI and angina?

The Systolic Hypertension in the Elderly Program (SHEP) demonstrated that a thiazide-based antihypertensive regimen (chlorthalidone, 12.5–25 mg/day, alone or combined with atenolol,

25–50 mg/day) reduces stroke risk by 36% and nonfatal MI plus coronary death by 27% in older (> 60 yr) patients with isolated systolic HTN (systolic BP > 160 mmHg/diastolic BP < 90 mmHg). Major cardiovascular events were reduced by 32%. As a result, overall all-cause mortality was 13% lower. Similar studies in younger hypertensive patients have shown a smaller beneficial effect or no effect of antihypertensive drug therapy on CAD events.

SHEP Cooperative Research Group: Prevention of stroke by anti-hypertensive drug treatment in older persons with isolated systolic hypertension. Final results of the Systolic Hypertension in the Elderly Program (SHEP). JAMA 265:3255–3264, 1991.

118. Are calcium blockers as effective as diuretics in isolated systolic hypertension?
A similarly designed multicenter clinical trial, the Systolic Hypertension in Europe (Syst-Eur) Trial, showed the same reduction in cardiac and stroke events in older (>60 yr) patients with systolic HTN (systolic BP > 160 mm Hg) and normal or mildly elevated diastolic BP (< 95 mm Hg) with a long-acting dihydropyridine calcium blocker, alone or in combination with an ACE inhibitor. The SHEP and Syst-Eur trials confirm a significant beneficial reduction in coronary heart disease (CHD) as well as stroke from lowering systolic BP in patients with isolated systolic HTN with either a diuretic or dihydropyridine calcium blocker–based therapy.

Staessen JA, Fagard R, Thijs L, et al: Randomised double-blind comparison of placebo and active treatment for older patients with isolated systolic hypertension. The Systolic Hypertension in Europe (Syst-Eur) Trial Investigators. Lancet 350:757–764, 1997.

119. A 42-year-old woman has an office BP reading of 150/90 mmHg. Should you initiate antihypertensive therapy?
Initiation of chronic antihypertensive drug therapy in a patient with a single office BP measurement of 150/90 mmHg is not recommended. Unlike diastolic BP, systolic BP is subject to wider variations between office visits and even between examiners during a single office visit.

120. What factors may affect systolic BP measurements and lead to an erroneous diagnosis of systemic HTN?
- Patient's anxiety level
- Ambient temperature at the doctor's office
- Examiner (physician or nurse)
- Time of day
- Physical activity preceding BP measurement
- Size of cuff used
- Patient's posture (supine, sitting, or standing)
- Coexistent medical problems (e.g., fever, thyrotoxicosis, anemia, AV fistula)

121. How many BP measurements are needed to initiate antihypertensive therapy?
Drug therapy for hypertension is generally recommended for sustained elevations of sitting BP exceeding 140/90 mmHg during at least two clinic visits. The exceptions are diabetics and patients with chronic renal disease, for whom antihypertensive drug therapy is recommended at a BP of 130/80 or higher.

122. Which antihypertensive drug classes are currently recommended as first-line drugs in the treatment of HTN in patients at high risk for CHD?
Four classes of antihypertensive drugs are recommended as first-line therapy in hypertensive patients at high risk for CHD because of associated risk factors such as old age, dyslipidemia, diabetes, or smoking history:
- Thiazide diuretics
- Beta blockers
- Calcium blockers
- ACE inhibitors

All of these drugs have now been conclusively demonstrated to reduce the incidence of stroke and CHD in high-risk, predominantly older hypertensive patients.

Seventh Report of the Joint National Committee on Prevention, Detection, Evaluation, and Treatment of High Blood Pressure: The JNC 7 report. JAMA 289:2560–2572, 2003.

ALLHAT Officers and Coordinators for the ALLHAT Collaborative Research Group: Major outcomes in high-risk hypertensive patients randomized to angiotensin-converting enzyme inhibitor or calcium channel blocker versus diuretic: The Antihypertensive and Lipid-Lowering Treatment to Prevent Heart Attack Trial (ALLHAT). JAMA 288:2981–2997, 2002.

Yusuf S, Sleight P, Pogue J, et al: Effects of an angiotensin-converting-enzyme inhibitor, ramipril, on cardiovascular events in high-risk patients. The Heart Outcomes Prevention Evaluation Study Investigators. N Engl J Med 342:145–153, 2000.

Staessen JA, Fagard R, Thijs L, et al, for the Systolic Hypertension–Europe (Syst-Eur) Trial Investigators: Morbidity and mortality in the placebo-controlled European Trial on Isolated Systolic Hypertension in the Elderly. Lancet 350:757–764, 1997.

123. What classes of antihypertensive drugs are preferred for use in a patient with a known history of CHF? Which drugs should you avoid?

- Vasodilators: direct vascular smooth muscle–relaxing drugs (hydralazine and minoxidil)
- ACE inhibitors (captopril, enalapril, lisinopril, ramipril or monopril)
- Angiotensin receptor blockers (losartan, irbesartan, valsartan, candesartan, telmisartan)
- Diuretics, such as thiazide diuretics (hydrochlorothiazide)

KEY POINTS: HYPERTENSION

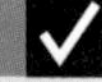

1. If blood pressure is > 160/100 mmHg, start two antihypertensive drugs to maximize control of HTN and prevention of hypertensive complications.
2. Systolic blood pressure is the more powerful and more consistent predictor of heart disease, stroke, and end-stage renal disease.
3. Thiazide diuretics and amlodipine are equally effective in preventing cardiovascular complications of HTN in patients who are at high risk for CHD and older than 55 yr.
4. Both thiazide diuretics and amlodipine are more effective than an ACE inhibitor as first-line antihypertensive therapy, particularly in older people and/or African Americans.

124. Which drugs should be avoided in patients with a known history of CHF?

Drugs with negative inotropic effects should be avoided:

- Calcium blockers of the nondihydropyridine class (verapamil, diltiazem)
- Beta blockers (e.g., propranolol, metoprolol, atenolol)

125. Are all calcium blockers contraindicated in patients with heart failure?

No. Amlodipine, a dihydropyridine calcium blocker with no clinically significant negative inotropic effects, has been extensively evaluated in two large, prospective, placebo-controlled clinical trials in patients with heart failure. Unlike nondihydropyridine calcium blockers, amlodipine can be used safely in patients with impaired systolic function who have an indication for the use of a calcium blocker, such as HTN or angina pectoris.

126. Do beta blockers ever have a role in patients with heart failure?

Although beta blockers are generally considered to be contraindicated in patients with heart failure, an increasing number of clinical trials with beta blockers such as carvedilol and metoprolol—

carefully and gradually titrated starting with very low doses—support a beneficial long-term effect in patients of New York Heart Association (NYHA) functional class II and III (mild-to-moderate symptomatic heart failure). The initiation of beta blockers even in low doses in patients with heart failure should be done very cautiously as a significant proportion of these patients (as high as 30–40%) may experience symptomatic hypotension or worsening heart failure symptoms in the first 4 weeks.

127. Explain the significance of the ALLHAT clinical trial.

The ALLHAT trial is the largest multicenter, double-blind, controlled clinical trial designed to evaluate the effects of four different classes of antihypertensive drugs (e.g., thiazide diuretics, ACE inhibitors, alpha blockers, and calcium blockers) on CHD and stroke risk. It showed no superiority of ACE inhibitors, calcium blockers, or alpha blockers over diuretics in preventing CHD events.

128. Summarize the comparative results of the ALLHAT trial.

- CHD risk was similar in all four groups.
- BP control was significantly better and systolic blood pressure was 2 mmHg lower in diuretic-treated patients than in ACE inhibitor–treated patients. This difference was even higher (about 4 mmHg) in African-Americans.
- No difference in BP control or BP levels between diuretic- and calcium blocker–treated patients.
- Between 10% and 15% higher risk of stroke and CHD events in ACE inhibitor–treated compared with diuretic-treated patients. African Americans expectedly had a 40% higher stroke risk and a 19% higher CV risk compared with those treated with a diuretic; this was associated with a 4-mm higher systolic BP.

129. What are the two key take-home messages from ALLHAT?

1. Control of HTN frequently requires multiple antihypertensive drugs used in combination. The recent JNC 7 report recommends initiation of *two* anti-hypertensive drugs whenever BP is > 160/100 mmHg (now called stage 2 HTN).
2. More effective reduction of SBP (even 2 mm lower) in a high-risk older hypertensive patient results in more effective cardiovascular prevention.

130. Which lifestyle modifications have proved beneficial to hypertensive patients?

- Lose weight if overweight
- Limit alcohol intake to 1 oz/day of ethanol (24 oz of beer, 8 oz of wine, or 2 oz of 100 proof whiskey)
- Exercise (aerobic) regularly
- Reduce sodium intake to < 100 mmol/day (< 2.3 gm of sodium or approximately 6 gm of NaCl)
- Maintain adequate dietary potassium, calcium, and magnesium intake
- Stop smoking
- Reduce dietary saturated fat and cholesterol intake for overall cardiovascular health (reducing fat intake also helps reduce caloric intake, which is important for control of weight and type II diabetes)

Seventh Report of the Joint National Committee on Prevention, Detection, Evaluation, and Treatment of High Blood Pressure: the JNC 7 report. JAMA 289:2560–2572, 2003.

CONGESTIVE HEART FAILURE

131. List common signs and symptoms of CHF.

In order of decreasing specificity:

Right heart failure

Jugular vein distention

Hepatomegaly

Increased prothrombin time

Peripheral edema

Increased aspartate aminotransferase, bilirubin

(continued)

Right heart failure	**Left heart failure**
Pleural effusion	Chest x-ray with redistribution of perfusion or interstitial edema
Decreased albumin	Third heart sound (S_3)
Abdominal discomfort	Cardiomegaly
Anorexia	Pulmonary rales
Proteinuria	Paroxysmal nocturnal dyspnea, orthopnea
	Dyspnea on exertion

132. What is the differential diagnosis of CHF?

Isolated right heart failure	**Left or biventricular failure**
Pulmonary embolus	Aortic stenosis
Tricuspid stenosis	Aortic insufficiency
Tricuspid regurgitation	Mitral stenosis
Right atrial tumor	Mitral regurgitation
Cardiac tamponade	Most cardiomyopathies
Constrictive pericarditis	Acute MI
Pulmonic insufficiency	Myxoma
RV infarction	Hypertensive heart disease
Intrinsic lung disease	Myocarditis
Ebstein's anomaly	Supraventricular arrhythmias
High cardiac output states (e.g., anemia, systemic fistulae, beriberi, Paget's disease, carcinoid, thyrotoxicosis)	LV aneurysm
	Cardiac shunts
	High cardiac output states

133. What factors can precipitate an exacerbation of formerly well-controlled chronic CHF?

When patients with well-controlled chronic CHF experience sudden exacerbations, in addition to worsening of the underlying condition(s) that led to the CHF, a precipitating factor must be searched for and corrected. These factors include:

Increased consumption of salt	Paget's disease
Fluid overload	Poor compliance with medications
Pulmonary emboli	Arrhythmias
Fever, infection	Elevated BP
Anemia	High environmental temperature
Renal failure	Cardiac ischemia or MI
Pregnancy	Thyrotoxicosis

134. A 78-year-old man with a long-standing history of CHF presents with weakness, anorexia, nausea, and dizziness. He has been receiving digoxin, 0.5 mg/day orally, and furosemide, 120 mg two times/day orally. What problem should you first suspect?

Any patient receiving digitalis who presents with GI symptoms, such as anorexia, nausea, or vomiting, should be suspected of having digitalis toxicity. The nausea and vomiting are thought to be mediated by stimulation of the area postrema in the medulla oblongata of the brain stem rather than by any direct effects of digitalis on the GI mucosa. These GI manifestations may also occur in patients receiving excessive parenteral doses of digitalis.

135. What are the less common causes of GI symptoms in patients with CHF?

Uncommonly, patients with chronic CHF complain of similar GI symptoms due to passive hepatic congestion or ascites. Differentiation of the various causes of nausea and vomiting in such patients, on clinical grounds alone, can be difficult.

136. List other manifestations of digitalis toxicity.

- **Neurologic symptoms:** headache, neuralgia, confusion, delirium, and seizures
- **Visual symptoms:** scotomata, halos, altered color perception
- **Cardiac toxicity:** ventricular or junctional tachyarrhythmias, AV block
- **Miscellaneous:** gynecomastia, skin rash

137. Describe the cardiac complications of digitalis intoxication.
Cardiac manifestations are by far the most life-threatening complications of digitalis intoxication. Almost any arrhythmia can be a manifestation of digitalis intoxication. Common examples include paroxysmal atrial tachycardia with AV block, junctional tachycardia with or without AV block, and first-degree or Mobitz I second-degree AV block. The coexistence of increased automaticity or ectopic pacemakers with impaired AV conduction is also highly suggestive of digitalis intoxication.

138. What laboratory test helps confirm the diagnosis of digitalis toxicity?
The single most useful laboratory test to confirm the clinical suspicion of digitalis intoxication is a serum digoxin level. However, even serum digoxin levels in the "therapeutic range" may be toxic in elderly patients and patients with hypokalemia, hypercalcemia, acid-base disorders, or thyroid disorders.

139. Which drugs are presently available for the treatment of CHF?
The drugs traditionally used to treat CHF include various classes of vasodilators (venodilators, such as nitrates and ACE inhibitors), inotropic drugs (such as digoxin), and diuretics (particularly loop diuretics).

140. Which drug has been proved to decrease mortality in patients with CHF?
ACE inhibitors have been shown in a large number of major clinical trials to reduce cardiovascular mortality in patients with systolic CHF NYHA FC II-IV and are now considered the standard cardioprotective therapy in patients with CHF. Angiotensin receptor blockers (e.g., valsartan) have been shown to reduce cardiovascular mortality and are recommended in patients who are intolerant of ACE inhibitors (particularly due to cough).

Consensus Trial Study Group: Effects of enalapril on mortality in severe congestive heart failure: Results of the Cooperative North Scandinavian Enalapril Survival Study (CONSENSUS). N Engl J Med 316:1429–1435, 1987.

141. Why are digoxin, diuretics, and nitrates still used to treat CHF?
Although digoxin, diuretics, and nitrates do not reduce mortality in patients with CHF, they are an important part of management because they decrease the number of hospitalizations for acute CHF exacerbations.

142. Discuss the role of beta blockers in the treatment of CHF.
Historically, beta blockers were contraindicated in patients with symptomatic heart failure because they may acutely worsen symptoms. However, over 12 large clinical trials have consistently demonstrated that the beta blockers metoprolol and carvedilol (started at very low doses and gradually titrated upward over several weeks) reduce cardiovascular mortality in patients with stable, well-compensated CHF treated with an ACE inhibitor. Recently carvedilol was shown to be superior to metoprolol in reducing cardiovascular mortality in patients with CHF and thus may be the preferred agent.

INFECTIONS

143. When is surgical intervention generally indicated in infectious endocarditis?
Most patients with infective endocarditis involving native heart valves can be successfully and effectively treated with a 4- to 6-week course of parenteral antibiotics. In contrast, patients with

infective endocarditis involving prosthetic heart valves commonly are candidates for valve replacement. In both patient groups, however, the need for valve replacement depends most importantly on the evolution of major complications of endocarditis that are not generally appropriately managed with antiobitics.

144. List the complications of endocarditis that require valve replacement.

- Heart failure refractory to adequate medical therapy
- More than one major systemic embolic episode
- Persistent bacteremia despite appropriate antibiotics
- Severe valvular dysfunction by echocardiography
- Ineffective antimicrobial therapy (e.g., fungal endocarditis)
- Resection of mycotic aneurysm
- Many cases of prosthetic valve endocarditis, especially with dehiscence or obstruction
- Development of persistent heart block or bundle branch block, usually seen in aortic valve involvement and unrelated to drug therapy or ischemic heart disease
- Extravalvular myocardial invasion, such as myocardial abscess or purulent pericarditis

145. What infectious pathogens may produce culture-negative endocarditis?

There are many potential reasons why blood cultures may be negative in the presence of infective endocarditis. They include prior administration of antibiotics, presence of uremia, and infection by fastidious organisms. Nutritionally deficient streptococci, *Brucella* sp., intracellular organisms (*Rickettsia* and *Chlamydia* spp.), fungi, anaerobes, and the HACEK organisms also must be considered when cultures are negative.

146. List the HACEK organisms.

- ***H****aemophilus* sp.
- ***A****ctinobacillus actinomycetemcomitans*
- ***C****ardiobacterium hominis*
- ***E****ikenella corrodens*
- ***K****ingella kingae*

147. What does the new onset of conduction system abnormalities in the setting of endocarditis imply?

Perivalvular and/or myocardial abscesses. Surgical drainage and valve replacement are usually necessary.

148. Explain the pathophysiology of the so-called immunologic manifestations of subacute bacterial endocarditis (SBE).

Immunologic manifestations of infective endocarditis are believed to be mediated by the deposition of immune complexes within extracardiac structures, such as the retina, joints, fingertips, pericardium, skin, and kidney, rather than direct bacterial invasion. Interestingly, these immunologic manifestations of endocarditis are reported almost exclusively in patients with a prolonged course of SBE.

149. List examples of the immunologic manifestations of SBE.

- **Roth spots:** cytoid bodies in the retina
- **Osler nodes:** tender nodular lesions in the terminal phalanges
- **Janeway lesions:** painless macular lesions on palms and soles
- **Petechiae** and purpuric lesions
- **Proliferative glomerulonephritis**

150. What are the most common causes of acute pericarditis in the outpatient settting?

In the outpatient setting, pericarditis is usually idiopathic. Many of these cases are probably due to viral infections. The coxsackie viruses A and B are highly cardiotropic and are two of the most common viruses that lead to pericarditis and myocarditis. Other responsible viruses include mumps, varicella-zoster, influenza, Epstein-Barr, and HIV.

151. What are the most common causes of acute pericarditis in the inpatient setting?
In the inpatient setting, some of the more common etiologies can be recalled with the mnemonic **TUMOR**, which also serves as a reminder that metastatic cancer is a frequent cause of pericarditis and pericardial effusion in hospitalized patients:
T = **T**rauma
U = **U**remia
M = **M**yocardial infarction (acute and post), **M**edications (e.g., hydralazine and procainamide)
O = **O**ther infections (bacterial, fungal, tuberculous)
R = **R**heumatoid arthritis and other autoimmune disorders, **R**adiation

152. What causes Lyme disease? How does it present?
Lyme disease is caused by the tick-borne spirochete, *Borrelia burgdorferi.* A rash, followed in weeks to months by involvement of other organ systems, including the heart, neurologic system, and joints, often marks the initial infection.

153. What is the major cardiac finding in Lyme disease?
About 1 in 10 patients manifests cardiac involvement, usually with severe AV block, which is often associated with syncope because of concomitant depression of ventricular escape rhythms. Temporary pacing is indicated (the AV block usually resolves), as is antibiotic treatment with high-dose IV penicillin or oral tetracycline.

CONGENITAL HEART DISEASE

154. Which congenital cardiac lesions most often present in adulthood?
Bicuspid aortic valve and ASD are the most common CHDs that present in adulthood. Congenital cyanotic cardiac lesions presenting in adulthood are distinctly uncommon. ASD alone accounts for about 30% of all CHD in adults.

155. List the types and frequencies of ASDs.
- Ostium secundum 70%
- Ostium primum 15%
- Sinus venosus 15%

156. *Coeur en sabot* is a term coined in 1888 by a French scientist in his first report of a congenital cardiac disease. Which congenital heart disease is it?
Coeur en sabot was first coined by E.L. Fallot in a case report of tetralogy of Fallot. It describes the typical configuration of the cardiac silhouette on chest x-ray in affected patients. The four components of this malformation are:
- Ventricular septal defect
- Obstruction to RV outflow
- Overriding of the aorta
- RV hypertrophy

157. Summarize the radiographic findings in tetralogy of Fallot.
The most distinctive radiographic finding in tetralogy of Fallot is RV hypertrophy, which results in a fairly classic boot-shaped (or wooden shoe–shaped) configuration of the cardiac silhouette, with prominence of the RV and a concavity in the region of the underdeveloped RV outflow tract and main pulmonary artery.

158. Which cardiac disease most commonly presents in adulthood with RBBB, first-degree AV block, and left axis deviation on ECG?
The presence of complete or incomplete RBBB is an ECG hallmark of RV volume overload, often accompanied by rightward deviation of the QRS axis, except in patients with ostium primum ASD. Because of hypoplastic changes in the left anterior fascicle, patients with ostium primum ASD have left axis QRS deviation. Thus, the combination of RBBB and left axis QRS deviation is a fairly distinctive feature of ostium primum ASD, and it is often accompanied by first-degree AV block.

CARDIAC SYNDROMES AND OTHER ENTITIES

159. How common are cardiac manifestations of ankylosing spondylitis (AS)?
The incidence of cardiovascular involvement in AS ranges from 3% to 10%, depending on the duration of the disease.

160. What valvular dysfunction is commonly encountered in AS?
The characteristic cardiac involvement consists of dilatation of the aortic valve ring and the sinuses of Valsalva as well as inflammatory changes in the aortic valve ring. The resultant clinical hallmark is aortic root dilatation and aortic regurgitation, often rapidly progressive and ultimately requiring aortic valve replacement. Echocardiography is the diagnostic technique of choice in the evaluation and follow-up of these patients.

161. What is the ECG triad of Wolff-Parkinson-White (WPW) syndrome?
- Short PR interval (< 0.12 sec)
- Wide QRS complex (> 0.12 sec)
- Delta wave or slurred upstroke of QRS complex (Fig. 3-4)

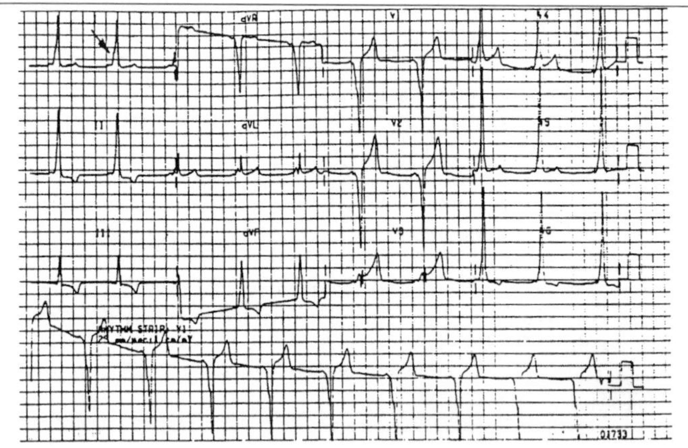

Figure 3-4. Right anteroseptal accessory pathway in WPW. The 12-lead ECG characteristically exhibits a normal to inferior axis. The delta wave is negative in V1 and V2; upright in leads I, II, aVL (augmented voltage for left arm) and aVF (augmented voltage for the foot); isoelectric in lead III; and negative I aVR (augmented voltage for the right arm). The arrow indicates delta wave (lead I). (From Braunwald E [ed]: Heart Disease: A Textbook of Cardiovascular Medicine, 3rd ed. Philadelphia, W.B. Saunders, 1988, p 686.)

162. Discuss the mechanism underlying sudden cardiac death in patients with WPW syndrome.
Patients with a pre-excitation syndrome such as WPW are at risk for developing AF with antegrade conduction along the accessory pathway. This tachycardia presents a serious risk because of its propensity to degenerate into VF due to very rapid conduction over the accessory pathway. Patients with accessory pathways and short refractory periods (< 200 msec) are at highest risk for this antegrade conduction AF and therefore sudden cardiac death.

163. Are patients with intermittent pre-excitation during sinus rhythm at risk for sudden cardiac death?
Intermittent pre-excitation during sinus rhythm and loss of conduction along the accessory pathway during exercise or during administration of ajmaline or procainamide suggest that the refractory period of the accessory pathway is long (> 250 msec). These patients are not at risk of developing very rapid ventricular rates when AF or atrial flutter occurs and are therefore not at risk for sudden cardiac death.

164. What is Marfan syndrome?
Marfan syndrome is a generalized disorder of connective tissue that is inherited as an autosomal dominant trait. Cardiac abnormalities occur in over 60% of patients and are almost always responsible for early death when it occurs.

165. What is the most common cardiac lesion in Marfan syndrome?
The most common cardiac lesion is dilatation of the aortic ring, sinuses of Valsalva, and ascending aorta. This dilatation leads to progressive aortic regurgitation and may be complicated by acute aortic dissection. The risk of dissection is markedly increased during pregnancy.

166. Describe another common valvular dysfunction in Marfan syndrome.
Another common valvular dysfunction in Marfan syndrome is mitral regurgitation due to a redundant myxomatous mitral valve (called "floppy" prolapsed mitral valve). In contrast to adults, children with Marfan syndrome are much more likely to have severe isolated mitral regurgitation than aortic root or aortic valve disease.

167. To what does the term *Marfan syndrome–forme fruste* refer?
Mitral valve prolapse (MVP) in the absence of other systemic manifestations of Marfan's syndrome has been called Marfan syndrome–forme fruste, in view of the similar pathologic appearance of the myxomatous mitral valve in both disorders. Isolated mitral valve prolapse is more common than Marfan syndrome.

168. What are the three types of Takayasu's arteritis?
Type I involves primarily the aortic arch and brachiocephalic vessels. **Type II** affects the thoracoabdominal aorta and particularly the renal arteries. **Type III** combines features of both types I and II (Fig. 3-5). Types I and III may be complicated by aortic regurgitation.

169. Which age and gender groups most commonly present with Takayasu's arteritis? How does this distribution differ from atherosclerosis and giant cell arteritis?
Takayasu's arteritis typically affects young women, with a female:male ratio of 8:1. In about three fourths of all cases, onset is in the teenage years. In sharp contrast, atherosclerotic aortic disease usually affects older men, and giant cell arteritis usually affects women over age 50 years (Table 3-8).

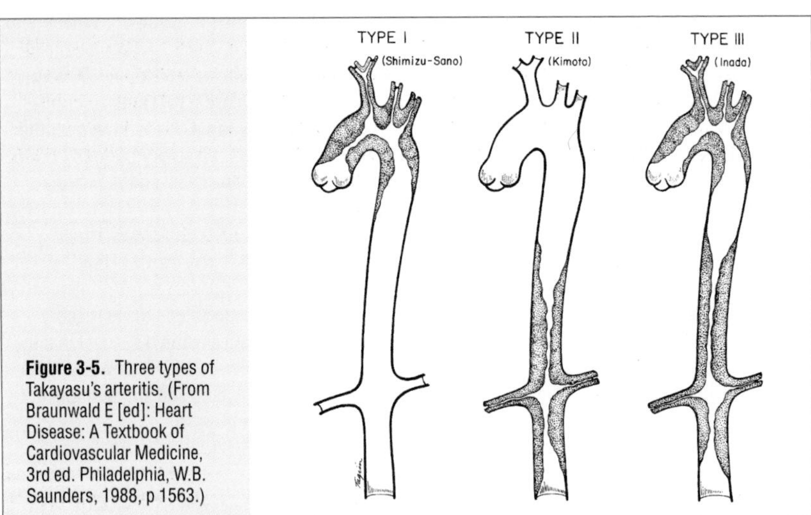

Figure 3-5. Three types of Takayasu's arteritis. (From Braunwald E [ed]: Heart Disease: A Textbook of Cardiovascular Medicine, 3rd ed. Philadelphia, W.B. Saunders, 1988, p 1563.)

TABLE 3-8. COMPARISON OF TAKAYASU'S ARTERITIS, ATHEROSCLEROSIS, AND GIANT CELL ARTERITIS

	Takayasu's Arteritis	Atherosclerosis	Giant Cell Arteritis
Synonyms	Pulseless disease, reversed coarctation	—	Granulomatous arteritis
Age at onset	15–25 yrs	> 50 yrs	> 50 yrs
F:M ratio	8:1	1:4	2–3:1
Systemic prodrome	Fever, weight loss	None	Headache, fever
Site of involvement	Aortic arch, thoracoabdominal	Large arteries	Temporal arteries
Complications	Pulseless arms, aortic hypertension	Stroke, MI, claudication (leg)	Blindness, jaw or arm claudication, polymyalgia

170. **Describe the classic clinical prodrome associated with Takayasu's arteritis.**
Patients with Takayasu's arteritis commonly present with a number of systemic manifestations. The classic clinical prodrome associated with Takayasu's arteritis consists of the following clinical features:

1. Fever and night sweats
2. Anorexia and weight loss
3. Malaise and fatigue
4. Arthralgias
5. Pleuritic pain

171. What is the holiday heart syndrome?
The holiday heart syndrome is characterized by the presence of supraventricular arrhythmias in alcoholic patients following an acute alcoholic binge, sometimes associated with holiday parties or long weekends. These arrhythmias are often transient and do not require long-term antiarrhythmic drug therapy. The most common arrhythmias are AF and atrial flutter. Digitalis and beta blockers produce an effective and rapid therapeutic response. Supportive care is also essential to prevent alcohol withdrawal symptoms in these patients.

172. Which of the cardiac chambers is most frequently involved in an atrial myxoma?
- Left atrium: 86%
- Right atrium: 10%
- Left ventricle: 2%
- Right ventricle: 2%
- Multiple locations: 10%

173. What technique is used to prevent recurrence of myxoma?
The most common site of origin of atrial myxomas is the fossa ovalis. To prevent recurrence of myxoma, a wide resection of the fossa ovalis area of the interatrial septum is performed during surgical excision.

174. What is the most common cause of chronic mitral regurgitation in the United States?
Mitral valve prolapse, which has replaced rheumatic heart disease (the most common cause of chronic mitral regurgitation in the 1950s and 1960s).

175. What are the physical examination findings in mitral regurgitation?
Mitral regurgitation is associated with an apical holosystolic murmur. The intensity and radiation of the murmur vary with the cause and severity. Physical examination also may reveal an S_3, peripheral pulses with a quick upstroke and short duration, a widened pulse pressure, and a hyperdynamic precordium.

176. How is mitral regurgitation treated?
Medical management includes afterload reduction (to maximize "forward" cardiac output), salt restriction and diuretics (in the face of CHF), and digitalis (in the face of AF). Surgical mitral valve replacement should be performed in patients refractory to medical management before they enter the severely symptomatic stage, or in asymptomatic patients before they develop irreversible ventricular dysfunction as evidenced by LV ejection fraction of less than 40% or progressive ventricular dilatation.

PACING

177. Describe the three-letter code used to indicate the essential functions of a cardiac pacemaker.
First letter: chamber(s) paced (A = atrial, V = ventricle, D = dual chamber)
Second letter: chamber(s) sensed (A = atrial, V = ventricle, D = dual chamber)
Third letter: mode of response to sensed event (0 = no response, I = inhibition, T = triggering, and D = dual response

178. What are the two most commonly used pacemakers today?
- **VVI**, a pacemaker that can pace and sense the right ventricle (VV) and has an inhibited mode of response (I).

- **DDD**, the so-called dual-chamber AV sequential pacemaker, can pace and sense either right ventricle or right atrium (DD) and has both inhibited and triggered modes of response (D).

179. What do the different modes of response indicate?

I = Inhibited: Pacemakers with an inhibited mode of response do not pace when a spontaneous depolarization (atrial or ventricular) is sensed by the pacemaker. Following a fixed interval, if no spontaneous depolarization is sensed, pacing occurs. The inhibited mode of response is most commonly used.

T = Triggered: These pacemakers pace shortly after a spontaneous depolarization is sensed. After a fixed interval, pacing will occur if no spontaneous depolarization is sensed.

D = Dual-response: The pacemakers have both inhibited and triggered modes of response.

180. Who generally receives dual-chamber pacemakers?

Dual-chamber pacemakers (DDD) are more expensive, are more difficult to implant, and require greater expertise from the clinician in charge of the patient's follow-up compared with ventricular-demand pacemakers (VVI). Insertion of a dual-chamber pacemaker is therefore reserved for patients who are not good candidates for ventricular-demand pacemakers. Examples include older patients, patients with CHF or LV hypertrophy, and physically active young adults who would not tolerate fixed-rate ventricular pacing.

181. Who is not a good candidate for dual-chamber pacemakers?

Patients who have a history of recurrent SVT are not good candidates for any pacing modality that involves atrial sensing, such as dual-chamber pacemakers. They are better served by a simpler VVI pacemaker.

182. Describe the manifestations and pathophysiology of pacemaker syndrome.

Patients suffering from symptomatic bradyarrhythmias who receive VVI pacemakers sometimes report dizziness, palpitations, a pounding sensation in the chest or neck, and/or dyspnea associated with ventricular pacing. The underlying mechanism is the loss of the normal AV synchrony during ventricular pacing.

183. How is pacemaker syndrome managed?

An improvement in cardiac output has been documented in various studies when the pacing modality was changed from ventricular to dual-chamber or AV sequential pacing. It is likely that patients with LV hypertrophy or LV failure or older patients who have a large atrial contribution to LV filling are most prone to develop pacemaker syndrome. They may be better candidates for AV sequential pacing using a DDD pacemaker.

AORTA

184. What are the causes of acute, severe aortic regurgitation (AR)?

- Infective endocarditis
- Dissecting aneurysm
- Rupture or prolapse of aortic leaflet(s)
- Traumatic rupture
- Spontaneous rupture of myxomatous valve
- Spontaneous rupture of leaflet fenestrations
- Sudden sagging of a "normal" leaflet
- Postoperative—faulty incision of a stenotic aortic valve

Morganroth J, et al: Acute severe aortic regurgitation. Ann Intern Med 87:225, 1977.

185. Why is a wide pulse pressure, typically present in chronic severe AR, unlikely to be observed in patients with acute AR?
The absence of a wide pulse pressure and of the characteristic arterial auscultatory signs of chronic AR in patients with acute AR is thought to be due to the much higher LV end-diastolic pressure (LVEDP) in the acute form. The acute development of a severe aortic valvular leak causes a much higher LVEDP in the normal-sized LV of patients with acute AR. Patients with chronic AR commonly have a dilated LV with increased compliance capable of accommodating large blood volumes without a significant rise of LVEDP.

186. Explain the effects of the rapid elevtion of LVEDP in acute AR.
As a result of the rapid elevation of LVEDP in acute AR and its rapid equilibration with aortic pressure, the diastolic rumble of acute AR is much shorter and softer than that of chronic AR. Another auscultatory manifestation of the rapid rise of LVEDP is premature mitral valve closure. This finding is considered a reliable echocardiographic sign of acute AR.

187. Summarize the hemodynamic features of AR.
See Table 3-9.

TABLE 3-9. SALIENT HEMODYNAMIC FEATURES OF SEVERE AORTIC REGURGITATION

	Acute	Chronic
LV compliance	Not ↑	↑
Regurgitant volume	↑	↑
LV end-diastolic pressure	Markedly ↑	May be normal
LV ejection velocity	Not significantly ↑	Markedly ↑
Aortic systolic pressure	Not ↑	↑
Aortic diastolic pressure	→ to ↑	Markedly ↓
Systemic arterial pulse pressure	Slightly to moderately ↑	Markedly ↑
Ejection fraction	Not ↑	↑
Effective stroke volume	↓	↔
Effective cardiac output	↓	↔
Heart rate	↑	↔
Peripheral vascular resistance	↑	Not ↑

↔ = unchanged, ↑ = increased, ↓ = decreased.
Data from Morganroth J, et al: Acute severe aortic regurgitation. Ann Intern Med 87:225, 1977.

188. What are the hemodynamic signs of chronic AR?
Chronic AR is characterized by a dilated LV due to long-standing volume overload, with a large stroke volume and a wide pulse pressure. The peripheral arterial auscultatory signs of chronic regurgitation are primarily due to this wide pulse pressure of chronic AR.

189. List the peripheral arterial signs of chronic AR.
- **de Musset's sign:** bobbing of the head with each heartbeat
- **Corrigan's pulse:** abrupt distention and quick collapse of femoral pulses (also called water-hammer pulse)

- **Traube's sign:** booming, "pistol-shot" systolic and diastolic sounds heard over the femoral pulse
- **Müller's sign:** systolic pulsations of the uvula
- **Duroziez's sign:** systolic murmur over the femoral artery when compressed proximally and diastolic murmur when compressed distally
- **Quincke's sign:** capillary pulsations of fingertips
- **Hill's sign:** popliteal cuff systolic pressure exceeding brachial cuff pressure by > 60 mmHg

190. What are the three types of aortic dissection according to the DeBakey classification? Explain their clinical and therapeutic significance.

The DeBakey classification divides aortic dissections into three groups based on location, with each type requiring a different therapeutic approach. In general, **type I** and **type II** are best managed surgically, whereas **type III** is best managed medically. These differences are based largely on the disparate natural history of proximal (types I and II) and distal (type III) dissections (Fig. 3-6). Even minimal progression of a proximal dissection can cause potentially fatal complications, such as cardiac tamponade, acute aortic regurgitation, or neurologic compromise. On the other hand, patients with distal aortic dissections often have advanced cardiovascular and cardiopulmonary disease and are therefore poor surgical candidates.

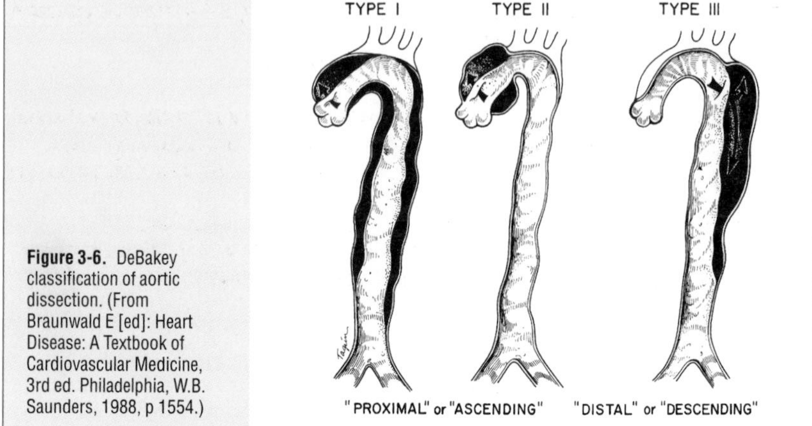

Figure 3-6. DeBakey classification of aortic dissection. (From Braunwald E [ed]: Heart Disease: A Textbook of Cardiovascular Medicine, 3rd ed. Philadelphia, W.B. Saunders, 1988, p 1554.)

191. What are the most common sites of aortic coarctation?

In descending order of frequency:

1. Postductal (adult-type coarctation)
2. Localized juxtaductal coarctation
3. Preductal (infantile-type coarctation)
4. Ascending thoracic aorta
5. Distal descending thoracic aorta
6. Abdominal aorta

192. Which congenital cardiac lesions are associated with coarctation of the aorta?

Aortic coarctation is frequently associated with other congenital cardiac lesions, including:

- Bicuspid aortic valve
- Patent ductus arteriosus

- Ventricular septal defect
- Berry aneurysms of circle of Willis

DRUG THERAPY

193. What are the third-generation thrombolytic drugs?

Third-generation thrombolytics (better called *fibrinolytics* because they basically degrade fibrin) are mutants of wild-type tissue plasminogen activator. There are three extensively evaluated third-generation thrombolytics:

1. Recombinant tissue plasminogen activator (r-PA; Retavase or Reteplase)
2. TNK tissue plasminogen activator (TNK–t-PA; Tenecteplase)
3. Novel plasminogen activator (n-PA; Lanoteplase)

Only r-PA and TNK–t-PA are currently FDA approved and commercially available; n-PA was found to cause an unacceptably high risk of intracranial hemorrhage and is not approved by the FDA for general use in the United States.

194. Explain the advantages of the third-generation thrombolytics.

Both r-PA and n-PA are deletion mutants of wild-type t-PA. They lack the finger moiety of wild-type t-PA. Deletion of the finger moiety makes the drug less "sticky" to the fibrin on the surface of the clot. This ability of the drug to "stick" to the outer clot surface is called "fibrin affinity." Deletion of the finger moiety confers less fibrin affinity to the drug and is believed to potentiate the clot dissolving effect of r-PA and n-PA.

The main advantages of third-generation thrombolytic drugs are:

- Greater clot lytic effect.
- Convenience: longer half-life makes these drugs "bolus-able" thrombolytics. Both r-PA and TNK–t-PA have longer half-lives than t-PA and can be given as bolus injections; r-PA is administered as a double bolus (10 U IV every 30 minutes) and TNK–t-PA is administered as a single 5-second IV bolus.
- Greater fibrin specificity: TNK–t-PA is 80-fold more fibrin specific than t-PA.
- Greater resistance to plasminogen activator inhibitor 1 (PAI-1), making it more resistant to breakdown by naturally occurring inhibitors of plasminogen activator. This is the case for TNK–t-PA.

195. Give the mechanisms of action and usual doses of vasodilator drugs.

See Table 3-10.

196. What is the mechanism of action of digitalis?

Digitalis and all cardiac glycosides act by inhibiting Na^+-K^+ ATPase activity (the sodium pump). This blocks the transport of sodium and potassium across cell membranes, leading to an intracellular increase in sodium and decrease in potassium. The increase in intracellular sodium in turn leads to an exchange for calcium. The increased intracellular calcium, the contractile element of muscle, leads to increased contractility (positive inotropic effect). The antiarrhythmic effects of cardiac glycosides are probably not due to any direct effect of the drugs. Rather, they are mediated by an increase in vagal tone in the atria and AV junction.

197. What factors contribute to digitalis toxicity?

- Hypokalemia
- Hypercalcemia
- Hypomagnesemia
- Renal insufficiency (digoxin)
- Hepatic insufficiency (digitoxin)
- Drugs (quinidine, verapamil, amiodarone, others)

TABLE 3-10. EFFECTS AND DOSAGES OF MAJOR VASODILATORS

Agent	Mechanism of Action	Venous Dilating Effect	Arteriolar Dilating Effect	Usual Dosage
Nitroglycerin	Direct	+++	+	25–500 μg/min IV
Isosorbide dinitrate	Direct	+++	+	5–20 mg q2h subling 10–60 mg q4h po
Hydralazine	Direct	—	+++	10–100 mg q6h po
Minoxidil	Direct	—	+++	10–40 mg/day po
Sodium nitroprusside	Direct	+++	+++	5–150 μg/min IV
Epoprostenol (prostacyclin)	Direct	+++	+++	5–15 ng/kg/min IV
Phenoxybenzamine	α-blockade	++	+	10–20 mg q8h po
Phentolamine	α-blockade	++	+	50 mg q4–6h po
Prazosin	α-blockade	+++	++	1–10 mg q8h po
Captopril	Inhibition of ACE	+++	++	6.25–50.0 mg q6–8h po
Enalapril	Inhibition of ACE	+++	+++	5–20 mg b.i.d. po
Lisinopril	Inhibition of ACE	+++	++	10–40 mg/day po
Quinapril	Inhibition of ACE	+++	++	10–40 mg/day po

Data from Rubenstein E, Federman D (eds): Scientific American Medicine. New York, Scientific American, 1988.

198. Name four classes of pharmacologic drugs that have proved effective in improving survival in acute MI.

In 188 randomized controlled prospective trials conducted over three and a half decades in over 350,000 patients, 10 pharmacologic classes of drugs were evaluated in patients with acute MI. Four classes of drugs proved effective in improving survival:

- Thrombolytics
- Beta blockers
- Anticoagulants (warfarin)
- Antiplatelet drugs (aspirin)

Mortality is reduced about 15–25% with these drugs. This amounts to saving 20–40 lives per 1000 treated patients. The single most life-saving pharmacologic therapy in acute MI is thrombolytic drug therapy, which saves 40 lives per 1000 treated patients and 60–80 lives for every 1000 patients treated within the first hour after symptom onset.

Guidelines for management of patients with acute myocardial infarction. Circulation 100:1016–1030, 1999.

199. Which two classes of drugs showed inconsistent results?

Nitrates and early use of ACE inhibitors improve survival but not drastically or consistently in various clinical trials.

200. Which four classes of drug demonstrate no beneficial effect or may even cause an increase in mortality?

- Magnesium
- Lidocaine (which is no longer routinely recommended in MI)
- Immediate- and short-acting calcium blockers, especially nifedipine
- Antiarrhythmic drugs

These drugs are no longer routinely recommended in survivors of acute MI in the most recently published guidelines for management of acute MI.

201. Patients maintained on digitalis commonly exhibit some changes on ECG referred to as the "digitalis effect." What are these changes?

Digitalis is to the ECG what syphilis once was to medicine, a great imitator. Digitalis can cause a variety of ECG abnormalities depending on the serum digoxin level. Administered in therapeutic doses, digoxin causes a characteristic sagging of the ST segment and flattening and inversion of the T waves. These changes typically occur in the inferolateral ECG leads.

202. How do they compare with the ECG changes in myocardial ischemia?

These ST and T-wave changes are difficult to distinguish from those of subendocardial myocardial ischemia; however, some subtle differences exist. Typically, horizontal or down-sloping ST-segment depression, sharp-angled ST-T junctions, and U-wave inversion are present in patients with subendocardial ischemia (coronary insufficiency). Less commonly, tall T waves may be a subtle ECG sign of myocardial ischemia.

203. In primary prevention trials aimed at reducing cardiovascular mortality with cholesterol-lowering statin drugs, which drugs have been shown to lower the risk of death from cardiac causes?

Three primary coronary prevention trials–the West of Scotland (WOSCOPS), the AFCAPS/TXCAPS, and the Anglo-Scandinavian Cardiac Outcome Trial (ASCOT)–have demonstrated that pravastatin, lovastatin, and atorvastatin reduce coronary and cardiovascular fatal and nonfatal events in patients with baseline LDL cholesterol levels ranging from 190 to 130 mg/dL. These three clinical trials provide compelling evidence that reduction of LDL cholesterol to 100 mg/dL or below is effective in preventing heart disease and stroke in patients with no known vascular disease.

Downs JR, Clearfield M, Weis S, et al: Primary prevention of acute coronary events with lovastatin in men and women with average cholesterol levels: Results of AFCAPS/TexCAPS. Air Force/Texas Coronary Atherosclerosis Prevention Study. JAMA 279:1615–1622, 1998.

Sever PS, Dahlof B, Poulter NR, et al, for the ASCOT investigators: Prevention of coronary and stroke events with atorvastatin in hypertensive patients who have average or lower-than-average cholesterol concentrations, in the Anglo-Scandinavian Cardiac Outcomes Trial–Lipid Lowering Arm (ASCOT-LLA): A multicentre randomised controlled trial. Lancet 361:1149–1158, 2003.

204. Most lipid-lowering drugs lower serum cholesterol levels by reducing the LDL fraction, but some are capable of raising the serum HDL cholesterol level as well. Which lipid-lowering drug is most effective in raising HDL cholesterol levels? Does this affect coronary mortality?

Among all available lipid-lowering drugs, **gemfibrozil** results in the most marked increase in HDL-cholesterol levels. A 600-mg dose was given twice daily in the Helsinki Heart Study. Unlike patients in the Lipid Research Clinics Coronary Primary Prevention Trial (LRC–CPPT), who received cholestyramine and experienced almost no change in the serum HDL level, gemfibrozil-treated patients experienced a 10% increase in HDL and a remarkable 34% reduction in coronary mortality. Cholestyramine-treated patients had only a 19% reduction in mortality. In the more recent HIT Trial (High-Density Lipoprotein Cholesterol Intervention Trial), gemfibrozil resulted in a modest increase in HDL of 6% and no significant change in LDL. There was a 24% reduction in the combined outcome of death from CHD, nonfatal MI, and stroke ($p < .001$). These findings suggest that raising HDL cholesterol levels and lowering levels of triglycerides without lowering LDL cholesterol levels would reduce recurrent coronary events in patients with known coronary artery disease.

Lipid Research Clinics Program: The Lipid Research Clinics Coronary Primary Prevention Trial results: Reduction in incidence of coronary heart disease. JAMA 251:351, 1984.

Frick MH, et al: Helsinki Heart Study: Primary prevention trial with dyslipidemia. N Engl J Med 317:1237–1245, 1987.

Rubins HB, Robins SJ, Collins D, et al: Gemfibrozil for the secondary prevention of coronary heart disease in men with low levels of high-density lipoprotein cholesterol. Veterans Affairs High-Density Lipoprotein Cholesterol Intervention Trial Study Group. N Engl J Med 341:410–418, 1999.

205. What is the "HDL hypothesis"?

The 10% increase in HDL-cholesterol levels induced by gemfibrozil in the Helsinki Heart Study probably accounted for the additional 15% reduction in CHD mortality. This led to the so-called HDL hypothesis—that is, an increase in HDL alone can decrease the risk of death from CAD.

206. What is the goal BP in most hypertensive patients without diabetes mellitus or chronic kidney disease?

The goal BP in most hypertensive patients is <140/90 mmHg. However, it is important to recognize that the cardiovascular and renal complications of hypertension continue to decrease as BP is lowered even below the arbitrary cut-off of 140/90 mmHg.

207. What is the goal blood pressure in hypertensive patients with diabetes mellitus or chronic kidney disease?

In patients with chronic kidney disease or diabetes mellitus, the goal BP is < 130/80 mmHg.

208. What are the goals in patients with prehypertension?

Patients with prehypertension (BP between 120/80 and 140/90 mmHg) are at a higher risk for cardiovascular complications than patients with a BP of < 120/80 mmHg. Thus, therapeutic lifestyle changes—weight reduction, reduction of dietary saturated fat and regular exercise—are recommended in patients with prehypertension to prevent the future development of HTN.

The Seventh Report of the Joint National Committee on Prevention, Detection, Evaluation, and Treatment of High Blood Pressure: the JNC 7 report. JAMA 2003 May 21; 289:2560–2572.

209. What does cardioselectivity of a beta-blocking drug mean? Summarize the clinical implications of this pharmacologic property.

Cardioselectivity refers to the predominant blockade of the $beta_1$-adrenergic receptors, which are mostly present in the heart. Cardioselective beta blockers, in low doses, have minimal blocking effects on $beta_2$-receptors, the predominant beta receptors in the lungs. However, cardioselectivity is only relative; when drugs are administered in large doses, cardioselectivity is markedly diminished. Despite these limitations, cardioselective beta blockers are much safer than noncardioselective beta blockers in patients with obstructive lung disease.

210. Which beta blockers are cardioselective?

- Atenolol (Tenormin)
- Metoprolol (Lopressor)
- Acebutolol (Sectral)

211. What is the importance of intrinsic sympathomimetic activity (ISA) as it applies to beta blockers?
ISA refers to the partial beta-adrenergic agonist properties of some beta blockers. When sympathetic activity is low (at rest), these beta blockers produce low-grade beta stimulation. However, under conditions of stress (exercise), beta blockers with ISA behave essentially as conventional beta blockers without ISA. The clinical significance of ISA is not clearly established.

212. Which beta blockers possess ISA?
Pindolol and acebutolol demonstrate ISA. All other beta blockers currently available have no significant ISA.

213. Is anticoagulation recommended before elective cardioversion of a patient with AF?
A 4-week course of adequate anticoagulation decreases the risk of thromboembolic events during and shortly after cardioversion. The risks and benefits of cardioversion and anticoagulation, however, must be weighed very carefully prior to elective cardioversion. The most important question is the urgency of cardioversion.

214. Is anticoagulation similarly required in a patient with AF with a fast ventricular rate of 230 bpm and systolic BP of 70 mmHg?
With clinical evidence of hemodynamic compromise (such as CHF, hypotension or systemic hypoperfusion, acute anginal symptoms, or acute MI), urgent cardioversion should be administered immediately, regardless of LA or LV size, systolic LV function, or prior anticoagulation. In AF with a fast ventricular response rate of 230 bpm and severe hypotension, cardioversion absolutely should not be delayed.

215. How is acute pulmonary edema managed?
The therapeutic approach to any patient with acute pulmonary edema must be individualized, but general guidelines include:

- IV diuresis
- IV, cutaneous, or oral preload-reducing drug therapy
- IV digitalization (in patients with acute pulmonary edema with or without associated AF)
- Oxygen therapy (depending on results of arterial blood gas measurements)
- Bed rest and salt restriction
- Afterload-reducing drugs

216. Describe the effect of IV diuresis.
IV diuresis with a loop diuretic, such as furosemide (20–60 mg IV push, to be repeated as necessary), lowers venous tone and thus lowers pulmonary wedge pressure even before inducing effective diuresis.

217. Which drugs are useful for reducing preload?
Nitrates are effective venodilators. In single oral doses of 40–60 mg (to be repeated three or four times daily), they are effective in lowering pulmonary capillary wedge pressure and thus improving congestive symptoms of dyspnea, orthopnea, paroxysmal nocturnal dyspnea, and nocturnal cough.

218. Describe the effects of afterload-reducing drugs.
Afterload-reducing drugs are effective in alleviating the signs and symptoms of CHF. ACE inhibitors such as captopril, enalapril, or lisinopril are effective afterload- and preload-reducing drugs and can be administered orally in patients with overt CHF. Unlike other drugs that effectively improve the symptoms of heart failure (such as diuretics and digoxin), ACE inhibitors

(and adrenergic receptor binders in ACE inhibitor–intolerant patients) are the only class of vasodilators that have been demonstrated in a large number of randomized, placebo-controlled clinical trials to reduce cardiovascular mortality in patients with heart failure and depressed LV systolic function.

219. Summarize the role of beta blockers in CHF treatment.
Beta blockers (carvedilol and metoprolol) are recommended in the long-term chronic treatment of CHF rather than in the acute CHF exacerbation phase when beta blocker use remains contraindicated.

BIBLIOGRAPHY

1. Braunwald E (ed): Heart Disease: A Textbook of Cardiovascular Medicine, 6th ed. Philadelphia, W.B. Saunders, 2001.
2. Isselbacher KJ, et al (eds): Harrison's Principles of Internal Medicine, 15th ed. New York, McGraw-Hill, 2001.
3. Marriott HJL: Practical Electrocardiography, 10th ed. Baltimore, Williams & Wilkins, 2000.

INFECTIOUS DISEASES

*Samuel A. Shelbourne III, M.D., and Richard J. Hamill, M.D.**

CHAPTER 4

Men take diseases, one of another. Therefore let me take heed of their company.

William Shakespeare, *Henry IV*

Throughout nature, infection without disease is the rule rather than the exception.

Rene Dubos, *Man Adapting*

1. **What are the most common causes of drug-induced aseptic meningitis?**
   - Nonsteroidal anti-inflammatory drugs (NSAIDs)
   - Antibiotics (especially trimethoprim/sulfamethoxazole)
   - Intravenous immunoglobulin
   - OKT3 antibodies

   Morris G, et al: The challenge of drug-induced aspetic meningitis. Arch Intern Med 159: 1185–1194, 1999.

2. **What is Vincent's angina?**
   This is a necrotizing pharyngitis caused by a mixture of anaerobes and spirochetes. *Streptococcus pyogenes* and *Staphylococcus aureus* may also play a role. Symptoms include an extremely sore throat, fever, and foul breath. Physical examination reveals pharyngeal ulcerations that are covered with a purulent exudate. Treatment with penicillin is curative.

3. **List the tick-borne infectious diseases in the U.S. along with the causative organism.**
   - Lyme disease (*Borrelia burgdorferi)*
   - Q fever *(Coxiella burnetii)*
   - Human ehrlichiosis (*Ehrlichia chaffeensis, Ehrlichia ewingii, Anasplasma phagocytophila)*
   - Rocky Mountain spotted fever (*Rickettsia rickettsii)*
   - Tularemia *(Francisella tularensis)*
   - Babesiosis *(Babesia microti)*
   - Relapsing fever *(Borrelia hermsii)*
   - Tick-borne encephalitis (flavivirus)
   - Colorado tick fever (orbivirus)

   Taege AJ: Tick trouble: Overview of tick-borne diseases. Cleve Clin J Med 67:245–249, 2000.

4. **Postsplenectomy sepsis is caused by what organisms?**
   Splenectomy predisposes patients to sepsis by encapsulated organisms, including:
   Streptococcus pneumoniae *Neisseria meningitidis*
   Haemophilus influenzae *Escherichia coli*
   Occasional cases due to *S. aureus* and *Capnocytophaga canimorsus* (DF-2) have been described.

5. Among immunocompetent adults, what are the major etiologic agents for community-acquired pneumonia (CAP)?

No etiologic agent is identified in over half the cases of CAP. When an etiology is found the major organisms include:

S. pneumoniae	*H. influenzae*
Mycoplasma pneumoniae	*Legionella pneumophila*
Chlamydia pneumoniae	*Respiratory viruses*
Anaerobic bacteria	*Staphylococcus aureus*

6. Infective endocarditis due to *Pseudomonas aeruginosa* occurs almost always in what risk group?

P. aeruginosa causes infective endocarditis on native heart valves in IV drug abusers. Rarely, it is a cause of prosthetic valve endocarditis. The occurrence of *P. aeruginosa* endocarditis varies regionally. The source of the organism is thought to be standing water that contaminates drug paraphernalia.

7. What are the causative organisms of native and prosthetic valve endocarditis (PVE) and their time of appearance relative to valve replacement surgery in the case of PVE?

Traditionally, PVE has been classified according to the time of onset with respect to the replacement surgery, with 2 months being the division between early- and late-onset endocarditis (Table 4-1).

TABLE 4-1. CAUSES OF VALVULAR ENDOCARDITIS

Organism	Native Valve (%)	Early PVE (%)	Late PVE (%)
Staphylococci			
S. epidermidis	4	35	26
S. aureus	28	17	12
Streptococci			
Group D and enterococci	8	3	9
Viridans streptcoocci	24	4	25
Other streptococci	18		
Gram-negative bacilli	4	16	12
Diphtheroids	1	10	4
Other bacteria	4	1	2
Candida	4	8	4
Aspergillus	1	2	1
Other fungi	1	1	<1
Culture negative	5	1	4

Data from Cabell CH, et al: Progress towards a global understanding of infective endocarditis: Early lessons from the International Collaboration on Endocarditis Investigation. Infect Dis Clin North Am 16:255–272, 2002.

8. **What are the causes of a biologic false-positive rapid plasma reagent (RPR) tests?**
The causes of biologic false-positive rapid plasma reagent (RPR) tests for syphilis can be divided into those of acute or chronic duration:

Acute (positive < 6 months)	**Chronic (> 6 months' duration)**
Acute febrile illnesses	Chronic infections (lepromatous leprosy)
Recent immunizations	Autoimmune diseases (e.g., lupus)
Pregnancy	IV drug addiction

When false-positive tests occur, the titer is usually low (< 1:8).

9. **Do the specific treponemal serologic tests for syphilis (i.e., MHA-TP, FTA-ABS) return to undetectable levels after appropriate antimicrobial therapy for syphilis?**
No. The treponemal tests remain positive for life after initial infection. These tests should not be used to assess response to therapy.

10. **Which drugs are most commonly associated with causing fever?**

Amphotericin B	Anticonvulsants
Neuroleptics	Anesthetics
Sulfonamides	NSAIDs
Antiretrovirals	Rifamycins

11. **List the clinical settings and risk factors associated with *Candida* infections.**
- **Chronic mucocutaneous infections:** defects in T-lymphocyte immunity, congenital (e.g., chronic mucocutaneous candidiasis) or acquired (e.g., AIDS)
- **Deeply invasive, disseminated infections:** peripheral neutrophil count < 500/mm^3; mucosal barrier breakdown (burn, cytotoxic agents, GI surgery, IV catheter sites); candidal overgrowth (broad-spectrum antibiotics)
- **Colonization of a catheter, with fever:** indwelling catheter

The difference between the first two categories may be difficult to distinguish clinically; if there is doubt, the patient should be treated for disseminated disease.

Pappas PG, et al: Guidelines for the treatment of candidiasis. Clin Infect Dis 38:161–189, 2004.

12. **What are the infusion-related syndromes associated with IV vancomycin administration?**
- **Red-man syndrome** is a histamine-mediated phenomenon that occurs with too rapid an infusion of vancomycin. It is characterized by the development of erythema, hives, and pruritus across the upper trunk and face.
- **Pain and spasm syndrome** is characterized by throbbing chest pain that resolves when the antibiotic infusion is stopped. The pain is not secondary to myocardial ischemia.
- **Hypotension**, a very rare infusion-related syndrome, can usually be treated with antihistamines, although pressor agents are occasionally needed.

13. **The commercial Monospot test for detection of heterophile antibodies is reactive in what percentage of patients with acute infectious mononucleosis?**
Heterophile antibodies, as detected by the Monospot test, are present in approximately 90% of cases at some point in the illness.

14. **What is the differential diagnosis of exudative pharyngitis?**

Groups A, C, and G streptococci	*Yersinia enterocolitica*
Arcanobacterium hemolyticum	*Mycoplasma pneumoniae*
Corynebacterium diphtheriae	Adenovirus
Anaerobic bacteria	Herpes simplex virus
HIV-1	Epstein-Barr virus

15. **Patients with multiple myeloma are prone to develop infections due to what types of organisms?**
Infections in patients with myeloma demonstrate a biphasic pattern. Infections with *Str. pneumoniae* and *H. influenzae* occur at the time of initial presentation of myeloma, early in the disease, and during response to chemotherapy. Infections with *S. aureus* and gram-negative bacilli (including *E. coli, P. aeruginosa, Klebsiella pneumoniae, Enterobacter* sp. and *Serratia marcescens*) cause approximately 80% of infections seen after diagnosis of myeloma and 92% of infectious deaths. These latter infections occur in patients with active and advancing disease and in those responding to chemotherapy in the period in which they are neutropenic.
Savage DG, et al: Biphasic pattern of bacterial infection in multiple myeloma. Ann Intern Med 96:47–50, 1982.

16. **When examining a sputum specimen, how can you determine if a specimen originates from the lower respiratory tract and is adequate for culture?**
Generally, a sputum is considered adequate when there are < 10 epithelial cells and > 25 polymorphonuclear leukocytes per low-power (× 100) field.

17. **Describe the three clinical presentations of tetanus in adults.**
- **Generalized tetanus**, the most common form of the disease, is characterized by trismus, nuchal rigidity, dysphagia, irritability, and rigidity of the abdominal muscles.
- **Localized tetanus** is manifested by persistent rigidity of a group of muscles close to the site of injury. It occasionally progresses to generalized tetanus.
- **Cephalic tetanus** is a severe form of localized tetanus that occurs when the injury is on the head or neck. It usually presents with cranial motor nerve dysfunction (most commonly CN VII) and has a poor prognosis.

Bleck TP: Tetanus: Dealing with the continuing clinical challenge. J Crit Illness 2:41–52, 1987.

18. **If a patient with no prior history of tetanus vaccination recovers from an episode of tetanus, is he or she at risk for a second episode?**
Yes. The occurrence of tetanus does not prevent second episodes of clinical disease from occurring because the amount of toxin needed to produce the clinical syndrome is so small that it is usually not immunogenic. Hence, persons recovering from tetanus should be vaccinated with tetanus toxoid against future episodes of the disease.

19. **What are the different types of clinically important antimicrobial resistance mechanisms displayed by *S. aureus*?**
    1. Plasmid-mediated production of extracellular enzymes (beta-lactamases) that act on the beta-lactam ring, causing resistance to penicillin and ampicillin.
    2. Chromosomally mediated resistance (methicillin-resistance or intrinsic resistance) that results from production of penicillin-binding proteins with altered affinity for beta-lactam antibiotics. This mechanism is mediated by *mecA* gene and is increasingly prevalent among community-associated methicillin-resistant *S. aureus* (CA-MRSA).
    3. Increasing reports of *S. aureus* strains with intermediate resistance to vancomycin have appeared. These organisms have been called VISA (vancomycin-intermediate *S. aureus*) or GISA (glycopeptide-intermediate *S. aureus*) strains. The minimal inhibitory concentrations for vancomycin are typically in the range of 8–16 μg/ML; the mechanism of resistance has not been delineated but may involve alterations in the cell wall and capture of antibiotic molecules distant from sites of cell wall synthesis.
    4. Vancomycin-resistant *S. aureus* (VRSA) have also been reported. They contain the *vanA* gene found in vancomycin-resistant enterococci.

Hiramatsu K, et al: New trends in *Staphylococcus aureus* infections: Glycopeptide resistance in hospital and methicillin resistance in the community. Curr Opin Infect Dis 15:407–413, 2002.

20. *Staphylococcus saprophyticus* is most commonly associated with what infectious problem?
Urinary tract infections (UTI), usually in young women. There is a high correlation between genitourinary mucosal colonization with this organism and the subsequent development of UTI. Symptoms and urinalysis findings are indistinguishable from those of infections due to enteric organisms. This bacterium accounts for 20% of UTIs in women 16–35 years old.

21. What are the two major organisms causing toxic shock syndrome (TSS)?
S. aureus and *Str.. pyogenes* are the two main causes.

22. How is the diagnosis of staphyloccal TSS made?
TSS is a clinical diagnosis based on the presence of certain signs and symptoms. For a definite diagnosis, all of the following criteria must be present:

- Temperature ≥ 38.9°C (102°F)
- Rash (diffuse or palmar erythroderma) with desquamation of palms or soles 1–2 weeks after onset of illness.
- Hypotension, manifested by one of the following: systolic BP < 90 mmHg; orthostatic decrease in systolic BP > 15 mmHg; orthostatic dizziness or syncope
- Clinical or laboratory abnormalities in three or more organ systems: mucous membrane, GI, hepatic, central nervous system (CNS), renal, muscular, cardiovascular.
- Isolation of *S. aureus* from sterile or nonsterile site

Tofte RW, et al: Toxic shock syndrome in the United States: Evidence of a broad clinical spectrum. JAMA 246:2163–2167, 1981.

23. List the criteria for a definite diagnosis of streptococcal TSS:

- Isolation of *S. pyogenes* from sterile site (only considered probable if isolated from nonsterile site)
- Hypotension
- Two or more of the following: renal impairment, hepatic involvement, erythematous rash, coagulopathy, adult respiratory distress syndrome, soft tissue necrosis.

Working Group on Severe Streptococcal Infections: Defining the group A streptococcal toxic shock syndrome: Rationale and consensus definitions. JAMA 269:390–391, 1993.

24. What is the significance of bacteremia or endocarditis due to *Streptococcus bovis*?
A strong association exists between lesions of the GI tract, particularly bowel carcinoma, and *S. bovis* bacteremia or endocarditis. Patients in whom this organism is identified should have a thorough evaluation of the GI tract.

25. How can the West Nile virus (WNV) polio-like syndrome and Guillain-Barré syndrome (GBS) be differentiated clinically?
See Table 4-2.

26. Name five different disease manifestations in humans secondary to the dimorphic fungus *Histoplasma capsulatum.*

1. Acute pulmonary histoplasmosis
2. Disseminated histoplasmosis
3. Mediastinal granuloma or fibrosis
4. Chronic cavitary pulmonary histoplasmosis
5. Histoplasmoma

TABLE 4-2. WNV POLIO-LIKE SYNDROME VERSUS GUILLAIN-BARRÉ SYNDROME

	WNV Polio-Like Syndrome	GBS
Fever	+	–
Acute illness	+	–
Signs of meningeal infection	+	–
Symmetrical paralysis	–	–
Motor loss	+	+
Sensory loss	Rare	80%
Pattern of progression of paralysis	No pattern	Ascending
Duration of progression of paralysis	3–4 days	Up to 2 weeks in stages

Data from Gordon SM, et al: West Nile viral fever: Lessons from the 2002 season. Cleve Clin J Med 70:449-454, 2003.

27. **What sexually transmitted diseases commonly cause genital ulceration with regional adenopathy?**
   - Syphilis
   - Chancroid
   - Granuloma inguinale (donovanosis)
   - Genital herpes
   - Lymphogranuloma venereum

   Krockta WP, Barnes RC: Genital ulceration with regional adenopathy. Infect Dis Clin North Am 1:217–233, 1987.

28. **What animal vectors are involved in human rabies?**
   Dogs account for > 90% of reported human cases of rabies in areas of the world where domestic rabies is not well controlled. Other domestic animals contribute 5–10% worldwide; these include cats, cattle, horses, sheep, and pigs. In the U.S., the principal vectors are wild mammals, including the striped skunk, raccoon, foxes, and insectivorous bats. Small rodents, birds, and reptiles are not known to be reservoirs of rabies.

   Rupprecht CE: The ascension of wildlife rabies: A cause for public health concern or intervention? Emerging Infect Dis 1:107–114, 1995.

29. **Which organisms are likely to cause a chronic UTI with urinary pH ≥ 7.5?**
   Urinary pH is elevated in chronic UTIs caused by organisms that are urease-producers. *Proteus* sp. are the most common organisms that cause this clinical presentation. Others include *Corynebacterium urealyticum*, *S. saprophyticus*, *Ureaplasma urealyticum*, and *Providencia* sp. *Klebsiella* and *Serratia* sp. are rare causes.

   O'Leary JJ, et al: The importance of urinalysis in infectious diseases. Hosp Physician 27:25–30, 1991.

30. **Linear calcifications seen in the wall of the urinary bladder on a roentgenogram are indicative of what chronic infection?**
   Schistosoma haematobium infection may result in bladder wall calcifications due to the deposition of eggs in the submucosa and mucosa of the bladder. The consequent inflammatory response leads to scarring and calcium deposition.

31. **Which organism appears as delicate, weakly gram-positive, beaded filaments that also are acid-fast if 1% sulfuric acid is used to decolorize instead of acid-alcohol (i.e., weakly acid fast)?**
Nocardia species (e.g., *Nocardia asteroides*).
McNeil MM: The medically important aerobic actinomycetes: Epidemiology and microbiology. Clin Microbiol Rev 7:359–379, 1994.

32. **What are the most common etiologic agents in acute sinusitis syndrome in adults?**
Bacteria
- *S. pneumoniae:* 31% (20–35%)
- *H. influenzae* (unencapsulated): 21% (6–26%)
- Anaerobic bacteria (*Bacteroides, Peptococcus, Fusobacterium* spp.): 6% (0–10%)
- Mixed *S. pneumoniae* and *H. influenzae:* 5% (1–9%)
- *S. aureus:* 4% (0–8%)
- *S. pyogenes:* 2% (1–3%)
- *M. catarrhalis:* 2%
- Gram-negative bacteria 0% (0–24%)

Viruses
- Rhinovirus: 15%
- Influenza virus: 5%
- Parainfluenza virus: 3%

33. **What are the most common etiologic agents in acute sinusitis syndrome in children?**
Bacteria
- *S. pneumoniae:* 36%
- *H. influenzae:* 23%
- *Moraxella catarrhalis:* 19%
- *S. pyogenes:* 2%
- Gram-negative bacteria: 2%

Viruses
- Parainfluenza virus: 2%
- Adenovirus: 2%

Brook I: Acute and chronic frontal sinusitis. Curr Opin Pulm Med 9:171–174, 2003.

34. **How reliable are sinus tract cultures for determining the etiologic agent of chronic osteomyelitis?**
The likelihood that a sinus-tract isolate corresponds with an operative isolate is high if *S. aureus* is the organism isolated from a sinus tract culture (78%); however, only 44% of sinus tract cultures from patients with biopsy-proven *S. aureus* osteomyelitis yield this organism. The predictive values for the *Enterobacteriaceae*, *P. aeruginosa*, and mixed cultures of *Streptococcus* species isolated from sinus tracts are < 50%, and only a small number of cultures from sinus tracts of patients with chronic osteomyelitis caused by these organisms will yield the causative pathogen.
Zuluaga AF, et al: Lack of microbiological concordance between bone and non-bone specimens in chronic osteomyelitis: An observational study. BMC Infect Dis 2:8, 2002.

35. **In a young, healthy patient who presents with *P. aeruginosa* osteomyelitis of the calcaneus bone, what is the most likely cause?**
A puncture wound to the foot. Almost 90% of cases of osteomyelitis that result from puncture wounds to the feet are due to *P. aeruginosa*; the remaining 10% are due to various other gram-negative organisms, staphylococci, streptococci, and atypical mycobacteria.

Riley HD: Puncture wounds of the foot: Their importance and potential for complications. J Okla State Med Assoc 77:3–6, 1984.

36. What is the most common cause of nonepidemic viral encephalitis in the U.S.?
Herpes simplex type 1, which causes a focal encephalitis.

37. Who should receive prophylaxis after exposure to persons with *N.meningitidis* meningitis?

- Household contacts
- People in closed populations, such as military barracks, nursery schools, college dormitories, and chronic care hospitals
- Hospital personnel who have intimate exposure to infected patients (but not other personnel without such exposure)

38. Define fever of undetermined origin (FUO).
The classic definition of FUO is as follows:

- Illness of > 3 weeks' duration: This eliminates any acute, self-limited illnesses.
- Documented fever > 101°F or 38.3°C on several occasions.
- Uncertain diagnosis after two clinic visits or 3 days in the hospital.

39. List the causes of FUO.

- Infection (generalized or localized)
- Cancer (hematologic and tumors)
- Rheumatologic disorders (rheumatoid arthritis, systemic lupus erythematosus, vasculitis)
- Drug-induced fever
- Alcoholic hepatitis
- Granulomatous hepatitis
- Inflammatory bowel disease,Whipple's disease
- Recurrent pulmonary emboli
- Factitious fever
- Undiagnosed

Larson EB, et al: Fever of undetermined origin: Diagnosis and follow-up of 105 cases, 1970–1980. Medicine 61:269–292, 1982.

40. Which infections may cause FUO?

- **Generalized:** tuberculosis, histoplasmosis, typhoid fever, cytomegalovirus, Epstein-Barr virus, syphillis, brucellosis, malaria
- **Localized:** infective endocarditis, empyema, peritonitis, cholangitis, intra-abdominal abscess, urinary tract infection (pyelonephritis)

41. Which types of cancer may cause FUO?

- **Hematologic cancers:** lymphoma, Hodgkin's disease, acute leukemia
- **Tumors:** hepatoma, renal cell carcinoma, atrial myxoma

42. What is a Simon focus?
During primary infection with *Mycobacterium tuberculosis*, apical and subapical pulmonary foci may undergo necrosis when delayed hypersensitivity develops. These foci then develop tiny calcific deposits, within which latent but viable mycobacteria persist. These foci can later reactivate.

43. What is Pott's disease?
Spinal tuberculosis. Percival Pott, an English surgeon, in 1779 first wrote the classic description of the disease that bears his name.

44. **List the clinical features of genitourinary tuberculosis.**
- Sterile pyuria (50%)
- Painless hematuria (40%)
- Fever (10%)
- Perinephric abscess (10%)
- Positive sputum culture (20–40%)
- Positive urine culture (80%)
Christensen WI: Genitourinary tuberculosis: Review of 102 cases. Medicine 53:377–390, 1974.

45. **What is the differential diagnosis of eosinophilic meningitis?**
- CNS infection caused by parasites
- *M. tuberculosis*
- *Treponema pallidum*
- Fungi (*Coccidioides immitis, H. capsulatum*)
- Viruses (lymphocytic choriomeningitis virus, coxsackie B4)
- *Rickettsia* sp.
- Neoplasia (leukemia, lymphoma, meningeal tumors)
- Multiple sclerosis
- Hypereosinophilic syndrome
- Collagen vascular disease
- Allergic reaction to foreign body or direct instillation of drugs or contrast agent into the cerebrospinal fluid (CSF)
- Drug allergy (e.g., ibuprofen, ciprofloxacin)
Lo R, et al: Eosinophlic meningitis. Am J Med 114:217–223, 2003.

46. **Which CNS parasites are likely to cause eosinophilic meningitis?**
- *Angiostrongylus cantonensis*
- *Toxoplasma gondii*
- *Trypanosoma* sp.
- *Trichinella spiralis*
- *Toxocara canis, Toxocara cati*
- *Taenia solium*
- *Fasciola hepatica*
- *Paragonimus westermani*
- *Gnathostoma spinigerum*
- *Bayliascariasis procyonis*

47. **Most cases of Rocky Mountain spotted fever (RMSF) occur in what regions of the United States?**
The south Atlantic states and south-central region (e.g., Oklahoma, Missouri, Arkansas). Despite its name, few cases of RMSF occur in the Rocky Mountain states (Fig. 4-1).

48. **What are the major pulmonary syndromes associated with *Aspergillus* sp.?**
- **Allergic bronchopulmonary aspergillosis** (ABPA) occurs in patients with asthma who have eosinophilia, transient pulmonary infiltrates thought to be due to bronchial plugging, and elevated total serum IgE and IgG antibody to aspergillus.
- **Aspergilloma** (fungus ball) results from colonization and growth of aspergillus, usually within a preexisting pulmonary cavity.
- **Invasive aspergillosis** usually occurs in individuals with profound granulocytopenia and is also being described more frequently in people with AIDS.
- **Chronic necrotizing aspergillosis** is a slowly progressive form of invasive aspergillosis that occurs in patients who have some underlying pulmonary disease (chronic obstructive pulmonary disease, sarcoidosis, pneumoconiosis, or inactive TB) or mild systemic

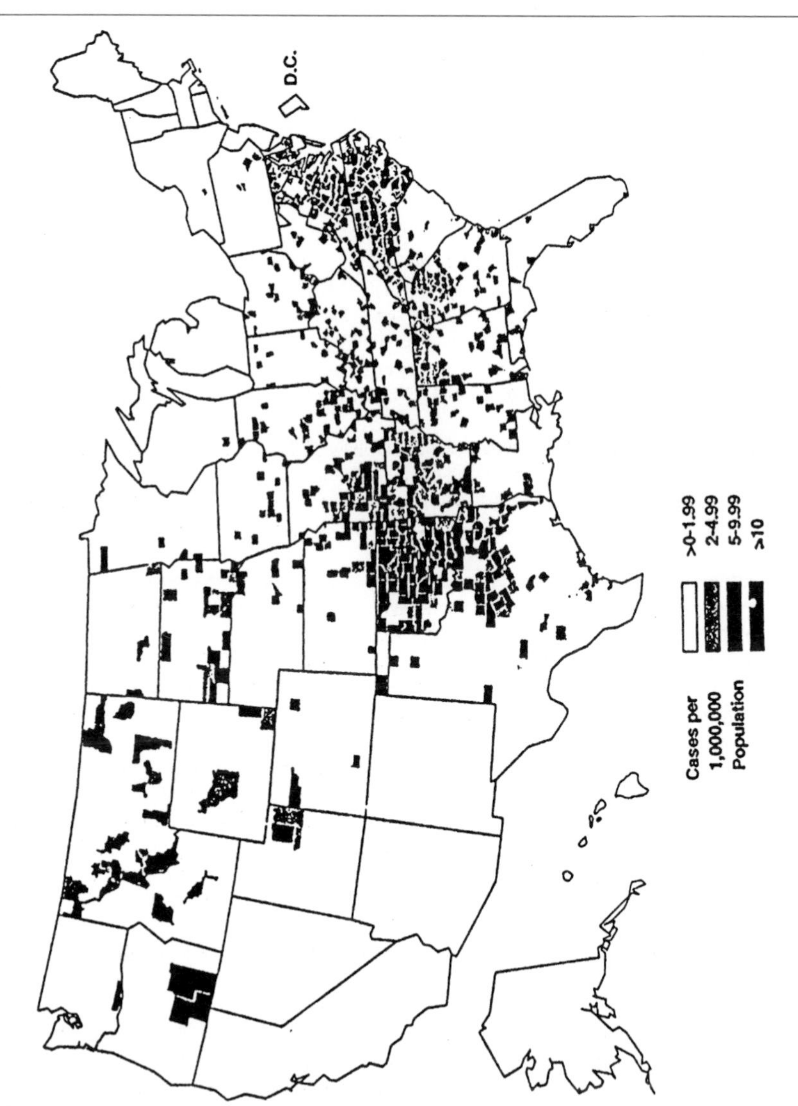

Figure 4-1. Distribution of Rocky Mountain spotted fever. (From Dalton MJ, et al: National surveillance for Rocky Mountain spotted fever, 1981–1992: Epidemiologic summary and evaluation of risk factors for fatal outcome. Am J Trop Med Hyg 52:405–413, 1995, with permission.)

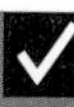

KEY POINTS: MANIFESTATIONS OF THE SYSTEMIC INFLAMMATORY RESPONSE SYNDROME

1. Temperature > 38°C or < 36°C
2. Respiratory rate > 20 breaths/min or arterial $pCO_2 < 32$ mmHg
3. Heart rate > 90 beats/min
4. White blood cell count > 12,000 cells/mm^3, < 4000 cells/mm^3, or > 10% band forms

immunocompromising illness (low-dose corticosteroids, diabetes mellitus, alcoholism). Patients have a chronic infiltrate that may slowly progress to cavitation or aspergilloma formation.

Latgé J-P: *Aspergillus fumigatus* and aspergillosis. Clin Microbiol Rev 12:310–350, 1999.

49. How are pulmonary syndromes associated with *Aspergillus* sp. treated?

- **ABPA:** Corticosteroids have been used, although anecdotal reports suggest itraconazole may have a role.
- **Aspergilloma:** No specific treatment is usually given unless significant hemoptysis occurs, in which case surgical excision is performed.
- **Invasive aspergillosis:** Amphotericin B or one of the newer liposomal preparations, caspofungin or voriconazole, with or without surgical excision, are options for therapy.

50. What is the Fitz-Hugh–Curtis syndrome? What organisms cause it?

The Fitz-Hugh–Curtis syndrome is a perihepatitis usually caused by either *Neisseria gonorrhoeae* or *Chlamydia trachomatis.* It is thought to occur by spread of organisms from the fallopian tubes to the surface of the liver. This should be considered one of the causes of right-upper-quadrant pain in young, sexually active persons. It occasionally has been reported in males, probably as a result of bacteremic spread.

51. Which organisms most commonly cause infectious complications after bites?

Streptococci (alpha and group A beta-hemolytic), *S. aureus, Eikenella corrodens, Peptostreptococcus* sp., *Bacteroides* sp., and *Fusobacterium* sp. are the most common organisms cultured from human bite wounds. *Pasteurella multocida* and *C. canimorsus* (DF-2) commonly cause infections after dog or cat bites. Several other pathogens have been transmitted after bites by these animals, including rabies, tularemia (cats), brucellosis (dogs), EF-4 (dogs), and blastomycosis (dogs).

Goldstein EJC: Bite wounds and infection. Clin Infect Dis 14:633–640, 1992.

52. What is the Jarisch-Herxheimer reaction?

It is a self-limited systemic reaction that occurs within 1–2 hours after the initial treatment of syphilis with antimicrobial agents. It is particularly common in patients treated for secondary syphilis but can occur when any stage is treated. The reaction consists of the abrupt onset of chills, fever, myalgias, tachycardia, hyperventilation, vasodilatation with associated flushing, and mild hypotension. It is probably due to the release of pyrogens from the spirochetes.

53. What is typhlitis?

Typhlitis, also known as necrotizing enterocolitis or neutropenic enterocolitis, is a fulminate, necrotizing process that occurs in the GI tract of individuals with profound neutropenia. The disease is manifested by fever, abdominal pain and distention, rebound tenderness in the right lower quadrant, and diarrhea. Involvement of the cecum and terminal ileum is characteristic.

54. Which species of malaria is associated with the occurrence of febrile paroxysms every 72 hours?

Plasmodium malariae. The other species of malaria that infect humans—*Plasmodium vivax*, *P. ovale*, and *P. falciparum*—have 48-hour erythrocyte cycles and, therefore, a 48-hour fever pattern.

Hoffman SL: Diagnosis, treatment and prevention of malaria. Med Clin North Am 76:1327–1355, 1992.

55. Which species of malaria have exoerythrocytic stages from which late relapses may occur if treatment is not adequate?

P. vivax and *P. ovale* have exoerythrocytic stages in the liver. Relapse may occur months to years later.

Zucker JR, et al: Malaria: Principles of prevention and treatment. Infect Dis Clin North Am 7:546–567, 1993.

56. Extrusion of "sulfur granules" from a draining wound is characteristic of which infection?

Infections with *Actinomyces* sp. characteristically form external sinuses, which discharge "sulfur granules." These consist of conglomerate masses of branching filaments of the organism cemented together and mineralized by host calcium phosphate stimulated by tissue inflammation. They do not contain sulfur.

57. What is the causative agent of Whipple's disease?

Tropheryma whippelii, a gram-positive actinomycete that is not closely related to any other known bacterial genus. Whipple's disease is a multisystemic disorder characterized by migratory polyarthritis, diarrhea, malabsorption, weight loss, generalized lymphadenopathy, hyperpigmentation, and occasional neurologic abnormalities.

Relman DA, et al: Identification of the uncultured bacillus of Whipple's disease. N Engl J Med 327:293–301, 1992.

58. How often is the Gram stain likely to be positive in patients with bacterial meningitis?

The Gram stain of the CSF in patients with bacterial meningitis demonstrates the etiologic agent in most cases. The following list demonstrates the sensitivity of the Gram stain for each pathogen:

- *N. meningitidis:* 66%
- *Str.. pneumoniae:* 83%
- *H. influenzae:* 76%
- *Listeria monocytogenes:* 42%

59. Rhinocerebral mucormycosis occurs most commonly in what setting?

Rhinocerebral mucormycosis occurs almost exclusively in patients with diabetes mellitus, particularly when poorly controlled or with ketoacidosis. Occasional cases have been described in patients with hematologic neoplasms or renal insufficiency and in infants with severe diarrhea. The disease is characterized by black, necrotic lesions of the palate or nasal mucous membranes that rapidly involve the paranasal sinuses with extension into the brain. The organism has a particular predisposition to invade vascular structures.

Sugar AM: Mucormycosis. Clin Infect Dis 14:S126–S129, 1992.

60. The intermediate stage of which tapeworm causes the clinical syndrome of cysticercosis?

Cysticercus cellulosae is the intermediate stage of *Taenia solium*, the pork tapeworm, and causes the clinical syndrome of cysticercosis.

61. What is the most common cause of secondary pneumonia following illness due to influenza?

Str. pneumoniae most commonly causes pneumonia after influenza virus infection. However, the incidence of pneumonia caused by *S. aureus* is also increased, and so this agent must also be considered when treating a patient with this clinical syndrome.

62. What diseases are associated with consumption of contaminated fish and shellfish?

Several viral, bacterial, and parasitic infections can result from ingestion of contaminated fish and shellfish. They include:

Hepatitis A	Norwalk virus gastroenteritis
Vibrio cholerae 0 group 1	*Vibrio cholerae* non-01
Vibrio parahaemolyticus	*Vibrio vulnificus*
Clostridium botulinum	*Giardia lamblia*
Diphyllobothriasis	Anisakiasis

In addition, disease due to seafood toxin consumption can occur:

Ciguatera poisoning	Paralytic shellfish poisoning due to *Gonyaulax* species of dinoflagellates
Scombroid poisoning	
Tetrodotoxication due to eating puffer fish, *Fugu*	Neurotoxic shellfish poisoning due to the toxic dinoflagellate, *Ptychodiscus brevis*

Eastaugh J, Shepherd S: Infectious and toxic syndromes from fish and shellfish consumption: A review. Arch Intern Med 149:1735–1740, 1989.

KEY POINTS: CARDINAL FEATURES OF BOTULISM 

1. Symmetric descending paralysis (diplopia, dysarthria, dysphonia & dysphagia)
2. Absence of fever
3. Responsive patient
4. Normal or slow heart rate
5. Absence of sensory deficits

63. What is the significance of infection due to *E. coli* O157:H7?

E. coli O157:H7 has emerged as a major cause of both sporadic cases and outbreaks of diarrheal disease in North America. Most outbreaks have been associated with the consumption of beef, most commonly undercooked ground beef. Other outbreaks have been associated with fecally contaminated drinking water supplies. It can cause either bloody or nonbloody diarrhea.

In addition, *E. coli* O157:H7 is responsible for most cases of hemolytic-uremic syndrome, a major cause of acute renal failure in children.

Boyce TG, et al: *Escherichia coli* O157:H7 and the hemolytic-uremic syndrome. N Engl J Med 333:364–368, 1995.

64. What is the "hyperinfection" syndrome associated with *Strongyloides stercoralis*?

Hyperinfection syndrome due to *S. stercoralis* is the result of systemic dissemination by the filariform larval stage of the organism. This usually occurs in individuals who are immunocompromised, primarily due to defects in cell-mediated immunity. Patients present with abdominal pain, diarrhea, vomiting, shock, fever, cough, and decreased mental status. Bacteremia is a frequent accompanying event, usually with enteric organisms that are thought to accompany the larvae as they migrate through the bowel wall.

65. Which infection occurs in nursery workers who handle sphagnum moss?

Outbreaks of lymphocutaneous infection due to *Sporothrix schenckii* have occurred in nursery and forestry workers who handle seedlings packed in sphagnum moss. Disease has also been associated with contaminated hay, timbers, and thorny bushes, such as roses.

Coles FB, et al: A multistate outbreak of sporotrichosis associated with sphagnum moss. Am J Epidemiol 136:475–487, 1992.

66. What are the infectious causes of parotitis?

Acute viral parotitis	Acute suppurative parotitis
Mumps virus	*S. aureus*
Influenza	*Str. pneumoniae*
Parainfluenza types 1 and 3	Enteric gram-negative bacilli
Coxsackievirus A and B	*H. influenzae*
ECHO virus	*Actinomyces* sp.
Lymphocytic choriomeningitis	*M. tuberculosis*
Anaerobic organisms	*Salmonella typhi*
HIV	*Burkholderia pseudomallei*

67. What are the most common pathogens seen in months 2–6 after solid organ transplantation?

They are more typical of the pathogens seen in immunocompromised hosts:

Viruses	Others
Cytomegalovirus	Aspergillus
Epstein-Barr virus	Nocardia
Varicella-zoster virus	Toxoplasma
Papovavirus (BK and JC)	Cryptococcus
Adenovirus	*Pneumocystis jiroveci*
Herpes simplex virus	Legionella
Non-A, non-B hepatitis	*L. monocytogenes*

68. Which infectious agents have been reported to be transmitted by blood transfusion?

The most common transmissible pathogens are viruses, but others have been implicated.

Hepatitis A, hepatitis B, hepatitis C,	*T. pallidum*
Hepatitis D	*B. microti*
Hepatitis G virus/GB virus C	*Plasmodium* sp. (malaria)
TT virus	*Trypanosoma cruzi* (Chagas' disease)
SEN viruses	*Leishmania* sp.
HIV-1 and HIV-2, HTLV I and II	*Toxoplasma gondii*
Cytomegalovirus,	*Y. enterocolitica*
Epstein-Barr virus	*Serratia* and *Pseudomonas* spp.
Human herpesvirus 8	*Staphylococcal* sp.
Parvovirus B19	*Bacillus cereus*
West Nile virus	

Chamberland ME: Emerging infectious agents: Do they pose a risk to the safety of transfused blood and blood products? Clin Infect Dis 34:E797–E805, 2002.

69. *Vibrio vulnificus* has been described primarily with which two clinical syndromes?

- Cutaneous cellulitis after a localized inoculation
- High-mortality sepsis syndrome with bacteremia, usually occurring after raw oyster ingestion and seen in immunocompromised patients, particularly cirrhotics.

70. What organism shares a common epidemiologic niche and the same tick vector as *B. burgdorferi*?

B. microti, a protozoan that parasitizes human erythrocytes, shares some of the same geographic distribution as *B. burgdorferi* (Lyme disease). *Ixodes scapularis* is the most important tick vector, with *Dermacentor variabilis* being a less frequent vector. Some of this same geographic distribution is also shared by one of the agents causing human granulocyte ehrlichiosis, *A. phagocytophilum*, for which *I. scapularis* (the black-legged tick) is also the vector. Consequently, it is theoretically possible to see simultaneous infection with all three agents.

71. Which infectious agents have been implicated in cervical carcinoma?

Cancer of the cervix behaves epidemiologically as if it were a sexually transmitted disease (STD). Strong epidemiologic associations exist between cervical infections with herpes simplex virus and *C. trachomatis*, but the strongest association exists with infection with human papillomavirus (HPV). HPV types 16 and 18 have the strongest link with subsequent malignancy.

Kiviat N, et al: Cervical neoplasia and other STD-related genital tract neoplasia. In Holmes KK, et al (eds): Sexually Transmitted Diseases, 3rd ed. New York, McGraw-Hill, 1999, pp 811–831.

72. An immigrant from Mexico who presents with a seizure disorder and has multiple small ring-like lesions on a head CT scan is likely to have what disorder?

Neurocysticercosis. This is invasion of the CNS by the larval form of the pork tapeworm, *T. solium*. CT scans typically show cystic lesions that do not usually enhance with contrast and, in many cases, hydrocephalus. It is the most common cerebral parasitic infection in humans.

73. Name the etiologic agents of the STDs chancroid, lymphogranuloma venereum, and granuloma inguinale.

Chancroid	*Haemophilus ducreyi*
Lymphogranuloma venereum	*C. trachomatis*, serovars L1–3
Granuloma inguinale (donovanosis)	*Calymmatobacterium granulomatis*

74. What percentage of older patients with *Salmonella* bacteremia have an endovascular source of infection?

Approximately 25% of patients over age 50 have an endovascular source. *Salmonella* organisms tend to "seed" abnormal tissues (e.g., hematomas, tumors, cysts, stones, and altered endothelium such as aortic aneurysms) during bacteremia.

Cohen PS: The risk of endothelial infection in adults with *Salmonella* bacteremia. Ann Intern Med 89:931–932, 1978.

75. Infection with *Chlamydia psittaci* should be considered an occupational hazard for what group of people?

Pet shop employees, pigeon fanciers, zoo workers, veterinarians, and poultry processors. It causes an atypical pneumonia.

76. Describe the serologic response to Epstein-Barr virus infections.
See Figure 4-2.

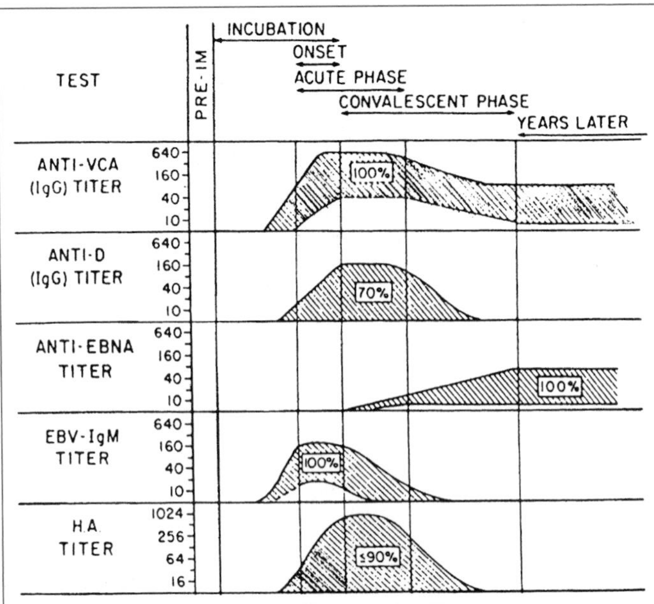

Figure 4-2. The typical sequence of serologic events after exposure to EBV. The incubation period ranges from 30 to 50 days. Antibody to viral capsid antigen (anti-VCA, difficult to detect in some labs) can be demonstrated at the time of clinical presentation and is diagnostic of acute infection. The EBV nuclear antigen (anti-EBNA) characteristically appears 3–4 weeks after the onset of clinical illness. Both anti-VCA and anti-EBNA antibodies are present lifelong after infection. (HA = heterophile antibody, anti-D = antibody to early antigen.) (From Schooley RT: Chronic fatigue syndrome: A manifestation of Epstein-Barr virus infection? In Remington JS, Swartz MN [eds]: Current Clinical Topics in Infectious Diseases, vol 9. New York, McGraw-Hill, 1988, pp. 126–146, with permission.)

77. What is the differential diagnosis of infectious causes of monocytosis?

Infectious causes	**Noninfectious causes**
Tuberculosis	Myeloproliferative disorders
Epstein-Barr virus mononucleosis	Lymphomas
Rocky Mountain spotted fever	Solid tumors
Diphtheria	Gaucher's disease
Subacute bacterial endocarditis	Regional enteritis
Histoplasmosis	Ulcerative colitis
Typhus	Sprue
Brucellosis	Rheumatoid arthritis
Kala-azar	Systemic lupus erythematosus
Malaria	Polyarteritis nodosa
Syphilis	Post-splenectomy
Recovery from neutropenia	Sarcoidosis
Recovery from chronic infection	

Calubiran O, et al: The significance of lymphocytes, monocytes, and platelets in infectious diseases. Hosp Physician 26:10–12, 1990.

78. What is the differential diagnosis of atypical lymphocytosis in patients with > 20% atypical lymphocytes?

- Epstein-Barr mononucleosis
- Viral hepatitis
- Cytomegalovirus mononucleosis

79. What is the differential diagnosis of atypical lymphocytosis in patients with < 20% atypical lymphocytes?

Infections	Noninfectious causes
Varicella	Drug hypersensitivity reactions
Rubella	Drug fever
Herpes simplex	Dermatitis herpetiformis
Varicella-zoster	Radiation therapy
Tuberculosis	Stress
Brucellosis	Lead intoxication
Smallpox	
Babesiosis	
Ehrlichiosis	
Rubeola	
Roseola infantum (HHV-6)	
Influenza	
Syphilis	
Toxoplasmosis	
Malaria	
Rocky Mountain spotted fever	

Calubiran O, et al: The significance of lymphocytes, monocytes, and platelets in infectious diseases. Hosp Physician 26:10–12, 1990.

80. What causes hand-foot and mouth disease? Describe the clinical findings of this disease.

Hand-foot and mouth disease may be caused by a number of viruses in the picornavirus family. It has been most often associated with coxsackievirus A16, but outbreaks have also been attributed to coxsackieviruses A4, A5, A9, A10, B2, and B5 and enterovirus 71. It is characterized by an ulcerative exanthem, usually occurring on the buccal mucosa, which is followed by a vesicular exanthem on the hands and feet.

81. What precautions are needed when administering rifampin?

- Rifampin has a significant first-pass effect after ingestion. Consequently, drug levels are optimal if the total daily dose is taken once instead of divided.
- Rifampin stains secretions orange-red; individuals who wear soft contact lenses should be warned about staining of the lenses.
- Rifampin reduces the serum concentration of a number of drugs because of its potent induction of hepatic microsomal enzymes.

82. Summarize the clinically important consequences of reduced serum concentrations of drugs affected by rifampin.

- Decreased digoxin levels can result in decompensated heart failure.
- Decreased warfarin levels can result in inadequate anticoagulation.
- Exacerbation of hyperglycemia may result from decreased serum concentrations of oral hypoglycemic agents.
- Decreased efficacy of oral contraceptive agents may occur.
- Ketoconazole and itraconazole levels are substantially reduced.

- Thyroid replacement therapy may be inadequate due to decreased levels of L-thyroxine in patients with hypothyroidism.
- Rejection of solid organ transplants may result from decreased cyclosporine concentrations.
- Asthma or Addison's disease may relapse during glucocorticosteroid therapy.
  Baciewicz AM, et al: Rifampin drug interactions. Arch Intern Med 144:1667–1671, 1984.

83. **List the candidates for pneumococcal immunization.**
    - Immunocompetent persons aged 2–64 years at increased risk for pneumococcal disease or its complications because of chronic illnesses (cardiovascular disease, pulmonary disease, diabetes mellitus, alcoholism, cirrhosis, CSF leaks)
    - Immunocompetent people > 65 years old
    - Immunocompromised people ≥ 2 years old at increased risk for pneumococcal disease or its complications because of anatomic or functional asplenia (including sickle cell anemia), leukemia or lymphoma, nephrotic syndrome, multiple myeloma, conditions associated with immunosuppression (e.g., organ transplantation or immunosuppressive chemotherapy), Hodgkin's disease, and chronic renal failure
    - HIV-infected people, asymptomatic or symptomatic
    - Persons living in special environments or social settings with an identified increased risk of pneumococcal disease or its complications (e.g., certain Native American populations)

    CDC: Prevention of Pneumococcal Disease. Recommendations of the Immunization Practices Advisory Committee. MMWR 46(RR-08):1–24, 1997.

84. **What is ecthyma gangrenosum?**
    Ecthyma gangrenosum consists of skin lesions that occur in association with gram-negative bacteremia, most commonly in neutropenic patients. *P. aeruginosa* is the most commonly implicated bacteria, but other species have produced this lesion, including *Aeromonas hydrophila* and *E. coli.* The lesions typically begin as painless erythematous macules that rapidly progress to papules and develop central vesicles or bullae. Eventually, they ulcerate to form gangrenous ulcers. The characteristic histologic appearance demonstrates large numbers of bacteria in and around blood vessels, but with an absence of an inflammatory response.

85. **What animal is the reservoir for the agent causing the hantavirus pulmonary syndrome?**
    The deer mouse, *Peromyscus maniculatus*, is the reservoir for the Sin Nombre virus that causes the hantavirus pulmonary syndrome.

    Childs JE, et al: Serologic and genetic identification of *Peromyscus maniculatus* as the primary rodent reservoir for a new hantavirus in the southwestern United States. J Infect Dis 169:1271–1280, 1994.

86. **List the diseases caused by the various *Bartonella* species.**
    - *B. bacilliformis:* veruga peruana
    - *B. quintana:* Oroya fever (Carrion's disease), trench fever, bacillary angiomatosis/visceral peliosis, fever/bacteremia, endocarditis
    - *B. henselae:* lymphadenopathy, fever/bacteremia, bacillary angiomatosis/visceral peliosis, cat-scratch disease, endocarditis
    - *B. elizabethae:* endocarditis
    - *B. clarridgeiae:* cat-stratch disease
    - *B. vinsonii* subsp. *berkhoffi:* endocarditis
    - *B. vinsonii* subsp. *arupensis:* fever
    - *B. grahamii:* neuroretinitis

    Daly JS: *Bartonella* species. In Gorbach SL, Bartlett JG, Blacklow NR (eds): Infectious Diseases, 3rd ed. Philadelphia, Lippincott Williams & Wilkins, 2004, p 1847.

87. What are the "flesh-eating" bacteria?
"Flesh-eating" bacteria is the term coined by the British press to describe invasive necrotizing infections caused by *Str. pyogenes* (group A streptococci). These infections are characterized by aggressive soft-tissue infection, shock, adult respiratory distress syndrome, and renal failure. The mortality is 30–70%. The pathophysiology of these infections is thought to involve bacterial production of pyrogenic exotoxins, which function as superantigens to stimulate T-cell production of cytokines responsible for many of the clinical manifestations.

Stevens DL: Streptococcal toxic-shock syndrome: Spectrum of disease, pathogenesis, and new concepts in treatment. Emerging Infect Dis 1:69–78, 1995.

88. Which upper GI lesions are assocaited with *Helicobacter pylori*? Which are not?
See Table 4-3.

TABLE 4-3. ASSOCIATION OF HELICOBACTER PYLORI WITH COMMON PATHOLOGIC LESIONS OF THE UPPER GASTROINTESTINAL TRACT

Lesion	Association with *H. pylori*
Chronic diffuse superficial gastritis	Nearly always associated
Type A (pernicious anemia) gastritis	Negative association
NSAID gastropathy	Negative or no association
Acute erosive gastritis (e.g., alcohol, aspirin)	No association
Gastric ulceration	Commonly observed in patients who are not ingesting NSAIDs or aspirin
Duodenal ulceration	Usually associated with idiopathic lesions (non–drug-induced, non–Zollinger-Ellison syndrome)
Gastric adenocarcinoma	Positively associated with (noncardia) cancers of the body and antrum
Gastric lymphoma	Strongly associated with MALT-type B-cell lymphomas
Gastroesophageal reflux disease	Presence of *cag*+ strains has protective association
Barrett's esophagus	May colonize distal-most gastric epithelium in patients with gastric colonization; presence of *cag*+ strains has protective association
Adenocarcinoma of the esophagus	Presence of *cag*+ strains has protective association

From Blaser MJ: *Helicobacter pylori* and related organisms. In Mandell GL, Bennett JE, Dolin R (eds): Principles and Practice of Infectious Diseases, 5th ed., New York, Churchill Livingstone, 2000, p 2288.

89. Which conditions predispose patients to the development of cellulitis due to group A streptococci?

Cellulitis due to the group A streptococci (and sometimes B, C, or G) has been described in a number of clinical settings in which there has been **impairment of venous and lymphatic drainage**. These situations include:

- Extremities from which the saphenous vein has been harvested for coronary artery bypass grafting
- Following mastectomy with axillary lymph node dissection for breast cancer
- Following vulvectomy and inguinal lymphadenectomy for cancer of the vulva
- After regional lymph node dissection for melanoma
- Following traumatic injuries to extremities
- Following retroperitoneal lymph node dissections for genitourinary tumors

Simon MS, et al: Cellulitis after axillary lymph node dissection for carcinoma of the breast. Am J Med 93:543–548, 1992.

90. List the infectious causes of adrenal insufficiency.

- *M. tuberculosis*
- *H. capsulatum*
- Other fungi (*Cryptococcus neoformans, C. immitis, S. schenckii, Blastomyces dermatitidis, Paracoccidioides brasiliensis*)
- *N. meningitidis* (in Waterhouse-Friderichsen syndrome) and other organisms causing shock
- In HIV infection, *Mycobacterium avium* complex and cytomegalovirus

Painter BF: Infectious causes of adrenal insufficiency. Infect Med 11:515–520, 1994.

KEY POINTS: CLINICAL CHARACTERISTICS OF "LADY WINDERMERE SYNDROME" DUE TO *MYCOBACTERIUM AVIUM* COMPLEX

1. Elderly white women
2. No significant underlying disease
3. Multifocal, nodular bronchiectasis involving middle lobes and lingula
4. Nonsmokers
5. Isolation of *M. avium* complex in low numbers from sputum specimens

91. What is the significance of *Clostridium septicum* infection?

There is a strong association between *C. septicum* infection and underlying malignancy. Approximately 40% of cases involve a hematologic malignancy, and 34% involve colorectal carcinoma. Patients frequently present with myonecrosis, often at sites distant from the presumed source of entry.

Kornbluth AA, et al: *Clostridium septicum* infection and associated malignancy: Report of 2 cases and review of the literature. Medicine 68:30–37, 1989.

92. How many blood cultures should be done for patients with suspected bacteremia or endocarditis in order to make a diagnosis?

If 20–30 mL of blood is drawn during each venipuncture (to be divided between one aerobic and one anaerobic blood culture bottle or between two aerobic bottles), one set of blood cultures will identify the offending pathogen approximately 91.5% of the time and two sets will be positive in > 99%. Consequently, two separate sets of blood cultures are normally recommended.

Smith-Elekes S, et al: Blood cultures. Infect Dis Clin North Am 7:221–234, 1993.

93. What is erythema nodosum leprosum?

This complication of therapy is seen in patients with the full lepromatous form of leprosy and most commonly occurs within the first year of treatment. It is manifested as nodular skin lesions that histopathologically resemble arthus-type reactions, with localized vasculitis in the veins and arteries characterized by polymorphonuclear neutrophil (PMN) and eosinophilic infiltrates. It may also be associated with neuritis, polyarthritis, and immune-complex glomerulonephritis.

Jacobson RR, et al: The diagnosis and treatment of leprosy. South Med J 69:979–985, 1976.

94. What infectious diseases result from human louse infestations?

The body louse, *Pediculus humanus humanus*, which is a strict human parasite, is responsible for transmission of three different bacterial species to humans:

- *Borrelia recurrentis*, which causes relapsing fever.
- *Bartonella quintana,* which is recognized as the cause of bacillary angiomatosis, bacteremia, trench fever, endocarditis and chronic lymphadenopathy, particularly among homeless individuals.
- *Rickettsia prowazekii*, which is the cause of epidemic typhus.

Raoult D, Roux V: The body louse as a vector of reemerging human diseases. Clin Infect Dis 29:888–911, 1999.

95. What organisms are responsible for most infections in patients with cystic fibrosis?

Chronic lung infection in patients with cystic fibrosis is usually caused by a limited number of organisms.

- *S. aureus* and *P. aeruginosa* are the most frequently isolated pathogens.
- *Burkholderia cepacia* is also commonly seen, particularly in adult patients with cystic fibrosis.
- Various other bacteria, including non-typeable *H. influenzae*, *Str. pneumoniae* and some of the *Enterobacteriaceae,* are occasionally isolated.
- The most important fungal pathogen is *Aspergillus fumigatus*, which causes allergic bronchopulmonary aspergillosis in this patient population.

Gilligan PH: Microbiology of airway disease in patients with cystic fibrosis. Clin Microbiol Rev 4:35–51, 1991.

96. What is xanthogranulomatous pyelonephritis?

Xanthogranulomatous pyelonephritis is a chronic infection of the renal parenchyma and surrounding tissues that occurs most commonly in the presence of renal lithiasis or urinary tract obstruction. It most commonly occurs in middle-aged females and is usually due to *Proteus mirabilis* or *E. coli*. The renal parenchyma becomes replaced by characteristic foamy histiocytes, which may also be found in urine cytologic specimens.

Goodman M, et al: Xanthogranulomatous pyelonephritis (XGP): A local disease with systemic manifestations. Medicine 58:171–181, 1979.

97. What species of *Ehrlichia* have been associated with human disease?

Several species of *Ehrlichia* have been recognized as causes of human tick-borne zoonotic infections. The species associated with human diseases include:

- *E. chaffeensis* causes human monocytic ehrlichiosis
- *E. ewingii* and *A. phagocytophilum* have been identified as causes of human granulocytic ehrlichiosis
- *E. sennetsu* causes a mononucleosis-like illness in Japan and Malaysia
- *E. canis* has been reported in one patient in Venezuela

98. What is Lemierre's syndrome?

Lemierre's syndrome is suppurative thrombophlebitis of the internal jugular vein that results from acute oropharyngeal infection. This may lead to septic embolization, most often to the lungs. Anaerobic bacteria, particularly *Fusobacterium necrophorum*, are usually involved.

Sinave CP, Hardy GJ, Fardy PW: The Lemierre syndrome: Suppurative thrombophlebitis of the internal jugular vein secondary to oropharyngeal infection. Medicine 68:85–93, 1989.

99. What are Koch postulates?

Koch postulates, which were actually proposed by Henle, are used to establish a causal relation between a specific agent and a specific disease:

1. The agent must be present in every case of the disease.
2. The agent must be isolated from the diseased host and grown in pure culture.
3. The specific disease must be reproduced when a portion of the culture is inoculated into a healthy susceptible host.
4. The organism must be recovered again from the experimentally infected host.

100. The use of medicinal leeches is associated with infection due to what organism?

A. hydrophila, which has the same freshwater habitat as the medicinal leech, *Hirudo medicinalis*, may complicate microvascular surgical infections where leeches are used because of their anticoagulant properties.

Abrutyn E: Hospital-associated infection from leeches. Ann Intern Med 109:356–358, 1988.

101. How does human disease due to *Dirofilaria immitis* usually present?

D. immitis, the dog heartworm, usually presents as a solitary, noncalcified pulmonary nodule in humans. Because humans are an unsuitable host for this worm, larvae that mature in subcutaneous tissues after inoculation by infected mosquitoes enter veins and travel to the heart and act as emboli into the pulmonary arteries, resulting in infarcts.

Nicholson CP, et al: *Dirofilaria immitis*: A rare, increasing cause of pulmonary nodules. Mayo Clin Proc 67:646–650, 1992.

102. With what syndromes are the various herpesviruses associated?

- **Herpes simplex virus:** mucocutaneous lesions, encephalitis
- **Varicella zoster virus:** chickenpox, shingles

  Cytomegalovirus: mononucleosis syndrome, meningoencephalitis, transverse myelitis, hepatitis, myocarditis, pneumonitis, esophagitis, colitis, and retinitis, usually in immunocompromised patients
- **Epstein-Barr virus**: infectious mononucleosis, Burkitt's lymphoma, nasopharyngeal carcinoma, Epstien-Barr virus–related lymphoproliferative syndromes
- **Human herpesvirus 6:** roseola (exanthem subitum) and nonspecific febrile illnesses in young children, mononucleosis-like syndrome in adults, febrile seizures, meningoencephalitis and encephalitis, hepatitis, opportunistic infections (interstitial pneumonitis) in immunocompromised patients; possible associations: chronic fatigue syndrome, lymphoproliferative disorders, and histiocytic necrotizing lymphadenitis (Kikuchi's syndrome)
- **Human herpesvirus 7:** possibly exanthum subitum-like illness, hepatitis, and encephalitis
- **Human herpesvirus 8:** Kaposi's sarcoma, primary effusion (body cavity-based) lymphoma, multicentric Castleman's disease; possible association: primary pulmonary hypertension
- **Herpes B virus:** myelitis and hemorrhagic encephalitis following primate bites and scratches

103. What are the six classic exanthems of childhood and their causes?
See Table 4-4.

TABLE 4-4. SIX CLASSIC EXANTHEMS OF CHILDHOOD

Order	Exanthems	Causative Agents
First	Rubeola (measles)	Measles virus
Second	Scarlet fever	*Str. pyogenes*
Third	Rubella (German measles)	Rubella virus
Fourth	Filatov-Dukes disease (variant of scarlet fever)	*Str. pyogenes*
Fifth	Erythema infectiosum	Parvovirus B19
Sixth	Exanthem subitum (roseola)	Human herpes virus 6

104. List the common infectious causes of nodular lymphangitis.

- *S. schenckii*
- *Mycobacterium marinum*
- *Nocardia brasiliensis*
- *Leishmania brasiliensis*
- *Francisella tularensis*

105. List the less common causes of nodular lymphangitis.
Unusual causes: *Nocardia asteroides, Mycobacterium chelonae, Leishmania major*
Rare causes: *Mycobacterium kansasii, B. dermatitidis, C. neoformans, H. capsulatum, Str. pyogenes, S. aureus, Pseudomonas pseudomallei, Bacillus anthracis,* cowpox

Kostman JR, DiNubile MJ: Nodular lymphangitis: A distinctive but often unrecognized syndrome. Ann Intern Med 118:883–888, 1993.

106. What types of infections occur principally in patients with diabetes mellitus?

- Invasive otitis externa due to *P. aeruginosa*
- Rhinocerebral mucormycosis
- Emphysematous cholecystitis
- Emphysematous cystitis and pyelonephritis

Joshi N, et al: Infections in patients with diabetes mellitus. N Engl J Med 341:1906–1912, 2000.

107. What are the clinical manifestations of anthrax?
The clinical manifestations of anthrax are initiated after the introduction into the body of the endospores of the causative organism, *B. anthracis.* The most common manifestations include:

- Cutaneous anthrax, which accounts for 95% of all anthrax in the United States.
- GI and oropharyngeal anthrax, which occur after ingestion of the endospores.
- Inhalational anthrax, which usually occurs after inhalation of the endospores that have contaminated animal hides or products.
- Anthrax meningitis, which occurs after bacteremic spread, usually from a skin focus.

Swartz MN: Recognition and management of anthrax: An update. N Engl J Med 345: 1621–1626, 2001.

KEY POINTS: CLINICAL CLUES FOR DIPHTHERIA

1. Mildly painful tonsillitis and/or pharyngitis with associated gray palatal membrane
2. Cervical lymphadenopathy and neck swelling
3. Hoarseness and stridor
4. Unilateral palatal paralysis
5. Moderate temperature elevation
6. Serosanguinous nasal discharge with associated mucosal membrane

108. What are the neurologic complications of Lyme disease?

The neurologic manifestations of Lyme disease are extremely variable and may include:

- Bell's palsy and other cranial neuropathies, particularly involving cranial nerves III, IV, and VI
- Radiculopathy that can involve any distribution
- Mononeuritis multiplex
- Aseptic meningitis, usually with a lymphocytic pleocytosis
- Encephalitis syndromes
- Transverse myelitis
- Demyelinating polyneuropathy

Finkel MF: Lyme disease and its neurologic complications. Arch Neurol 45:99–104, 1988.

109. What microbial agents are traditionally considered potential biologic warfare agents?

B. anthracis
Brucella suis
C. burnetii
F. tularensis
Smallpox virus
Yersinia pestis
Viral encephalitides (e.g., Venezuelan equine encephalitis)
Viral hemorrhagic fevers (e.g., Lassa fever, Rift Valley fever, Crimean Congo hemorrhagic fever, Ebola, Marburg)

Kortepeter MG, Parker GW: Potential biological weapons threats. Emerging Infect Dis 5:523–527, 1999.

110. What are the clinical manifestations of infection due to parvovirus B19?

- Ertythema infectiousum ("Fifth's disease")
- Arthropathy (particularly in adults)
- Transient aplastic crisis (e.g., in patients with sickle cell anemia)
- Pure red cell aplasia (e.g., in patients with AIDS)
- Virus-associated hemophagocytic syndrome
- Hydrops fetalis

111. Which microbial pathogens cause traveler's diarrhea?

No pathogen is identified in about 40% of cases. Identified pathogens are listed below with their frequency:

- Enterotoxigenic *E. coli* (40–60%)
- Enteroadherent *E. coli* (15%)
- Invasive *E. coli* (< 5%)

- *Shigella* sp. (10%)
- *Salmonella* sp. (< 5%)
- *Campylobacter* sp. (< 5%)
- *Vibrio* sp. (< 5%)
- *Aeromonas* sp. (< 5%)
- Rotavirus (5%)
- *G. lamblia* (< 5%)
- *Entamoeba histolytica* (< 5%)
- *Cryptosporidium* sp. (< 5%)

Gorbach SL: Traveler's diarrhea. In Gorbach SL, Bartlett JG , Blacklow NR (eds): Infectious Diseases, 3rd ed. Philadelphia, Lippincott Williams & Wilkins, 2004, pp.681–688.

KEY PONTS: MOST COMMON PATHOGENS RESPONSIBLE FOR FOOD-BORNE ILLNESS

1. *Campylobacter*
2. *Salmonella*
3. *Shigella*
4. *E. coli* O157:H7
5. *Cryptosporidium*

112. Describe the most common adverse effects associated with infusion of amphotericin B.

- Acute, infusion-related effects ("shake and bake"): rigors, nausea and vomiting, fevers, headache
- Renal effects: azotemia, hypokalemia, hypomagnesemia, renal tubular acidosis
- Anemia due to suppression of release of erythropoietin

BIBLIOGRAPHY

1. Gorbach SL, Bartlett JG, Blacklow NR (eds): Infectious Diseases, 3rd ed. Philadelphia, Lippincott Williams & Wilkins, 2004.
2. Holmes KK, et al (eds): Sexually Transmitted Diseases, 3rd ed. New York, McGraw-Hill, 1999.
3. Mandell GL, Bennett JE, Dolin R (eds): Principles and Practice of Infectious Diseases, 5th ed. New York, Churchill Livingstone, 2000.

GASTROENTEROLOGY

Rhonda A. Cole, MD

CHAPTER 5

GASTROINTESTINAL BLEEDING

1. **List the five ways in which gastrointestinal (GI) bleeding presents.**
   - **Hematemesis:** vomiting of blood. The blood may be a fresh, bright red in color or like coffee grounds.
   - **Melena:** black, tarry, foul-smelling stool.
   - **Hematochezia:** bright red blood per rectum, blood mixed with stool, bloody diarrhea, or clots.
   - **Occult GI blood loss:** normal-appearing stool that is hemoccult-positive.
   - **Symptoms only:** syncope, dyspnea, angina, palpitations, or shock.

2. **Describe the initial approach to the patient who presents with acute GI bleeding.**
   In any patient presenting with acute GI bleeding, the key word is *resuscitation!* The initial approach should include a rapid assessment to gauge the urgency of the situation, especially whether the patient is hemodynamically stable or unstable (blood pressure, pressure, and signs of orthostasis must be obtained). Venous access should be obtained with a large-bore IV cannula, and fluids such as normal saline should be begun immediately. Blood should be obtained for a complete blood count, clotting studies, platelets, routine chemistry, and type and cross-match.

3. **Describe the management of a hemodynamically unstable patient.**
   If there are signs of an acute, life-threatening bleed and an unstable condition, aggressive resuscitation and evaluation for the source must be under taken immediately. Placement of a nasogastric (NG) tube to assess for evidence of an upper GI source and, if present, to document the rapidity of bleeding should be done at this time. Close monitoring of vital signs and urinary output in an ICU setting is imperative. The patient must be also be monitored for signs of concomitant heart, lung, renal, or central nervous system disease.

4. **Give a good rule of thumb for blood transfusions.**
   A good rule of thumb is that blood transfusions should be given as quickly as the patient has lost blood. For example, if the patient presents with massive hematochezia and is hemodynamically compromised, packed red blood cells should be given as quickly as possible. On the other hand, the patient who presents with iron deficiency anemia, hemoccult positive stools, and stable vital signs may not require blood transfusions at all. Once the patient has been stabilized, a search can be carried out to localize the source of bleeding and perform any indicated endoscopic therapy.

5. **How is the site of bleeding determined?**
   The presence of a GI bleed should be confirmed by inspecting the stool for melena or hematochezia and the NG tube aspirate for blood. The site of bleeding can frequently be determined from the patient's complaints. Upper GI bleeding often presents with hematemesis combined with melena; hematochezia with a negative NG aspirate suggests a lower GI source.

6. **List the common causes of upper GI bleeding.**
   - Duodenal and gastric ulcers
   - Esophageal or gastric varices in the cirrhotic patient
   - Mallory-Weiss tears (most commonly seen in alcoholic patients or patients with forceful vomiting)
   - Erosive gastritis as a result of nonsteroidal anti-inflammatory drugs (NSAIDs) or in intubated ICU patients

7. **Is examination of the skin helpful in identifying the source of an upper GI bleed?**
   The skin examination can be helpful for suggesting a potential source if certain stigmata are present. Lymphadenopathy or abdominal masses may suggest sources for intra-abdominal pathology (Table 5-1).

TABLE 5-1. SKIN FINDINGS IN CONDITIONS THAT CAUSE GI BLEEDING

Disease	Associated skin findings
Peutz-Jeghers	Pigmented macules on lips, palms, soles
Malignant melanoma	Melanoma
Hereditary hemorrhagic telangiectasias	Telangiectasias on lips, mouth, palms, soles (Osler-Weber-Rendu)
Blue rubber bleb nevus	Dark, blue soft nodules
Bullous pemphigoid	Oral and skin bullae
Neurofibromatosis	Café-au-lait spots, axillary freckles, neurofibromas
Cronkhite-Canada	Alopecia; hyperpigmentation of creases, hands, and face
Cirrhosis	Spider angiomata, Dupuytren's contracture
Neoplasm	Acanthosis nigricans
Kaposi's sarcoma	Cutaneous Kaposi's sarcoma
Ehlers-Danlos	Skin fragility, keloids, paper thin scars
Pseudoxanthoma elasticum	Yellow "chicken fat" papules and plaques in flexural areas
Turner's	Webbing of neck, purpura, skin nodules

From Berger T, Silverman S: Oral and cutaneous manifestations of gastrointestinal disease. In Sleisenger MH, Fordtran JS (eds): Gastrointestinal Disease, 5th ed. Philadelphia, W.B. Saunders, 1994, pp 268–285.

8. **What are predictors of poor outcome in patients presenting with bleeding ulcers?**
   - Elderly patients (age > 60yr)
   - Patients with fresh blood per NG tube or rectum
   - Patients who remain hemodynamically unstable despite aggressive resuscitative measures
   - Patients who have four or more comorbid illnesses (e.g., cardiac disease, liver disease, diabetes) NSAID use

9. **List the common causes of lower GI bleeding.**
   - Hemorrhoids are the most common cause but rarely present with massive bleeding requiring hospitalization.
   - Diverticulosis accounts for a significant percentage of cases. Diverticular bleeding may occur from either the right or left colon.
   - Angiodysplasia or vascular ectasias are among of the more common well-recognized causes in older patients. They are commonly found in the cecum and ascending colon.
   - Neoplasms of the large bowel usually present with chronic occult bleeding but occasionally bleed acutely.

10. **What are the less common causes of lower GI bleeding?**
Less common causes include Meckel's diverticulum, ischemic or inflammatory bowel disease, and solitary ulcers of the cecum and rectum.

11. **Does melena indicate a right-sided colonic source and hematochezia a left-sided source?**
Usually. The color of stool depends on colonic transit time. If the stool remains in contact with bacteria that degrade hemoglobin, the resulting stool is melanic. Although right-sided lesions are usually associated with melena (dark, tarry stools) and left-sided lesions with hematochezia (the passage of bright red blood per rectum), the opposite can also be seen. Therefore, the evaluation of a patient with hematochezia must include examination of the proximal colon.

12. **What are the possible causes of esophageal varices?**
Elevation of pressure in the hepatic portal system leads to the development of varices. The normal portal venous pressure is ~ 10 mmHg but increases to > 20 mmHg in portal hypertension. The causes of portal hypertension are classified as presinusoidal, sinusoidal, and postsinusoidal. The most common cause in the Western world is alcohol-related cirrhosis.

13. **List the presinusoidal cause of esophageal varices.**
   - Portal vein thrombosis
   - Splenic vein thrombosis
   - Primary biliary cirrhosis
   - Schistosomiasis

14. **What are the sinusoidal causes of esophageal varices?**
Cirrhosis and idiopathic disease.

15. **List the postsinusoidal cause of esophageal varices.**
   - Heart failure
   - Constrictive pericarditis
   - Hepatic vein thrombosis (Budd-Chiari syndrome)
   - Veno-occlusive disease

16. **Which two factors determine whether esophageal varices will develop and whether they will bleed?**
Portal pressure and variceal size. The portal to hepatic vein pressure gradient must be > 12 mmHg (normal = 3–6 mmHg) for varices to develop. Beyond this level, there is poor correlation between portal pressure and likelihood of bleeding. The best predictor of impending variceal hemorrhage is size. When varices reach a large size (> 5 mm in diameter), they are more likely to rupture and bleed. At any given pressure, the wall of a large varix is under greater tension than that of a small varix and must be thicker to withstand the pressure.

17. **List the classic features of Meckel's diverticulum.**
    - Occurs in 1–3% population
    - Usually found within 100 cm of the ileocecal valve
    - Cause of 50% lower GI bleeding in children
    - Rare etiology for bleeding in patients older than 40 years
    - Gastric mucosa is present in ~ 40%

18. **In the patient who has undergone multiple evaluations for the localization of recurrent occult GI bleeding without identification of a source, what test needs to be performed?**
    In patients who have had multiple upper GI endoscopies, colonoscopies, barium studies, and RBC scans without identification of the source of blood loss, enteroscopy needs to be performed. Enteroscopy can be performed either with push enteroscopy or wireless capsule endoscopy. The source of bleeding is most likely from AVMs (or angiodysplasias), usually hiding in the small intestine. Of particular note is that before a patient undergoes enteroscopy the hemoglobin should be 10 or higher to aid in detecting these tiny vessels.

LIVER AND HEPATITIS

19. **What is Budd-Chiari syndrome?**
    Partial or complete obstruction of blood flow out of the liver, usually involving the hepatic veins. The patient characteristically presents with hepatomegaly, ascites, and abdominal pain. Underlying etiologies include myeloproliferative disorders (~50%), malignancy, infections of the liver, oral contraceptive pills, pregnancy, collagen vascular diseases, and hypercoagulable states.

20. **Which of the hepatitides is of major health concern?**
    Hepatitis C. It is estimated that as many as 1 in 10 persons are at risk for this potentially chronic liver disease for which there is currently no cure. Over 50% of people who have served in the U.S. armed forces are positive for hepatitis C, making the illness a priority in the federal health system. In addition to the known sources of risk, at least one third of all infected patients have no known risks for this potentially debilitating illness.

21. **What complications are associated with hepatitis C?**
    The frequency of patients presenting with complications associated with hepatitis C virus (HCV) infection is expected to triple within the next 20 years. This corresponds to a 61% increase in incidence of cirrhosis, a 68% increase in the incidence of hepatocellular carcinoma, a 279% increase in decompensated liver disease, and a 528% increase in the demand for liver transplantation.

22. **What are the differences among hepatitis A, B, and C?**
    Hepatitis A, called infectious hepatitis, is easily spread by the fecal/oral route. The hepatitis A virus (HAV) causes a short-lived, benign, acute hepatitis that is not followed by chronic liver disease. IgG antibodies to HAV remain positive for life. To determine if the hepatitis is acute, one must look for IgM antibodies in the serum.

    Hepatitis B, called serum hepatitis, is contracted by contact with blood or other bodily secretions from an infected individual, usually through a break in the skin or use of a contaminated needle. Unlike hepatitis A, hepatitis B may cause chronic disease and cirrhosis. It also predisposes to hepatocellular carcinoma (hepatoma). A carrier state is possible in which patients demonstrate persistent hepatitis B surface antigenemia (HBsAg) without clinically evident disease but are able to transmit the disease.

Hepatitis C had been previously included in the non-A, non-B hepatitis category. It is the form of hepatitis most commonly contracted from blood transfusion. It also is the most common viral cause of chronic liver disease and increases the patient's risk for developing hepatoma (hepatocellular carcinoma).

23. **Who should receive the hepatitis A vaccine?**
Infants > 2 years who are at risk, travelers to endemic areas, military personnel and others with occupational exposure, IV drug abusers, people with high-risk sexual practices, Native Americans and Alaskans (ethnic groups with high rates of HAV), people in communities with outbreaks of HAV, and patients with clotting factor disorders and chronic liver disease.

24. **How is the Havrix vaccine administered?**
Children 2–18 years: 360 EL.U/0.5 cc, two doses 1 month apart; then 0.5 cc 6–12 months after primary series
Adults: 720 EL.U/0.5 cc, one dose; then 0.5 cc 6–12 months after primary series

25. **How is the Vaqta vaccine administered?**
Children: 2–17 years: 25 U/0.5 cc, one dose; then 0.5 cc, one dose 6–18 months after primary dose
Adults: 50 U/cc, one dose; then 50 U/cc, one dose 6 months after primary dose
Viral hepatitis guide for practicing physicians. Cleve Clin J Med 67(Suppl 1), 2000.

26. **Summarize the usual serologic response to naturally acquired hepatitis B infection.**
See Figure 5-1.

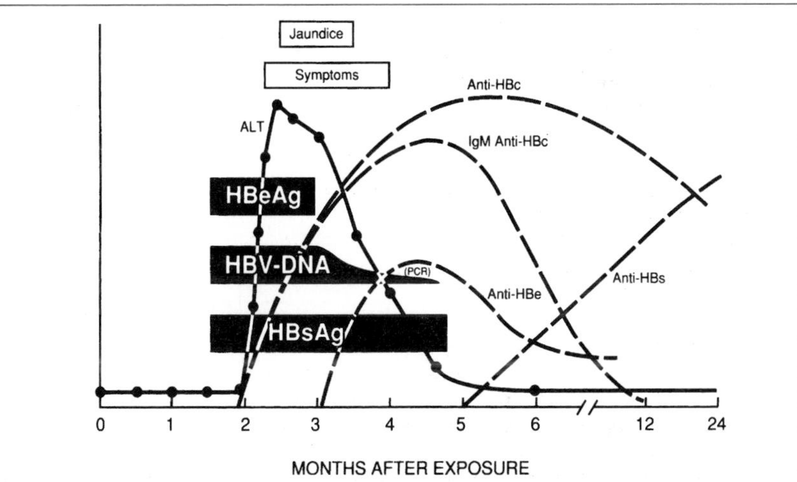

Figure 5-1. Clinical and serologic course of a typical case of acute hepatitis B. HBsAg = hepatitis B surface antigen, HBeAg = hepatitis B e antigen, DNA-p = DNA polymerase, HBV-DNA = hepatitis B virus DNA, ALT = alanine aminotransferase, anti-HBC = antibody to hepatitis B core antigen, anti-HBe = antibody to HBeAg, anti-HBs = antibody to HbsAg. (From Hoofnagle JH: Acute viral hepatitis. In Mandell GL, et al [eds]: Principles and Practice of Infectious Diseases, 4th ed. New York, Churchill Livingstone, 1995, p 1143.)

27. How should you treat a health care worker with a recent (< 48 hours) needlestick exposure to hepatitis B?
The worker should receive hepatitis immunoglobulin, 0.06 ml/kg IM, as soon as possible and within 7 days of exposure. If the worker has not previously received the hepatitis B vaccine, the vaccination program should be initiated with the usual three doses—the first dose within 14 days after exposure and again at 1 and 6 months.

28. How is HCV transmitted? What are the possible courses of the disease?
Blood transfusions, shared and/or contaminated needles among IV drug abusers, intransal drugs, high-risk sexual behavior, tattoos, and (albeit low) vertical transmission from infected mothers to unborn children (accounts for 3–6%). Nearly 30% of persons infected with hepatitis C have no known risk exposure. Significant liver disease develops in 50% of persons infected, and they are at risk for the development of hepatocellular carcinoma. Detection of HCV-RNA by polymerase chain reaction is the definitive test for active hepatitis C.

29. How is hepatitis D virus (delta virus) transmitted?
Hepatitis D virus (HDV) is a very small RNA virus that contains a defective genome and requires HBsAg to become pathogenic. Infection may occur under two circumstances:

- In conjunction with simultaneous infection with hepatitis B in a previously unexposed patient (coinfection)
- In the chronic carrier of HBsAg (superinfection).

Hepatitis D is diagnosed by detecting IgM antibody to HDV in acute serum or an increase in IgG antibody to HDV in convalescent serum.

30. What is hepatitis E?
Hepatitis E virus (HEV) causes enterically (fecal-oral) transmitted non-A, non-B hepatitis. It is endemic to Southeast and Central Asia, Africa, and Mexico but is rare in the U.S. It is also responsible for large epidemics of acute hepatitis. It is possible that zoonotic HEV infection may occur in areas where animal hosts are abundant, including pig farming areas in the U.S. This illness is particularly severe in pregnant women in whom mortality rates from acute liver failure may reach 20%.

31. What is hepatitis G?
Hepatitis G is an RNA virus that is transmitted primarily through blood and blood products. It frequently occurs as a coinfection with hepatitis C or other hepatitis viruses as a result of common modes of transmission. Currently no data support any role for hepatitis G in chronic or serious liver disease.

32. When should the patient with acute viral hepatitis be admitted for hospitalization?

Older age	Pregnancy
Underlying systemic illnesses	Underlying chronic hepatitis of another etiology
Encephalopathy	Volume depletion or inability to hold down fluids
Ascites	Prothrombin time (PT) > 15 sec
Bilirubin > 15 mg/dL	Albumin < 3 mg/dL
Hypoglycemia	Worsening PT or bilirubin with improving transaminases = *fulminant hepatic failure*
Social problems that may result in loss to follow-up	

33. What three conditions result in very high transaminases (> 1000)?

- Ischemia
- Viral hepatitis
- Drug-induced hepatitis

34. What causes chronic liver disease?

- Viral hepatitis B, C, and D
- Wilson's disease
- Alcohol
- Drug-induced disease
- Autoimmune hepatitis
- $Alpha_1$ antitrypsin

35. What is fulminant hepatic failure?

Characteristically this entity involves a previously healthy patient who undergoes acute and progressive liver failure. The mortality rate is ~ 80% if untreated. Fulminant hepatic failure usually begins as malaise, anorexia, and low-grade fever, followed by signs and symptoms of liver failure (e.g., jaundice, encephalopathy). The most common cause of death in fulminant hepatic failure is either brain edema or sepsis. The most definitive therapy is liver transplantation.

36. List the common causes of fulminant hepatic failure.

- Viral hepatitides A,B,C,D,E
- Drugs: acetaminophen, antituberculosis drugs, troglitazone, Ectasy
- Herbal medications: Jin bu huan, comfrey
- Toxins: *Amanita phalloides*, carbontetrachloride, trichloroethylene
- Vascular: Budd-Chiari syndrome, veno-occlusive disease, ischemia or hypoxia, heatstroke
- Miscellaneous: malignant infiltration, Wilson's disease, acute fatty liver of pregnancy, Reye's syndrome

37. What is Wilson's disease?

It is an autosomal recessive genetic disorder characterized by an accumulation of copper in the liver and brain. The Wilson's gene is ATP7B, which is either absent or markedly diminished in Wilson's disease. The lack of the gene results in diminished synthesis of ceruloplasmin and/or defective transport of hepatocellular copper into bile for excretion.

38. What is $alpha_1$ antitrypsin (A_1AT) deficiency?

A_1AT is a relatively common autosomal recessive disease resulting from a defect in the gene for the q arm of chromosome 14. The disease is characterized by hepatic involvement, pulmonary emphysema, panniculitis, and arterial aneurysms.

NUTRITION

39. Name six common vitamins and trace minerals and the clinical manifestations of their respective deficiency states.

- Thiamine: beriberi, muscle weakness, tachycardia, heart failure
- Niacin: pellagra, glossitis
- Vitamin A: xerophthalmia, hyperkeratosis of skin
- Vitamin E: cerebellar ataxia, areflexia
- Zinc: hypogeusia, acrodermatitis
- Chromium: glucose intolerance

40. Name the two most common nutritional deficiencies seen in patients with intestinal disease.
Deficiencies of calcium and folate. When the small bowel is diseased, intestinal loss of calcium is excessive, and the rate of bone resorption is insufficient to maintain serum calcium.

41. With what is severe folate deficiency most often associated?
Severe folate deficiency occurs most often in association with chronic alcoholism, celiac sprue, tropical sprue, and blind loop syndrome. Minor deficiencies can be found in Crohn's disease and following partial gastrectomy. Since folate absorption is largely completed in the upper small intestine, malabsorption is worse in disorders that affect the upper gut. However, any intestinal disorder accompanied by a decrease in dietary intake or rapid transport may result in folate deficiency.

42. An elderly man presents with profound peripheral neuropathy and a markedly low serum level of vitamin B_{12}. Physical examination reveals an abdominal scar consistent with previous laparotomy, but the patient does not remember what kind of surgery was done. What two operations may result in B_{12} deficiency? Why?
Gastrectomy. Vitamin B_{12} absorption starts in the stomach, where it binds to intrinsic factor and R proteins produced there. In the duodenum, the R proteins are hydrolyzed off the vitamin B_{12} in the presence of an alkaline environment, which then allows for further binding of B_{12} with intrinsic factor. Vitamin B_{12} cannot be absorbed unless it is bound to intrinsic factor. If the patient's stomach was completely or partially removed, he would have insufficient intrinsic factor.

Terminal ileal resection. This patient may have had Crohn's disease and undergone resection of a large portion (> 100 cm) of terminal ileum, the site of absorption of the vitamin B_{12}–intrinsic factor complex.

43. How are both mechanisms of deficiency treated?
Both mechanisms of deficiency can be easily treated with supplemental intramuscular vitamin B_{12} injections.

44. What is the most common disorder of carbohydrate digestion in humans?
Lactase deficiency. Lactase-deficient adults retain 10–30% of intestinal lactose activity and develop symptoms (diarrhea, bloating, and gas) only when they ingest sufficient lactose. Symptoms result from the colonic bacteria metabolizing lactose to methane, CO_2, and short-chain fatty acids.

45. After avoiding dairy products, the patient's symptoms have disappeared. Does this confirm the diagnosis of lactose deficiency?
No. The diagnosis cannot be made simply by advising the patient to avoid dairy products for 2 weeks to determine if the altered bowel habits revert to normal because many patients who respond to these manipulations are actually not lactase deficient. The diagnostic test to be used is the lactose hydrogen breath test.

46. Outline the fundamental principles of total parenteral nutrition (TPN).
1. Patients generally require 25–35 kcal/kg for maintenance.
2. The optimal calorie/nitrogen ratio appears to be about 160 cal/gm N.
3. The average adult requires about 30 mL water/kg body weight/day.
4. IV lipid emulsions are a suitable source of nonprotein calories that contribute to conservation of body protein. A regimen in which calories are supplied by both dextrose solution and lipid emulsions, with fat providing 20–30% of the total calories, appears to be the most effective form of parenteral nutrition.

47. What are the most common complications of TPN?
The most common complications are related to catheter placement and management. Examples include infections, thrombosis, nonthrombotic occlusion, and other mechanical complications during line placement. Catheter-related complications can be minimized by maintaining strict and reproducible technique as well as meticulous line care.

48. What long-term complications may arise?

- In prolonged TPN, especially when excessive carbohydrate calories are given, patients frequently develop liver tenderness and transaminase elevations. The increased liver values are thought to reflect hepatic steatosis. Aspartate aminotransferase (AST) and alanine aminotransferase (ALT) abnormalities should return to normal when TPN is discontinued. If TPN is continued, one should decrease the dextrose infusion and increase the amount of fat calories provided.
- A complication of long-term (home) TPN is metabolic bone disease, which is similar to osteomalacia and osteoporosis. The addition of acetate or phosphate may offset the urinary calcium losses and restore positive calcium balance in these patients.
- An increased incidence of cholecystitis and cholelithiasis related to gallbladder stasis is seen in patients on TPN.

49. Which vitamin deficiencies might develop in a patient maintained on long-term TPN (> 6 mo) containing only Na^+, K^+, Cl^-, $HCO3^-$, glucose, and amino acids?
This TPN solution clearly is lacking in vitamins and trace minerals. In a matter of weeks, the patient would be expected to develop deficiencies in magnesium, zinc, essential fatty acids, and water-soluble vitamins (with the exception of B_{12}). Over several months, vitamin K and copper deficiencies would develop. Over a period of years, deficiencies in the fat-soluble vitamins A and D as well as selenium, chromium, and vitamin B_{12} would result.

50. What is body mass index (BMI)?
BMI measures weight as it relates to height and is an accurate indicator of categories of obesity.

51. Summarize the standards of weight and obesity according to BMI.

BMI	Category
18 – 24.9 kg/m^2	Normal
25 – 29.9 kg/m^2	Overweight
> 30 kg/m^2	Obese
≥ 40 kg/m^2	Severe or morbid obesity
≥ 50 kg/m^2	Super obesity

52. Define obesity. What is its impact on American society?
Obesity is defined as a chronic disease of excess body fat. More than 30% of all Americans are categorized as obese. Obesity is at epidemic proportions among school-age children. Ten percent of all African-American women ages 40–60 years old are morbidly obese. Three hundred thousand deaths annually are attributable to obesity. Obesity is second only to smoking as a leading cause of preventable death.

53. What comorbid diseases are directly attributable to obesity?
Type 2 diabetes mellitus, coronary artery disease, hypertension, deep venous thrombosis, pulmonary embolus, lymphedema thrombophlebitis, weight-bearing osteoarthritis (involving the hip, knees, ankles, and feet), low back syndrome, herniated disk, lower extremity edema, gallbladder disease, gastroesophageal reflux disease (GERD), asthma, sleep apnea, pseudotumor cerebri, cirrhosis, varicosities, intertriginous dermatitis, breast cancer, uterine cancer, prostrate cancer, and Pickwickian syndrome.

CANCER

54. When should screening for colorectal cancer (CRC) begin?

In asymptomatic people of normal risk status, screening should begin at age 50.

55. What are appropriate methods for colon cancer screening?

Beginning at age 50, everyone should have an annual digital rectal examination with testing of the stool obtained for trace blood. Alternatively, the patient can submit three stool samples to his physician to check for blood. If the test is positive, the patient should be referred for examination of the entire colon. Examination of the colon can be completed by an air contrast barium enema, followed by flexible sigmoidoscopy or by colonoscopy with biopsy/removal of any abnormal lesions.

56. What dietary factors increase the risk of CRC?

- Low intake of fiber, fruits, vitamins E and C, beta-carotene, calcium
- High intake of fat, meat, animal protein

57. List the other risk factors for CRC.

Colon cancer in a first-degree relative < 60 years old
Familial adenomatous polyposis
Personal history of uterine, endometrial, breast cancer
Cancer family syndrome
Chronic ulcerative colitis affecting left colon more than right
Hereditary nonpolyposis colon cancer (HNPCC)
Lynch syndrome I or Lynch syndrome II
Personal history of CRC or adenomatous polyp > 1 cm
Advanced age (> 80 yr)

58. What is the significance of an adenomatous polyp?

Adenomatous polyps are neoplastic polyps, found most often in the colon, that give rise to symptoms only when they become large. They are frequently detected incidentally on colonoscopic exam or barium enema. Their importance relates to their malignant potential; nearly all colonic carcinomas arise from adenomatous polyps. About 75% of adenomatous polyps are tubular adenomas, 15% are tubulovillous adenomas, and the rest are villous adenomas.

59. What factors increase the likelihood that a polyp is malignant?

Villous tumors are more likely to be malignant than tubular adenomas. Other factors that relate to malignant potential include tumor size > 1 cm, degree of cellular atypia, and number of polyps present.

60. How are adenamatous polyps managed?

Adenomatous polyps should be removed with endoscopic polypectomy. Patients should undergo colonoscopy at routine intervals so that additional polyps may be removed before they progress to malignancy.

61. Summarize the guidelines for surveillance of patients after polypectomy.

- Hyperplastic polyps: no follow-up (unless polyp is > 2 cm or > 20 polyps are found throughout the colon).
- 1–2 adenomatous polyps < 1 cm, negative family history: 5 years.
- 2 adenomatous polyps or adenomatous polyp > 1 cm: 3 years.
- Villous histology or high-grade dysplasia: 3 years.
- Polyps in a patient with a positive family history: 3 years.
- Large, sessile, or numerous adenomatous polyps: although 1–2 years is usual, follow-up is based on clinical judgment and should be individualized for each patient.
- Dirty prep: clinical judgment.

- Piecemeal resection of > 2 cm sessile adenoma: look at site within 3–6 months and biopsy to exclude dysplasia of the flat mucosa. Follow-up then based on clinical judgment.
- Once follow-up is negative for new polyps: every 5 years.

62. Summarize the guidelines for surveillance of patients after CRC resection.
Colonoscopy should be performed in the perioperative period to clear the colon of any synchronous lesions. The next colonoscopy following clearing should be 3 years postoperatively *or* according to postpolypectomy surveillance guidelines if a polyp is detected. An alternative approach is to perform a screening colonoscopy 1 year postoperatively, then follow polypectomy guidelines as indicated. In the patient who has a history compatible with HNPCC, follow-up should be every 1–2 years. In patients with rectal cancer, a flexible sigmoidscopy or rectal endoscopic ultrasound should be performed every 3–6 months for 2 years because rectal cancer has a greater tendency to recur locally.

63. Name the most common malignant neoplasms of the small intestine.
- Adenocarcinoma (45%)
- Carcinoid (34%)
- Leiomyosarcoma (18%)
- Lymphoma (3%)

64. List, in order of frequency, the most common benign neoplasms of the small intestine.
Leiomyoma > lipoma > adenoma > hemangioma

INFLAMMATORY BOWEL DISEASE

65. How do Crohn's disease and ulcerative colitis differ?
See Table 5-2.

TABLE 5-2. DISTINGUISHING FEATURES OF CROHN'S DISEASE AND ULCERATIVE COLITIS

	Crohn's Disease	Ulcerative Colitis
Symptoms	Pain is more common; bleeding is uncommon	Diarrhea with a bloody-mucosal discharge, cramping
Location	Can affect GI tract from mouth to anus	Limited to colon
Pattern of colonic involvement	Skip lesions	Continuous involvement
Histology	Transmural inflammation, granulomas, focal ulceration	Mucosal inflammation, crypt abscesses, crypt distortion
Radiologic	Terminal ileal involvement, deep ulcerations, normal haustra between involved areas, strictures, fistulas	Rectum involved, shortened colon, absence of haustra (lead-pipe sign)
Complications	Obstruction, fistulas, abscesses, kidney stones, gallstones, B_{12} deficiency	Bleeding, toxic megacolon, colon cancer

66. What are the pathologic gold standards for differentiating between Crohn's disease and ulcerative colitis?
The finding of a granuloma = Crohn's disease. The finding of crypt abscesses = ulcerative colitis. Again, these findings are documented in fewer than one third of patients, but when found, they are considered pathognomic for these diseases.

67. What are the extraintestinal manifestations of inflammatory bowel disease?
Arthritis, ankylosing spondylitis, sacroileitis, osteoporosis, erythema nodosum, pyoderma gangrenosum, aphthous ulcers, iritis, uveitis, episcleritis, fatty liver, gallstones, pericholangitis, sclerosing cholangitis, cholangiocarcinoma, kidney stones, venous thrombosis, weight loss, hypoalbuminemia, anemia, vitamin and electrolyte disturbances.

ULCERS

68. What are the two major functions of acid secretion in the stomach?
- Acid activates the enzyme pepsin by converting pepsinogen to pepsin, initiating the first stages of protein digestion.
- Acid serves as an antibacterial barrier to protect the stomach from colonization.

69. List the factors that lead to recurrent ulcer after ulcer surgery.
- Untreated *Helicobacter pylori* infection
- NSAIDs use
- Incomplete vagotomy
- Adjacent nonabsorbable suture that acts as an irritant
- "Retained antrum" syndrome, in which antral tissue left behind at surgery produces a continued source of gastric production
- Antral G-cell hyperplasia (uncommon)
- Zollinger-Ellison syndrome (gastrinoma)
- Gastric cancer

Other factors that may contribute to recurrent ulcers but have not necessarily been implicated as primary causes include smoking, enterogastric reflex (bile acid reflex), primary hyperparathyroidism, and gastric bezoar.

70. List the most common causes of peptic ulcer disease in order of frequency.
- *H. pylori* infection (duodenal >> gastric)
- Traditional NSAIDs (gastric >> duodenal)
- Hyperacidity states (e.g., Zollinger-Ellison syndrome)

71. How common is *H. pylori* infection?
H. pylori infection is the most infectious disease worldwide. It is estimated that 1 in 10 persons are infected. This microaerophilic spiral bacterium inhabits the mucus layer of the stomach. It is associated with the development of peptic ulcer disease, ocurring in up to 90+% of patients with duodenal ulcers. Although millions are infected, only ~10% develop peptic ulcer disease.

72. Which diseases are strongly associated with *H. pylori* infection?
- Peptic ulcer disease (duodenal >> gastric)
- Chronic active gastritis
- MALToma (mucosa-associated lymphoid tissue)
- Gastric carcinoma

73. How is *H. pylori* infection treated?
Over 60 treatment regimens for *H. pylori* have been used. Triple therapy (two antibiotics plus a proton pump inhibitor) is the gold standard, resulting in eradication of > 90% of the organism. At present no regimen results in 100% cure. It is prudent to know the resistance rates to antibiotics in the population being treated so that adjustments may be made. In addition, no resistance to bismuth has yet been documented. The following is a typical regimen resulting in an eradication rate of 90–95%:

- Clarithromycin, 500 mg twice daily
- Amoxicillin, 1000 mg twice daily
- Proton pump inhibitor, maximum dose twice daily

74. What is the clinical triad of Zollinger-Ellison syndrome (ZES)?
Gastric acid hypersecretion, severe ulcer disease of the upper GI tract as a direct result of acid hypersecretion, and a non-beta cell tumor of the pancreas that secretes the hormone gastrin (gastrinoma).

75. What other clues help to diagnose ZES?
The other common feature of ZES is diarrhea, which may precede the diagnosis of ZES by many years. The diagnosis should be suspected in patients with a compatible clinical history and gastric acid hypersecretion.

PANCREATITIS

76. What are the most common causes of acute pancreatitis in the U.S.?
In the U.S. 90% of cases of acute pancreatitis are due to choledocholithiasis, ethanol abuse, or idiopathic causes. Most patients who previously were thought to have an idiopathic etiology actually have been found to have diminutive gallstones (microlithiasis). In the private hospital setting, 50% of patients with acute pancreatitis have gallstones (gallstone pancreatitis). In public hospitals, up to 66% of first episodes are caused by excessive alcohol consumption.

77. Which drugs have the strongest association with acute pancreatitis?
Asparaginase, azathioprine, 6-mercaptopurine, dideoxyinosine, pentamadine, and vinca alkaloids.

78. List other drugs that may be associated with acute pancreatitis.

- Analgesics: acetaminophen, piroxicam, NSAIDs, morphine
- Diuretics: furosemide, thiazides, metolazone
- Antibiotics: sulfonamides, tetracyclines, erythromycin, ceftriaxone
- Anti-inflammatory agents: salicylates, 5-ASA products, sulfasalazine, corticosteroids, cyclosporine
- Toxins: ethanol, methanol
- Hormones: estrogens, oral contraceptive pills
- Others: octreotide, cimetidine, valproic acid, ergotamine, methyldopa, propofol, alpha interferons, zalcitabine, isotretinoin, ritonavir, ranitidine

79. List Ranson's criteria for the prognosis in acute pancreatitis.
See Table 5-3.

80. How are Ranson's criteria used to make a prognosis?
When there are fewer than three positive signs, the patient has mild disease and an excellent prognosis. The mortality rate is 10–20% with three to five signs and > 50% with six or more signs.

TABLE 5-3. RANSON'S CRITERIA FOR PROGNOSIS IN ACUTE PANCREATITIS

On Admission	In Initial 48 Hours
Age > 55 yrs	Hematocrit decrease of > 10%
WBC > 16,000/mm^3	BUN rise of > 5 mg/dL
Serum LDH > 350 IU/L	Serum calcium < 8 mg/dL
Blood glucose > 200 mg/dL	Arterial PO_2 < 60 mmHg
SGOT/AST > 250 IU/L	Base deficit > 4 mEq/L
	Estimated fluid sequestration > 6 L

WBC = white blood cell, LDH = lactate dehydrogenase, SGOT/AST = aspartate aminotransferase, BUN = blood urea nitrogen.
Ranson JH: Etiologic and prognostic factors in human acute pancreatitis: A review. Am J Gastroenterol 77:633, 1982.

81. **What conditions may cause an increase in serum amylase other than acute pancreatitis?**

Macroamylasemia
Renal failure
Mesenteric infarction
Parotitis
Burns
Cholecystitis
Post–endoscopic retrograde cholangiopancreatography
Perforated peptic ulcer disease
Ruptured ectopic pregnancy
Diabetic ketoacidosis
Peritonitis
Tumors of pancreas, salivary glands, ovary, lung, prostate
Pancreatitis complications (pseudocyst, abscess, ascites)

82. **When is surgery indicated in the management of pancreatic pseudocysts?**
Onset of symptoms, increasing size, onset of complications, and a suspicion that a cystic malignancy is present.

83. **What may be a serious vascular complication of pancreatitis?**
Splenic vein thrombosis, which is associated with pancreatic or peripancreatic inflammation and/or tumors. Splenic vein thrombosis classically results in gastric varices without accompanying esophageal varices. The definitive therapy is surgical splenectomy.

VASCULAR DISEASE

84. **What is intestinal angina?**
When occlusive vascular disease, usually atherosclerosis, affects two of the three major arteries supplying the gut (Fig. 5-2), it may be associated with a syndrome of intermittent, cramping, midabdominal pain commonly called intestinal angina. Symptoms worsen during eating, often causing patients to lose weight simply by avoiding meals or eating small ones.

85. **How is intestinal angina diagnosed and treated?**
The diagnosis is facilitated by angiography, which documents significant stenosis of vessels. Treatment for patients with a significant gradient across the stenosis is surgical bypass, endarterectomy, or percutaneous transluminal angioplasty.

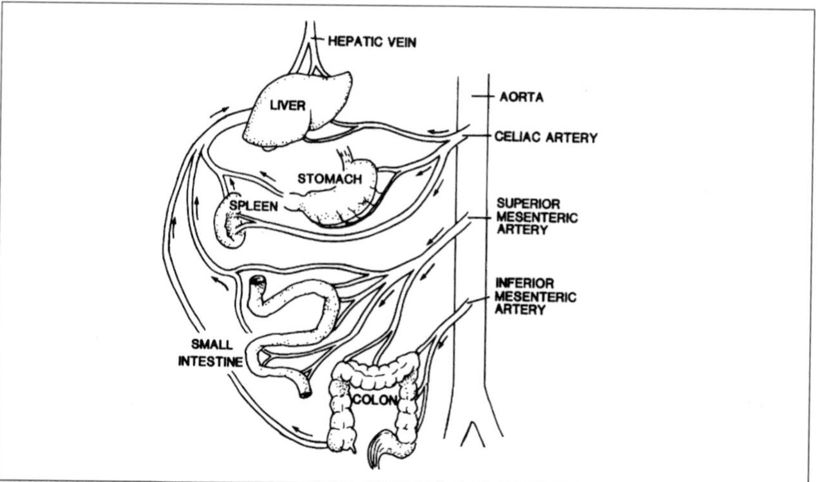

Figure 5-2. Major splanchnic organs and vessels. (From McNally PR [ed]: GI/Liver Secrets. Philadelphia, Hanley & Belfus, 1996.)

86. **Which two colonic segments are most commonly involved in ischemic colitis? Why?**
Ischemic colitis most commonly occurs in the regions lying in the "watershed" areas between two adjacent arterial supplies. These are the splenic flexure, which lies between the inferior and superior mesenteric arteries, and the rectosigmoid junction, which lies between the inferior mesenteric and interior iliac arteries.

87. **Describe the presentation of hepatic hemangioma.**
A hepatic hemangioma is a benign blood vessel tumor that is most commonly found incidentally on imaging examinations of the liver. Hemangiomas are usually single and asymptomatic and measure < 5 cm. The incidence is thought to range from 0.4 % to 20%.

88. **Define superior mesenteric artery syndrome.**
Because of its anatomic position anterior to the aorta and posterior to the superior mesenteric vessels, the third portion of the duodenum is prone to luminal compression by these vessels. Processes that result in narrowing of the aortomesenteric angle may lead to compression of the duodenum. Causes include sudden weight loss, immobilization, scleroderma, neuropathies that reduce duodenal peristalsis (e.g., diabetes), and use of narcotics.

DIARRHEA

89. **What are the four pathophysiologic mechanisms of diarrhea?**
- **Osmotic:** An osmotically active agent in the intestinal lumen cannot be absorbed and therefore draws fluid in the intestinal lumen.
- **Exudative:** Due to infection, food allergy, celiac sprue, inflammatory bowel disease, collagenous colitis, graft-versus-host disease

- **Secretory:** Mucosal stimulation of active chlorine ion secretion is seen with *E. coli, Vibrio cholerae*, hormone-producing tumors, bile acids, and long-chain fatty acids.
- **Altered intestinal transit**

90. What causes osmotic diarrhea?
Osmotic diarrhea is caused by ingestion of excessive amounts of a poorly absorbable but osmotically active solute. Commonly implicated substances include mannitol or sorbitol (seen in patients chewing large quantities of sugar-free gum), magnesium sulfate (Epsom salt), and some magnesium-containing antacids. Carbohydrate malabsorption also may cause osmotic diarrhea through the action of unabsorbed sugars (lactulose). Clinically, osmotic diarrhea stops when the patient fasts (or stops ingesting the poorly absorbable solute).

91. Explain the mechanism of secretory diarrhea.
Secretory diarrhea involves a disruption of normal bowel function. Small intestinal epithelial cells normally secrete less than they absorb, ultimately leading to a net absorption of fluid and electrolytes. If this process is interrupted by a pathologic process that stimulates increased secretion or inhibits absorption, secretory diarrhea may occur.

92. Which three diagnostic features can distinguish secretory from osmotic diarrhea?

1. The stool osmolar gap is < 50 mOsm/kg in secretory diarrhea but is > 50 mOsm/kg in osmotic diarrhea.
2. Secretory diarrhea is typically unrelated to ingested foods or solutes and persists during a 24–72-hour fast, whereas osmotic diarreha stops when ingestion of the offending solute ends.
3. Patients with a pure secretory diarrhea do not have WBCs, RBCs, or fat in their stool.

93. What organisms are responsible for bacillary dysentery?
The term *dysentery* refers to a diarrheal stool that contains inflammatory exudate (pus) and blood. *Bacillary dysentery* refers to infectious diarrhea caused by invasive pathogens, most commonly, *Shigella, Salmonella, Campylobacter,* and enteroinvasive or enterohemorrhagic *Escherichia coli.*

94. A 50-year-old woman complains of 6–8 loose stools per day for 1 month. The cause is not immediately evident after a careful history and physical exam. What diagnostic tests should be performed at this stage?
If performed early in the disease course, a complete blood count, serum chemistry profile, and urinalysis may help pinpoint the likely causes of diarrhea. For example, the patient who has an anemia with a very high MCV may be suspected of having malabsorption and diarrhea based on the presence of ileal disease and inability to absorb vitamin B_{12}. Basic stool studies, including bacterial culture and sensitivity, Sudan stain for fat, Wright's stain for WBCs, test for occult blood, and a phenolphthalein test for the presence of laxative ingestion, are simple and quickly obtainable tests that may give valuable results.

95. Discuss the role of proctosigmoidoscopy in the diagnosis of diarrhea.
Proctosigmoidoscopy is a very important part of the examination in most patients with chronic and recurrent diarrhea. In the patient aged 50 and older this should be expanded to a full colonoscopy so as to allow screening for polyps. Examination of the rectal mucosa may reveal pseudomembranes seen with antibiotic-associated diarrhea, discrete ulceration typical of amebiasis, or a diffusely inflamed granular mucosa seen in ulcerative colitis. Biopsy specimens can be obtained through the scope for histologic examination, and fresh stool samples can be collected for cultures.

96. What is traveler's diarrhea?

Traveler's diarrhea is a common term given to the onset of diarrhea in patients who have traveled to other countries, usually in the third world, where the enteric flora are different. Eighty percent of cases are caused by bacteria that can be transmitted via a fecal-oral route. Viruses account for 10% of cases, and parasites cause 2–3%. In the remainder of cases the cause is unknown.

97. How can traveler's diarrhea be prevented?

Travelers should carefully select, handle and prepare food and dairy products. Everything should be washed thoroughly and freshly cooked. Commercially bottled water, carbonated beverages, and beer are safe—but ice is not!

98. What are most common organisms implicated in traveler's diarrhea?

Enterotoxigenic *E. coli*
Enteroaggregative *E. coli*
Shigella sp.
Salmonella sp.
Campylobacter jejuni
Aeromonas sp.
Plesiomonas sp.
Norwalk virus
Rotavirus
Giardia sp.
Cryptosporidium sp.
Cyclospora sp.

99. What prophylactic regimens are recommended for traveler's diarrhea?

- Ciprofloxacin , 500 mg twice daily for 5 days (or one of the other fluoroquinolones)
- Bismuth subsalicyate (Pepto-Bismol), 2 tablets with every meal and at bedtime for 5 days
- Bactrim DS, one tablet twice daily for 3 days (*Note:* Many organisms are now resistant to Bactrim.)

100. How does the time of onset of illness relate to the possible causes of food poisoning?

See Table 5-4.

NONHEPATITIS LIVER DISEASE

101. Explain the Child-Pugh system for staging cirrhosis.

See Table 5-5.

102. Summarize the clinical manifestations of liver disease and their pathogenetic basis.

See Table 5-6.

103. A patient with known cirrhosis of the liver presents with massive swelling of the abdomen. A fluid wave can be elicited on examination of the abdomen by striking one flank and feeling the transmitted wave on the opposite flank. What is the appropriate diagnostic procedure at this point?

After the diagnosis of new-onset ascites on physical examination, all patients should undergo abdominal paracentesis and ascitic fluid analysis. A small amount of fluid is aspirated from the midline of the abdomen between the umbilicus and pubis with a small-gauge needle. The most important tests to order are the serum albumin value and cell count.

104. Explain the significance of the serum albumin value.

The serum albumin value should be measured within a few hours of the paracentesis to ensure accuracy. Ascitic fluid with a serum: ascitic fluid albumin gradient (S-A AG) > 1.1 gm/dL is designated as high-gradient ascites. Fluids with values < 1.1 gm/dL are designated as

TABLE 5-4. CAUSES OF FOOD POISONING

Onset	Symptoms and Signs	Agents
1 h	Nausea, vomiting, abdominal cramps	Heavy metal poisoning (copper, zinc, tin, cadmium)
1 h	Paresthesias	Scrombroid poisoning, shellfish poisoning, Chinese restaurant syndrome (MSG), niacin poisoning
1–6 h	Nausea and vomiting	Preformed toxins of *Staphylococcus aureus* and *Bacillus cereus*
2 h	Delirium, parasympathetic hyperactivity, hallucinations, disulfiram reaction, or gastroenteritis	Toxic mushroom ingestion
8–16 h	Abdominal cramps, diarrhea	In vivo production of enterotoxins by *Clostridium perfringens* and *B. cereus*
6–24 h	Abdominal cramps, diarrhea, followed by hepatorenal failure	Toxic mushroom ingestion (*Amanita* sp.)
16–48 h	Fever, abdominal cramps, diarrhea	*Salmonella, Shigella, Clostridium jejuni,* invasive *E. coli, Yersinia enterocolitica, Vibrio parahemolyticus*
16–72 h	Abdominal cramps, diarrhea	Norwalk agent and related viruses, enterotoxins produced by *Vibrio* sp., *E. coli*, and occasionally *Salmonella, Shigella*, and *C. jejuni*
18–36 h	Nausea, vomiting, diarrhea, paralysis	Food-borne botulism
72–100 h	Bloody diarrhea without fever	Enterotoxigenic *E. coli*, most frequently serotype 0157:H7
1–3 wk	Chronic diarrhea	Raw milk ingestion

Mandell GL, et al (eds): Principles and Practice of Infectious Diseases, 4th ed. New York, Churchill Livingstone, 1995.

TABLE 5-5. CHILD-PUGH STAGING OF CIRRHOSIS

Parameter	Score 1	Score 2	Score 3
Albumin	> 3.5	3.0–3.5	< 3.0
Bilirubin	< 2.0	2.0–3.0	> 3.0
Prologation of PT	< 4 sec	4–6 sec	> 6 sec
Ascites	None	Moderate	Massive
Encephalopathy	None	Moderate	Severe
Child's score:	A = 5–6	B = 7–9	C = > 9

TABLE 5-6. CLINICAL MANIFESTATIONS OF LIVER DISEASE

Sign/Symptom	Pathogenesis	Liver Disease
Constitutional		
Fatigue, anorexia, malaise, weight loss	Liver failure	Severe acute or chronic hepatitis Cirrhosis
Fever	Hepatic inflammation or infection	Liver abscess Alcoholic hepatitis Viral hepatitis
Fetor hepaticus	Abnormal methionine metabolism	Acute or chronic liver failure
Cutaneous		
Spider telangiectasias, palmar erythema	Altered estrogen and androgen metabolism	Cirrhosis
Jaundice	Diminished bilirubin excretion	Biliary obstruction Severe liver disease
Pruritus		Biliary obstruction
Xanthomas and xanthelasma	Increased serum lipids	Biliary obstruction/cholestasis
Endocrine		
Gynecomastia, testicular atrophy, diminished libido	Altered estrogen and androgen metabolism	Cirrhosis
Hypoglycemia	Decreased glycogen stores and gluconeogenesis	Liver failure
Gastrointestinal		
RUQ abdominal pain	Liver swelling, infection	Acute hepatitis Hepatocellular carcinoma Liver congestion (heart failure) Acute cholecystitis Liver abscess
Abdominal swelling	Ascites	Cirrhosis, portal hypertension
GI bleeding	Esophageal varices	Portal hypertension
Hematologic		
Decreased RBCs, WBCs, platelets	Hypersplenism	Cirrhosis, portal hypertension
Ecchymoses	Decreased synthesis of clotting factors	Liver failure
Neurologic		
Altered sleep pattern, subtle behavioral changes, somnolence confusion, ataxia, asterixis, obtundation	Hepatic encephalopathy	Liver failure, portosystemic shunting of blood

RUQ = right upper quadrant.
From Andreoli TE, et al: Cecil Essentials of Medicine, 2nd ed. Philadelphia, W.B. Saunders, 1990, p 312.

low-gradient ascites. The terms *high-albumin gradient* and *low-albumin gradient* should replace the terms *transudative* and *exudative* in the description of ascites.

105. **Which diseases are associated with high-gradient ascites?**
Portal hypertension (i.e., cirrhosis), congestive heart failure, constrictive pericarditis, inferior vena cava obstruction, hypoalbuminemia, Meigs' syndrome, myxedema, fulminant hepatic failure, nephrotic syndrome (occasionally), and mixed ascites.

106. **Which diseases are associated with low-gradient ascites?**
Peritoneal neoplasms, pancreatic ascites, tuberculosis, nephrotic syndrome, ascites due to bowel obstruction or infarction, and ascites in connective tissue diseases.

107. **Explain the significance of the blood cell count.**
A large number of RBCs in the fluid or grossly bloody ascites suggests neoplasm. An ascitic fluid and WBC count of > 500/mL is strongly suggestive of a peritoneal infection or an inflammatory process.

108. **What other tests should be considered in the diagnosis of ascites?**
Other tests to be ordered in the appropriate clinical settings include cytologic examination, lactic dehydrogenase, specific tumor markers, glucose, and cultures for bacteria, mycobacteria, and fungi.

109. **List the benign primary hepatic lesions.**
- Focal nodular hyperplasia
- Hepatic adenoma
- Bile duct adenoma
- Bile duct hamartoma
- Biliary cyst
- Hemangioma
- Focal fat

110. **List the malignant primary hepatic lesions.**
- Hepatocellular carcinoma
- Hepatoblastoma
- Cholangiocarcinoma
- Angiosarcoma
- Biliary crystadenoma and/or carcinoma
- Sarcoma

111. **How is acetaminophen toxic to the liver?**
Acetaminophen is toxic to the liver only in excessive doses or when the protective detoxifying pathway in the liver is overwhelmed. Accumulation of the toxic metabolic, N-acetyl-p-benzoquinone, is responsible for death of hepatocytes. Acetaminophen is the second most common cause of death from poisoning in the United States.

112. **At what doses does acetaminophen become toxic to the liver?**
Hepatotoxicity of acetaminophen occurs in nonalcoholic patients at doses > 7.5 gm. A potentially lethal effect is seen with ingestion of > 140 mg/kg (10 gm in a 70-kg man). Chronic alcoholics are at greater risk of acetaminophen injury due to alcohol induction of the cytochrome P450 system and attendant malnutrition and low levels of glutathione. Glutathione is an intracellular protectant naturally found in the hepatocyte.

113. **What are the absolute contraindications to liver transplantation?**
Extrahepatic malignancy, AIDS, active/ongoing substance abuse, uncontrolled systemic infection, inability to comply with the posttransplant immunosuppression regimen and advanced cardiopulmonary disease.

114. **What is the most prevalent liver disease in the U.S.?**
Nonalcoholic steatohepatitis (NASH), also known as nonalcoholic fatty liver disease. This disease is present in ~20% of the American population and perhaps as high as 30–80% of people who are obese. NASH is clinically silent except for abnormal liver tests and is most often discovered incidentally. Imaging studies usually show steatosis of the liver.

ESOPHAGEAL DISEASE

115. **Describe the approach to treatment of GERD.**
See Table 5-7.

TABLE 5-7. TREATMENT OF GASTROESOPHAGEAL REFLUX DISEASE

Dietary and lifestyle changes
- Postural therapy: elevate head of bed 6–8 inches; avoid lying down after eating; remain upright at least 2 h after eating (most important lifestyle change)
- Limit intake of foods and drink that reduce lower esophageal sphincter (LES) pressure: fatty foods, peppermint, acidic foods, onions, chocolate, caffeine, alcohol
- Avoid medications that reduce LES pressure: theophylline, nitrates, tranquilizers, progesterone, calcium blockers, anticolinergic agens, beta-adrenergic agonists
- Stop smoking
- Decrease the size of meals
- Weight reduction if obese
- Avoid tight-fitting garments around abdomen

Proton pump inhibitor
- Most potent single agent for treating severe reflux esophagitis (e.g., omeprazole, lansoprazole, rabeprazole, pantoprazole, and esomeprazole)
- Acts to increase the pH of gastric contents and heal erosive esophagitis

Endoscopic therapy: to increase LES pressure

Surgery (endoscopic or open): aimed at restoring LES competence or preventing reflux

116. **What are the extraesophageal manifestations of GERD?**
- Cardiac: atypical chest pain, arrythmias, ischemia
- Vocal cords: laryngitis, granuloma, polyps, ulcers, neoplasm
- Respiratory: adult-onset asthma, recurrent bronchitis, aspiration or chronic interstitial pneumonia, irreversible airway disease, pulmonary fibrosis, sleep apnea
- Chronic or recurrent cough

- Pharyngeal: globus, pharyngitis, recurrent sore throat, hoarseness
- Oral: burning mouth syndrome, dental erosions
- Other: sudden infant death syndrome, otitis media

117. How is extra-esophageal GERD treated?
Treatment for extraesophageal manifestations requires high doses of proton pump inhibitors twice daily for a minimum of 3 months.

118. What is Barrett's esophagus?
Barrett's esophagus is a complication that develops in patients with long-standing reflux peptic esophagitis. It represents a unique reparative process in which the original squamous epithelial cell lining of the esophagus is replaced by a metaplastic columnar-type epithelium. In most adults, this epithelium resembles intestinal mucosa, complete with goblet cells.

119. Summarize the clinical significance of Barrett's esophagus.
The clinical significance lies primarily in its malignant potential. There is an increased risk (30–1253 above the general population) of esophageal adenocarcinoma arising in Barrett's epithelium. The actual incidence is unknown, but the average is about 10%. Currently adenocarcinoma of the junction, which primarily arises from Barrett's epithelium, is the fastest growing GI cancer among white men in the U.S.

120. How is Barrett's esophagus managed?
The management of Barrett's esophagus is the same as the treatment of GERD. Acid suppression with proton pump inhibitors in high doses controls symptoms and heals esophageal damage. Although the inflammatory changes associated with Barrett's epithelium can be healed, once Barrett's epithelium has developed, the process cannot be reversed by any form of antireflux therapy.

121. Is routine surveillance for esophageal cancer necessary in patients with Barrett's esophagus?
The benefits of periodic endoscopic screening for dysplasia have not been shown, but endoscopic surveillance and four-quadrant biopsies of each 2-cm segment of the esophagus at 1- to 2-year intervals are advocated by most.

122. Name the three types of esophageal dysphagia. How can a patient's history be used to distinguish between them?

- **Transfer:** pathologic alteration in the neuromotor mechanism of the oropharyngeal phase.
- **Transit:** abnormal peristalsis and LES function. Transit dysphagia is due to motor disorders in which the primary peristaltic pump of the esophagus fails.
- **Obstructive:** mechanical narrowing of the esophagus. Obstructive dysphagia may be due to intrinsic lesions blocking the esophagus (e.g., peptic strictures, esophageal webs, carcinoma) or to extrinsic lesions (e.g., mediastinal tumors) compressing the esophagus.

123. Describe the typical history of a patient with transfer dysphagia.
Patients give a history of difficulty in swallowing liquids, while solids pass normally. These patients may have stroke, myasthenia gravis, amyotrophic lateral sclerosis, or botulism.

124. What is the typical history of a patient with transit dysphagia?
Motor disorders often begin with dysphagia to both solids and liquids. Transit dysphagia is commonly seen in such entities as achalasia and scleroderma. Dysphagia that worsens on ingesting cold liquids and improves with warm liquids suggests a motor disorder.

125. How does obstructive dysphagia typically present?
Obstructive dysphagia typically presents as dysphagia to solid food that may progress to include liquids. Patients usually give a history of eating only soft foods, chewing foods longer, and avoiding steak, apples, and fresh bread. Solid-food dysphagia associated with a long history of heartburn and regurgitation suggests a peptic stricture. If the bolus can be dislodged by repeated swallowing or drinking water, a motor disorder is usually the cause.

126. What is the initial diagnostic step after a thorough history and examination?
The initial diagnostic step is a barium swallow. The barium swallow is then quickly followed by an upper GI endoscopy.

127. Define achalasia.
Achalasia is the best-known motor disorder of the esophagus. Its usual onset is in patients aged 25–60 years, with an equal frequency between the sexes. Symptoms include dysphagia (solids and liquids), regurgitation of undigested foods, heartburn, and chest pain.

128. How is achalasia diagnosed?
The diagnosis can be made by esophageal manometry, which yields the following characteristic findings:

- Loss of peristalsis (absolute requirement)
- Failure of the LES to relax
- Increased LES pressure

129. Define pseudoachalasia.
Pseudoachalasia refers to other esophageal conditions that mimic the clinical and x-ray findings of achalasia. The majority of causes are neoplasms that either obstruct the LES directly by tumor or as a paraneoplastic disorder. Common causes are amyloidosis, sarcoidosis, Chagas' disease, eosiniphilic gastroenteritis, neurofibromatosis, idiopathic intestinal pseudo-obstruction, Anderson-Fabry's disease and multiple endocrine neoplasia type IIB.

130. How is 24-hour pH monitoring endoscopy used to assess patients with suspected esophageal disease?
24-Hour ambulatory pH monitoring of the esophagus provides a temporal profile of acid reflux events and acid clearance and correlates these events with symptoms. Specific variables measured include the number of reflux episodes in 24 hours, acid clearance times from the esophagus, and esophageal exposure to acid. These values can be determined while the patient is in the upright or recumbent position. This is the gold standard for documenting or excluding GERD and determining whether atypical GERD symptoms are a result of acid reflux. Anyone who undergoes surgery for GERD must have a 24-hour pH probe and esophageal manometry.

131. Summarize the role of esophageal manometry in the assessment of esophageal disease.
Esophageal manometry is useful in evaluating patients with noncardiac chest pain and a history suggestive of esophageal motor disorder, achalasia, or esophageal reflux disease.

132. Why is endoscopy useful in assessing esophageal disorders?
Endoscopy provides a direct view of the esophageal mucosa and allows directed biopsy when necessary. Endoscopy and biopsy are necessary to make a definitive diagnosis of many esophageal diseases (e.g., malignancy). The benefits of endoscopy include the ability to perform therapeutic intervention such as biopsy, cytology, brushing, dilations, and stent placement.

MALABSORPTION

133. What causes Whipple's disease?
Whipple's disease is a systemic disease that may affect almost any organ system of the body, but in most cases it involves the small intestine. The causative agent is the bacterium *Tropheryma whippelii.* Patients present with intestinal malabsorption, weight loss, diarrhea, abdominal pain, fever, anemia, lymphadenopathy, and arthralgias. Nervous system symptoms, pericarditis, or endocarditis may also be present.

134. How is Whipple's disease diagnosed?
The major pathologic feature is infiltration of involved tissues with large glycoprotein-containing macrophages that stain strongly positive with a periodic acid–Schiff stain. This diagnosis is most often made by biopsy of the small intestine. One can also see characteristic rod-shaped, gram-positive bacilli that are not acid-fast.

135. How is Whipple's disease treated?
Effective treatment includes prolonged antibiotic therapy, usually with double-strength trimethoprim/sulfamethoxazole given for a minimum of 1 year. Repeat intestinal biopsy should document the disappearance of the Whipple bacillus before therapy is discontinued. Relapses are not uncommon and are treated for a minimum of 6–12 months. Patients allergic to sulfonamides should receive parenteral penicillin.

136. In a small-bowel biopsy, the mucosa shows flat villa with markedly hyperplastic crypts. What is the diagnosis?
Celiac sprue, also called gluten enteropathy, is an allergic disease characterized by malabsorption of nutrients secondary to the damaged small intestinal mucosa. The responsible antigen is gluten, a water-insoluble protein found in cereal grains such as wheat, barley, oats, and rye. Withdrawal of gluten from the diet results in complete remission of both the clinical symptoms and mucosal lesions. Although this disease is present worldwide, the distribution varies; the highest prevalence is in western Ireland.

137. What is dermatitis herpetiformis?
Dermatitis herpetiformis is a pruritic skin condition that also may be reversed with dietary therapy (gluten restriction). It is characterized by papulovesicular lesions in a symmetrical distribution on the elbows, knees, buttocks, face, scalp, neck, and trunk.

138. How does dermatitis herpetiformis relate to celiac sprue?
Although most patients with celiac sprue do not develop skin lesions of dermatitis herpetiformis, patients with dermatitis herpetiformis usually have the sprue-like mucosal lesion in the small bowel. The two diseases appear to be distinct entities that respond to the same dietary restrictions. Unlike the intestinal disease, the skin lesions can be treated with the antibiotic dapsone, with a clinical response within 1–2 weeks.

139. What is the blind-loop syndrome?
The blind-loop syndrome is a constellation of symptoms and laboratory abnormalities that include malabsorption of vitamin B_{12}, steatorrhea, hypoproteinemia, weight loss, and diarrhea. These symptoms are attributed to overgrowth of bacteria within the small intestine and have been associated with a number of diseases and surgical abnormalities. The common link between these conditions is abnormal motility of a segment of small intestine, resulting in stasis. The aim of therapy is to reduce the bacterial overgrowth and consists of antibiotics and, when feasible, correction of the small intestinal abnormality that led to the condition.

KEY POINTS: GASTROENTEROLOGY ✓

1. Proton pump inhibitors should be given 15–30 minutes prior to a meal to be most effective.
2. CT scan with contrast is the most accurate radiographic test to diagnose pancreatitis.
3. Hepatocellular carcinoma is the fifth most common malignancy worldwide—accounting for 1 million deaths per year.
4. The mechanism for GERD is inappropriate, transient relaxation of the lower esophageal sphincter
5. Irritable bowel syndrome is more common in men in areas outside the U.S.
6. The two most common symptoms of GERD are heartburn (burning sensation that patients feel behind the breast bone area) and regurgitation (effortless passage of fluid into back of mouth or throat).
7. The majority of children who experience GERD below the age of 10 will outgrow their symptoms.
8. The most common benign liver lesion is focal nodular hyperplasia.

140. Describe the process of normal fat absorption.

Normal fat absorption requires all phases of digestion to be intact. The process begins with secretion of pancreatic lipase and colipase. These enzymes are activated intraluminally and require an optimal pH of 6–8. Both enzymes are necessary for triglyceride hydrolysis in the duodenum. The products of triglyceride hydrolysis (i.e., fatty acids and monoglycerides) then must be solubilized by bile salts to form micelles, which are subsequently absorbed by the small intestinal epithelium.

141. What mechanisms may lead to fat malabsorption?

- Any disorder that causes deficiencies of pancreatic enzyme secretion or leads to an acidic intraluminal environment may lead to fat malabsorption.
- Any disorder that interrupts the enterohepatic circulation or secretion of bile salts may impair micelle formation and therefore result in fat malabsorption.
- If the intestinal epithelial cell is in some way diseased, monoglyceride absorption and processing into chylomicrons for transport out of the small intestine may be impaired, leading to fat malabsorption.
- Disease of the intestinal lymphatics with impaired chylomicron transport has also been reported to result in fat malabsorption.

142. Which diseases can affect fat absorption?

- Chronic pancreatitis
- Cystic fibrosis
- Pancreatic carcinoma
- Postgastrectomy syndrome
- Biliary tract obstruction
- Terminal ileal resection or disease
- Cholestatic liver disease
- Intestinal epithelial disease (e.g., Whipple's disease, sprue, eosinophilic gastroenteritis)

- Lymphatic disease (e.g., abetalipoproteinemia, intestinal lymphangiectasia, lymphoma, tuberculous adenitis)
- Small bowel bacterial overgrowth (bile salts are deconjugated and inactivated by bacteria)
- ZES (low intraluminal pH)

143. Summarize the pathologic mechanism of small bowel bacteria overgrowth. How is it diagnosed?

Any abnormality of the small intestine that results in local stasis or recirculation of intestinal contents is likely to be associated with marked proliferation of intraluminal bacteria. The gold standard for diagnosing bacterial overgrowth is culture of the upper small bowel of > 100,000 cfu/mL.

144. What disorders may be associated disorders with small bowel bacteria overgrowth?

- Gastric proliferation of bacteria as seen in hypochlorhydric or achlorhydric states, particularly when in combination with motor or anatomic disturbances
- Small intestinal stagnation associated with anatomic alterations following surgery, such as afferent loop syndrome after a Billroth II procedure
- Duodenal and jejunal diverticulosis, particularly as seen in scleroderma
- Surgically created blind loops, such as end-to-side anastomoses
- Chronic low-grade obstruction secondary to small intestinal strictures, adhesions, inflammation, or carcinoma
- Motor disturbances of the small intestine (e.g., scleroderma, idiopathic pseudo-obstruction, diabetic neuropathy)
- Abnormal communication between the proximal small intestine and the distal intestinal tract, as seen in gastrocolic or jejunocolic fistulas or resection of the ileocecal valve
- Immunodeficiency syndromes (e.g., AIDS, primary immunodeficiency states, malnutrition)

145. How does bacterial overgrowth of the small bowel result in fat malabsorption?

The bacterial enzymes deconjugate intraluminal bile salts to free bile acids, which are unable to solubilize monoglycerides and free fatty acids into micelles for absorption by the epithelial cells. The result is impaired absorption of fat and fat-soluble vitamins.

146. What constitutes a normal fecal fat concentration? What is steatorrhea?

The typical U.S. diet consists of 100–150 gm of fat per day. Fat absorption is extremely efficient, and most of the ingested fat is absorbed with very little excretion into the stool. The average fecal fat concentration for the normal person is 4–6 gm/day, ranging to an upper limit of normal of approximately 7 gm. Patients with steatorrhea, or increased excretion of fecal fat, may have up to 10 times this amount in the stool.

147. How is steatorrhea detected?

A 72-hour stool sample is collected while the patient is on a defined dietary fat intake of > 100 gm/day. Chemical analysis of the stool collection measures the amount of fat present. This test is highly reliable but neither specific nor sensitive in determining the etiology of steatorrhea.

OBSTRUCTION

148. Name the four most common causes of mechanical small bowel obstruction in adults.

- Adhesions (about 74%)
- Hernias (8%)
- Malignancies of the small bowel (8%)
- Inflammatory bowel disease with stricture formation

149. Define small bowel ileus.
Paralytic ileus is a relatively common disorder and occurs when neural, humoral, and metabolic factors combine to stimulate reflexes that inhibit intestinal motility. The result is small bowel and/or colonic distention due to intestinal muscle paralysis.

150. What seven entities may cause small bowel ileus?
- Abdominal surgery
- Peritonitis
- Generalized sepsis
- Electrolyte imbalance (especially hypokalemia)
- Retroperitoneal hemorrhage
- Spinal fractures
- Pelvic fractures

151. What role do drugs play in small bowel ileus?
Drugs such as phenothiazines and narcotics inhibit small bowel motility and also may contribute to paralysis.

152. How is small bowel ileus treated?
Treatment consists of NG suction to relieve distention and IV fluids to replace losses, followed by correction of the underlying disorder.

153. What conditions may aggravate or be associated with colonic pseudo-obstruction?
See Table 5-8.

TABLE 5-8. CONDITIONS ASSOCIATED WITH COLONIC PSEUDO-OBSTRUCTION
1. Trauma (nonoperative) and surgery (gynecologic, orthopedic, urologic)
2. Inflammatory processes (pancreatitis, cholecystitis)
3. Infections
4. Malignancy
5. Radiation therapy
6. Drugs (narcotics, antidepressants, clonidine, anticholinergics)
7. Cardiovascular disease
8. Neurologic disease
9. Respiratory failure
10. Metabolic disease (diabetes, hypothyroidism, electrolyte imbalance, uremia)
11. Alcoholism

154. What are bezoars?
Bezoars are clusters of food or foreign matter that have undergone partial digestion in the stomach, failed to pass through the pylorus into the small bowel, and formed a mass in the stomach. Substances typically comprising bezoars include hair (trichobezoars) and, more commonly, plant matter (phytobezoars).

155. How do patients with bezoars present?
Bezoars may become quite large and can present with abdominal mass, gastric outlet obstruction, attacks of nausea and vomiting, and peptic ulceration. Factors important in the formation of bezoars include the amount of indigestible materials in the diet (pulpy, fibrous fruit or vegetables such as oranges), the quality of the chewing mechanism, and loss of pyloric function, which limits the size of food particles that may enter the duodenum.

BILIARY TRACT DISEASE

156. Which U.S. ethnic groups have the highest prevalence of cholesterol gallstone formation?
American Indians and Mexican Americans.

157. List the types of gallstones.
- Cholesterol: 70–80% of all stones in Western countries; risks are female gender, obesity, age over 40 years, and multiparity
- Pigmented (20–30%)
- Black calcium bilibrubinate: risks are cirrhosis, chronic hemolytic syndromes
- Brown calcium salts: can form de novo in bile ducts; associated with infections of biliary system

158. What is Charcot's triad?
Right-upper-quadrant pain, jaundice, and fever. This triad is present in ~50% of patients with bacterial cholangitis.

159. Which tests are used in the initial diagnostic evaluation of a patient with suspected obstructive jaundice?
The cause of jaundice can be determined in many cases from clinical data and routine laboratory tests. The only special study that is routinely useful in the early evaluation of obstructive jaundice is an ultrasound scan of the gallbladder, bile ducts, and liver. Ultrasound is fairly specific for detecting gallstones and ductal dilatation (the latter signifying ductal obstruction). However, a negative scan does not prove the absence of stones or obstruction, since the sensitivity of ultrasound in detecting obstruction is only about 90%.

160. What are the advantages of endoscopic ultrasound (EUS)?
EUS is an excellent noninvasive method of assessing the patient with obstructive jaundice. It can image the entire pancreaticobiliary system and document the presence of tumors, stones, or strictures. More advanced EUS systems are equipped to guide biopsies and obtain tissue samples via fine-needle aspiration. The primary limitation of EUS is that it is not yet widely available.

161. Discuss the role of CT in the evaluation of obstructive jaundice.
Abdominal CT is fairly sensitive for detecting ductal dilatation and can be useful in localizing the site of ductal obstruction. A CT scan is less able to detect stones of the gallbladder and common bile duct than ultrasound, but it is better able to image mass lesions and to evaluate the pancreas.

162. Is magnetic retrograde cholangiopancreatiography (MRCP) useful in the evaluation of obstructive jaundice?
MRCP is a useful diagnostic tool in the evaluation of jaundice. MRCP can reveal the size of the ducts and document presence of stones, although it has not supplanted the ultrasound.

163. Are liver scans helpful in the evaluation of jaundice?
Liver biopsy in the patient with extrahepatic ductal obstruction is not routinely useful. It may reveal evidence of cholestasis and cholangitis but will not help to determine the cause. A liver scan using technetium sulfur colloid is of very little value in the jaundiced patient.

164. What causes air in the biliary system?
Previous surgery or endoscopic procedure is the most common cause. Other causes include penetrating ulcers, erosion of gallstone into the bowel lumen, traumatic fistula, neoplasms, and bowel obstruction.

IRRITABLE BOWEL SYNDROME

165. What is irritable bowel syndrome (IBS)?
IBS is defined as a functional bowel disorder that is characterized by at least 3 months, which does not have to be consecutive, in the past 12 months of abdominal discomfort or pain that has two or three of the Rome II criteria:

- Relief with defecation
- Onset associated with a change in frequency of stool
- Onset associated with a change in form or appearance of stool

166. What findings suggest organic disease instead of IBS?
New onset of symptoms in an elderly patient
Pain that interferes with normal sleep patterns
Weight loss
Anemia
Blood in the stools
Pain on awakening from sleep
Diarrhea that awakens the patient
Fever
Steatorrhea
Physical exam abnormalities

167. What is the differential diagnosis of IBS?
Psychiatric disorders (depression, anxiety, somatization)
Diabetes
Scleroderma
Inflammatory bowel disease
Chronic pancreatitis
Postgrastrectomy syndromes
Medications
Hypothryoidism
Lactose malabsorption
Endocrine disorders
Celiac sprue
Infectious diarrhea

BIBLIOGRAPHY

1. Feczko PJ, Halpert RD (eds): Case Review: Gastrointestinal Imaging. St. Louis, Mosby, 2000.
2. Lichetenstein GR, Wu GD (eds): The Requisites in Gastroenterology: Vol 2: Small and Large Intestines. St. Louis, Mosby, 2003.
3. Reddy KR, Long WB (eds): The Requisites in Gastroenterology: Vol 3: Hepatobiliary Tract and Pancreas. St. Louis, Mosby, 2003.
4. Rustgi AK (ed): The Requisites in Gastroenterology: Vol 1: Esophagus and Stomach. St. Louis, Mosby, 2003.
5. Sleisenger MH, Fordtran JS (eds): Gastrointestinal Disease: Pathophysiology, Diagnosis, and Management, 7th ed. Philadelphia, W.B. Saunders, 2003.
6. Tytgat GNJ, Classen M, Waye JD, Nakazawa S: Practice of Therapeutic Endoscopy, 2nd ed. London, W. B. Saunders, 2000.

ONCOLOGY

Teresa G. Hayes, M.D., Ph.D.

CHAPTER 6

While there are several chronic diseases more destructive to life than cancer, none is more feared.

Charles H. Mayo (1865–1939)
Annals of Surgery 83:357, 1926

GENERAL ISSUES

1. **Define carcinogenesis.**
Carcinogenesis is the alteration of normal cells into malignant cells. It is generally a multistage evolution of genetic and epigenetic alterations that causes cells to escape the normal growth constraints of their host.

2. **What are the known genetically related mechanisms of neoplasia?**
Four broad categories of genes can influence the origin and progression of neoplasia:
   - Oncogenes
   - Tumor suppressor genes
   - Regulators of cell death
   - Mutation control genes

3. **Describe the effects of oncogenes.**
Oncogenes in humans and other animals have the capacity to transform normal cells into malignant ones. These genes, acquired at conception or mutated during life, make the patient susceptible to cancer by altering or impairing several processes:
   - Production of nuclear transcription factors that control cell growth (e.g., *myc*).
   - Signal transduction within cells (e.g., *ras*).
   - Interaction of growth factors and their receptors (e.g., *her/neu*).

   More than 100 different oncogenes have been identified, but only some have been associated with human cancers exclusively. Mutations convert proto-oncogenes to oncogenes by amplification, translocation, and point mutation.

4. **How do tumor suppressor genes affect carcinogenesis?**
Mutations of tumor suppressor genes must occur in both alleles to cause loss of function and thus affect tumor growth. Multiple tumor suppressor genes have been identified (e.g., *p53* and *rb*) and are found in many different types of cancers. These mutations are the basis of the inherited predispositions to cancers and are inherited in the heterozygous state.

5. **Describe the role of regulators of cell death.**
The cell death genes are involved in the programmed death (**apoptosis**) of cells no longer needed by the body. Mutation in one of these genes (e.g., *bcl-2*) allows cells to live that should have died, causing excessive accumulation of cells. Activation of the **telomerase** gene, which controls cell senescence, is thought to cause cells to become immortal by turning off the normal aging process.

6. **What are mutation control genes?**
Genes such as *hMSH2* and *hMLH1* are responsible for ensuring the fidelity of the DNA duplication process. Microsatellite instability results from the faulty DNA editing process. Subsequently, the mutation rate increases and cancers occur.

7. **List common environmental causes of cancer.**
   - Social agent (e.g., tobacco, alcohol)
   - Occupational exposure: arsenic, benzene, CCl_4, chromium, combustion byproducts (engine exhaust), polycyclic hydrocarbons (coal byproducts)
   - Ionizing radiation: UV-B (sunlight), mining, others
   - Dietary factor: aflatoxin B, high-fat diet, nitrates/nitrites (converted endogenously to nitrosamines), smoked foods, diet low in fresh fruits and vegetables
   - Foreign body reactants (e.g., asbestos fiber)
   - Chronic inflammation (e.g., ulcerative colitis)
   - Infectious agents (e.g., Epstein-Barr virus, hepatitis B and C viruses, human papillomavirus, human T-lymphotropic virus, *Helicobacter pylori*
   - Iatrogenic agents (e.g., cancer chemotherapeutic drugs, DES, estrogens, Thoratrast)

8. **Summarize dietary "protective" factors.**
Diets high in antioxidants and lycopene, including many fruits and vegetables (such as tomatoes and broccoli), are thought to protect against cancer development by scavenging for free radicals. Some vitamins may modify the effect of chemical carcinogenesis: vitamin A (which promotes the differentiation of epithelial tissues), vitamin C (which blocks the formation of N-nitrosocarcinogens from nitrite and secondary amines), and vitamin E (which is a free-radical scavenger).

9. **Which cancers tend to cluster in families?**
Some common cancers (e.g., breast, endometrial, colon, prostate, lung, melanoma, and stomach) have a 2–3 times increased risk of development in first-degree relatives. This cluster may be due to hereditary factors, shared exposures to environmental carcinogens, chance associations, or a combination of all three.

10. **Summarize the familial clustering of breast cancer.**
The familial clustering of breast cancer may be due, in about 10–15% of cases, to a genetic locus (*BRCA1* or *BRCA2*, several others) that is predictive of familial breast and/or ovarian cancer.

KEY POINTS: FAMILIAL CANCER

1. Up to 15% of cancers are familial, due to inherited chromosomal alterations.
2. A careful family history is essential.
3. Screening of family members is indicated in autosomal dominant conditions.
4. Chemoprevention (e.g., tamoxifen for breast cancer) or prophylactic removal of the tissue at risk may be considered in very high-risk families.

11. **Describe the Lynch cancer family syndrome.**
The Lynch cancer family syndrome is associated with an autosomal dominant pattern of predisposition to nonpolyposis colorectal cancer as well as an increased incidence of other cancers, including endometrial, ovarian, breast, stomach, small intestine, pancreatic, urinary tract, and

biliary tract. This syndrome is associated with mutations in the mismatch repair genes *MLH1*, *MSH2*, and *MSH6*.

12. **What is Li-Fraumeni syndrome?**
Li-Fraumeni syndrome is a familial cancer syndrome with an autosomal dominant pattern of inheritance and a varied spectrum of mesenchymal and epithelial tumors, and multiple primary neoplasms in children and young adults. The gene for this cancer *(p53)* is located on the short arm of chromosome 17.

13. **Describe MEN I.**
Multiple endocrine neoplasia type 1 (MEN I), associated with a gene on chromosome 11, causes parathyroid, pituitary, and islet cell tumors.

14. **Summarize the two phenotypes of MEN II.**
MEN II has two phenotypes: type A (medullary thyroid carcinoma, pheochromocytoma, and parathyroid hyperplasia) and type B (medullary thyroid carcinoma, pheochromocytoma, marfanoid habitus, mucosal neuromas). Germ-line point mutations of the *RET* proto-oncogene on chromosome 10 are responsible for both types, which develop medullary thyroid carcinoma and pheochromocytoma.

15. **What are tumor markers?**
Tumor markers include enzymes, hormones, gene loci, and oncofetal antigens that are associated with particular tumors. The markers reflect the presence of the tumor or the quantity of the tumor (tumor burden). Many cancers do not produce tumor markers, and tumors known to produce markers may sometimes fail to do so, particularly if they are very poorly differentiated.

16. **How are tumor markers used?**
Some of the markers, such as prostate-specific antigen (PSA) and alpha-fetoprotein (AFP), are highly sensitive, highly specific, and of high predictive value. Others, such as lactic dehydrogenase (LDH) or carcinoembryonic antigen (CEA), are nonspecific and may be elevated in many conditions besides malignancies. The most important use of these markers is in following the effects of therapy on tumor burden and in detecting recurrent disease after initial therapy.

17. **Summarize the significance of CEA.**
CEA is a glycoprotein of 200,000 daltons that is found in gastrointestinal (GI) mucosal cells and pancreaticobiliary secretions. Elevations occur with breaks in the mucosal basement membrane by a tumor but can also occur in smokers and with cirrhosis, pancreatitis, inflammatory bowel disease, and rectal polyps. CEA is most useful in monitoring the activity of disease in recurrent colorectal cancer if it was elevated prior to treatment.

18. **Why is PSA important?**
PSA is a serine protease found only in the prostate. Its normal function is liquefaction of seminal gel. The serum level of PSA may be elevated in any type of prostate disease, including benign prostatic hypertrophy, prostatitis, and prostate cancer. However, high levels of PSA, especially in patients with small volume prostates, are a strong indicator of probable prostate cancer. Very elevated PSA levels (> 100 ng/mL) correlate with metastatic disease.

19. **Discuss the role of AFP as a tumor marker.**
AFP is an alpha-globulin of 70,000 daltons that is made by the yolk sac and liver of the human fetus. It is elevated in hepatomas and certain germ cell neoplasms and has been found to be a highly sensitive marker for disease activity. Although AFP is rather nonspecific and can be elevated in acute viral and chronic hepatitis, very high levels (> 1000) correlate with the presence of these malignancies.

20. **What is human chorionic gonadotropin (HCG)?**
HCG is a glycoprotein normally secreted by the trophoblastic epithelium of the placenta. It is used as a sensitive and specific marker for germ cell tumors of the testes and ovary and extra-gonadal presentations of these tumors.

KEY POINTS: TUMOR MARKERS

1. Other than PSA, most tumor markers are not useful in screening for malignancies in the general population.
2. Tumor markers are generally nonspecific and can be elevated in a variety of conditions.
3. They are used to assist in diagnosis and therapy in patients suspected to have malignancy by clinical parameters.
4. CEA and CA-125 have clinical utility in patients diagnosed with colorectal and ovarian cancer, respectively, only if the level was elevated before treatment of the cancer.
5. CA 19-9 can be highly elevated in cases of benign biliary tract obstruction.
6. PSA levels over 10 ng/mL have a 60% probability of prostate cancer; levels over 100 ng/mL correlate with metastatic disease.

21. **List the principles used in formulating combination chemotherapy regimens.**
- Drugs used should have activity against the tumor.
- Drugs should be selected with dissimilar toxicities.
- Drugs with different mechanisms of action should be used.
- Several cycles of therapy, with adequate biologic effect, should be used before determining efficacy.
- Recovery of normal tissues should be allowed before starting the next cycle.

22. **What are the mechanisms of tumor resistance to chemotherapeutic agents?**
- Intrinsic cytokinetic or biochemical resistance
- Impaired transport of the drug into the cell or active extrusion from the cell
- Altered drug affinity for the target enzyme
- Amplification of genes
- Membrane alterations from overproduction of high-weight glycoproteins

23. **Summarize the toxic effects of chemotherapy.**
The most common immediate effects are nausea and vomiting, which vary in presence and degree with the type of drug. Some medications, such as cisplatin, are very emetogenic, whereas others, like fludarabine, are unlikely to cause emesis. Many chemotherapy drugs cause myelosuppression. Leukopenia predisposes to acute and serious infections; thrombocytopenia predisposes to bleeding; and anemia may worsen symptoms from other problems, such as chronic obstructive pulmonary disease and atherosclerotic cardiovascular disease (Table 6-1).

24. **Which chemotherapeutic drugs are associated with cardiotoxicity?**
Cardiotoxicity is most frequently associated with **doxorubicin** (Adriamycin) and other drugs of the anthracycline class, which cause a progressive loss of cardiac muscle cells. In previously normal hearts, toxicity is dose related and does not become clinically important until a total dose of approximately 450 mg/m^2 of doxorubicin is administered. In patients with already compromised cardiac function, toxicity may occur at lower dosages.

TABLE 6-1. TOXICITIES OF CHEMOTHERAPEUTIC AGENTS

Drug	Acute Toxicity	Delayed Toxicity
Bleomycin (Blenoxane)	Nausea/vomiting, fever, hypersensitivity reactions	**Pneumonitis, pulmonary fibrosis,*** rash and hyperpigmentation, stomatitis, alopecia, Raynaud's phenomenon, cavitating granulomas
Carboplatin (Paraplatin)	Nausea/vomiting	**Myelosuppression*** peripheral neuropathy (uncommon), hearing loss, hemolytic anemia, transient cortical blindness
Capecitabine (Xeloda)	Nausea, diarrhea, stomatitis	**Hand-foot syndrome*** (palmar-plantar erythrodysesthesia), hyperbilirubinemia
Chlorambucil (Leukeran)	Seizures, nausea/vomiting	**Myelosuppression,*** pulmonary infiltrates and fibrosis, leukemia, hepatic toxicity, sterility
Cisplatin (Platinol)	Nausea/vomiting, anaphylactic reaction	**Renal damage,*** ototoxicity, myelosuppression, hemolysis, ↓$Mg^{2+}/Ca^{2+}/K^{+}$, peripheral neuropathy, Raynaud's, sterility
Cytarabine (ara-C)	Nausea/vomiting, diarrhea, anaphylaxis	**Myelosuppression,*** oral ulceration, conjunctivitis, hepatic damage, fever, pulmonary edema, neurotoxicity (high dose), rhabdomyolysis, pancreatitis with asparaginase, bladder cancer, SIADH
Dacarbazine (DTIC)	Nausea/vomiting, diarrhea, anaphylaxis, pain on administration	**Myelosuppression,*** cardiotoxicity,* alopecia, flulike syndrome, renal impairment, hepatic necrosis, facial flushing, paresthesias, photosensitivity, urticarial rash
Daunorubicin (Cerubidine)	Nausea/vomiting, diarrhea, red urine, severe local tissue necrosis on extravasation, transient ECG changes, anaphylactoid reaction	**Myelosuppression,*** cardiotoxicity,* alopecia, stomatitis, anorexia, diarrhea, fever and chills, dermatitis in previously irradiated areas, skin and nail pigmentation
Doxorubicin (Adriamycin)	Nausea/vomiting, red urine, severe local tissue necrosis on extravasation, diarrhea, fever, transient ECG changes, ventricular arrhythmia, anaphylactoid reaction	**Myelosuppression,*** cardiotoxicity,* alopecia, stomatitis, anorexia, conjunctivitis, acral pigmentation, dermatitis in previously irradiated areas, acral erythrodysesthesia, mucositis
Etoposide (VP16)	Nausea/vomiting, diarrhea, fever, hypotension, allergic reaction	**Myelosuppression,*** alopecia, peripheral neuropathy, mucositis and hepatic damage with high doses, leukemia

(*continued*)

TABLE 6-1. TOXICITIES OF CHEMOTHERAPEUTIC AGENTS *(continued)*

Drug	Acute Toxicity	Delayed Toxicity
Floxuridine (FUDR)	Nausea/vomiting, diarrhea	**Oral and GI ulceration**,* **myelosuppression**,* alopecia, dermatitis, hepatic dysfunction with infusion
Fluorouracil (5-FU)	Nausea/vomiting, diarrhea, hypersensitivity, photosensitivity	**Oral and GI ulcers**, **myelosuppression**,* diarrhea, ataxia, arrhythmias, angina, hyperpigmentation, hand-foot syndrome, conjunctivitis, CHF
Gemcitabine (Gemzar)	Fatigue, nausea and vomiting	**Bone marrow depression**, especially thrombocytopenia; edema; pulmonary toxicity; anal pruritus
Ifosfamide (Ifex)	Nausea/vomiting, confusion, nephrotoxicity, metabolic acidosis, **cardiac toxicity with higher doses***	**Myelosuppression**,* **hemorrhagic cystitis**, alopecia, SIADH, neurotoxicity
Irinotecan (Camptosar)	Nausea and vomiting, diarrhea, fever	**Diarrhea, anorexia**, stomatitis, bone marrow depression, alopecia, abdominal cramping
Mechlorethamine (nitrogen mustard)	Nausea/vomiting, local reaction and phlebitis	**Myelosuppression**,* alopecia, diarrhea, oral ulcers, leukemia, amenorrhea, sterility
Methotrexate	Nausea/vomiting, diarrhea, fever, anaphylaxis, hepatic necrosis	**Oral/GI ulceration**,* **myelosuppression**,* hepatic toxicity, renal toxicity, **pulmonary infiltrates and fibrosis**,* osteoporosis, conjunctivitis, alopecia, depigmentation
Mitoxantrone (Novantrone)	Blue-green sclera and pigment in urine, nausea/vomiting, stomatitis	**Myelosuppression**,* cardiotoxicity, alopecia, white hair, skin lesions, hepatic damage, renal failure
Paclitaxel (Taxol), docetaxel (Taxotere)	Hypersensitivity, hypotension, nausea, pain on extravasation	**Myelosuppression**,* alopecia, peripheral neuropathy, rash and edema (docetaxel)
Topotecan (Hycamtin)	Nausea/vomiting, diarrhea, headache	**Myelosuppression**,* alopecia, transient elevations in hepatic enzymes
Vinblastine (Velban)	Nausea/vomiting, local reaction and phlebitis with extravasation	**Myelosuppression**,* alopecia, stomatitis, loss of DTRs, jaw pain, muscle pain, paralytic ileus
Vincristine (Oncovin)	Local reaction with extravasation	**Peripheral neuropathy**,* alopecia, mild myelosuppression, constipation, paralytic ileus, jaw pain, SIADH

TABLE 6-1. TOXICITIES OF CHEMOTHERAPEUTIC AGENTS *(continued)*

Drug	Acute Toxicity	Delayed Toxicity
Vinorelbine (Navelbine)	Local reaction with extravasation	**Granulocytopenia**,* anemia, fatigue

* Dose-limiting effects.
SIADH = syndrome of inappropriate antidiuretic hormone, ECG = electrocardiographic, CHF = chronic heart failure, DTR = deep tendon reflexes.
Modified from Drugs of choice for cancer chemotherapy. Med Lett 42:83–92, 2000.

25. How is doxorubicin-related cardiotoxicity monitored?
Cardiac radionuclide gated wall motion studies (multiple-gated acquisition scans) or echocardiograms measuring ejection fraction are used to monitor changes in cardiac function.

26. Distinguish between neoadjuvant therapy and adjuvant therapy.
Neoadjuvant therapy means treatment such as chemotherapy or hormonal therapy prior to definitive surgery or radiotherapy. Patients given neoadjuvant therapy often have large or fixed tumors, and the idea is to shrink these tumors to make subsequent surgical removal or radiotherapy easier and more effective. This differs from *adjuvant therapy*, in which the tumor has been grossly removed by surgery, and chemotherapy and/or radiotherapy is then administered to eradicate micrometastatic disease and therefore prevent recurrence.

27. What are radiosensitizers?
Radiosensitizers are chemical agents that increase the sensitivity of cells in vitro to radiation and are usually classified as nonhypoxic cell sensitizers. This class of compounds includes drugs such as halogenated pyrimidine nucleoside analogs, 3-amino-benzamide, taxanes, and various platinum compounds. Radiosensitization by these compounds may be mediated by a variety of mechanisms, none of which is precisely understood. However, it is often assumed that effects on the induction and/or repair of radiation-induced damage may be involved.

28. Define tumor doubling time.
Tumor doubling time refers to the time required for the tumor to double in size. The doubling time varies greatly among cancers. Primary cancers of the lung, for example, may be ranked with respect to the doubling time: adenocarcinoma doubles within 21 weeks, squamous cell carcinoma within 12 weeks, and small cell carcinoma within 11 weeks. Primary breast cancer doubles within 14 weeks and primary colorectal cancer within 90 weeks.

29. How is the doubling time of tumors calculated from x-rays?
The doubling time of tumors can be roughly calculated from x-rays by measuring the diameter of the lesion (assuming that it is approximately spherical) and calculating its volume with the formula: volume = $4/3\ \pi r^3$, where π is the constant *pi* and r is the radius of the lesion. After the volume is calculated on two separate occasions, doubling time can be extracted from a plot of volume versus time.

30. What is the Gompertz equation?
The calculation in question 29 is a rough estimate because it assumes very simple growth kinetics and the absence of other factors affecting the growth, which is rarely, if ever, the case.

Tumor cell populations exhibit a reduction in net fractional growth rate with increasing population size. The Gompertz equation describes this slowing of growth with size and takes into account various other factors, such as decreasing blood supply with increasing size of tumor.

31. **What is the most common cause of cancer death in the U.S. today, excluding skin cancer?**
Lung cancer, for both men and women. See cancer incidence and mortality percentages in Figure 6-1.

COMPLICATIONS OF CANCER

32. **What are the causes of anemia in patients with cancer?**
Anemia in cancer patients is often multifactorial. Anemia may result from blood loss due to bleeding from tumors or from gastritis due to the use of nonsteroidal anti-inflammatory agents (NSAIDs). It may also be caused by hemolysis (secondary to antibodies associated with the tumor), disseminated intravascular coagulation (DIC), sepsis, or a paraneoplastic syndrome. Anemia is frequently caused by bone marrow suppression by chemotherapy or by marrow involvement by the tumor.

33. **Define anemia of chronic disease.**
Anemia of chronic disease is common in cancer patients. The diagnosis is made when no other cause of anemia can be found and plasma iron is < 60 mg/dL, total iron-binding capacity is 100–250 mg/dL, and ferritin is > 60 ng/mL. The hematocrit is generally 25–30%. An inadequate erythropoietin response to anemia and a blunted response to treatment with recombinant human erythropoietin have been demonstrated in some patients.

34. **What are the predisposing factors for infection in patients with cancer?**
Predisposing factors for infection include defects in cellular and humoral immunity, organ compromise due to tumor-related obstruction, chemotherapy-related granulocytopenia, disruption of mucosal (e.g., respiratory and alimentary tract) and integumental surfaces, iatrogenic procedures or placement of prosthetic devices, central nervous system dysfunction, and hyposplenic or postsplenectomy states.

35. **Discuss the sources of infection in patients with cancer.**
The vast majority of infections originate from the patients' own endogenous flora. Sources of infection in neutropenic patients include the lungs, urinary tract, skin, upper aerodigestive tract (mouth, skin, teeth), central nervous system, rectum, perirectum, biopsy sites, and GI tract (appendicitis, cholecystitis, perforations). In investigating the cause of an infection, cultures should include blood, urine, sputum, and, if appropriate to the patient's clinical status, stool, pleural fluid, or peritoneal fluid.

36. **Which tumors spread to bone most commonly?**
Cancers of the lung, breast, kidney, prostate, and thyroid as well as multiple myeloma and malignant melanoma spread to bone most commonly.

37. **Are metastatic bone lesions osteoblastic or osteolytic?**
Renal cell carcinoma and multiple myeloma tend to be purely lytic, prostate carcinoma tends to be mainly blastic, and the others are mixed. Tumors that are lytic are most often associated with hypercalcemia, whereas blastic metastases are not generally associated with this complication.

38. **To which bones does cancer most often metastasize?**
The most frequently involved bones are the spine, ribs, pelvis, and long bones.

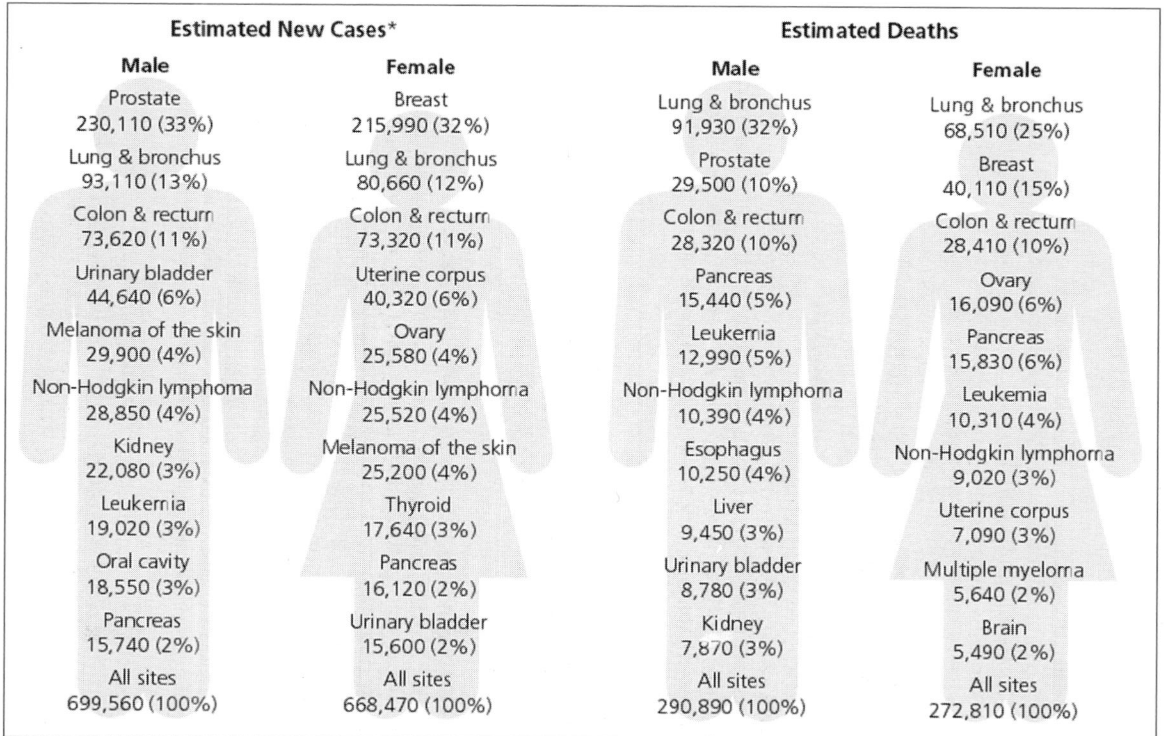

Estimated New Cases*		Estimated Deaths	
Male	**Female**	**Male**	**Female**
Prostate 230,110 (33%)	Breast 215,990 (32%)	Lung & bronchus 91,930 (32%)	Lung & bronchus 68,510 (25%)
Lung & bronchus 93,110 (13%)	Lung & bronchus 80,660 (12%)	Prostate 29,500 (10%)	Breast 40,110 (15%)
Colon & rectum 73,620 (11%)	Colon & rectum 73,320 (11%)	Colon & rectum 28,320 (10%)	Colon & rectum 28,410 (10%)
Urinary bladder 44,640 (6%)	Uterine corpus 40,320 (6%)	Pancreas 15,440 (5%)	Ovary 16,090 (6%)
Melanoma of the skin 29,900 (4%)	Ovary 25,580 (4%)	Leukemia 12,990 (5%)	Pancreas 15,830 (6%)
Non-Hodgkin lymphoma 28,850 (4%)	Non-Hodgkin lymphoma 25,520 (4%)	Non-Hodgkin lymphoma 10,390 (4%)	Leukemia 10,310 (4%)
Kidney 22,080 (3%)	Melanoma of the skin 25,200 (4%)	Esophagus 10,250 (4%)	Non-Hodgkin lymphoma 9,020 (3%)
Leukemia 19,020 (3%)	Thyroid 17,640 (3%)	Liver 9,450 (3%)	Uterine corpus 7,090 (3%)
Oral cavity 18,550 (3%)	Pancreas 16,120 (2%)	Urinary bladder 8,780 (3%)	Multiple myeloma 5,640 (2%)
Pancreas 15,740 (2%)	Urinary bladder 15,600 (2%)	Kidney 7,870 (3%)	Brain 5,490 (2%)
All sites 699,560 (100%)	All sites 668,470 (100%)	All sites 290,890 (100%)	All sites 272,810 (100%)

Figure 6-1. Leading sites of new cancer cases and deaths. Excludes basal and squamous cell skin cancers and in situ carcinoma except urinary bladder. Percentages may not total 100% due to rounding. (From American Cancer Society: Statistics for 2004. Available at http://www.cancer.org/docroot/ stt/stt_0.asp.)

39. **Characterize the pain associated with bone metastases.**
The pain of bone metastases is characterized by a dull, aching discomfort that is worse at night and may improve with physical activity.

40. **Which tumors metastasize to the lungs?**
Most types of tumors can metastasize to the lungs. Therefore, the more common the tumor, the more commonly it is found to have spread to the lung (e.g., breast cancers). Although they also can spread to the lungs, GI cancers tend to first metastasize locally and to the liver before pulmonary involvement is seen. Tumors that spread via the bloodstream, such as sarcomas, renal cell carcinoma, and colon cancer, tend to produce nodular lung lesions. Those that spread via lymphatic routes, such as cancers of the breast, pancreas, stomach, and liver, often manifest a pattern of lymphangitic spread.

41. **Discuss the symptoms of intracranial metastases.**
Headache occurs in up to 50% of patients with intracranial metastases. It is classically described as occurring early in the morning, disappearing or decreasing after arising, and may be associated with nausea and/or projectile vomiting. Other symptoms include focal signs such as unilateral weakness, numbness, seizures, or cranial nerve abnormalities. Nonfocal complaints such as mental status changes or ataxia may occur.

42. **How are intracranial metastases diagnosed and treated?**
The diagnosis is made by contrast-enhanced computed tomography (CT) or magnetic resonance imaging (MRI) of the brain. Treatment consists of decreasing intracranial pressure with steroids, followed by radiotherapy. Surgery is recommended for patients with single intracranial lesions.

43. **What are the signs and symptoms of malignant pericardial effusion?**
The presentation of malignant pericardial effusion can resemble heart failure, with dyspnea, peripheral edema, and an enlarged heart on chest x-ray. However, the dyspnea is often out of proportion to the degree of pulmonary congestion seen on the x-ray. Kussmaul's sign, or jugulovenous distention with inspiration, and pulsus paradoxus of > 10 mmHg with distant heart sounds are clues to the presence of a pericardial effusion.

44. **How is the diagnosis of malignant pericardial effusion confirmed?**
Confirmation of the clinical diagnosis is made by echocardiogram or CT scan. Malignant effusions are usually exudates and are often hemorrhagic. Cytology is helpful if positive but does not exclude cancer if negative.

45. **Discuss the treatment of malignant pericardial effusion.**
Treatment depends on the patient's condition but should include drainage of the fluid for diagnostic as well as therapeutic reasons. A nonsurgical approach is preferred, with catheter drainage followed by sclerosis of the pericardium, sometimes with a sclerosing agent such as doxycycline. Other approaches include subxiphoid pericardiectomy, balloon pericardiectomy, pericardial window, and pericardial stripping for patients with prolonged life expectancy.

46. **What are the presenting symptoms and signs of spinal cord compression?**
Ninety-five percent of cancer patients with spinal cord compression present with back pain. Other symptoms include lower extremity weakness, bowel or bladder incontinence, or increased deep tendon reflexes in the lower extremities.

47. **How is spinal cord compression diagnosed?**
The diagnosis is made by MRI or by myelography with CT, which will demonstrate blockage of the spinal canal.

48. **How is spinal cord compression treated?**
Treatment is directed first at relieving spinal cord swelling and pain, using high-dose steroids and adequate pain medication. However, definitive treatment must be carried out emergently to prevent further neurologic deterioration, which may be irreversible. Radiotherapy and/or surgery should be initiated immediately. Preservation of neurologic function is generally better with surgery.

49. **Which tumors most commonly cause spinal cord compression?**
The most common tumors causing cord compression are lung cancer, breast cancer, prostate cancer, carcinoma of unknown primary, lymphoma, and multiple myeloma. The most common site of cord compression is the thoracic spine, followed by the lumbosacral spine and the cervical spine.

50. **Which tumors are associated with nonbacterial thrombotic endocarditis?**
Also known as marantic endocarditis, this paraneoplastic syndrome is associated with **mucinous adenocarcinomas**, most commonly of the lung, stomach, or ovary, but has been described in other types of cancers as well.

51. **How does nonbacterial thrombotic endocarditis present?**
It is manifested by the appearance of embolic peripheral or cerebral vascular events causing arterial insufficiency, encephalopathy, or focal neurologic defects. Heart murmurs are often not present.

52. **How is nonbacterial thrombotic endocarditis diagnosed and treated?**
Echocardiograms may be negative, and the diagnosis is usually made post mortem. Treatment with anticoagulants or antiplatelet drugs has been tried with little success.

53. **What are the tumor-related causes of hypercalcemia?**
- **Lytic bone metastases**, which release calcium into the bloodstream. This is the most common cause in solid tumors with bony metastases.
- **Humoral hypercalcemia of malignancy** (HHM) occurs in patients without bony metastases. Cancers associated with this syndrome secrete a non-PTH substance with activity similar to parathyroid hormone. HHM is associated most commonly with squamous cell cancers of the lung, esophagus, or head and neck but can also be found in renal cell carcinoma, transitional cell carcinoma of the bladder, and ovarian carcinoma.
- Formerly known as **osteoclast-activating factor**, osteolytic substances such as interleukin 1 (IL-1), IL-6, and TNF-alpha (lymphotoxin) may cause hypercalcemia in plasma cell dyscrasias.
- **Vitamin D metabolites** produced by some lymphomas may promote intestinal calcium absorption.

54. **What is tumor lysis syndrome?**
When rapidly growing tumors are effectively treated with chemotherapy, breakdown products of tumor lysis are released into the bloodstream in large amounts. This process may cause hyperkalemia, hyperuricemia, hyperphosphatemia, and hypocalcemia. Renal failure can result from the hyperuricemia. This complication is seen within hours to days after treatment of tumors such as acute leukemia, Burkitt's lymphoma, and other rapidly proliferating lymphomas. It is rarely, if ever, seen with solid tumors, but has been described in small cell carcinoma of the lung.

55. **How is tumor lysis syndrome treated?**
Treatment is the same as for renal failure, with vigorous hydration, dialysis if necessary, and appropriate treatment of electrolyte disorders. Prophylactic treatment with aggressive hydration and allopurinol prior to administering chemotherapy in susceptible patients can prevent this serious complication.

56. Which medications are commonly used for cancer pain?

As elucidated in the World Health Organization guidelines, pain medications are to be administered in a three-step ladder according to the intensity and pathophysiology of symptoms and individual requirements. For mild pain, the recommended baseline drugs are NSAIDs (Table 6-2). Patients with moderate-to-severe pain generally require an opioid agent such as codeine or oxycodone; severe pain requires a stronger opioid such as morphine (Table 6-3).

TABLE 6-2. NONOPIOID AND ADJUVANT ANALGESIC DRUGS FOR CANCER PAIN

Class/Drug	Indications	Starting Oral Dose (mg/day and range/day)	Comments
NSAIDs			
Aspirin	Soft-tissue and bone pain	650 650–1000	GI and hematologic effects when used with opioids, avoid combining with steroids
Acetaminophen	Soft-tissue and bone pain	650 650–1000	Fewer GI effects than aspirin, no effects on platelet function, no significant anti-inflammatory effects
Ibuprofen	Soft-tissue and bone pain	400 200–800	Higher analgesic potential than aspirin, fewer GI and hematologic effects than aspirin
Choline magnesium trisalicylate	Soft tissue and bone pain	1500 1000–4000	Anti-inflammatory and analgesic effects, similar to aspirin without hematologic effects
Fenoprofen	Soft-tissue and bone pain	200 200–400	Like ibuprofen
Diflunisal	Soft-tissue and bone pain	500 500–1000	Longer duration of action than ibuprofen, higher analgesic potential than aspirin
Naproxen	Soft-tissue and bone pain	250 250–500	Like diflunisal
Celecoxib	For mild to moderate pain, osteoarthritis, rheumatoid arthritis	100–600	Less GI and renal toxicity; not evaluated in patients with cancer
Rofecoxib	For mild to moderate acute pain, osteoarthritis	12.5–60	Less GI and renal toxicity; not evaluated in patients with cancer

TABLE 6-2. NONOPIOID AND ADJUVANT ANALGESIC DRUGS FOR CANCER PAIN *(continued)*

Class/Drug	Indications	Starting Oral Dose (mg/day and range/day)	Comments
Anticonvulsants			
Phenytoin	Neuropathic pain (acute lancinating type)	100 100–300	Start with low dose, titrate slowly
Carbamazepine	Neuropathic	100 200–800	Useful in paroxysmal nerve pain
Gabapentin	Neuropathic pain, lancinating and burning pain	300–1800	Titrate to effect; sedation is a major side effect
Antidepressants			
Amitriptyline Imipramine Desipramine Nortriptyline Paroxetine	Neuropathic pain (e.g., postherpetic neuralgia, diabetic neuropathy, tumor- and radiation-induced plexopathy, neuropathy	10–200 10–150 10–150 10–150 10–40	Start at a low dose and titrate slowly; drug selection based on patient's ability to tolerate drug
Antihistamine			
Hydroxyzine	Somatic and visceral pain	25 25–100	Additive analgesia in combination with opioids; antiemetic and antianxiety effects
Phenothiazine			
Methotrimeprazine	Somatic and visceral pain	5–15 IM	Anxiolytic and antiemetic effects, available only in IM preparation, useful in opioid-tolerant patients with GI obstruction and pain
Steroids			
Prednisone	Somatic and neuropathic pain (e.g., inflammatory bone pain)	5 5–60	Anti-inflammatory, antiemetic, and analgesic effects
Dexamethasone	Reflex sympathetic dystrophy, brachial and lumbar plexopathy, bone and nerve pain	0.5 0.5–16	Analgesic and anti-inflammatory effects in epidural compression and brain metastases

(*continued*)

TABLE 6-2. NONOPIOID AND ADJUVANT ANALGESIC DRUGS FOR CANCER PAIN *(continued)*

Class/Drug	Indications	Starting Oral Dose (mg/day and range/day)	Comments
Neurostimulants			
Dextroamphetamine	Somatic and visceral pain (e.g., postoperative pain)	2.5 2.5–10	Additive analgesia in combination with opioids, reduces sedative effects
Methylphenidate	Opioid-induced sedation	5 5–15	Additive analgesia in combination with opioids, reduces sedative effects
Caffeine	Somatic and visceral pain, opioid-induced sedation	300 300–600	Additive analgesia in combination with opioids, reduces sedative effects

IM = intramuscular.
Adapted from Foley KM: Controlling cancer pain. Hosp Pract (Off Ed) 35(4):101–108, 111–112, 2000.

TABLE 6-3. OPIOID DRUGS COMMONLY USED IN CANCER PAIN MANAGEMENT

Drug	Equianalgesic Doses (mg)		Half-Life (h)	Duration of Action (h)
	Intramuscular	Oral		
Codeine	130	100	2–3	2–4
Oxycodone[1]	15	30	2–3	2–4
Propoxyphene	50	100	2–3	2–4
Morphine[1]	10	60 (single dose) 30 (repeated dose)	2–3	3–4
Hydromorphone[1]	1.5	7.5	2–3	2–4
Methadone	10	20	15–30	4–8
Oxymorphone	1	10 (per rectum)	2–3	3–4
Levorphanol	2	4	12–15	4–8
Fentanyl (parenteral)	0.1		1–2	1–3
Fentanyl (transdermal)[2]	–	–	1–2	48–72
Fentanyl (transmucosal)	–	–	1–2	1–2

[1]Oxycodone, morphine, and hydromorphone are also available in slow-release preparations.
[2]100 μg/hr transdermal fentanyl approximately equal to 4 mg/h IM morphine.
Adapted from Foley KM: Controlling cancer pain. Hosp Pract (Off Ed) 35(4):101–108, 111–112, 2000.

57. **What are the neuromuscular complications of cancer?**
See Table 6-4.

TABLE 6-4. NEUROMUSCULAR COMPLICATIONS OF CANCER

Site	Paraneoplastic Syndrome	Autoantibodies (Associated Cancer)
Brain and cranial nerves	Paraneoplastic cerebellar degeneration	Anti-Yo (GYN cancer) Anti-Hu (SCLC) Anti-Tr (HD) Anti-Ri (breast cancer)
	Opsoclonus-myoclonus (breast cancer)	Anti-Ri
	Carcinoma-associated retinopathy	Anti-recoverin (SCLC)
	Optic neuritis	
	Limbic encephalitis	Anti-Hu (SCLC)
	Brain stem encephalitis	Anti-Hu (SCLC)
Spinal cord	Myelitis	Anti-Hu (SCLC)
	Subacute motor neuronopathy	Anti-Hu (SCLC)
	Motor neuron disease/ALS	Anti-Hu (rarely)
	Necrotizing myelopathy	
	Stiff-man syndrome	Anti-amphiphisin (breast, SCLC)
Peripheral nerves and dorsal root ganglia	Subacute or chronic sensorimotor neuropathy	
	Acute polyradiculopathy (GBS)	
	Neuropathy associated with plasma cell dyscrasias	Anti-MAG
	Brachial neuritis	
	Mononeuritis multiplex	
	Sensory neuronopathy	
	Autonomic neuronopathy	
Neuromuscular junction	Lambert-Eaton myasthenic syndrome	Anti-VGCC
	Myasthenia gravis	Acetylcholine receptor Ab
Muscle	Dermatomyositis/polymyositis	
	Acute necrotizing myopathy	
	Carcinoid myopathy	
	Neuromyopathy	
	Neuromyotonia	Ab to potassium channels

These syndromes frequently occur together as part of paraneoplastic encephalomyelitis/sensory neuronopathy with anti-Hu antibody.
GYN = gynecologic, SCLC = small cell lung cancer, HD = Hodgkin's disease, ALS = amyotrophic lateral sclerosis, MAG = myelin-associated glycoprotein, Ab = antibody, VGCC = voltage-gated calcium channel, GBS = Guillain-Barré syndrome,
From Schiff D, et al: Neurologic emergencies in cancer patients. Neurol Clin 16:449–481, 1998, with permission.

GASTROINTESTINAL AND LIVER CANCERS

58. Who gets esophageal cancer?

Squamous cell cancer of the esophagus occurs in the 40- to 60-year-old age group and is seen mainly in men. The incidence is increased in Africa, China, Russia, Japan, Scotland, and the Caspian region of Iran. In the U.S. the nonwhite male population is at increased risk. Adenocarcinoma of the esophagus tends to occur in obese white men.

59. List the risk factors for esophageal cancer.

- Excessive alcohol and/or tobacco use
- Native Bantu beer (southern Africa)
- Chronic hot beverage ingestion
- Lye ingestion: > 30% of cases develop esophageal cancer
- Tylosis: > 40% of cases develop esophageal cancer
- Achalasia
- Plummer-Vinson syndrome
- Nontropical sprue
- Prior oral and pharyngeal cancer
- Occupational exposure to asbestos, combustion products, ionizing radiation
- Other occupational exposure: waiters, bartenders, metal workers, and construction workers
- Decreased dietary intake of fruits and vegetables throughout adulthood

60. Discuss the incidence of adenocarcinoma of the esophagus.

The incidence of esophageal adenocarcinoma has greatly increased over the past two decades. Adenocarcinoma of the esophagus is now more prevalent than squamous cell carcinoma in the United States and Western Europe, with most tumors located in the distal esophagus and esophagogastric junction.

61. What are the risk factors for adenocarcinoma of the esophagus?

Adenocarcinoma of the esophagus in a younger population without the traditional risk factors has been associated with chronic esophagitis, reflux disease, and Barrett's esophagus.

Devesa SS, et al: Changing patterns in the incidence of esophageal and gastric carcinoma in the United States. Cancer 83:2049–2053, 1998.

62. How does esophageal cancer present?

Dysphagia: first with solids, then with liquids
Weight loss
Regurgitation
Occult GI bleeding
Aspiration pneumonia
Cough
Fever
Choking
Hoarseness
Chest pain on swallowing
Gastroesophageal reflux disease (GERD)

63. How should esophageal cancer be treated?

The only curative procedure is surgery. However, fewer than half of patients are operable at the time of presentation, and of these, only one half to two thirds have tumors that are resectable. Nonsurgical patients are treated with combined chemoradiotherapy or palliative measures alone if their performance status is too poor for active therapy. Some evidence indicates that survival in patients with adenocarcinoma of the esophagus is improved with preoperative combined chemotherapy and radiotherapy. Ongoing trials are investigating whether the outcome with chemoradiotherapy is equivalent to that of surgery.

64. **List the risk factors for gastric cancer.**

Precursor conditions	Genetic and environmental factors
Chronic atrophic gastritis and intestinal metaplasia	Family history of gastric cancer
Pernicious anemia	Blood type A
Partial gastrectomy for benign disease	Hereditary nonpolyposis colon cancer syndrome
H. pylori infection	Low socioeconomic status
Ménétrier's disease	Low consumption of fruits and vegetables
Gastric adenomatous polyps	Consumption of salted, smoked, or poorly preserved foods
Barrett's esophagus	Cigarette smoking (?)

65. **Discuss the role of oncogenes and tumor-suppressor genes in gastric cancer.**
The role of oncogenes and tumor suppressor genes is currently being elucidated. Allelic deletions of the *MCC, APC*, and *p53* tumor-suppressor genes have been reported in 33, 34, and 64% of gastric cancers, respectively. Disparities between mutations associated with the intestinal and diffuse types of gastric cancers may account for their different natural histories.

66. **List the symptoms of gastric cancer at the time of diagnosis.**

Symptoms	Frequency (%)
Weight loss	61.6
Abdominal pain	51.6
Nausea	34.3
Anorexia	32.0
Dysphagia	26.1
Melena	20.2
Early satiety	17.5
Ulcer-type pain	17.1
Lower-extremity edema	5.9

Fuchs CS, et al: Gastric carcinoma. N Engl J Med 333:32–41, 1995.

67. **List the risk factors for pancreatic cancer.**
- Smoking (2–3 times increased risk)
- Diet high in calories, fat, and protein, low in fruits and vegetables
- Diabetes mellitus
- Chronic pancreatitis
- Surgery for peptic ulcer disease
- Occupational exposure to 2-naphthylamine and petroleum products (> 10 yr increases risk to 5:1), dichlorodiphenyltrichloroethane (DDT)

68. **What hereditary syndromes increase the risk for pancreatic cancer?**
Familial pancreatic cancer, hereditary pancreatitis, familial adenomatous polyposis syndrome, familial atypical multiple mole melanoma syndrome (hereditary dysplastic nevus syndrome), ***BRCA2***, and Peutz-Jeghers syndrome.

69. **Do gender and ethnicity affect the risk for pancreatic cancer?**
- Males > females
- Blacks > whites

Evans DB, et al: Cancer of the pancreas. In DeVita, et al (eds): Cancer: Principles and Practice of Oncology, 6th ed. Philadelphia, Lippincott Williams & Wilkins, 2001.

70. List the symptoms and signs of pancreatic cancer based on tumor location.

Symptoms/Signs	Head	Body/Tail
Weight loss	92%	100%
Jaundice	82%	7%
Pain	72%	87%
Anorexia	64%	33%
Nausea	45%	43%
Vomiting	37%	37%
Weakness	35%	43%
Palpable liver	83%	—
Palpable gallbladder	29%	—
Tenderness	26%	27%
Ascites	19%	20%

Adapted from Moossa AR, et al: Tumors of the pancreas. In Moossa AR, et al (eds): Comprehensive Textbook of Oncology, 2nd ed. Baltimore, Williams & Wilkins, 1991, p 964.

71. Describe the diagnostic and staging evaluation for patients suspected of having pancreatic cancer.

Endoscopic ultrasound (EUS), helical CT, and gadolinium-enhanced MRI are useful diagnostic modalities for suspected carcinoma of the pancreas. These techniques allow accurate depiction of local tumor extent, involvement of adjacent vascular structures, and distant metastases.

Test	Diagnostic Yield (Various Series)
CA19-9 level > 200 U/mL	97%
CT scan of abdomen	74–94%
ERCP	91–94%
EUS	94%
Angiography	88–90%
Ultrasound of abdomen	69–90%
MRI of abdomen	NA

ERCP = endoscopic retrograde cholangiopancreatography, NA = not applicable.

A high level of CA 19-9 is specific for pancreatic cancer only if the bilirubin is not elevated, because biliary tract obstruction can cause high levels of CA 19-9.

72. How is the diagnosis of pancreatic cancer confirmed?

If a lesion in the pancreas is seen, CT or EUS-guided fine-needle aspirate can confirm the diagnosis of malignancy. Additional staging includes routine laboratory studies, chest x-ray, and other tests as directed by the history and physical. If there is bone pain or elevated alkaline phosphatase, then bone scan should be done.

Forsmark CE, et al: Diagnosis of pancreatic cancer and prediction of unresectability using the tumor-associated antigen CA19-9. Pancreas 9:731–734, 1994.

Kahl S, et al: Endoscopic ultrasound in pancreatic diseases. Dig Dis 20:120–126, 2002.

73. What is the most important risk factor for hepatocellular carcinoma?

Underlying cirrhosis appears to be the most important risk factor for the development of hepatocellular carcinoma. Macronodular cirrhosis is found in 85% of patients with hepatocellular carcinoma. In the United States, alcoholic cirrhosis is an important cause. Chronic infection with hepatitis B or C viruses is the major etiologic agent for human hepatocellular carcinoma around the world, since it causes development of cirrhosis.

74. What other risk factors may be involved?

Extensive studies of aflatoxins in human foods in Africa suggest a quantitative relationship between average human aflatoxin consumption and the incidence of hepatocellular carcinoma. In a small proportion of hepatocellular carcinomas, the cause appears to be related to other factors, including other hepatotropic viruses, chemicals, mycotoxins, and hepatic parasites. The relative importance of these factors seems to vary among populations.

75. List the common presenting features of primary tumors of the liver.

- Asthenia (85–90%)
- Hepatomegaly (50–100%)
- Abdominal pain (50–70%)
- Jaundice (45–80%)
- Fever (9.5%)

76. List the unusual ways in which hepatomas may present.

- Hemoptysis secondary to pulmonary metastases
- Rib mass secondary to bony metastasis
- Encephalitis-like picture secondary to brain metastasis
- Heart failure secondary to cardiac metastasis and thrombosis of the inferior vena cava
- Priapism secondary to soft-tissue metastasis
- Bone pain and pathologic fractures secondary to bony metastases

77. What are the systemic manifestations of hepatocellular carcinoma?

Endocrine: erythrocytosis, hypercalcemia

Nonendocrine: hypoglycemia, porphyria cutanea tarda, cryofibrinogenemia, osteoporosis, hyperlipidemia, dysfibrinogenemia, alpha fetoprotein synthesis

Margolis S, et al: Systemic manifestations of hepatoma. Medicine 51:381–390, 1972.

78. Which environmental factors are thought to be related to the development of colon cancer?

Abundant epidemiologic data support the link between environmental factors and colorectal cancer:

- A diet high in fat and red meat increases the risk of developing colon cancer.
- Consuming fresh fruits and vegetables decreases the risk.
- Physical inactivity and central obesity increase the risk of developing colon cancer.
- Regular use of NSAIDs, especially aspirin, may lessen the risk of developing colorectal cancer.

Nevertheless, as with all epidemiologic data, confounding factors not identified may be significant.

79. Besides environmental factors, what other risk factors are associated with the development of colon cancer?

Up to 15% of patients with colorectal cancer have a family history of the disease, suggesting the involvement of a genetic factor or factors. Among the genes identified for involvement in colorectal carcinogenesis are K-*ras, APC, DCC, hMSH2, hMLH1, hPMS1*, and *p53*. Patients who have had polyps or whose first-degree family members had polyps are at a moderately increased risk. Patients with inflammatory bowel disease, especially ulcerative colitis, are at very high risk for developing colorectal cancer.

80. What syndromes are associated with colon cancer?

Familial adenomatous polyposis, Gardner's syndrome, and hereditary nonpolyposis colorectal cancer are autosomal dominant syndromes. The first two account for < 1% of all colorectal cancers, and the last for 6–15%. Hereditary nonpolyposis colorectal cancer is a familial cancer syndrome that differs in natural history and genetic characteristics from sporadic colorectal cancer.

81. What is familial polyposis coli?
Familial polyposis coli is characterized by thousands of adenomatous polyps throughout the large bowel. If left untreated, cancer will develop in all patients with this syndrome. The cancer will usually manifest before age 40. The more common nonpolyposis syndrome also involves the proximal large bowel. The median age at presentation is < 50 years, and patients with a strong family history should be intensively screened.

82. What other nonenvironmental risk factors may be involved in colorectal cancer?
- **Age** > 40 yrs in symptomatic patients
- **Associated diseases:** ulcerative colitis, granulomatous colitis, Peutz-Jeghers syndrome
- **Past history:** colon cancer or polyps, female genital or breast cancer

Winawer S: Early diagnosis of colorectal cancer. Curr Conc Oncol March/April 1981, p 8.

83. What are the presenting symptoms of colon cancer?
The presenting symptoms depend on the location of the lesion. Lesions in the **ascending colon**, where the stool is still quite liquid, do not present with mass effects. However, these tumors frequently ulcerate, leading to chronic blood loss. Patients present with symptoms of anemia or with guaiac-positive stools on screening tests. In the **transverse bowel**, the stool is more concentrated and formed, so that symptoms of obstruction such as abdominal cramping, abdominal pain, or perforation may occur. Cancers in the **rectosigmoid** present with tenesmus, decreased stool caliber, and hematochezia.

84. What are the uses and limitations for CEA level testing?
CEA is an antigen produced by many colon cancers. It should not be used for cancer screening because it is very nonspecific and not sensitive enough to pick up early cancers. It is usually (85% of cases) normal in patients with stage I disease, those who are most amenable to curative surgery. It has also been found to be elevated in cancers of the stomach, pancreas, breast, ovary, and lung and with various nonmalignant conditions such as alcoholic liver disease, inflammatory bowel disease, heavy cigarette smoking, chronic bronchitis, and pancreatitis.

85. When should CEA testing be done?
Testing should be done preoperatively in patients undergoing resection for colon cancer, so that the data can be used to follow the course of the disease. The CEA level is only useful if it is high before treatment. CEA should return to normal in 30–45 days after complete resection of the cancer. A preoperative elevated level that returns to normal after surgery, but then subsequently becomes elevated, is a very reliable indicator of tumor recurrence. CEA can also be used as a marker for response to chemotherapy.

86. List the two roles of chemotherapy in the treatment of colon cancer.
- Treatment of metastatic disease
- Adjuvant treatment

87. Which agents are commonly used for treatment of metastatic disease?
5-Fluorouracil (5-FU), leucovorin, capecitabine, irinotecan (CPT-11), and oxaliplatin, alone or in combination, plus newer agents such as bevacizumab (Avastin). Response rates in metastatic disease are in the range of 20–40%.

88. How is chemotherapy used as an adjuvant treatment for colon cancer?
Patients who were treated with 5-FU and leucovorin after curative-intent resections of stage III colon cancer were found to have reduced recurrence rate and death rate compared to untreated controls. Chemotherapy is now considered standard postoperative therapy for stage III patients. In stage II disease, adjuvant treatment is sometimes given to patients at high risk for recurrence, as judged by pathologic features of the resected specimens.

GENITOURINARY CANCERS

89. What tests are available for the diagnosis and staging of prostate cancer? How do their results correlate with the stage?

See Table 6-5.

TABLE 6-5. DIAGNOSTIC EVALUATION AND STAGING OF PROSTATE CANCER

Prostate Stage	Histology of Biopsy Specimen	Urinary Symptoms	Noninvasive Assessment of Metastatic Disease: SAP	PSA	Bone Scan	Pelvic CT Scan	Surgical LN Sampling
I	Incidental histologic finding in 5% or less of resected tissue, well differentiated	Compatible with BPH	N	Often ↑	—	—	Usually not performed
II	Incidental histologic finding in > 5% of resected tissue, or tumor not well differentiated, or palpable nodule confined to prostate	Compatible with BPH	N	Often ↑	—	—	+ in 8–25% (indicating stage IV disease)
III	Extends through prostate capsule	Present	N	Usually ↑	—	—	+ in 40–50% (indicating stage IV disease)
IV	Invades other organs or metastatic	Present	Often ↑	Usually ↑	±	±	+ in 95% of patients with elevated SAP

SAP = serum alkaline phosphatase, PSA = prostate specific antigen, LN = lymph node, BPH = benign prostatic hypertrophy, ↑ = elevated, – = negative, + = positive.

90. What is the long-term survival of patients with prostate cancer?

TNM Stage	5-Year Survival (%)
I	85–93
II	74–82
III	56–68
IV	32–48

DeVita T Jr, Hellman S, Rosenberg SA (eds): Cancer: Principles and Practice of Oncology, 6th ed. Philadelphia, Lippincott Williams & Wilkins, 2001.

91. **How is PSA used in the diagnosis of prostate cancer?**
PSA is a glycoprotein found in the ductular epithelium of normal and malignant prostate tissue. It can be elevated in benign prostatic hyperplasia, prostatitis, and prostate cancer. Gram for gram, malignant prostate cells secrete more PSA than benign prostate tissue. PSA is currently used as a screening method for prostate cancer. If the PSA is > 10 ng/mL, the chance is almost 60% of having prostate cancer. The rate of rise of the PSA and the percentage of free PSA also can help to determine if an elevated PSA level is due to benign or malignant causes.

92. **How often should men be screened for prostate cancer?**
The America Cancer Society and the American Urological Association recommend yearly rectal exam and PSA in all men older than 50 and in men older than 40 in high-risk groups (e.g., blacks, strong family history).

93. **Summarize the effects and mechanisms of the various androgen-deprivation therapies for prostate cancer.**
See Figure 6-2.

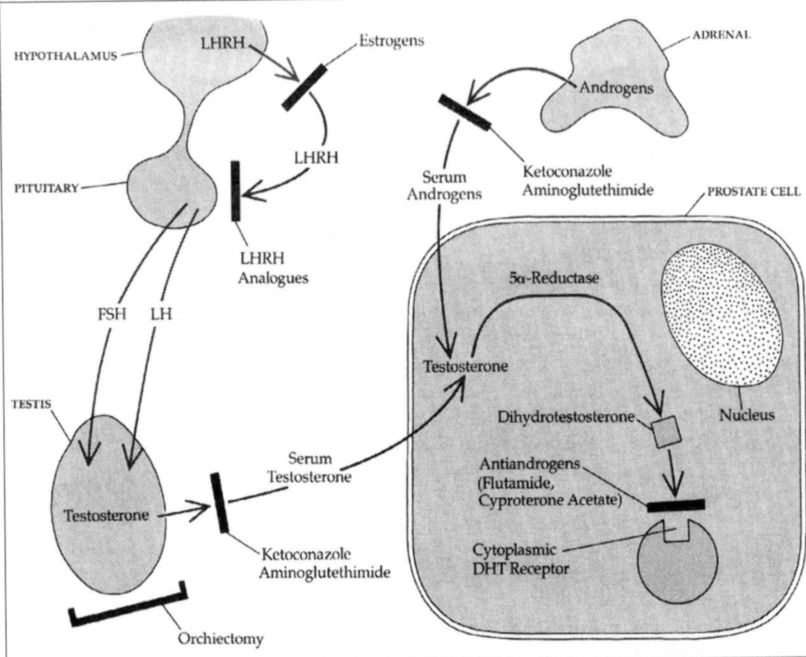

Figure 6-2. Androgen deprivation, which prevents the trophic influence of testosterone on the prostate in advanced prostate carcinoma, can be affected in a variety of ways. Estrogens such as diethylstilbestrol inhibit the release of luteinizing hormone–releasing hormone (LHRH) from the hypothalamus, thus diminishing the release of follicle-stimulating hormone (FSH) and luteinizing hormone (LH) from the anterior pituitary and reducing the signal that stimulates testosterone production by the testes. LHRH analogs such as leuprolide initially stimulate but ultimately inhibit the release of FSH and LH from the anterior pituitary and thus have an estrogen-like effect. The testes, which produce most of the testosterone, can be removed by orchiectomy. Ketoconazole and aminoglutethimide inhibit a variety of steroid synthetic pathways, including those that produce androgens in the testes and adrenal glands. In the prostate cells, testosterone is converted into dihydrotestosterone (DHT) by the enzyme 5α-reductase. Antiandrogens such as flutamide, cyproterone acetate, and certain progestational agents block the binding of DHT to its cytoplasmic receptor. (From Rubenstein E, Federman DD [eds]: Scientific American Medicine. New York, Scientific American, 1993, p 12[IXA]:8, with permission.)

94. What does the Gleason score mean in relation to prostate cancer?
The Gleason score on a prostate cancer biopsy is used to determine how aggressive a prostate cancer is likely to be, based on its appearance on light microscopy. The pathologist assigns a number from 1 to 5 to the two most common patterns of differentiation in the specimen, with 1 being the most well differentiated and 5 the most poorly differentiated pattern. The sum of the two numbers is the Gleason's score. Values of 2–4 represent the least aggressive cancers and 8–10 the most aggressive. Cancers with Gleason's scores of 5–7 are intermediate in their behavior.

95. What is appropriate therapy for stage I prostate cancer?
Watchful waiting, radical prostatectomy, external-beam radiation therapy, and transurethral prostatectomy (TURP) if needed for symptoms of benign prostatic hypertrophy (BPH) all can be appropriate choices, depending on the patient.

96. List the appropriate therapy options for stage II prostate cancer.
Radical prostatectomy, external-beam radiation therapy, brachytherapy, and watchful waiting for selected patients

97. List the appropriate therapy options for stage III prostate cancer.
Radiation therapy ± hormonal therapy, radical prostatectomy with pelvic lymphadenectomy ± hormonal therapy, and watchful waiting for selected patients

98. What is appropriate therapy for stage IV postate cancer?
- For urinary obstruction, TURP or radiation therapy
- For asymptomatic patients, endocrine manipulation or close observation
- For symptomatic disease, hormonal therapy
- For symptomatic areas, palliative radiation therapy
- For disease refractory to hormonal therapy, chemotherapy

99. List the environmental risk factors for the development of bladder cancer.
- Occupational hazards (e.g., workers in dye industry, hairdressers, painters, leather workers)
- Geographic factors (e.g., endemic schistosomiasis)
- Self-ingested toxins (e.g., tobacco, phenacetin, possibly artificial sweeteners)
- Alkylating agents (cyclophosphamide)
- Previous cancers, especially those of the urothelial tract

100. What cytogenetic abnormalities are risk factors for bladder cancer?
- Presence of the Ha-*ras* oncogene
- Alterations in the *p53* suppressor gene
- Methylation of the *myc* oncogene
- Abnormalities on chromosomes 1, 5, 7, 9, 11, 17

101. What is the classic triad of symptoms of renal cell cancer?
The classic triad of symptoms consists of gross hematuria, abdominal mass, and pain. All three symptoms, however, are present in only 9% of patients with renal cell cancer. Hematuria is seen in 59% of patients, abdominal mass in 45%, and pain in 41%.

102. List other symptoms of renal cell cancer along with their frequency.
- Weight loss (28%)
- Anemia (21%)
- Tumor calcification on x-ray (13%)
- Symptoms from metastases (10%)
- Fever (7%)
- Asymptomatic when diagnosed (7%)

- Hypercalcemia (3%)
- Acute varicocele (2%)

Skinner DG, et al: Diagnosis and management of renal cell carcinoma: A clinical and pathologic study of 309 cases. Cancer 28:1165, 1971.

103. Why is renal cell cancer called "the internist's tumor"?
Despite the classic triad of presenting features, renal cell cancer has been called "the internist's tumor" due to its various unusual presentations. Examples include amyloidosis, hypercalcemia, hypertension, hepatopathy without liver metastases, enteropathy, heart failure, and immune complex glomerulonephritis.

104. What determines the prognosis for renal cell cancer?
Survival depends on stage and grade of the tumor.

105. Give the 5-year survival rates for the four stages of renal cell cancer.

- Stage I (confined to the renal parenchyma, ≤ 7 cm in greatest dimension): 88–95%
- Stage II (confined to the renal parenchyma, > 7 cm in greatest dimension: 67–88%
- Stage III (involves the renal vein, inferior vena cava, or regional lymph nodes): 40–59%
- Stage IV (invades beyond Gerota's fascia or distant metastases): 2–20%

106. Give the 5-year survival rates for the various grades of renal cell cancer.

- Grade I (highly differentiated tumors, sharply demarcated from surrounding tissue): 100%
- Grade IIA (moderately differentiated tumors, locally well circumscribed but not necessarily provided with capsule): 59%
- Grade IIB (moderately differentiated tumors, poorly circumscribed but not diffusely infiltrating or markedly polymorphous and mitotic): 36%
- Grade III (poorly differentiated, markedly polymorphous tumors that are diffusely infiltrating; tumors with abundant growth in capillary vessels): 0%

American Joint Committee on Cancer: Cancer Staging Manual, 5th ed. Philadelphia, Lippincott, 1997.

DeVita T Jr, Hellman S, Rosenberg SA (eds): Cancer: Principles and Practice of Oncology, 6th ed. Philadelphia, Lippincott Williams & Wilkins, 2001.

107. What treatments are available for advanced stage renal cell cancer? How effective are they?
The most effective therapy is early diagnosis and surgery. Once the disease is widespread, there are few effective therapies. Biologic response modifiers such as interferon, interleukins, tumor necrosis factor, and activated lymphocytes are used. Under strict selection criteria, overall response rates of 15–30% have been achieved, but some durable responses occur. Megestrol acetate has been used with variable success, mainly resulting in responses of 10–15%. A few chemotherapeutic agents are slightly active, with response rates in the same range as the hormonal treatments; the most commonly used agent is vinblastine. Thalidomide and bevacizumab, a monoclonal antibody against vascular endothelial growth factor, have shown modest results in prolonging progression-free survival.

108. How common is testicular cancer in the U.S.?
Testicular cancer is responsible for approximately 1.3% of all cancers in U.S. males. The majority of these are men 29–35 years of age, with 8980 new cases annually. The incidence of testicular cancer is higher in patients with cryptorchidism, Klinefelter's syndrome, and testicular feminization syndrome.

109. What causes testicular cancer?
The cause is unknown, but age, genetic influences, repeated infection, radiation, and possible endocrine abnormalities have been suggested. Cytogenetic markers associated with germ cell

cancer of the testes include the presence of isochromosome 12p. When present in multiple copies, a poorer prognosis is indicated.

American Cancer Society, Statistics for 2004. Available at http://www.cancer.org/docroot/stt/stt_0.asp.

110. What are the presenting features of testicular cancer?

A tumor that presents locally is detected as a mass in the scrotum. The mass is often painless, although pain is noted in about 25% of reported cases. When the tumor has already spread (5–15%), symptoms of metastases to the lungs and liver are demonstrated. Other diagnostic possibilities of a scrotal mass include epididymitis, hydrocele, inguinal hernia, hematocele, hematoma, testicular torsion, spermatocele, varicocele, and gumma.

111. Which pathologic types are most commonly seen among testicular cancers?

Tumors of One Histologic Type

- Seminoma (germinoma)
  - Typical (35%)
  - Anaplastic (4%)
  - Spermatocytic (1%)
- Embryonal carcinoma (20%)
- Teratoma (10%)
- Choriocarcinoma (1%)

Tumors of Mixed Histologic Type

- Embryonal carcinoma and teratoma (teratocarcinoma) (24%)
- Other combinations (5%)

112. What are the stages of testicular cancer?

Stage I: no lymph node involvement or distant metastases
Stage II: regional lymph node metastasis
Stage III: distant metastasis to nonregional lymph nodes, lungs, or other sites

The stages are further subdivided based on the results of serum LDH and tumor marker studies (AFP and beta HCG).

113. What determines survival rate in testicular cancer?

Survival can no longer be determined on the basis of stage but depends much more on the response to therapy. In patients who respond, the survival curves plateau at about 90%.

114. How should stage I testicular cancer be treated?

Transinguinal orchiectomy is performed in all patients with testicular carcinoma. This procedure serves to make the pathologic diagnosis and is the treatment for stage I cancer.

115. How is pure seminoma treated?

Limited stage cases are treated with radiation to the retroperitoneal nodes or close observation followed by radiation if there is relapse. Disseminated disease is treated with combination chemotherapy.

116. How are nonseminomatous tumors treated?

For nonseminomatous tumors, retroperitoneal lymphadenectomy is most commonly done. If nodes are positive, patients may be treated with two to four cycles of adjuvant chemotherapy.

117. Describe the treatment for stage III disease.

For patients with stage III disease or earlier stage disease with bulky mediastinal or retroperitoneal masses, three to four courses of chemotherapy are given, followed by resection of any residual disease.

118. How are patients followed for recurrent disease?
Tumor markers—AFP and HCG—are followed for evidence of recurrent disease. These markers are quite sensitive for the presence of disease, although normal values do not rule out disease.

119. Describe the extragonadal germ cell syndrome.
The extragonadal germ cell syndrome is characterized by germ cell tumors found in the mediastinum, retroperitoneum, or pineal gland in relatively young males, with elevated HCG or AFP and marked elevation of LDH. Patients often respond to treatment with chemotherapy developed for testicular cancer. A careful search for an occult testicular primary tumor must be carried out, since the testis is thought to be a relative sanctuary from the effects of chemotherapy. Ultrasound evaluation is useful in this setting.

LUNG CANCER

120. What are the common presenting signs and symptoms of lung cancer?
Common symptoms of lung cancer fall into four categories:
- Secondary to central or endobronchial growth of the primary tumor
- Secondary to peripheral growth of the primary tumor
- Secondary to regional spread of the tumor in the thorax by contiguity or by metastasis to regional lymph nodes
- Secondary to distant metastases or systemic effects

121. List symptoms secondary to central or endobronchial growth of the primary tumor.
- Cough
- Dyspnea from obstruction
- Wheeze and stridor
- Pneumonitis from obstruction (fever, productive cough)
- Hemoptysis

122. Which symptoms may be secondary to peripheral growth of the primary tumor?
- Pain from pleural or chest wall involvement
- Dyspnea on a restrictive basis
- Lung abscess syndrome from tumor cavitation
- Cough

123. List symptoms related to regional spread of the tumor in the thorax by contiguity or by metastasis to regional lymph nodes.
Tracheal obstruction
Recurrent laryngeal nerve paralysis with hoarseness
Sympathetic nerve paralysis with Horner's syndrome
Superior vena cava syndrome from vascular obstruction
Lymphatic obstruction with pleural effusion
Esophageal compression with dysphagia
Phrenic nerve paralysis with elevation of the hemidiaphragm and dyspnea
C8 and T1 nerve compression with ulnar pain and Pancoast's syndrome
Pericardial and cardiac extension with resultant tamponade, arrhythmia, or cardiac failure
Lymphangitic spread through the lungs with hypoxemia and dyspnea

124. Which symptoms may be due to distant metastases or systemic effects?

Bone pain	Hemiparesis
Painful lymphadenopathy	Weight loss
Hypercalcemia	Fatigue, malaise

Cohen MH: Signs and symptoms of bronchogenic carcinoma. In Straus MJ (ed): Lung Cancer: Clinical Diagnosis and Treatment, 2nd ed. New York, Grune & Stratton, 1983, pp 97–111.

125. What are the accepted and proposed risk factors for lung cancer?

- **Cigarette smoking** causes 85% of lung cancers in men. In women, lung cancer has surpassed breast cancer as the leading cause of cancer death. Passive smoking also increases the risk of lung cancer, causing 25% of the lung cancers in nonsmokers.
- **Radon exposure** increases the risk of lung cancer, especially in smokers, who have a 10-fold higher risk. An estimated 25% of lung cancer in nonsmokers and 5% in smokers is attributed to radon daughter exposure in the home.
- **Marijuana smoking** increases the risk of lung cancer in smokers.
- **Emphysema**, which develops in smokers, is associated with an increased risk.
- **Other agents**: Bis-chloromethylether, arsenic, nickel, ionizing radiation, asbestos, chromates.

126. Which chromosomal defects are associated with lung cancer?

Deletion of 3p (usually 3pl4–23) is found in virtually all cases (93%) of small cell lung cancer (SCLC; both classic and variant), in 100% of bronchial carcinoids, and 25% of non-SCLC. Also seen are absent or reduced expression of the *rb* gene at 13ql4, increased production of the c-*jun* oncogene product, and constitutive expression of c-*raf*-1 gene on 3p25. More than 50% of all lung cancers contain a mutation of the *p53* tumor suppressor gene. A *ras* family oncogene is mutated in about 20% of non-SCLC, but not in SCLC.

127. Which tests are used for the evaluation of suspected lung cancer?

The primary evaluation should include a chest x-ray and sputum cytology. If the expectorated sputum cytology is negative, bronchoscopy with biopsy, percutaneous biopsy, or thoracoscopy may be done. Preoperative evaluation includes CT scanning of the chest and upper abdomen to evaluate for mediastinal and hilar nodes and for liver and/or adrenal metastases. Pulmonary function tests, mediastinoscopy, and positron emission tomography scan should be done if surgical resection is considered. In SCLC and advanced-stage non-SCLC, screening for the presence of brain metastases is recommended, using CT or MRI with contrast. Elevated alkaline phosphatase with normal liver CT suggests bony metastasis, and a bone scan should be done.

128. Which paraneoplastic syndromes are associated with lung cancer?

See Table 6-6.

129. Which treatment modalities are used to manage SCLC?

Because of early hematogenous spread, surgery is not generally an option for patients with SCLC. Chemotherapy (using combinations of drugs such as etoposide, cisplatin, carboplatin, or CPT-11) and radiotherapy are used concurrently or sequentially. These therapies in limited stage disease have resulted in complete remission rates of 40–60%, median survival of 16–24 months, and 5-year survivals of 5–10%. Prophylactic radiotherapy to the brain remains controversial, and timing, dose, and long-term complications continue to be argued.

130. How effective is the treatment of advanced stage (IV) SCLC?

Patients with advanced-stage SCLC often have good partial responses to chemotherapy, but the responses are not durable. Median survival for patients with extensive disease who respond to treatment is 6–12 months. However, this is a significant improvement over the survival of untreated patients, which is measured in weeks.

TABLE 6-6. PARANEOPLASTIC SYNDROMES IN LUNG CANCER

1. **Systemic symptoms**
   Anorexia-cachexia (31%)
   Fever (21%)
   Suppressed immunity
2. **Endocrine symptoms** (12%)
   Ectopic PTH: hypercalcemia (epidermoid)
   SIADH (SCLC)
   Ectopic secretion of ACTH: Cushing's syndrome
3. **Skeletal symptoms**
   Clubbing (29%)
   Hypertrophic pulmonary osteoarthropathy: periostitis (1–10%) (adenocarcinoma)
4. **Coagulation-thrombosis**
   Migratory thrombophlebitis, Trousseau's syndrome: venous thrombosis
   Nonbacterial thrombotic endocarditis: arterial emboli; DIC: hemorrhage
5. **Neurologic-myopathic symptoms**
   Lambert-Eaton syndrome (SCLC)
   Peripheral neuropathy
   Subacute cerebellar degeneration
   Cortical degeneration
   Polymyositis
   Retinal blindness
6. **Cutaneous symptoms**
   Dermatomyositis
   Acanthosis nigricans
7. **Hematologic symptoms** (8%)
   Anemia
   Granulocytosis
   Leukoerythroblastosis
8. **Renal symptoms** (1%)
   Nephrotic syndrome
   Glomerulonephritis

SIADH = syndrome of inapproriate antidiuretic hormone, ACTH = adrenocorticotropic hormone.
Data from Cohen MH: Signs and symptoms of bronchogenic carcinoma. In Straus MJ (ed): Lung Cancer: Clinical Diagnosis and Treatment. New York, Grune & Stratton, 1977, pp 85–94.

KEY POINTS: LUNG CANCER

1. The most common cause of cancer death in the United States for both men and women is lung cancer.
2. Eighty-five percent of lung cancer is caused by smoking; these deaths are entirely preventable.
3. Lung cancer is rarely curable unless it is diagnosed in a very early stage.
4. Patients should be counseled to quit all forms of tobacco use at every physician's visit.

131. What is the superior vena cava (SVC) syndrome? What is its significance in lung cancer?

SVC syndrome results when the flow of blood in the SVC is obstructed due to thrombosis within the vessel or external compression of the vein by tumor (Fig. 6-3). Lung cancer, especially SCLC, accounts for up to 80% of cases. Lymphoma and other mediastinal malignancies account for the remaining 20%.

132. Why is SVC syndrome significant?

Although obstruction of the vena cava has been considered a life-threatening oncologic emergency, only rarely does it progress to cause laryngeal edema, seizures, coma, and death. Usually, patients present with dyspnea, face and arm edema, a sense of fullness in the head, and cough. Typically, collateral circulation develops over time, limiting the severity of symptoms.

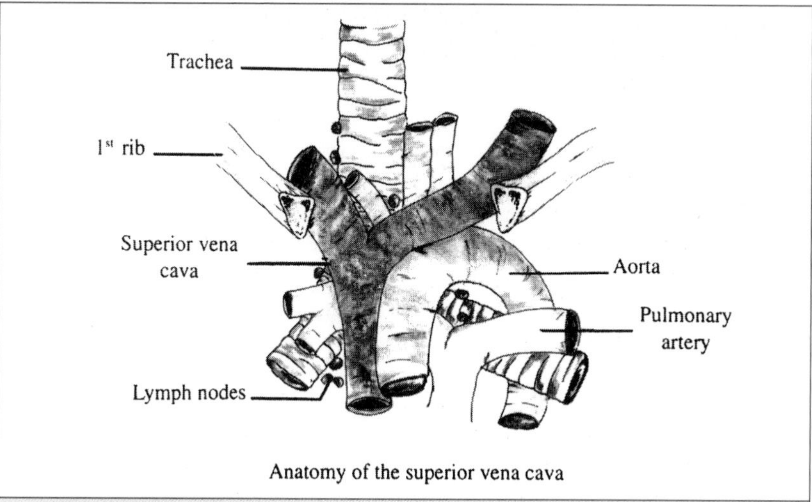

Figure 6-3. Anatomy of the superior vena cava. (From Wood ME, Bunn PA Jr: Hematology/Oncology Secrets. Philadelphia, Hanley & Belfus, 1994, p 240.)

Physical findings include prominent veins over the neck and chest, and failure of hand veins to collapse when the arms are lifted above the head. SVC syndrome can be treated by radiotherapy or stent placement. Patients with SVC syndrome should not be given intravenous medications in the upper extremities.

133. How is non-SCLC treated?

The first decision to be made is whether the patient is a candidate for resection. If the patient is medically able to undergo surgery, this is the procedure of choice. Resection should be performed if the following are *not* present:

- Distant metastases
- Malignant pleural effusion
- SVC obstruction
- Involvement of supraclavicular, cervical, or contralateral mediastinal nodes
- Recurrent laryngeal nerve paralysis
- Involvement of the mediastinum, tracheal wall, or mainstem bronchus < 2 cm from the carina
- Small cell carcinoma histology

134. How is stage IIIA non-SCLC treated?

In stage IIIA disease (large tumor or involvement of mediastinal nodes), preoperative chemotherapy and radiotherapy significantly improve survival. If patients are not able to undergo surgery or the tumor is locally advanced but inoperable, then combined chemotherapy and radiotherapy are indicated. In higher-stage disease, systemic chemotherapy or palliative care are options, depending on the performance status of the patient.

HEAD AND NECK CANCER

135. What are the presenting symptoms of head and neck cancer?

See Table 6-7.

TABLE 6-7. PRESENTING SYMPTOMS OF HEAD AND NECK CANCER

Site	Symptoms
Oral cavity: lips, buccal mucosa, alveolar ridge, retromolar trigone, floor of mouth, hard palate, anterior two thirds of tongue	Mass, ulcer, leukoplakia, erythroplasia bleeding, pain, loose teeth, earache, trismus, halitosis
Larynx: supraglottic (false cords, arytenoid), glottic (true vocal cords), subglottic	Hoarseness, bleeding, sore throat, thyroid cartilage pain
Pharynx: nasopharynx, oropharynx, soft palate, uvula, tonsil, base of tongue, hypopharynx, pyriform sinus	Sore throat, earache, epistaxis, nasal voice, dysphagia, masses, hearing loss, blood-streaked saliva
Maxillary sinus	Sinusitis, epistaxis, headache
All sites	Bleeding (oral or nasal), neck nodes, pain at site of tumor or referred pain

136. **What are the two major risk factors for squamous cell cancer of the head and neck area?**
Tobacco is the most significant contributing factor to the development of head and neck cancers. Nine of ten patients with cancer in this area are smokers. Snuff dipping and tobacco chewing are important causes of oral cancer. Smokers have an increased mortality related to head and neck cancer once it has been diagnosed, showing a two-fold increase in mortality over nonsmokers. **Alcohol** is also strongly correlated with the development of head and neck cancer. About half of the patients with these cancers have cirrhosis, and three quarters drink alcohol excessively.

137. **What other risk factors have been identified?**
Other factors include poor dental hygiene and viral and occupational exposures. The Epstein-Barr and Herpes simplex type I viruses have been implicated in up to 15% of cases. Woodworkers have an increased incidence of nasopharyngeal cancer. Syphilitic glossitis predisposes to tongue cancer, and nickel compounds to nasal sinus cancer.

138. **Describe the evaluation and initial staging of patients with head and neck cancer.**
Initial staging of head and neck cancer includes a thorough **triple endoscopy** of upper and lower airway and upper aerodigestive tract, with biopsy of any suspicious lesions. Measurement and biopsy, if indicated, of any cervical or supraclavicular nodes should be performed. A **CT scan** of the area helps to determine the extent of disease. CT of the chest should be done to evaluate for pulmonary or hepatic metastases.

139. **What are the most common sites of metastases of head and neck cancer?**
The most common sites of metastases are local lymphatics, followed by lung metastases. Bone metastases occur in about 15% of the patients. Brain metastases are rare and are seen mainly in patients with nasopharyngeal cancer. It is also important to remember that second primaries in the aerodigestive tract are not uncommon. Depending on tobacco and alcohol history, a second cancer of the head and neck, esophagus, or lung may occur in up to 20% of patients at some time in the course of their disease, especially if they continue to smoke and drink.

140. **What is the most appropriate treatment of head and neck cancer?**
Early-stage head and neck cancers are treated primarily with surgery, usually involving radical neck node dissection, sometimes accompanied by postoperative radiotherapy. Radiotherapy is

also used for recurrences that are not amenable to surgery. Depending on tumor location and stage, some head and neck cancers are treated with **multimodality therapy**, using chemotherapy in combination with radiotherapy, or prior to surgery or radiotherapy. For cancer of the larynx, vocal cord preservation with chemotherapy and radiotherapy is preferred whenever possible. Cessation of smoking and alcohol consumption is essential to decrease the occurrence of second primary cancers in the head and neck region.

141. Which chemotherapeutic agents are used in the treatment of squamous cell cancers of the head and neck? How effective are they?
Effective agents include 5-fluorouracil (5-FU) infusions with cisplatin or carboplatin, taxanes, methotrexate, bleomycin, and mitomycin C. Response rates for these agents vary from 25% to 80%, depending on the agent, schedule, tumor type, previous treatment, and performance status. Combination chemotherapy regimens usually show higher initial response rates but have yet to show an increase in survival rates.

BREAST CANCER

142. What are the current recommendations for screening for breast cancer?
There are currently several sets of recommendations from the various specialty organizations whose members are engaged in breast cancer screening (Table 6-8).

TABLE 6-8. RECOMMENDED FREQUENCY OF SCREENING FOR BREAST CANCER

	AGE > 50		AGE < 50	
Organization	Mammogram	Breast Exam	Mammogram	Breast Exam
ACS	Annual	Annual	Age 40–49, annual	Age 20–39, every 3 yr Age 40–49, annual
NCI	Annual	With every periodic physical	Starting at age 40, every 1–2 years*	With every periodic physical
ACOG	As determined by woman's doctor		Age 35–50, baseline*	Age 35–50, exams recommended
ACR	Annual	Annual	Age 40–49, annual	
ACP	Age 50–59, on "routine" basis Age > 60, as determined by doctor and patient	—	Not recommended	
USPSTF	Age 50–69, annual	Age 50–69, annual	Not recommended	Age 40–49, annual

ACS = American Cancer Society, NCI = National Cancer Institute, ACOG = American College of Obstetricians and Gynecologists, ACR = American College of Radiology, ACP = American College of Physicians, USPSTF = U.S. Preventive Services Task Force.
* Mammography recommended more frequently for women with high risk factors.

143. How are high-risk women identified?
The primary care physician must identify high-risk patients who may have a mutation in a dominant breast cancer susceptibility gene. Such families have a history of breast or ovarian cancer in as many as half of all female relatives, with early age of onset and/or bilateral or multifocal disease. These patients have been shown to have a high incidence of the *BRCA1* and *BRCA2* genes on chromosome 17 and 13, respectively. Patients with these gene mutations have been shown to have a cumulative lifetime risk of breast cancer ranging up to 87%.

144. How is the diagnosis of breast cancer established?
By tissue examination. This may be done by percutaneous fine-needle aspirate, with or without x-ray direction, or by incisional or excisional biopsy. While mammograms are essential in screening and localizing tumors, up to 15% of breast cancers may not be seen on mammogram, and the diagnosis cannot be made definitively without tissue confirmation. Any clinically suspicious mass must be biopsied.

145. At what age does the incidence rate of breast cancer peak?
See Figure 6-4.

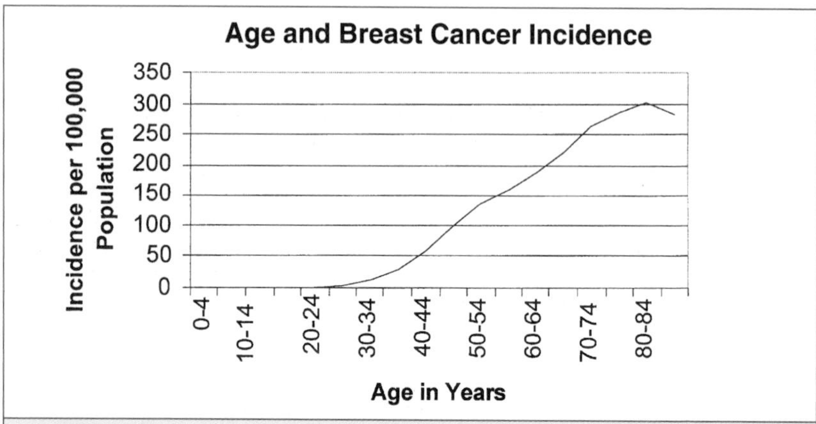

Figure 6-4. Annual age-specific incidence rates of breast cancer, 1993–1997. (From SEER Cancer Statististics Review, 1973–1997 at http://seer.cancer.org.gov/Publications/CSR1973_1997/breast.pdf.)

146. What factors place women at high risk for breast cancer?
Factors associated with a threefold or more increase in risk include the following:

- Age > 40 yr
- Previous cancer in one breast
- Breast cancer in a first- or second-degree family member
- History of multiple breast biopsies
- Parity: nulliparous, or first pregnancy after age 31 years
- Lobular carcinoma in situ
- Gene mutations: *BRCA1, BRCA2, hMSH2, hMLH1, hPMS1, p53*, others
- Radiation exposure to chest wall during childhood or adolescence

147. What factors place women at intermediate risk for breast cancer?
Factors associated with a 1.2- to 1.5-fold increase in risk include the following:

- Early menarche or late menopause
- Oral estrogens

- History of cancer of the ovary, uterus, or colon
- Alcoholic beverages (?)
- Obesity

148. What can women do to reduce their risk of breast cancer?
Recent studies have shown that for women at high risk for breast cancer due to a previous personal history of breast cancer, first-degree family members with breast cancer, and other factors, the use of tamoxifen can reduce the occurrence of new breast cancers by about half. Some women who are known to carry the *BRCA1* or *BRCA2* gene mutations choose to undergo prophylactic simple mastectomies, which reduce the incidence of breast cancer by about 90%.

Vogel VG: Breast cancer prevention: A review of current evidence. CA Cancer J Clin 50:156–170, 2000.

149. What are the poor prognostic factors in primary breast cancer?

1. Estrogen or progesterone receptors negative
2. Positive HER-2/neu status
3. Premenopausal patient
4. Large tumor size
5. Positive axillary nodes
6. Local skin involvement
7. Fixed axillary nodes
8. Distant metastasis
9. Aneuploidy and high cathepsin D
10. Nuclear grade 3 (poor)
11. High S-phase fraction

150. Describe the appropriate treatment of localized-regional breast cancer.
Although there is no single "right" way to treat localized breast cancer, and a great deal of controversy exists, the guidelines based on stage are available.

151. Summarize the guidelines for treatment of stage I breast cancer.
The two basic options are lumpectomy with axillary dissection and radiation or modified radical mastectomy. Lumpectomy/radiotherapy is used if cosmesis is important, complete excision is possible, and > 6000 rads can be delivered to the tumor bed. Modified radical mastectomy is used if cosmesis is unimportant, lesion size is large relative to breast size, or radiotherapy is not technically feasible.

152. What are the guidelines for stage II breast cancer?
Modified radical mastectomy with postoperative chemotherapy and/or hormonal therapy, depending on estrogen and progesterone receptor status of the tumor and menopausal status of the patient.

153. Summarize the guidelines for stage III breast cancer.
Modified radical mastectomy is performed with postoperative chemotherapy and/or hormonal therapy, depending on estrogen and progesterone receptor status of the tumor and menopausal status of the patient, followed by local radiotherapy. For very large or fixed tumors that are initially deemed to be inoperable, preoperative chemotherapy or hormonal therapy may render such cancers surgically removable.

154. How is stage IV breast cancer treated?
The basic choice is systemic chemotherapy or hormone therapy, depending on hormone receptor status, reserving surgery and radiotherapy for local control.

155. How is adjuvant therapy used in the management of breast cancer?
Table 6-9 summarizes current guidelines for premenopausal and postmenopausal women. In addition, postoperative chest wall and regional lymph node radiation therapy is given to patients considered to be at high risk for local recurrence. Risk factors for local recurrence include four or more positive axillary nodes, extracapsular nodal extension, large primary tumors, and positive or very close tumor resection margins.

TABLE 6-9. CURRENT RECOMMENDATIONS FOR THE USE OF ADJUVANT SYSTEMIC THERAPY IN BREAST CANCER

	Premenopausal	Postmenopausal
Node negative*		
ER and PR negative	Chemotherapy	Chemotherapy
ER or PR positive	Chemotherapy + TAM, ovarian ablation or LHRH agonist	Tamoxifen ± chemotherapy
Node positive†		
ER and PR negative	Chemotherapy	Chemotherapy
ER or PR positive	Chemotherapy + TAM, ovarian ablation or LHRH agonist	Tamoxifen ± chemotherapy

* Adjuvant treatment is recommended for patients with poor prognosis tumors: tumor size > 2 cm, poor nuclear grade, high S-phase fraction.
† Adjuvant treatment is recommended for all patients. ER = estrogen receptor, PR = progesterone receptor, TAM = tamoxifen, LHRH = luteinizing hormone-releasing hormone.

156. Discuss the role of aromatase inhibitors in adjuvant therapy for breast cancer.
Recent studies have shown that in hormone-positive cancers, aromatase inhibitors such as anastrozole may be more effective than tamoxifen, and the addition of letrozole after 5 years of adjuvant tamoxifen may be beneficial. These findings remain to be confirmed.

157. Which chemotherapy agents are used in the treatment of metastatic breast cancer?
Among the most effective chemotherapy agents for breast cancer are doxorubicin, epirubicin, paclitaxel, docetaxel, vinorelbine, cyclophosphamide, methotrexate, fluorouracil, capecitabine, and prednisone. These agents are used singly or in combination in the treatment of advanced or metastatic breast cancer. If the tumor overexpresses the *Her/neu* oncogene, trastuzumab (Herceptin) may be added to improve the effectiveness of chemotherapy.

158. How effective are chemotherapy agents in the treatment of metastatic breast cancer?
Overall induction response rates range from 55% to 65%. Median survival times are 14–18 months. The survival rates depend more on the site of the metastatic disease than on the treatment, with visceral disease faring more poorly than bony or soft tissue metastases. Most patients receive more than one treatment regimen, since the median time to failure of most programs is about 6 months.

159. What other drugs may be used to treat metastatic breast cancer?
For bony or soft tissue metastases in patients with estrogen or progesterone receptor-positive breast cancer, hormonal agents such as tamoxifen, anastrozole, letrozole, exemestane, or luteinizing hormone-releasing hormone agonists (in premenopausal women) can be used for effective palliation lasting many months. Newer drugs that target growth factor pathways in breast cancer are currently in development.

GYNECOLOGIC CANCERS

160. Define the risk groups on which current recommendations for cervical carcinoma screening are based.
Recommendations concerning periodic screening of women in the U.S. using Pap smears (Papanicolaou-Traut smears) have been developed for the various risk groups. **Low-risk** groups are those women who have never had sexual activity, have had a hysterectomy for nonmalignant reasons, or have reached the age of 60 and have never had a positive Pap smear. **High-risk** patients are those who are sexually active early, have had many partners, or are in low socioeconomic groups.

161. Summarize the current recommendations for cervical carcinoma screening.
The American Cancer Society and the American College of Obstetricians and Gynecologists recommend that asymptomatic women over 18 years of age and those under age 18 who are sexually active have annual screening for at least 3 years initially. Some groups recommend that women then be screened every 2–3 years until age 65, while others suggest yearly screening as long as the patient is sexually active. High-risk patients should be screened yearly.

162. Sumarize the appropriate management of a patient with an abnormal Pap smear.
A persistently abnormal Pap smear should lead to colposcopy and/or biopsy.

163. What should be done if carcinoma in situ or dysplasia is found?
Cryotherapy, laser therapy, cone biopsy, or hysterectomy should be performed, depending on the size and extent of the lesion.

164. What should be done if invasive cancer is found on biopsy?
A metastatic work-up is indicated. Stage I disease is treated with radical hysterectomy or radiation therapy, whereas all other stages are further evaluated with a CT scan. If the para-aortic nodes are enlarged, a needle biopsy should be done. Patients with a positive biopsy are treated with pelvic radiation therapy and concurrent chemotherapy. If nodes are normal on the CT scan or if the needle biopsy is negative, laparotomy with para-aortic node biopsies should be considered to determine the actual state of the nodes. If the biopsy is positive, then treatment should proceed as for other positive-node biopsies. If it is negative, treatment is external beam radiotherapy followed by intracavitary radioactive implants.

165. Which studies are used in the staging of carcinoma of the cervix?
- Pelvic exam
- Biochemical profile
- Chest x-ray
- CT scan or MRI (MRI is preferred)
- Lymphangiograms may be useful in selected cases
- Cystoscopy and proctosigmoidoscopy for advanced disease

166. What are the 5-year survival rates, relative to stage, for carcinoma of the cervix?
See Table 6-10.

167. How is stage I carcinoma of the cervix treated?
IA: Total or radical hysterectomy, conization, or intracavitary radiation.
IB: External-beam pelvic irradiation combined with two or more intracavitary applications; radical hysterectomy with bilateral pelvic lymphadenectomy ± postoperative total pelvic irradiation plus chemotherapy; radiation therapy plus chemotherapy with cisplatin or cisplatin/5-FU for patients with bulky tumors.

TABLE 6-10. FIVE-YEAR SURVIVAL RATES RELATIVE TO STAGE

Stage	Description	5-Year Survival Rate
I	Tumor strictly confined to the cervix	89–100%
II	Tumor extends beyond the uterus but not to the pelvic wall The tumor involves the vagina but not the lower third	67%
III	Tumor extends to the pelvic wall, and/or involves the lower third of the vagina, and/or causes hydronephrosis or nonfunctioning kidney	53%
IV	Tumor extends beyond the true pelvis, or has involved the bladder or rectal mucosa, or has distant metastases	5–24%

168. Summarize the treatment of stage II carcinoma of the cervix.
IIA: Same as stage IB.
IIB: Radiation therapy plus chemotherapy: intracavitary radiation and external-beam pelvic irradiation combined with cisplatin or cisplatin/fluorouracil.

169. How is stage III carcinoma of the cervix treated?
Same as stage IIB.

170. Summarize the treatment of stage IV carcinoma of the cervix.
IVA: Same as stage IIB and stage III.
IVB: Chemotherapy with agents such as cisplatin, paclitaxel, ifosfamide-cisplatin, or irinotecan. Radiotherapy may be used for palliation.

Cervical Cancer, PDQ Treatment Statements for Health Professionals, National Cancer Institute. Available at http://cancer.gov/cancerinfo/pdq/treatment/cervical/healthprofessional/.

171. Name the risk factors for carcinoma of the endometrium.
1. Infertility
2. Obesity
3. Failure of ovulation
4. Dysfunctional bleeding
5. Prolonged estrogen use
6. Diabetes mellitus
7. Hypertension
8. Polycystic ovaries
9. Familial cancer syndrome (Lynch)
10. Tamoxifen use

172. What are the 5-year survival rates for the various grades and stages of endometrial cancer?
See Table 6-11.

173. List the risk factors for ovarian cancer.
- Nulliparity or low parity
- Presence of basal cell nevus syndrome
- Family history of ovarian cancer or ovarian cancer syndromes
- Gonadal dysgenesis (46XY type)
- History of breast, endometrial, or colon cancer
- Asbestos exposure
- Presence of Peutz-Jeghers syndrome
- Use of fertility drugs (?)

NIH Consensus Development Panel on Ovarian Cancer: Ovarian cancer: Screening, treatment, and follow-up. JAMA 273:491–497, 1995.

TABLE 6-11. FIVE-YEAR SURVIVAL RATES FOR GRADES AND STAGES OF ENDOMETRIAL CANCER

	Description	5-Year Survival Rate
Grade		
I	Differentiated	81%
II	Intermediate	74%
III	Undifferentiated	50%
Stage		
I	Tumor confined to the corpus	92%
II	Tumor involves the corpus and cervix	78%
III	Tumor extends outside the corpus, but not outside the true pelvis (may involve the vaginal wall or parametrium but not the bladder or rectum)	42%
IV	Tumor involves the bladder or rectum, extends outside the pelvis, or has distant metastases	14%

174. Discuss the appropriate use of the CA-125 antigen.

CA-125 serum tumor marker, an antigenic determinant detected by radioimmunoassay, is elevated in 80% of epithelial ovarian cancers. Because it is high in only half of patients with stage I cancers and is increased in a significant proportion of healthy women and women with benign disease, it is not a sensitive or specific test and should not be used for screening in women with average risk for ovarian cancer. In high-risk patients or in patients suspected of having an ovarian cancer, it can be used in conjunction with bimanual rectovaginal pelvic examination and transvaginal ultrasonography. When the CA-125 value is elevated before treatment in a patient with an established diagnosis of ovarian cancer, it is useful as a marker of disease recurrence after surgical resection.

175. List the neurologic paraneoplastic syndromes associated with ovarian cancer.

- Peripheral neuropathy
- Organic brain syndrome
- Acute myelogenous leukemia–like syndrome
- Cerebellar ataxia (anti-Yo paraneoplastic cerebellar degeneration)
- Cancer-associated retinopathy
- Opsoclonus-myoclonus

176. What other paraneoplastic syndromes may be associated with ovarian cancer?

- Cross-matching of blood antigens
- Cushing's syndrome
- Hypercalcemia
- Thrombophlebitis
- Dermatomyositis
- Palmar fasciitis and polyarthritis

177. What are the 5-year survival rates for the various stages of carcinoma of the ovary?

Stage	5-Year Survival Rate
I: Growth limited to the ovaries	84%
II: Growth involving one or both ovaries with pelvic extension	63%
III: Tumor involving ovaries with peritoneal implants outside the pelvis and/or positive retroperitoneal or inguinal nodes	29%
IV: Distant metastases	17%

178. Describe the treatment for advanced-stage ovarian cancer.
Patients with stage III epithelial ovarian cancers are first treated with surgery, consisting of total abdominal hysterectomy and bilateral salpingo-oophorectomy with omentectomy and debulking of as much gross tumor as possible. This is followed by intravenous chemotherapy with cisplatin or carboplatin combined with taxol or cyclophosphamide. Patients with stage IV disease are given combination chemotherapy. The survival benefit of surgical debulking in patients with stage IV extra-abdominal disease is not yet known.

MISCELLANEOUS TOPICS

179. Which cancers are associated with AIDS? How is their incidence changing with the use of highly active antiretroviral therapy?
Kaposi's sarcoma, non-Hodgkin's lymphoma, and cervical cancer are all AIDS-defining conditions. The rates of Hodgkin's disease and anal carcinoma are also significantly increased in some populations of AIDS patients. The incidence of Kaposi's sarcoma has been falling over time. Although the absolute number of cases is falling in most (but not all) series, non-Hodgkin's lymphoma accounts for an increasing proportion of AIDS-defining illness.

Grulich AE: Update: Cancer risk in persons with HIV/AIDS in the era of combination antiretroviral therapy. AIDS Reader 10:341–346, 2000.

180. What phenotype is most highly associated with the development of melanoma?
Typical physical characteristics of patients with melanoma are fair skin, reddish hair, and freckles. Familial melanoma families have been described in which > 25% of the kindred are affected with a vertical distribution of disease. There is an early age of onset, from the third to fourth decades. The incidence of multiple primary melanomas is increased, as is the presence of atypical nevi (B-K moles or familial atypical multiple melanoma with melanocyte dysplasia). However, there is a superior overall survival, possibly related to earlier detection. Ocular melanoma is also seen in this group of patients. The gene for the dysplastic nevus syndrome/familial melanoma is located on chromosome 1.

181. Where does melanoma metastasize?
Melanoma can metastasize anywhere in the body, including lungs, liver, and bones. It is one of the few cancers that can cross the placenta and spread to a developing fetus. It often metastasizes to the bowel, where it causes obstruction and bleeding. Lesions seen on barium dye studies are ulcerated with a central crater and a surrounding heaped-up border, causing the barium to pool in a "target" configuration.

WEB SITES

1. *National Cancer Database: http://www.facs.org/cancer/ncdb/index.html*
2. National Guideline Clearinghouse: http://www.guideline.gov/
3. PDQ Cancer Information Summaries: http://www.cancer.gov/
4. SEER Cancer Statistics Review, 1975–2000: http://seer.cancer.gov/csr/1975_2000/

BIBLIOGRAPHY

1. American Joint Committee on Cancer: Cancer Staging Manual, 6th ed. New York, Springer-Verlag, 2002.
2. Calabresi P, Schein PS (eds): Basic Principles and Clinical Management of Cancer, 2nd ed. New York, Macmillan, 1993.
3. Casciato DA, Lowitz BB (eds): Manual of Clinical Oncology, 5th ed. Boston, Little, Brown, 2000.
4. DeVita T Jr, Hellman S, Rosenberg SA (eds): Cancer: Principles and Practice of Oncology, 6th ed. Philadelphia, Lippincott Williams & Wilkins, 2001.
5. Haskell CM: Cancer Treatment, 4th ed. Philadelphia, W.B. Saunders, 1995.
6. Holland JF, Frei E, et al (eds): Cancer Medicine, 6th ed. New York, BC Decker, 2003.
7. Tannock IF, Hill RP (eds): The Basic Science of Oncology, 3rd ed. New York, McGraw-Hill, 1998.

NEPHROLOGY

Sharma S. Prabhakar, M.D.

CHAPTER 7

ASSESSMENT OF RENAL FUNCTION

1. **What is the glomerular filtration rate (GFR)?**
GFR is the ultrafiltrate of plasma that exits the glomerular capillary tuft and enters Bowman's capsule to begin the journey along the tubule of the nephron. It is the initial step in the formation of urine and is usually expressed in milliliters per minute.

2. **How is the GFR measured clinically?**
The GFR is measured indirectly with a marker substance contained in glomerular filtrate, which is then excreted in the urine. The amount of this substance leaving the kidney (urinary mass excretion) must equal the amount of marker substance entering the kidney as glomerular filtrate; it must not be reabsorbed, secreted, or metabolized after entering the kidney tubule. The marker substance is chosen so that its concentration in the glomerular filtrate is equal to its concentration in the plasma (i.e., the substance is freely filterable across the glomerular capillary). Therefore, the amount of substance X entering the kidney equals the GFR multiplied by the plasma concentration of the substance (P_X). Likewise, the amount of the substance leaving the kidney in the urine equals the urinary concentration of the substance (U_X) multiplied by the urine flow in ml/min (V). Therefore, the formula for calculating GFR using our marker substance X becomes: $GFR \times P_X = U_X V$ *or* $GFR = U_X V / P_X$
A stable plasma concentration of the substance (steady-state situation) is required to make the above equation useful.

3. **Why is creatinine used as a marker substance for GFR determinations in clinical settings?**
Creatinine is an endogenous substance, derived from the metabolism of creatine in skeletal muscle, which fulfills almost all of the requirements for a marker substance: it is freely filterable, not metabolized, and not reabsorbed once filtered. A small amount of tubular secretion makes the creatinine clearance a slight overestimate of the GFR, but this overestimate becomes quantitatively important only at low levels of GFR. Creatinine is released from muscle at a constant rate, resulting in a stable plasma concentration. The creatinine clearance is commonly determined from a 24-hour collection of urine. This time period is used to average out the sometimes variable creatinine excretion that may occur from hour to hour. Creatinine is easily measured, making it a nearly ideal marker for GFR determination.

4. **Is any other substance used as a marker of GFR in laboratory settings?**
The polysaccharide **inulin** is often used in laboratory determinations of GFR. However, it requires constant intravenous infusion, making it somewhat impractical for routine clinical use in patients.

5. **Can the completeness of a 24-hour urine collection be judged?**
Since total creatinine excretion in the steady state is dependent on muscle mass, day-to-day creatinine excretion remains fairly constant for an individual and is related to lean body weight. In general, men excrete 20–25 mg creatinine/kg body weight/day, whereas women excrete 15–20

mg/kg/day. Therefore, a 70-kg man excretes ~1400 mg creatinine/day. Creatinine excretion levels measured on a 24-hour urine collection that are substantially less than the estimated value suggest an incomplete collection.

6. **What is the relationship between the plasma creatinine concentration and GFR?**
Because creatinine production and excretion remain constant and equal, the amount of creatinine entering and leaving the kidney remains constant. Thus:

$$GFR \times P_{Cr} = U_{Cr} \times V = \text{constant } \textbf{\textit{or}} \text{ } GFR = (1/P_{Cr}) \times \text{constant}$$

Creatinine excretion remains constant as GFR declines until the GFR reaches very low levels. Therefore, the GFR is a function of the reciprocal of the plasma creatinine concentration.

7. **Does a given plasma creatinine concentration reflect the same level of renal function in different patients?**
Not necessarily. Remember that creatinine production is directly proportional to muscle mass, and that the plasma creatinine concentration (P_{Cr}) is determined in part by creatinine production. Examination of the creatinine clearance (C_{Cr}) for an 80-kg man compared to that of a 40-kg woman, assuming both individuals have P_{Cr} of 1.0 mg/dL (0.01 mg/mL), shows the following:
For the 80-kg man, creatinine excretion should be:

$$80 \text{ kg} \times 20 \text{ mg/kg/day} = 1600 \text{ mg/day} = 1.11 \text{ mg/min}$$
$$GFR = (1.11 \text{ mg/min})/(0.01 \text{ mg/mL}) = 111 \text{ mL/min}$$

For the 40-kg woman, creatinine excretion should be:

$$40 \text{ kg} \times 15 \text{ mg/kg/day} = 600 \text{ mg/day} = 0.42 \text{ mg/min}$$
$$GFR = (0.42 \text{ mg/min})/(0.01 \text{ mg/mL}) = 42 \text{ mL/min}$$

This example demonstrates that the same P_{Cr} can represent markedly different GFRs in different individuals.

8. **What formula is used to estimate GFR when a measured C_{Cr} is not immediately available?**
The following formula was devised to provide a rough estimate of the GFR when a measured C_{Cr} is not immediately available:

$$C_{Cr} = (140 - [\text{age} \times \text{lean body wt in kg}])/(P_{Cr} \times 72)$$

If we use this formula to estimate the GFR of the above individuals and assume an age of 50 years for each, we get a GFR of 100 for the man and 50 for the woman. These estimates are in the range of those determined previously and serve to illustrate the relative differences in the GFR calculated for two individuals with the same P_{Cr}. Recognizing this fact and using this formula to estimate GFR could prevent a serious error when selecting the dose of a drug that is excreted by the kidneys.

9. **How does the blood urea nitrogen (BUN) relate to the GFR?**
BUN is excreted primarily by glomerular filtration. Its level in the plasma tends to vary inversely with GFR. BUN, however, is a much less ideal marker of GFR than is creatinine. Its production may not be constant, in that it varies with protein intake, liver function, and catabolic rate. In addition, urea can be reabsorbed once filtered into the kidney, and this reabsorption increases in conditions with low urine flow, such as volume depletion. This latter circumstance is one cause

of a high (> 15:1) BUN-to-creatinine ratio in plasma. Thus, creatinine is the better marker for GFR. But the plasma level of BUN can be used along with the C_{Cr} to indicate the presence of certain states, such as volume depletion.

10. **What is the difference between clearance and excretion?**
Urinary **excretion** of a substance is simply the total amount of a substance excreted per unit of time. It is usually expressed in mg/min. **Clearance** expresses the efficiency with which the kidney removes a substance from the plasma. The volume of plasma that must be completely cleared of a substance per unit of time accounts for the amount of that substance appearing in the urine per unit of time. It is expressed in volume per unit of time, usually mL/min.

11. **Give an example of clearance.**
Substance (X) with a plasma concentration (P_x) of 1.0 mg/ml, urine concentration (U_x) of = 10 mg/mL, and urine flow (V) of 1.0 mL/min has the following clearance:

$$Cl_x = (U_x/P_x) \times V = (10 \text{ mg/mL} \times 1 \text{ mL/min})/1.0 \text{ mg/min} = 10 \text{ mL/min}$$

The calculated clearance of 10 mL/min indicates that the amount of substance X appearing in the urine is the same as if 10 mL of plasma were completely cleared of the substance and excreted in the urine each minute. The urinary excretion of X is 10 mg/min, but this measurement does not indicate the efficiency with which the substance is removed from the plasma.

12. **How does measurement of urinary protein excretion help in the evaluation of renal disease?**
Normal urinary protein excretion is < 150 mg/day, with albumin constituting < 50% of this protein. Failure of the tubules to reabsorb the normally filtered small-molecular-weight (MW) proteins leads to **tubular proteinuria**. This occurs in diseases that affect tubular function, and the proteins are almost entirely of smaller MW rather than albumin. **Glomerular proteinuria** occurs when the normal glomerular barrier to the passage of plasma proteins is disrupted. This results in variable quantities of albumin and sometimes larger MW proteins spilling into the urine. Quantitatively, tubular proteinuria is usually < 1 g/24 h, and glomerular proteinuria is usually > 1 g/24 h. When the proteinuria is > 3.5 g/1.73 m^2 body surface area, it is said to be in the **nephrotic range**. Significant degrees of proteinuria (> 150 mg/day) could indicate intrinsic renal disease. Quantification and characterization of the proteinuria are useful in detecting the presence of renal disease and also in determining involvement of the tubule, glomerulus, or both.

13. **What information can be gained from examining urine sediment?**
Urine sediment is normally almost cell free, is usually crystal free, and contains a very low concentration of protein (< 1+ by dipstick). Examination of this sediment is an important part of the work-up of any patient with renal disease. The examination should be performed by the physician before diagnostic or therapeutic decisions are made. The information must be correlated with all other aspects of the patient's history, physical examination, and laboratory database. The examination can provide evidence of many conditions, including renal inflammation (cells, protein), infection (WBCs, bacteria), stone disease (crystals), and systemic diseases (e.g., bilirubin, myoglobin, hemoglobin).

ACUTE RENAL FAILURE

14. **What is acute renal failure (ARF)?**
ARF is a syndrome of many etiologies characterized by a sudden decrease in renal function leading to a compromise in the kidney's ability to regulate normal homeostasis. This inability is multifactorial. The kidney is unable to maintain the content and volume of the extracellular

fluid or perform its routine endocrine functions. In most cases, ARF is a potentially reversible process. The clinical manifestations of ARF are generally more severe than those associated with chronic renal failure (CRF) because of the rapidity of development of symptoms. Unlike CRF, a cause for ARF can usually be identified and must be addressed to prevent further kidney or other organ damage. ARF is a potentially reversible disorder if the causative factor or factors are identified and corrected, and appropriate supportive care must be given to optimize the chances for recovery of renal function.

15. **Define oliguria.**
Oliguria refers to a urine volume that is inadequate for the normal excretion of the body's metabolic waste products. Since the daily load of metabolic products amounts to approximately 600 mOsm and the maximal urine concentrating ability of the human kidney is about 1200 mOsm/kg H_2O, there is a minimal obligate urine volume of 500 mL/day for most people. Therefore, a 24-hour urine volume of < **500 mL/day** is said to represent oliguria. When associated with ARF, oliguria portends a poorer prognosis than does nonoliguric ARF.

16. **Define anuria.**
Anuria refers to a 24-hour urine volume of < 100 mL. It denotes a severe reduction in urine volume that is commonly associated with obstruction, renal cortical necrosis, or severe acute tubular necrosis (ATN). It is important to make the distinction between oliguria and anuria so that these diagnostic entities will be considered and appropriate therapy planned.

17. **How are the causes of ARF classified?**
The causes of ARF as classified as prerenal, renal, or postrenal.

18. **List the common prerenal causes of ARF in the U.S.**
- True volume depletion, as seen with GI losses (vomiting, diarrhea, bleeding), renal losses (diuretics, osmotic diuresis [glucose], hypoaldosteronism, salt-wasting nephropathy, diabetes insipidus), skin or respiratory losses (insensible losses, sweat, burns), and third-space sequestration (intestinal obstruction, crush injury or skeletal fracture, acute pancreatitis)
- Hypotension (shock)
- Edematous states (heart failure, hepatic cirrhosis, nephrosis)
- Selective renal ischemia (hepatorenal syndrome, NSAIDs, bilateral renal artery stenosis, calcium channel blockers)

19. **What are the renal causes of ARF?**
    1. **Ischemia** (all causes of severe prerenal disease, especially particularly hypotension)
    2. **Nephrotoxins**, such as drugs and exogenous toxins. Common examples include aminoglycoside antibiotics, radiocontrast media, cisplatin, and NSAIDs. Rare examples include cephalosporins, rifampin, amphotericin B, polymyxin B, methoxyflurane, acetaminophen overdose, heavy metals (mercury, arsenic, uranium), carbon tetrachloride, ethylenediamine tetraacetic acid, and tetracyclines. In addition, heme pigments may lead to rhabdomyolysis (myoglobinuria) and intravascular hemolysis (hemoglobinuria).

20. **What are the postrenal causes of ARF?**
Obstruction due to strictures, stones, malignancies, or prostatic enlargement.

21. **What is meant by prerenal failure?**
Prerenal failure refers to a decrease in renal function resulting from a decrease in renal perfusion. The decrease in renal perfusion leads to functional changes within the kidney, which in turn compromise the kidney's ability to perform its homeostatic functions. This disorder is potentially correctable by addressing the factors leading to renal hypoperfusion. In some cases, renal hypoperfusion can be severe and prolonged enough to result in structural damage and

hence can lead to the "renal" category of ARF. Therefore, it is important that the prerenal syndrome be identified and corrected promptly.

22. Define acute tubular necrosis (ATN).
ATN is a syndrome characterized by structural and functional damage of the renal tubules and a functional decrease of glomerular function. If the patient survives, ATN is self-limited, with most patients recovering renal function within 8 weeks. It is most commonly caused by ischemia, but there are a multitude of other causes.

23. How can the use of urinary indices help to distinguish prerenal failure from ATN?
Patients with prerenal azotemia have intact tubular function. The kidney, in this setting, is attempting to minimize solute and water excretion in an effort to preserve extracellular fluid volume. By contrast, the tubules of patients with ATN do not properly recover solutes and water that have been filtered into the kidney.

24. List the typical findings in the urine of patients with prerenal azotemia.
- Low urinary sodium concentration (< 20 mEq/L)
- Low fractional excretion of sodium (< 1.0%)
- Low free-water excretion (high urine osmolality > 500 and urine specific gravity > 1.015)

25. Contrast the urinary indices of patients with ATN.
The urinary indices of patients with ATN reveal the kidney's relative inability to reabsorb sodium (urinary Na > 40 mEq/L and fractional Na excretion of > 3.0%) and to reabsorb water (urine osmolality < 350 mOsm/L and urine specific gravity < 1.010). Remember that there is considerable crossover between renal and prerenal failure with regard to these indices, and hence no value absolutely indicates one or the other diagnosis. The indices should be used along with other data (i.e., history, physical examination) to arrive at a clinical impression.

26. What is meant by the fractional excretion of sodium (FE_{Na+})?
FE_{Na+} is calculated by using the following equation: $FE_{Na+} = (U_{Na+} \times P_{Cr} \times 100)/(P_{Na+} \times U_{Cr})$ where U_{Na+} and P_{Na+} = urinary and plasma sodium concentrations (in mEq/L) and U_{Cr} and P_{Cr} = urinary and plasma creatinine in mg/dL.

27. What is the relevance of FE_{Na+} to the diagnosis of ARF?
An FE_{Na+} value < 1% favors prerenal states, whereas a value > 1% indicates intrarenal states or ATN. The test is more accurate than urinary Na measurement in this differentiation. However, it should be noted that an FE_{Na+} < 1% is occasionally reported for various causes of ARF other than prerenal states. In addition, an intact sodium reabsorptive capacity is necessary for the use of this test. Thus, in conditions such as underlying chronic renal disease, hypoaldosteronism, diuretic therapy, or metabolic alkalosis with bicarbonaturia, the FE_{Na+} will be inappropriately high despite the presence of volume depletion.

28. What is renal dose dopamine?
It is a widespread practice, particularly in surgical ICUs, to use a low-dose dopamine intravenous infusion in critically sick patients with oliguria to prevent or treat ARF. This practice is based on the belief that dopamine increases the urine output through direct tubular effects. It may also help to increase the tubular delivery of diuretics and may even increase renal blood flow. However, in low doses, dopamine may cause tachycardia and myocardial ischemia. In extreme cases, dopamine may also predispose to digital and bowel ischemia. Hence, low-dose dopamine infusion is not an innocuous intervention.

Chertow GM, Sayegh MH, Lazarus JM: Is dopamine administration associated with adverse or favorable outcomes in ARF? Am J Med 101:49–53, 1996.

29. List the indications for dialysis in patients with ARF.

- Uncontrollable hyperkalemia
- Acute pulmonary edema
- Uremic pericarditis
- Uremia encephalopathy (seizures, coma)
- Bleeding diathesis due to uremia
- Refractory metabolic acidosis (HCO_3^- < 10 mEq/L)
- Severe azotemia (BUN > 100 mg/dL, serum Cr > 10 mg/dL)

30. What is the mortality rate of ARF?

The overall mortality in ARF is very high (40–60%) despite the availability of dialysis. The mortality is worse in the subcategory of patients with a history of surgery or trauma. The prognosis is better in the absence of respiratory failure, bleeding, or infection and also in patients with nonoliguric ATN. ARF in the obstetric setting also has a better prognosis, with only a 10–20% mortality rate.

31. Under what clinical situations do ACE inhibitors lead to ARF?

In bilateral renal artery stenosis and renal artery stenosis of the single kidney or transplant kidney. It is believed that ARF under these conditions is mediated by ACE inhibitor–induced poststenotic dilatation of efferent arterioles and consequent reduction of glomerular hydrostatic pressure. In normal persons, this effect is offset by dilatation of afferent sites and maintenance of GFR. There have been reports of reversible renal failure in patients with chronic essential hypertension treated with ACE inhibitors. In patients with severe nephrosclerosis, GFR depends on angiotensin-induced efferent arteriolar constriction. In patients with decreased effective renal blood flow, as in congestive heart failure, cirrhosis, or nephrosis, systemic hypotension and effective arteriolar dilatation caused by ACE inhibitors result in ARF.

Toto RD, et al: Reversible renal insufficiency due to angiotensin converting enzyme inhibitors in hypertensive nephrosclerosis. Ann Intern Med 115:513–519, 1991.

32. Name the important risk factors for contrast-induced ARF.

1. Azotemia (Cr > 1.5 mg/dL)
2. Albuminuria > 2+
3. Hypertension
4. Age > 60 yr
5. Dehydration
6. Uric acid > 8.0 mg/dL
7. Multiple radiologic studies
8. Solitary kidney
9. Contrast medium > 2 mL/kg
10. Multiple myeloma with renal insufficiency

Berns AS, et al: Nephrotoxicity of contrast media. Kidney Int 36:730–40, 1989.

CHRONIC RENAL FAILURE

33. List the five stages of chronic kidney disease (CKD).

- **Stage 1:** Kidney damage with normal renal reserve (GFR > 90 mL/min)
- **Stage 2:** Mild renal insufficiency (GFR 60–89 mL/min)
- **Stage 3:** Moderate renal failure (GFR 30–59 mL/min)
- **Stage 4:** Severe renal failure or uremic syndrome (GFR 15–29 mL/min)
- **Stage 5:** End-stage renal disease (ESRD) (GFR > 15 mL/min)

34. Summarize the evolution of CKD through the five stages.

Patients with normal renal function have nephron mass in excess of that necessary to maintain a normal GFR. Thus, with progressive loss of renal mass, that which is initially lost is the **renal reserve**, which is not reflected by a rise of BUN and creatinine or in a disturbance of homeostasis. If the progression continues, this stage is followed by a stage of mild **renal insufficiency**, which is associated with mild elevation of BUN and creatinine and very mild symptoms, including nocturia and easy fatigability. With further progression, moderate **renal failure** ensues. This stage is characterized by apparent abnormalities of renal excretory function, including disturbances in water, electrolyte, and acid-base metabolism. Continued worsening of renal function is followed by the stage of severe renal failure with **uremic syndrome**, which includes multiple dysfunction of major organ systems in addition to the abnormalities of excretory function described. Finally, **ESRD** appears, at which time renal replacement therapy (dialysis or transplantation) is required to sustain life.

35. How do the remaining intact nephrons adapt in the diseased kidney?
When nephron mass is lost, the remaining intact (functioning) nephrons compensate to maintain the same excretory function performed by the normal kidney. The individual nephrons accomplish this task by increasing the GFR and excretion of salt and water compared to levels when there was a full contingent of functioning nephrons. The increased excretory function is accomplished by reducing reabsorption of filtered salt and water, often resulting in polyuria and nocturia.

36. What happens to the adaptation process in patients with chronic renal insufficiency?
Patients with chronic renal insufficiency have a reduced ability to respond to changes in intake with appropriate changes in excretory function. The remaining functioning nephrons of persons with decreased GFR are chronically excreting a higher salt load and are thus much closer to their maximum salt-excreting ability. Hence, these patients are less able to adjust to an increased salt intake by increasing salt excretion. At the opposite extreme, the remaining nephrons of the patient with a decreased GFR are less able to reduce their high salt excretion to compensate for a reduction in salt intake. These patients are more at risk of becoming salt-depleted in response to salt restriction than are patients with normal renal function.

37. Why is the renal potassium excretory ability usually well-maintained down to very low (10–15 mL/min) levels of GFR in patients with progressive CRF?
As is the case for salt excretion, the remaining intact nephrons significantly increase potassium excretion such that the level of excretion per nephron is much higher than when there was a full contingent of nephrons. This allows for a total renal K^+ excretion that is nearly normal. In addition, there is evidence that the extrarenal K^+ excretion, especially by the colon, is increased in patients with CRF. By these mechanisms, patients with a significant decrease in GFR are unlikely to be hyperkalemic purely as a result of chronic renal insufficiency. In this clinical situation, if hyperkalemia is seen, consideration should be given to acute rather than chronic renal insufficiency, hormonal disorders (i.e., hyporenin hypoaldosteronism), or tubular disorders (i.e., obstructive uropathy).

38. Name the common causes of CRF.
- Diabetes mellitus (41%)
- Hypertension (30%)
- Glomerulonephritis (13%)
- Obstructive uropathy (2%)
- Polycystic kidney disease and other interstitial diseases (4%)
- Others (10%)

Source: United States Renal Data Systems, 2003.

39. Why are ACE inhibitors preferred in diabetic kidney disease?
By decreasing the tone of efferent arterioles, ACE inhibitors reduce intraglomerular hypertension and thereby reduce proteinuria. Sufficient data now exist supporting the use of ACE

inhibitors, especially in diabetic patients with clinical or subclinical renal involvement, to retard the progression of diabetic nephropathy (both in terms of proteinuria as well as renal failure). A recent, large-scale, multicenter, prospective study concluded that captopril treatment was associated with a 50% reduction in the risk of death, dialysis, or transplantation in diabetics, an effect independent of blood pressure control. It is therefore recommended to initiate therapy with ACE inhibitors in patients with insulin-dependent (DM) who have either microalbuminuria (30–300 mg/day in at least two of three measurements) or overt albuminuria (> 300 mg/day). ACE inhibitor therapy should be instituted in these circumstances regardless of the presence of hypertension or renal failure.

Lewis EJ, et al: The effect of angiotensin converting enzyme inhibition on diabetic nephropathy. N Engl J Med. 329:1456–1462, 1993.

DIALYSIS

40. What are the indications for dialysis in a patient with CRF?
Dialytic therapy should be started when conservative management fails to maintain the patient in reasonable comfort. Usually, dialysis is required when the GFR drops to 5–10 mL/min. It is both unnecessary and risky to adhere to strict biochemical indications. Broadly speaking, the development of uremic encephalopathy, neuropathy, pericarditis, and bleeding diathesis are indications to start dialysis immediately. Fluid overload, congestive heart failure, hyperkalemia, metabolic acidosis, and hypertension uncontrolled by conservative measures are also indications for starting patients on dialysis therapy.

41. What are the contraindications for dialysis?
The presence of potentially reversible abnormalities is a major contraindication for dialysis. These include volume depletion, urinary tract infection, urinary obstruction, hypercatabolic state, uncontrolled hypertension, hypercalcemia, nephrotoxic drugs, and low cardiac output state.

42. Which clinical manifestations of uremia (CRF) can be improved with dialysis? Which ones persist or worsen?

Improve	Persist	Develop or Worsen
Uremic encephalopathy	Renal osteodystrophy	Dialysis dementia
Seizures	Hypertriglyceridemia	Nephrogenic ascites
Pericarditis	Amenorrhea and infertility	Dialysis pericarditis
Fluid overload	Peripheral neuropathy	Dialysis bone disease
Electrolyte imbalances	Pruritus	Accelerated atherosclerosis
GI symptoms	Anemia	Carpal tunnel syndrome (amyloid-related)
Metabolic acidosis	Risk of hepatitis	

43. Which poisons and toxins are dialyzable?
The toxins that can be removed by hemodialysis include alcohols (ethanol, methanol, ethylene glycol), salicylates, heavy metals (Hg, As, Pb), and halides. In addition, hemoperfusion successfully removes barbiturates, sedatives (meprobamate, methaqualone, glutethimide), acetaminophen, digoxin, procainamide, quinidine, and theophylline.

44. What is chronic ambulatory peritoneal dialysis (CAPD)?
CAPD is a manual form of peritoneal dialysis, usually performed by the patient, in which 1–2 L of dialysate fluid are infused into the peritoneal space through a Tenckhoff catheter and then drained after a dwell time of 4–6 h. The exchanges are repeated four to five times a day. CAPD is indicated in any patient with ESRD.

45. **What are the indications and contraindicatons for CAPD?**
CAPD is the treatment of choice for diabetics with severe peripheral vascular disease, since hemodialysis is not a viable option for such patients. This method provides more independence and mobility, and it should be offered to all young patients leading active lives. The contraindications include blindness, severe disabling arthritis, colostomy, poor motivation, and quadriplegia.

46. **What are the common mechanical complications of CAPD?**
Pain, bleeding, leakage, inadequate drainage, intraperitoneal catheter loss, abdominal wall edema, scrotal edema, incisional hernia, other hernia, intestinal hematoma, intestinal perforation.

47. **What are the common metabolic complications of CAPD?**
Hyperglycemia, hyperosmolar nonketotic coma, postdialysis hypoglycemia, hyperkalemia, hypokalemia, hypernatremia, hyponatremia, metabolic alkalosis, protein depletion, hyperlipidemia, obesity.

48. **List other potential complications of CAPD.**
- **Infections, inflammation:** bacterial or fungal peritonitis, tunnel infection, exit-site infection, diverticulitis, sterile peritonitis, eosinophilic peritonitis, sclerosing peritonitis, pancreatitis.
- **Cardiovascular:** acute pulmonary edema, fluid overload, hypotension, arrhythmia, cardiac arrest, hypertension.
- **Pulmonary:** basal atelectasis, aspiration pneumonia, hydrothorax, respiratory arrest, decreased forced vital capacity (FVC).

49. **What are the causes of peritonitis in a patient on peritoneal dialysis?**
Peritonitis is an important complication of CAPD. The frequency of infection has decreased considerably since this dialysis method was introduced, to about one episode every 18–24 patient months. This decrease is mainly due to the addition of a Luer-Lok adapter between the catheter and tubing and institution of monthly tubing changes. Causative organisms include *Staphylococcus epidermidis* and *Staphylococcus aureus* (70%), gram-negative organisms (20%), and fungi and tuberculosis (5%).

50. **Discuss the new developments in the treatment of anemia of CRF.**
The most important development is the use of recombinant human erythropoietin. Studies have documented the efficacy of this agent in improving the anemia and minimizing the need for blood transfusion. More importantly, the significance of correcting the iron deficiency in these patients by not only restoring the iron stores but also decreasing the requirements of the more expensive erythropoietin has been recognized.

Eschbach JW, et al: Recombinant human erythropoietin in anemic patients with end stage renal disease: Ann Intern Med 111:992–1000, 1989.

51. **What is dialysis bone disease?**
The bone disease in uremic patients does not necessarily improve after initiation of chronic dialytic therapy. In fact, additional factors are added that promote and complicate osteodystrophy. For instance, exposure to aluminum (as phosphate binders or, less commonly, in dialysate) superimposes a form of osteomalacia on secondary hyperparathyroidism. The mechanism of the aluminum effect on bone is believed to be due to deposition of the metal along the mineralization front, leading to interference with mineralization. In addition, aluminum may impair the function of osteoblasts. Another important entity is adynamic bone disease manifesting as osteomalacia, which is often associated with low parathyroid hormone levels.

Sherrard DJ, et al: The spectrum of bone disease in end stage renal failure—an evolving disorder. Kidney Int 48:436–442, 1993.

52. What is dialysis-associated amyloidosis?
Long-term dialytic therapy is associated with accumulation and deposition of amyloid fibrils containing beta$_2$-microglobulins. It usually manifests after 5–7 years of chronic dialytic therapy and is seen in most patients after 10 years of dialysis. Clinically, it manifests as asymptomatic lytic bone lesions, carpal tunnel syndrome (often bilateral), tenosynovitis, scapulohumeral periarthritis, and destructive arthropathy. No satisfactory preventive measures are available.

Koch KM: Dialysis related amyloidosis. Kidney Int 41:1416–1429, 1992.

PROTEINURIA/NEPHROTIC SYNDROME

53. List the four general mechanisms by which abnormally increased urinary protein excretion (> 150 mg/day) occurs.
The four general mechanisms are glomerular, tubular, overflow, and secretory.

54. What causes glomerular proteinuria?
Glomerular proteinuria results from damage to the glomerular filtration barrier (in glomerulonephritis), leading to leakage of plasma proteins into the glomerular ultrafiltrate.

55. Describe the mechanism behind tubular proteinuria.
Tubular proteinuria occurs with suboptimal reabsorption of the normally filtered protein as a result of tubular disease. This recovery of the small amount of normally filtered protein (usually ~2 g/day) allows for the normal excretion of < 150 mg/day of protein.

56. Explain overflow proteinuria.
Overflow proteinuria results from disease states that lead to excessive levels of plasma proteins (such as in multiple myeloma). The proteins are filtered and overload the reabsorptive capacity of the renal tubules.

57. What is secretory proteinuria?
Secretory proteinuria describes the proteinuria that occurs because of the addition of protein to the urine after glomerular filtration. The protein may come from the renal tubules (erg: Tamm-Horsfall protein from the ascending limb of the loop of Henle) or from the lower GU tract.

58. What conditions are associated with heavy proteinuria despite severely reduced GFR?
Heavy proteinuria is generally indicative of glomerular disease. In most glomerular diseases, proteinuria tends to decrease with diminishing GFR as the filtration of proteins also tends to decrease. However, in certain conditions, such as diabetic nephropathy, amyloidosis, focal glomerulosclerosis, and probably reflex nephropathy, proteinuria (often in the nephrotic range) persists despite severely diminished GFR.

59. Define nephrotic syndrome.
Nephrotic syndrome, also called nephrosis, is a symptom complex resulting from various etiologies and characterized by heavy proteinuria (usually > 3.5 g/day), generalized edema, and lipiduria with hyperlipidemia. Because all the other features are a consequence of marked proteinuria, some authorities restrict the definition of "nephrosis" to heavy proteinuria alone.

60. Define nephritic syndrome.
Nephritic syndrome is a renal disorder that results from diffuse glomerular inflammation. It is characterized by the sudden onset of gross or microscopic hematuria, decreased GFR, low

urine output (oliguria), hypertension, and edema. It can result from many different etiologies but is traditionally represented by postinfectious glomerulonephritis following infections with certain strains of group A beta-hemolytic streptococci.

61. **What are the various causes of an acute nephritic syndrome?**
   - **Postinfectious glomerulonephritis:** bacterial (e.g., pneumococci, *Klebsiella* sp. staphylococci, gram-negative rods, meningococci), viral (e.g., varicella, infectious mononucleosis, mumps, measles, hepatitis B, coxsackievirus), rickettsial (Rocky Mountain spotted fever, typhus), and parasitic (e.g., *Falciparum* malaria, toxoplasmosis, trichinosis)
   - **Idiopathic glomerular diseases:** membranoproliferative glomerulonephritis, mesangial proliferative glomerulonephritis, IgA nephropathy.
   - **Multisystem diseases:** systemic lupus erythematosus (SLE), Henoch-Schönlein purpura, essential mixed cryoglobulinemia, infective endocarditis
   - **Miscellaneous:** Guillain-Barré syndrome, postirradiation of renal tumors

62. **What are the common causes of nephrotic syndrome in adults and children?**
   In **adults** the most common cause is diabetes nephropathy (most common secondary nephropathy). Membranous nephropathy is the most common primary glomerulopathy in adults. In **children** the most common cause of nephrotic syndrome is minimal change disease, also called lipoid nephrosis or nil lesion. Other causes of nephritic syndrome include focal and segmental glomerulosclerosis and proliferative glomerulonephritides.

63. **In evaluating patients with nephrotic syndrome, which diseases must you rule out before considering the syndrome to be due to a primary renal disease?**
   - Drugs that may result in excessive urinary protein excretion (e.g., gold, penicillamine)
   - Systemic infections (e.g., hepatitis B and C, HIV, malaria)
   - Neoplasia (lymphomas)
   - Multisystem collagen vascular diseases (e.g., SLE)
   - Diabetes (nephropathy is classically associated with nephrotic syndrome)
   - Heredofamilial diseases (e.g., Alport's syndrome)

64. **Why is it important to distinguish primary renal disease from the above conditions?**
   The distinction between the above causes and primary renal disease is important for a number of reasons. Diagnostically, identification of some of these processes may help to identify the renal lesion without the need for a renal biopsy (as in diabetes). Treatment of such disorders may involve simple discontinuation of the offending agent (such as a drug). Management may need to be directed at a systemic disease (infection) rather than at the renal lesion itself.

65. **Name the common complications of the nephrotic syndrome.**
   - **Edema and anasarca**
   - **Hypovolemia** with acute prerenal and/or parenchymal renal disease. In the nephrotic syndrome, decreased effective arterial blood volume can lead to various degrees of renal underperfusion, resulting in renal failure in severe cases.
   - **Protein malnutrition** due to massive protein losses in excess of dietary replacement.
   - **Hyperlipidemia**, which raises the risk of atherosclerotic cardiovascular disease.
   - **Increased susceptibility to bacterial infection**, which often involves the lungs, meninges (meningitis), and peritoneum. Common organisms include *Streptococcus* (including *S. pneumoniae*), *Haemophilus influenzae*, and *Klebsiella* sp.
   - **Proximal tubular dysfunction,** which may lead to Fanconi syndrome with urinary wasting of glucose, phosphate, amino acids, uric acid, potassium, and bicarbonate.

- **Hypercoagulable state** manifested by an increased incidence of venous thrombosis, particularly in the renal vein, which may be due to urinary loss of anti-thrombotic factors.

66. **Are the syndromes of nephritis and nephrosis mutually exclusive?**
Some forms of glomerular diseases are characteristically nephrotic in their presentation (e.g., nil lesion) while some aggressive forms of proliferative glomerulopathies present as nephritic syndrome. Some others manifest mixed features (Table 7-1).

TABLE 7-1. INTERRELATIONSHIP OF MORPHOLOGIC AND CLINICAL MANIFESTATIONS OF GLOMERULAR INJURY

	Nephrosis	
Minimal change glomerulopathy	++++	
Membranous glomerulopathy	+++	
Focal glomerulosclerosis	++	+
Mesangioproliferative glomerulopathy	++	++
Membranoproliferative glomerulopathy	++	+++
Proliferative glomerulonephritis	+	+++
Acute diffuse proliferate glomerulonephritis	+	++++
Crescentic glomerulonephritis		++++
		Nephritis

From Mandal AK, et al: Diagnosis and Management of Renal Disease and Hypertension. Philadelphia, Lea & Febiger, 1988, p 248, with permission.

67. **A 62-year-old man with nephrotic syndrome is found to have no systemic etiology. What is the differential diagnosis?**
As opposed to minimal lesion in children, minimal lesion on renal biopsy in an elderly patient warrants an extensive search to rule out underlying malignancy, especially lymphomas (both Hodgkin's and non-Hodgkin's) and other solid tumors (such as renal cell carcinoma). One third of elderly patients with membranous nephropathy have underlying malignancy (colon, stomach, or breast).

NEPHROLITHIASIS

68. **What three mechanisms are important in the development of nephrolithiasis?**
Urinary tract stones occur in a wide variety of diseases and as a consequence of a variety of physiologic and pathologic processes. The three mechanisms currently thought to contribute to urinary stone formation are:
    - Precipitation of a substance from supersaturated solutions to form stones depends on many factors, including solubility, concentration, and urine characteristics (e.g., pH).
    - Normal constituents of urine that inhibit stone formation include citrate, pyrophosphate, and magnesium. Reduced concentrations of these substances are thought to contribute to stone formation.

- Protein matrix contributes to the formation, growth, and/or aggregation of stones. This matrix derives in part from renal tubular epithelial cells and from the uroepithelium.

69. What are the common constituents of urinary stones in the U.S.?

- Calcium oxalate: 35%
- Calcium apatite: 35%
- Magnesium ammonium phosphate (struvite): 18%
- Uric acid: 6%
- Cystine: 3%

70. Summarize the conditions that favor the formation of each kind of stone.

In general, an alkaline urine pH favors precipitation of inorganic stones—calcium phosphate (which undergoes rearrangement into hydroxyapatite). Alkaline urine pH and high concentrations of urinary ammonia lead to supersaturation of magnesium ammonium phosphate (struvite). This environment is created by the presence of urea-splitting bacteria (commonly *Proteus*, *Pseudomonas*, *Klebsiella*, and *Staphylococcus*), which contain the enzyme urease and convert urea to ammonia and CO_2. An acid pH favors precipitation of organic stones—uric acid and cystine. Urine pH has little effect on calcium oxalate solubility and therefore little influence on formation of these stones.

71. List common metabolic conditions that predispose to the formation of urinary stones.

- **Idiopathic hypercalciuria** is present in approximately 50% of stone-forming patients in the U.S. It is divided into absorptive (due to excessive GI absorption of calcium) and renal (due to renal leak of calcium) types.
- **Hyperuricosuria** (with and without gout) is present in approximately 30% of stone-formers. Increased uric acid excretion can also contribute to the formation of calcium-containing stones.
- **Hyperoxaluria** of various causes is present in about 15%.
- **Low urinary citrate excretion** is present in about 50% and can contribute to stone formation in most states.

72. What are the less common causes of urinary stones?

Less common causes include chronic UTI, primary hyperparathyroidism, cystinuria, and distal RTA. Typically, more than one of the above conditions is present in a stone-forming patient.

73. What are the consequences of urinary obstruction by a stone?

A stone acutely lodged in the GU tract can cause severe, colicky pain that radiates toward the lower abdomen and genital area. The ureteropelvic junction, the mid-ureter as it crosses the iliac artery, and the ureterovesical junction are the common sites for urinary obstruction by stones. In women who have children, the pain is often described as more severe than the pain of labor. The increased pressure inside the collecting system decreases the net pressure for glomerular filtration, resulting in a decreased GFR. The resulting urinary stasis predisposes to infection.

74. Do the consequences of urinary obstruction have permanent effects?

All of these problems correct toward normal if the stone passes or is removed from the urinary tract within a few days. If the obstruction becomes chronic, permanent renal injury can ensue, with an irreversible reduction in GFR and chronic dilatation of the collection system. This dilated collecting system is less efficient in delivering urine to the bladder (because of compromised peristalsis), predisposing to urinary stasis and infection.

75. How should you manage the patient with acute urinary obstruction due to a stone?

Most stones pass spontaneously in a few hours to days. Supportive management with analgesics and oral fluids usually suffices. Serum chemistries should be done to document the

KEY POINTS: NEPHROLOGY

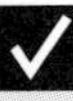

1. Maintenance of adequate hydration and minimizing the dose of contrast media, combined with the routine use of *N*-acetylcysteine, reduce the frequency of contrast-induced renal failure.
2. Despite the recent advances in dialysis and continuous filtration techniques, mortality remains high in ARF; hence the need for early detection and intervention, since half of these patients regain normal renal function.
3. Renal replacement therapy in the form of hemodialysis, CAPD, or renal transplantation should be considered once creatinine clearance drops to 10 mL/min (15 mL/min in diabetics).
4. Diabetic patients with microalbuminuria or over proteinuria should be treated with ACE inhibitors or ARBs even if BP is not elevated.
5. Reduction of proteinuria is critical in the management and prognosis of diabetic and nondiabetic glomerulopathies since proteinuria not only affects the progression of renal disease but is also an independent risk factor for cardiovascular complications.

degree of renal dysfunction (if any) and an imaging procedure (e.g., intravenous, pyelography, renal ultrasound) to locate the stone and estimate its size in order to help determine the possible need for surgical intervention.

76. **What should you do once the acute phase of obstruction ends?**
Once the acute phase ends with exit of the stone, evaluation should be aimed at identifying the condition that led to the formation of the stone, which will lead to a protocol for long-term management. A reasonable percentage of patients recover stone material from their urine. However, laboratory analysis is usually not readily available, and the approach to further management is more often empirical than based on analysis of recovered stones.

77. **Describe the general approach to avoidance of recurrent stones.**
In general, such patients should maintain a dilute urine, which can be accomplished by a high intake of hypotonic fluids. Recovery and characterization of stones, if possible, help to diagnose the predisposing condition and guide management. More specific management depends on the predisposing condition.

78. **What measures are appropriate for patients with absorptive or renal hypercalciuria?**
Absorptive hypercalciuria can be managed by reducing dietary calcium (type 2 only) or by using cellulose sodium phosphate, which binds intestinal calcium and prevents its absorption (type 1), or the diuretic thiazide, which promotes renal calcium reabsorption. **Renal** hypercalciuria can also be treated with thiazides.

79. **How is primary hyperparathyroidism treated?**
Primary hyperparathyroidism should be treated with parathyroidectomy.

80. **Summarize the management of uricosuric states.**
Uricosuric states resulting from the overproduction of uric acid should be treated with allopurinol or with potassium citrate if patients have hyperuricosuria associated with calcium oxalate stones.

81. **Describe the treatment of patients with excessive intestinal oxalate absorption.**
Conditions with excessive intestinal oxalate absorption can be treated with a low oxalate diet and use of magnesium or calcium salts, which bind oxalate and inhibit its reabsorption.

82. How is cystinuria treated?
Cystinuria can be managed conservatively (i.e., dilute or alkaline urine) or with penicillamine (increases the solubility of cysteine) if the conservative measures are ineffective.

83. How should you manage patients with struvite stones?
UTIs must be treated with antibiotics. Patients may also be given the urease inhibitor acetohydroxamic acid.

84. What are the three forms of lithotripsy?
Litho (stone or calculus) ***tripsy*** (crushing) is a way of breaking up stones by use of shock waves or ultrasound and may serve as an alternative to operation or cystoscopy for the removal of stones in the kidney and urinary tract. The three forms now available clinically are:

- Extracorporeal shock-wave lithotripsy
- Percutaneous ultrasonic lithotripsy
- Endoscopic ultrasonic lithotripsy

URINARY TRACT OBSTRUCTION

85. List the common causes of ureteric obstruction in adults.

- Renal stones
- Prostatic, bladder, or pelvic malignancy
- Retroperitoneal lymphoma, metastasis, or fibrosis
- Accidental surgical ligation
- Blood clot
- Pregnancy
- Stricture

86. How do unilateral and bilateral obstructions differ in their effects on the GFR?
Unilateral obstruction does not necessarily lead to a clinically measurable decrease in GFR in patients with normal renal funtion, but bilateral obstruction quite often leads to a decreased GFR in patients with both normal and abnormal renal function.

87. Describe in greater detail how unilateral obstruction affects the GFR.
In patients with normal renal function, unilateral obstruction with complete obliteration of ipsilateral function forces recruitment of the nephron reserve of the unaffected, contralateral kidney, resulting in no changes or only small changes in total GFR. Relatively large reductions in functioning nephron mass (about 40%) are necessary to elicit an appreciable rise in the plasma creatinine (P_{Cr}) concentrations when baseline renal function is normal (P_{Cr} 0.8–1.2 mg/dL). The relatively small change in GFR in patients with normal baseline renal function who are subjected to unilateral obstruction probably will not be reflected by a rise in P_{Cr}. The response is different for patients with baseline renal insufficiency. Such patients have already lost their reserve nephron mass and are likely using compensatory mechanisms to maintain their GFR. Unilateral obstruction in such patients may result in a significant fall in GFR and is more likely to be associated with a rise in P_{Cr}.

88. Describe the differences in clinical presentation between acute and chronic obstruction of the urinary tract.
Partial or complete obstruction of the urinary tract compromises urine passage whether it is acute or chronic. Nevertheless, the urinary findings and clinical consequences differ depending on the duration of the obstruction. After release of an **acute (> 24 h) obstruction**, there is commonly a decrease in excretion of sodium, potassium, and water. This results in excretion of a urine low in sodium and with increased osmolarity, a situation also seen with volume depletion.

In contrast, release of **chronic obstruction** commonly results in increased excretion of sodium and water and decreased excretion of acid (with urinary loss of bicarbonate) and potassium. These abnormalities can lead to volume depletion, free-water deficit (reflected by hypernatremia), and hyperkalemic non–anion-gap metabolic acidosis.

89. **What abnormalities of tubular function can occur with chronic obstruction?**
Chronic obstruction affects primarily distal rather than proximal nephron functions, including reabsorption of sodium and water and secretion of acid and potassium. The decreased **water** reabsorption results from decreased responsiveness of the collecting tubule to antidiuretic hormone, yielding a form of nephrogenic diabetes insipidus. The **acid** secretory defect results in incomplete bicarbonate recovery from the urine and a non–anion-gap metabolic acidosis. The **potassium** secretory defect results in potassium retention and hyperkalemia. Therefore, obstructive nephropathy is a common cause of hyperkalemic, hyperchloremic, non-anion-gap metabolic acidosis. These abnormalities usually resolve after correction of the obstruction but may require weeks or months to do so. In addition to the decrease in GFR and the potential tubular abnormalities, the resulting urinary stasis can predispose to infection, renal stones, and papillary necrosis. The salt and water retention can lead to hypertension.

90. **Which components of polyuria (postobstructive diuresis) are seen immediately after correction of chronic obstruction?**
The patient with obstruction and compromised renal function accumulates solute and water that are ordinarily excreted by the normally functioning kidney. Correction of the obstruction results in appropriate excretion of the accumulated urea, NaCl, and water in an effort to return the volume and content of the extracellular fluid to normal. This polyuria is physiologic. However, a minority of such patients have a pathologic polyuria, resulting from poor salt and/or water reabsorption. These abnormalities commonly resolve within a few hours but may last for days. Usually the polyuria is physiologic, but the patient must be observed. Pathologic polyuria may occur because of either salt or water loss (or both). Pathologic salt loss is reflected by continued excretion of a large amount of urinary sodium in the setting of volume depletion. Pathologic water loss is reflected by excretion of large volumes of dilute urine in spite of rising serum osmolality.

91. **Should the polyuria after correction of obstruction be treated?**
In pathologic polyuria, appropriate fluid replacement therapy should be instituted. If replacement is instituted during the physiologic polyuria, one will "chase" the patient's volume status so that polyuria continues as a result of the fluids that are administered.

92. **Explain "functional" obstruction of the urinary tract.**
This term refers to abnormalities that compromise the exit of urine from the kidney in the absence of anatomic obstruction of the outflow tract. Two examples are an atonic bladder and vesicoureteral reflux.

93. **What is an atonic bladder?**
An atonic bladder is unable to empty itself completely and hence contains urine, continuously yielding a higher than normal hydrostatic pressure. This high bladder pressure is transmitted via the ureters and may cause the abnormalities described above.

94. **What causes vesicoureteral reflux?**
Patients with vesicoureteral reflux have retrograde flow of urine into the ureter and/or kidney during voiding. This occurs because of an incompetent vesicoureteral valve. The transmitted pressure is felt to contribute to the renal abnormalities. Both of these conditions also predispose to infection.

95. How is the diagnosis of lower urinary tract obstruction (LTO) made?
The history, clinical setting, and the laboratory findings provide important clues. A palpable urinary bladder on examination is strong evidence for LTO or an atonic bladder. A post-void residual urine of > 100 mL on Foley catheter insertion is supportive of LTO. Imaging studies help confirm the diagnosis.

96. Which imaging studies are helpful in the diagnosis of LTO?
The distended bladder as well as large kidneys can be seen on plain abdominal x-rays. Renal ultrasound is a relatively sensitive, noninvasive procedure that is commonly used to investigate the possibility of LTO. Retrograde pyelography (selective catheterization and insertion of contrast dye into both ureters via cystoscopy) is occasionally necessary when the above studies do not yield a diagnosis and clinical suspicion remains strong for obstruction. Intravenous pyelograms should be avoided due to the risk of additional renal injury from the contrast dye. Abdominal CT scan is helpful but is more expensive than ultrasound. Radionuclide renal scans suggest LTO when there is prompt uptake of the dye with prolonged excretion.

GLOMERULAR DISORDERS

97. Define primary glomerulopathy.
Primary glomerular disease (or *primary glomerulopathy*) denotes a heterogeneous group of kidney diseases in which the glomeruli are the predominantly involved elements. Extrarenal involvement, if present, is usually secondary to consequences of the glomerular insult. Most of these disorders are idiopathic. The cardinal manifestations of the primary glomerular disorders are proteinuria, hematuria, alterations in GFR, and salt retention leading to edema, hypertension, and pulmonary congestion.

98. Which clinical syndromes are manifested by the primary glomerulopathies?
The clinical features of the primary glomerulopathies appear in various combinations in any given glomerular disorder and present as one of the following clinical syndromes:

1. **Acute glomerulonephritis**: An acute illness of abrupt onset characterized by variable degrees of hematuria, proteinuria, decreased GFR, and fluid and salt retention. It is usually associated with an infectious agent and tends to resolve spontaneously.
2. **Nephrotic syndrome:** An illness of insidious onset characterized primarily by heavy proteinuria of usually > 3.5 g/day in an adult and usually associated with hypoalbuminemia, lipidemia, and anasarca.
3. **Chronic glomerulonephritis:** A vague illness of insidious onset characterized primarily by progressive renal insufficiency, with a protracted downhill course of 5–10 years' duration. Varying degrees of proteinuria, hematuria, and hypertension are present.
4. **Rapidly progressive glomerulonephritis** (RPGN): A clinical disorder of rather subacute onset but with rapid progression to renal failure and no tendency toward spontaneous recovery. Patients are usually hypertensive, hematuric, and oliguric.
5. **Asymptomatic urinary abnormalities:** Patients have microscopic hematuria and/or proteinuria (usually < 3 g/day) but with no clinical symptoms.

99. Which strains of streptococci cause poststreptococcal glomerulonephritis (PSGN)?
Only certain serotypes of group A (beta-hemolytic) streptococci are nephritogenic. Type 12 is the most common type, but types 1, 2, 3, 18, 25, 49, 55, 57, and 60 are also nephritogenic. In contrast, all strains of streptococci can cause acute rheumatic fever, which is why the incidence of nephritis differs from that of rheumatic fever in outbreaks of streptococcal infection. The M-protein in streptococci is poorly linked to nephritogenicity. Recent evidence indicates that

nephritogenicity is more closely related to endostreptosin, a cell membrane antigen. Other streptococcal cytoplasmic antigens and autologous antigens also have been implicated.

100. What abnormalities are seen in patients with PSGN?
The urinalysis in PSGN is characterized by a nephritic sediment, high specific gravity, and non-selective proteinuria. The proteinuria is < 3 g/day in > 75% of patients, although proteinuria in the nephrotic range is occasionally seen. Pyuria is often noted, indicating glomerulitis. Hematuria is almost always present in either gross (smoky urine) or microscopic form. Red blood cell casts, if present, are very diagnostic. Dysmorphic erythrocytes are found in abundance. However, a benign urinary sediment does not rule out acute PSGN if clinical features are suggestive. In some cases, biopsy studies have confirmed PSGN.

101. What is the prognosis in acute PSGN? What are the poor prognostic signs?
In **children**, the immediate and late prognosis is quite favorable in both epidemic and sporadic cases. A diuresis occurs in 1 week, and serum creatinine returns to normal in 3–4 weeks. The mortality in acute cases is < 1%, and chronic sequelae are uncommon. Microscopic hematuria may last 6 months, and proteinuria may persist for as long as 3 years in 15% of patients. In **adults**, the prognosis is good in epidemic forms but less predictable in sporadic cases.

102. What are the poor prognostic signs in PSGN?
In **children** the factors indicating a poor prognosis include persistent heavy proteinuria, extensive crescents or atypical humps in initial biopsy, and severe disease in the acute phase requiring hospitalization. In **adults** severe impairment of renal function at the onset, persistent proteinuria, elderly age, and crescent formation on biopsy are poor prognostic factors.

103. What is rapidly progressive glomerulonephritis (RPGN)?
RPGN denotes the clinical syndrome associated with rapid and progressive deterioration of renal function, often terminating, if untreated, in ESRD within a period of weeks to months. Histologically, it is characterized by extensive glomerular crescent formation, in most cases involving over 75% of glomeruli. The cells of the crescents are thought to be derived from blood-borne monocytes.

104. Is RPGN synonymous with crescentic nephritis?
RPGN is strictly a clinical expression, whereas crescentic nephritis denotes the histologic picture in such patients. Several primary glomerulopathies demonstrate variable degrees of crescent formation, but they do not progress as rapidly as in RPGN.

105. How does routine urinalysis help in the evaluation of a primary glomerular disease?
In glomerular disease, the urinary sediment usually conforms to one of three different forms:

Nephrotic	**Nephritic**	**Chronic**
Heavy proteinuria	Red cells	Less proteinuria and hematuria
Free fat droplets	Red cell casts	Broad, waxy casts
Oval fat bodies	Variable proteinuria	Pigmented granular casts
Fatty casts	Frequent white cell and granular cells	
Variable hematuria		

Schreiner GE: The identification and clinical significance of casts. Arch Intern Med 99:356–369, 1957. With pemission.

106. Define fibrillary and immunotactoid glomerulonephritis.

These are two related yet distinct glomerular diseases characterized by deposition of Congo red-negative fibrils and characterized by a variety of light microscopic features and progressive clinical course. Fibrillary GN is defined as Congo red-negative fibrils < 30 nm in diameter, while immunotactoid nephritis is defined by glomerular deposition of hollow stacked microtubules > 30 nm in diameter. Both entities are relatively uncommon, accounting for less than 1% of native renal biopsies. Recurrence of these diseases is common after transplantation.

Rosenstock JL, Markowitz GS, Valeri AM, et al: Fibrillary and immunotactoid glomerulonephritis: distinct entities with different clinical and pathologic features. Kidney Int 63:1450–1461, 2003.

107. What are the renal manifestations of HIV disease?

The most common chronic renal disease from HIV infection is a type of focal glomerulosclerosis, the so-called HIV nephropathy. Typically, nephrotic proteinuria, large echogenic kidneys, minimal or modest hypertension, and rapidly progressive renal failure characterize the disease. Dialysis is well tolerated; however, the mean survival is less than 1 year in patients with full-blown AIDS. Transplantation is contraindicated in HIV nephropathy. The other renal manifestations include hyponatremia, hyperkalemia (often secondary to adrenal disease or hyporenin hypoaldosteronism), hypouricemia, and ARF, often due to anti-HIV medications.

108. Define the World Health Organization (WHO) nomenclature of lupus nephritis.

WHO recently categorized renal involvement in SLE into the following classes:

- Class I: Normal glomeruli
- Class II: Mesangial hypercellularity and proliferation
- Class III: Focal segmental glomerulonephritis
- Class IV: Diffuse proliferative glomerulonephritis
- Class V: Diffuse membranous glomerulonephritis
- Class VI: Advanced sclerosing glomerulonephritis

109. What are the current strategies for treatment of lupus nephritis?

Active treatment of hypertension, especially with ACE inhibitors, delays the progression of all classes of lupus nephritis. In general, class II and V lesions are amenable to therapy and are associated with better prognosis. A combination of cyclophosphamide (oral or IV) with oral low-dose steroids is effective in improving the prognosis of class III and IV lupus nephritis. IV pulse cyclophosphamide has become popular in view of less gonadal and bladder toxicities. Azathioprine and mycophenolate mofetil are used as alternates to cyclophosphamide. Treatment is generally ineffective in class VI lesions.

Berden JHM: Lupus nephritis. Kidney Int 52:538–558, 1997.

110. How is a patient with recurrent hematuria evaluated?

The first step is to exclude urinary stones and other structural lesions such as tumors of the upper and lower urinary tract. This step may involve renal imaging and urinary instrumentation. The presence of dysmorphic erythrocytes or red cell casts helps to distinguish glomerular bleeding from lower tract bleeding. Glomerular bleeding accounts for recurrent hematuria in over a quarter of patients younger than age 40 years.

111. What are the main causes of recurrent isolated glomerular hematuria?

The main causes of recurrent isolated glomerular hematuria include IgA nephropathy or Berger's disease (the most common primary glomerulopathy worldwide), thin basement membrane nephropathy, and idiopathic hypercalciuria. Demonstration of the first two entities may require renal biopsy. Berger's disease is primary IgA nephropathy. It is characterized by recurrent episodes of painless hematuria, often gross, and presence of RBC casts in urine. Hypertension and proteinuria are often minimal or modest. Only 25% of the patients progress to ESRD.

RENAL BONE DISEASE

112. What is Bricker's "trade-off" hypothesis?
The trade-off hypothesis propounded by Neil Bricker is the basis for the secondary hyperparathyroidism seen in renal failure.

113. Explain the trade-off hypothesis.
Early in the course of renal failure, the kidney fails to excrete phosphorus, leading to a transient and often undetectable rise in serum phosphorus. This tends to lower the serum level of ionized calcium temporarily, leading to stimulation of parathyroid hormone (PTH) secretion. The increased levels of PTH reduce tubular reabsorption of phosphate, leading to phosphate excretion and thereby tending to normalize the serum calcium and phosphorus levels. However, this process occurs at the expense of an elevated PTH level. With further declines in renal function, the serum phosphorus tends to rise, and the whole cycle is repeated. With advancing renal failure, these changes tend to keep serum calcium and phosphorus levels below normal at the expense of increasing serum PTH levels. The serum level of PTH is increased in an attempt to normalize serum phosphate and calcium levels, but the "trade-off" is the bone disease caused by the elevated PTH levels (osteitis fibrosa cystica).

114. List the three major bone histologic subtypes found in renal osteodystrophy.
Osteitis fibrosa cystica, which is a result of high bone turnover (bone changes due to secondary hyperparathyroidism), **osteomalacia**, and, occasionally, **osteosclerosis**. With better management of patients with ESRD, the long-term course of renal bone disease and its clinical features have changed, and newer entities have emerged. Adynamic or aplastic bone disease or low bone turnover has become a fairly common bone disease. Aluminum accumulation causes osteomalacia, which is one cause of adynamic bone disease. Decreased vitamin D, diabetes, and iron accumulation are other factors associated with adynamic bone disease.

115. Why do patients with CRF and marked hypocalcemia often fail to manifest tetany?
Tetany is a clinical manifestation of severe hypocalcemia in adults. Ionized calcium is decreased in the presence of alkalemia, so that tetany usually manifests only in the presence of an alkalemic pH. The degree of ionization is favorably increased by the acidemia seen in CRF, the result being that the ionic calcium is usually not reduced enough to cause tetany. However, if the acidosis is excessively treated with alkalizing agents, tetany may become manifest.

116. How do you manage secondary hyperparathyroidism in patients with CRF?
The cornerstone of treatment of secondary hyperparathyroidism involves measures to reduce serum parathormone levels. This reduction is accomplished by use of vitamin D analogs. However, it should not be attempted before the serum phosphorus level is normalized or the product of calcium and phosphorus is lowered to less than 70. The most commonly used vitamin D preparation is calcitriol (1,25 dihydroxycholecalciferol) either orally or intravenously. More recently, other analogs of vitamin D such as 19-nor-cholecalciferol (Zemplar) and 1-alpha calcidiol (Hectoral) have been successfully used and are claimed to be less hypercalcemic.

117. Does bone disease improve with dialysis or renal transplantation?
Renal osteodystrophy is not always improved with dialytic therapy. Indeed, the symptoms may worsen or progress because a number of additional factors are introduced that either directly or indirectly influence the severity of renal bone disease, including the aluminum content of dialysate, heparin administration, and administration of large amounts of acetate.

118. Does renal transplantion improve bone disease?
In patients who undergo renal transplantation, the uremic bone disease improves to a great extent. Increased osteoclastic and osteoblastic activities are noted within a few weeks after transplantation. However, in some patients, osteoporosis and the effects of secondary hyperparathyroidism may persist for as long as 1–2 years. In addition, steroid therapy may be responsible for osteoporosis and osteonecrosis that complicate the later phases of the post-transplant period. Another abnormality that may develop in the post-transplant phase is a renal phosphate leak, which if severe, may contribute to osseous abnormalities.

RENAL TRANSPLANTATION

119. Who is a potential candidate for renal transplantation?
Renal transplantation should be considered in all patients with ESRD who need some form of renal replacement therapy.

120. What are the absolute contraindications to renal transplantation?
- Reversible renal disease
- Active infection
- Recent malignant disease
- Active glomerulonephritis
- Presensitization to donor class I major transplantation antigens
- AIDS

121. List the relative contraindications to renal transplantation.
- Fabry's disease
- Oxalosis
- Advanced age
- Psychiatric problems
- Presence of anatomic urologic abnormality
- Iliofemoral occlusion
- Chronic active hepatitis

122. What are the donor-selection criteria in living-related transplantation?
Donors should have a normal physical examination, be under age 65 years and have the same ABO blood group as the recipient (or be type O). An angiogram is necessary to exclude the presence of multiple or abnormal renal arteries, because such abnormalities make the surgery prolonged and difficult. In general, the left kidney is preferred because of the longer renal vein. Some relative contraindications for kidney donation include severe hypertension, diabetes mellitus, HIV positivity, active medical illness, urologic abnormalities, persistently abnormal urinalyses, and family history of nephritis, polycystic kidney disease, or other renal disease.

123. What factors are considered important in evaluating suitability of a cadaver kidney?
The donor should have been free of neoplastic or infectious disease, *preferably* under 60 years of age, and have had good urine output and a normal serum creatinine before death. Urinalyses should be normal, and urine cultures should be negative. The kidney should be transplanted as early after harvesting as possible. The graft function tends to be worse 24 hours after harvesting. Of course, the donor should be free of infection with hepatitis B and HIV.

124. **Give the current survival figures for renal transplant recipients in the U.S.**
The 1-year patient survival rate for living-related renal transplantation is now around 95–100%, and for cadaveric transplantation, about 90%. With cyclosporine therapy, graft survivals are 90% and 80%, respectively, for living and cadaveric kidney transplants.

DIABETIC RENAL DISEASE

125. **What is the incidence of renal involvement in diabetes mellitus?**
CRF is an important cause of morbidity and mortality in all diabetics. Diabetes contributes up to 40% of all cases of ESRD in the U.S. Among type 1 diabetics, 40–60% develop CRF between 10 and 30 years after onset of diabetes. Although about one third of type 2 diabetics develop proteinuria, only 4% develop nephrotic syndrome and 6% develop ESRD. However, due to the large number of type 2 diabetics, they constitute the majority of diabetics on dialysis.

126. **What is the earliest evidence of renal involvement in diabetes mellitus?**
The earliest renal changes in diabetes consist of an increase in GFR of 25–50% and a slight enlargement of the kidney that persists for 5–10 years. At this stage, there may be a slight increase in albumin excretion rate (microalbuminuria), but the total protein excretion remains in the normal range. Studies indicate that patients with this "microalbuminuria" (> 20 μg/min of albumin) are more likely to develop overt diabetic nephropathy than those who do not exhibit microalbuminuria. The clinical phase starts with the appearance of proteinuria (corresponds to > 300 mg /day) on urine dipstick.

127. **Why is diabetic nephropathy associated with large kidneys?**
Diabetic nephropathy is one of the causes of CRF associated with large kidneys. Renal size is increased early in the course of diabetic renal disease and involves hypertrophy and hyperplasia. Elevated levels of growth hormone, often seen with uncontrolled hyperglycemia, are incriminated in this renal hypertrophy. However, the exact etiology remains unknown.

128. **What interventions are used for renal protection in diabetic nephropathy?**
Control of blood pressure, blood sugar levels, and dietary protein restriction have been shown to decrease proteinuria and retard the progression of renal failure. The hyperfiltration and hypertrophy seen early in the course of diabetic nephropathy can be corrected with insulin treatment. Strict glycemic control can reverse the elevated GFR and renal hypertrophy and also can decrease the spontaneous or exercise-induced microalbuminuria seen in the preclinical phase.

129. **What are the goals of glucose and blood pressure control?**
The goal is to maintain a blood glucose level within or close to the normal range while avoiding hypoglycemic attacks. However, once overt nephropathy begins and progressive renal insufficiency ensues, the benefit of tight glycemic control is still observed, although less pronounced than in the preclinical phase. Hypertesnion control slows the progression of diabetic nephropathy significantly. ACE inhibitors have been shown to accomplish the same, even in normotensive diabetic subjects. Recent evidence suggests that ARBs also accomplish the same objective.

Diabetes Control and Complications Trial Research Group: N Engl J Med 329:977–986, 1993.

130. **What are the agents of choice to treat hypertension in DM?**
ACE inhibitors should be the first-line agents in therapy for hypertension in DM. Shortly after ACE inhibitors are started, serum creatinine and potassium should be monitored to detect patients who develop hyperkalemia or an abrupt reduction in GFR. If no adverse effects are

seen for at least 2 weeks, ACE inhibitors can be safely continued. ARB can be used in place of ACE inhibitors when the latter are not tolerated.

131. What other agents may be considered?
It is unclear whether calcium channel blockers are as effective as ACE inhibitors in achieving these objectives, but they are effective in controlling the blood pressure in renal failure. Beta blockers may be effective, but their effects on the lipid profile and need for dose modification in renal failure and dialysis make them less desirable. Other agents, while being effective, may not offer any advantages over ACE inhibitors or calcium channel blockers.

Parving et al: Early aggressive anti-hypertensive treatment in diabetic nephropathy. Am J Kidney Dis 22:188–195, 1993.

132. Do diabetics with renal failure tolerate dialysis as well as nondiabetics?
Several years ago, it was thought that diabetics were not good candidates for dialytic therapy because about 80% of diabetics with ESRD who were placed on hemodialysis died in the first year. Over the past 15 years, results have improved significantly. One recent report indicates a 1-year survival of 85% and a 3-year survival of 60% in diabetics on hemodialysis. However, even today, diabetics tend to do poorly compared to nondiabetics. Their 3-year survival is 20–30% less, and their mortality is 2.25 times higher than that of nondiabetics. Atherosclerotic cardiac disease is the most common cause of death, with infections a close second.

MISCELLANEOUS RENAL DISORDERS

133. What are the risk factors associated with aminoglycoside nephrotoxicity?
Risk factors include dose and duration of drug therapy, recent aminoglycoside therapy, preexistent renal or liver failure, elderly age, volume depletion, concurrent nephrotoxin administration, and potassium and/or magnesium depletion.

Fumes D: Aminoglycoside nephrotoxicity. Kidney Int 33:900–911, 1988.

134. How should antibiotic doses be adjusted in patients with renal failure?
Several antibiotics need dosage modification in the presence of renal failure, notably aminoglycosides, most cephalosporins, many penicillins, and vancomycin. The adjustments can be made by maintaining the usual dose and varying the dosing interval, maintaining the dosing interval and varying the dose, or a combination of the two. The objective is to obtain a therapeutic drug concentration–time profile that is therapeutic and not toxic. For most commonly used antibiotics, dosing guidelines are established and readily accessible. No adjustment is needed for erythromycin, doxycycline, rifampin, and oral vancomycin. Tetracyclines, nitrofurantoin, nalidixic acid, and bacitracin should be totally avoided in renal failure.

Benett WM: Drug Prescribing in Renal Failure. Philadelphia, American College of Physicians, 1993, pp 15–35.

135. How do drugs interfere with assessment of renal function?
Cimetidine, trimethoprim, and acetylsalicylic acid increase serum creatinine by interfereing with the tubular creatinine secretion while methyldopa and cefoxitin interfere with creatinine assay, artificially elevating the serum creatinine level.Tolbutamide, penicillins, cephalosporins, sulfonamides, and contrast media can cause a false-positive reaction for protein in the urine.

136. Explain the interaction of digoxin with other drugs in renal failure.
Drug interactions are fairly common in patients with renal failure. Concomitant use of **metoclopramide** with digoxin decreases the absorption of the digoxin due to decreased gastric motility.

The digoxin dose may have to be increased. On the other hand, **quinidine** impairs renal excretion of digoxin, and hence the digoxin dose may have to be decreased.

137. **How do antacids interact with other drugs in cases of renal failure?**
Antacids impair the gastric absorption of **beta blockers** and **ferrous sulfate**. It is recommended to allow 1–2 hours between the two agents.

138. **With what drug may Scholl's solution interact in patients with renal failure?**
An important interaction occurs between Scholl's solution, an alkali that contains sodium citrate, and **aluminum hydroxide**. Citrate increases aluminum absorption so that aluminum toxicity may result. The combination has to be avoided.

139. **Explain the interaction between azathioprine and allopurinol.**
Azathioprine levels in the blood are elevated when used in conjunction with allopurinol due to decreased xanthine oxidase metabolism of azathioprine. The azathioprine dose therefore has to be decreased and leukocyte counts followed.

140. **Which drugs alter cyclosporine levels in the plasma?**
Phenytoin, phenobarbital, and **rifampin** increase cyclosporine clearance by the liver, and higher doses may be needed. On the other hand, **erythromycin, amphotericin B,** and **ketoconazole** decrease cyclosporine clearance by the liver; thus, the dose needs to be decreased.

141. **How does pregnancy affect healthy kidneys?**
Due to increased blood volume and hyperdynamic circulation in pregnancy, renal hemodynamics are altered. Most importantly, clearances of urea, creatinine, and uric acid are increased, leading to a decrease in the serum concentrations of these compounds. Urine protein excretion rates are increased. There is some dilation of the collecting system, including the ureters, partially due to the pressure from the gravid uterus but mainly due to the effect of progestational hormones on the muscular tone of the ureters. All of these changes revert to normalcy once the patient delivers.

142. **How does pregnancy affect diseased kidneys?**
Most renal diseases with proteinuria demonstrate increases in proteinuria during pregnancy. In diabetics with no renal disease, pregnancy does not adversely affect the renal function. However, there are no data about effects of pregnancy on renal function in patients with advanced diabetic nephropathy. Lupus nephritis is associated with an increased rate of spontaneous abortion and increased fetal loss. However, there is no evidence that pregnancy affects the long-term prognosis of lupus nephritis.

143. **What is a simple renal cyst?**
Simple cysts represent 60–70% of renal masses. They are common after age 50, most often asymptomatic, and usually detected as incidental findings in radiologic procedures done for other reasons.

144. **How is a simple renal cyst distinguished from a malignant cyst?**
On sonography, a simple cyst has smooth, sharply delineated margins, no echoes within the mass, and a strong posterior wall echo indicating good transmission through the cyst. These features generally exclude the possibility of malignancy. However, if there is any further suspicion, a CT scan should be done. CT findings consistent with a simple cyst include fluid that is homogeneous with a density of 0–20 Hounsfield units and no enhancement of the cyst fluid following the administration of radiocontrast media. Characteristics of renal cysts are summarized in Table 7-2.

TABLE 7-2. CHARACTERISTICS OF RENAL CYSTIC DISORDERS

Feature	Cysts	ADPKD	ARPKD	ACKD	MCD	MSK
Inheritance pattern	None	Autosomal dominant	Autosomal recessive	None	Often present, variable pattern	None
Incidence or prevalence	Common, increasing with age	1/200 to 1/1000	Rare	40% in patients on dialysis	Rare	Common
Age of onset	Adult	Usually adults	Neonates, children	Older adults	Adolescents, young adults	Adults
Presenting symptom	Incidental finding, hematuria	Pain, hematuria, infection, family screening	Abdominal mass, renal failure, failure to thrive	Hematuria	Polyuria, polydipsia, enuresis, renal failure, failure to thrive	Incidental, UTIs, hematuria, renal calculi
Hematuria	Occurs	Common	Occurs	Occurs	Rare	Common
Recurrent infections	Rare	Common	Occurs	No	Rare	Common
Renal calculi	No	Common	No	No	No	Common
Hypertension	Rare	Common	Common	Present from underlying disease	Rare	No
Diagnosis	Ultrasound	Ultrasound, gene linkage analysis	Ultrasound	CT scan	None reliable	Excretory urogram
Renal size	Normal	Normal to very large	Large initially	Small to normal, occ. large	Small	Normal

ADPKD = autosomal dominant polycystic kidney disease, ARPDK = autosomal recessive polycystic kidney disease, ACKD = acquired cystic kidney disease, MCD = medullary cystic disease, MSK = medullary sponge kidney.
Adapted from Grantham JJ: Cystic diseases of kidney. In Goldman K, Bennett JC, et al (eds): Cecil Textbook of Medicine, 21st ed. Philadelphia, W.B. Saunders, 2000.

145. You are asked to examine a 53-year-old man admitted to the hospital with fever, chills, right flank pain, and dysuria. Two years ago when he was evaluated for newly detected hypertension, he was noted to have polycystic kidney disease. Urinalysis showed 15–20 RBC, plenty of WBCs, and 3+ bacteria. An abdominal ultrasound is unremarkable except for bilateral polycystic kidneys, showing one of the renal cysts in the right kidney filled with highly echogenic material. At this point, your next step in management is to:

1. Order a urine culture
2. Start intravenous ampicillin
3. Start IV ciprofloxacin
4. Begin surgical drainage of the cyst.

The correct response is 3. The urinalysis is clearly indicative of an active urinary infection. Hence, although urine culture would be ordered, results would not affect the immediate management. The ultrasound is suggestive of an infected cyst. Since ampicillin does not penetrate the cyst wall and reach adequate concentrations to clear the infection, ciprofloxacin is the appropriate antibiotic of choice. Surgical drainage is needed only in cases resistant to intravenous antibiotics.

146. What are the renal manifestations of infective endocarditis?

Renal manifestations in infective endocarditis include incidental microscopic or gross hematuria and proteinuria. Renal failure is usually mild or absent. The histologic exam in these cases reveals focal proliferative glomerulonephritis. Rarely, a rapidly progressive renal failure with extensive crescent formation is reported. Nephrotic syndrome is rare. Serum IgG and C3 levels are often decreased, and immunofluorescence often demonstrates IgG, IgM, and in subendothelial and subepithelial deposits, suggesting an immune-complex etiology.

147. Describe the major differences between fibromuscular dysplasia (FMD) and atherosclerotic renal artery stenosis.

	FMD	**Atherosclerosis**
Age at onset	< 40 years	> 45 years
Gender	80% female	Primarily males
Distribution of lesion	Distal main renal artery	Aortic orifice and proximal main renal artery and intrarenal branches
Progression	Uncommon	Common; may progress to complete occlusion

148. How do you diagnose renovascular HTN?

Onset of HTN before age 20 or after age 50 should suggest the possibility of renovascular HTN. Similarly, the development of a refractory phase in a previously stable hypertensive patient, the presence of spontaneous hypokalemia, and the presence of an abdominal bruit are also suggestive.

149. What laboratory tests are useful in screening for renovascular HTN?

A **high plasma renin** profile is seen in approximately 80% of patients with renovascular HTN, as opposed to 15% in essential HTN. Another screening test often used is the **captopril test**. The administration of oral captopril causes a reactive rise of renin that is greater in patients with renovascular as opposed to essential HTN. The overall sensitivity is 74% and specificity 89%.

150. What imaging techniques are useful in screening for renovascular HTN?

Ultrasound determination of renal size (a difference of > 1.5 cm between the two kidneys) is very important in suggesting renal artery stenosis. **Captopril renography** has now replaced isotope renography as the screening procedure of choice, since the sensitivity is 92% and specificity 93%. The rationale for this test is that the GFR and renal blood flow of an ischemic kidney are dependent on the effects of angiotensin on the efferent glomerular arterioles and

hence fall markedly with ACE inhibition. Thus, captopril causes decreased isotope uptake by the ischemic kidney. The confirmation of renal artery stenosis is by renal angiography
Mann SJ, Pickering TG: Detection of renovascular hypertension. Ann Intern Med 117:845–853, 1992.

151. What is ANCA?
Antineutrophil cytoplasmic antibodies (ANCAs) are autoantibodies directed against intracellular neutrophils antigens, which produce one of the two immunoflorescence patterns cytoplasmic (c-ANCA) or perinuclear (p-ANCA) staining. c-ANCAs are directed toward proteinase-3, while p-ANCAs are specific for myeloperoxidase (MPO).

152. How do ANCAs help in distinguishing glomerular disorders?
ANCAs are often positive in pauci-immune vasculitidis. About 85–90% patients with Wegeners's granulomatosis are positive for c-ANCA while 50–80% with microscopic polyarteritis are positive for p-ANCA. However, many other autoimmune disorders with small vessel vasculitis, such as SLE, rheumatoid arthritis, and Sjögren's syndrome, are also positive for p-ANCA. It is highly recommended to obtain tissue biopsy in ANCA-positive vasculitis before immunosuppresssive therapy is begun.
Jeaneete JC, Falk RJ: Small vessel vasculitis. N Engl J Med 337:1512–1523, 1997.

153. What causes ARF secondary to rhabdomyolysis?
Rhabdomyolysis can cause ARF due to ATN. It occurs in various clinical conditions, including trauma, ischemic tissue damage after a drug overdose, alcoholism, seizures, and heat stroke (especially in untrained subjects or those with sickle cell trait). Hypokalemia and severe hypophosphatemia can also precipitate rhabdomyolysis. It is the most common cause of ARF in patients abusing illicit IV drugs.

154. Summarize the signs and symptoms of ARF secondary to rhabdomyolysis.
Typical patients have pigmented granular casts in urine sediment, a positive orthotolidine test in the urine supernatant (indicating the presence of heme), and markedly elevated plasma creatine kinase and other muscle enzymes, owing to their release from damaged muscle tissue. Other characteristics of ARF due to rhabdomyolysis include hyperphosphatemia, hyperkalemia, and a disproportionate increase in plasma creatinine (all of these being due to release of cellular constituents). A high anion-gap metabolic acidosis and severe hyperuricemia are also characteristic, and oliguria or anuria is common.

155. What is the mechanism of renal failure in rhabdomyolysis?
The mechanism of renal failure is not completely understood. Although myoglobin is not directly nephrotoxic, concurrent vasoconstriction or volume depletion decreases the renal perfusion and rate of urine flow in tubules, thereby promoting the precipitation of these pigment casts.

BIBLIOGRAPHY

1. Brenner EM (ed): Brenner & Rector's The Kidney, 7th ed. Philadelphia, W.B. Saunders, 2004.
2. Goldman L, Ausiello D (eds): Cecil Textbook of Medicine, 22nd ed. Philadelphia, W.B. Saunders, 2004.
3. Greenberg A: Primer on Kidney Diseases—National Kidney Foundation, 2nd ed. San Diego, Academic Press, 1998.
4. Rose BF: Pathophysiology of Renal Disease, 2nd ed. New York, McGraw-Hill, 1987.
5. Schrier RW (ed): Diseases of the Kidney, 6th ed. Boston, Little, Brown, 1997.
6. Schrier RW (ed): Renal and Electrolyte Disorders, 5th ed. Philadelphia, Lippincoot-Raven, 1997.

ACID/BASE AND ELECTROLYTES

Sharma S. Prabhakar, M.D.

CHAPTER 8

In all things you shall find everywhere the Acid and the Alcaly.
Otto Tachenius (1670)
Hyppocrates Chymacus, Ch. 21.

Hence if too much salt is used in food, the pulse hardens.
Huang Ti (The Yellow Emperor) (2697–2597 B.C.)
Nei Chung Su Wen, Bk. 3, Sect. 10, tr. by Ilza Veith,
in The Yellow Emperor's Classic of Internal Medicine.

REGULATION OF SODIUM, WATER, AND VOLUME STATUS

1. **List the osmolality and electrolyte concentrations of serum and commonly used intravenous (IV) solutions.**
See Table 8-1.

TABLE 8-1. OSMOLALITY AND ELECTROLYTE CONCENTRATIONS OF COMMONLY USED IV SOLUTIONS

Serum and Solutions	Osmolality (mOsm/kg)	Glucose (g/l)	Sodium (mEq/L)	Chloride (mEq/L)
Serum	285–295	65–110	135–145	97–110
5% D/W	252	50	0	0
10% D/W	505	100	0	0
50% D/W	2520	500	0	0
1/2 NS (0.45% NaCl)	154	0	77	77
NS (0.9% NaCl)	308	0	154	154
3% NS	1026	0	513	513
Ringer's lactate	272	0	130	109

D/W = dextrose in water, NS = normal saline. Ringer's lactate also contains 28 mEq/L lactate, 4 mEq/L K^+, and 4.5 mEq/L Ca^{2+}.

2. **How do you estimate a patient's serum osmolality?**
A close estimate can be derived from measurements of the serum sodium (Na^+), glucose, and blood urea nitrogen (BUN), using the following equation:

$$\text{Osmolality} = 1.86 \times [Na^+] + \frac{\text{Glucose}}{18} + \frac{\text{BUN}}{2.8} + 9$$

3. What percentage of the adult human body consists of water? What percentage of the water content is intracellular versus extracellular?

Approximately 60% of the adult man and 50% of the adult woman are water. About two thirds of this volume is intracellular, and one third is extracellular. About 20% of the extracellular fluid volume is plasma water.

4. What are the sources and daily amounts of water gain and loss?

The average adult male gains and loses 2600 mL of water each day. The gains occur from direct fluid ingestion (1400 mL/day), from the fluid content of ingested food (850 mL/day), and as a product of water produced by oxidation reactions (350 mL/day). Water losses occur through urine (1500 mL/day), perspiration (500 mL/day), respiration (400 mL/day), and feces (200 mL/day).

5. List the factors necessary to allow the kidney to excrete free water.

1. A filtrate must be formed to allow renal excretion of free water.
2. Glomerular filtrate must escape reabsorption in the proximal tubule to reach the diluting segment (ascending loop of Henle), where free water is created.
3. An adequately functioning diluting segment must be present.
4. The free water formed by the diluting segment must leave the nephron without being reabsorbed by the collecting tubule. This nephron segment is intrinsically impermeable to water but is made permeable by antidiuretic hormone (ADH).

6. Summarize the relationship between glomerular filtration rate (GFR) and excretion of free water.

The lower the GFR, the lower the kidney's ability to respond rapidly to a free-water challenge with excretion of free water.

7. What pathologic states can affect fluid reabsorption in the proximal tubule?

Pathologic states involving vigorous fluid reabsorption in the proximal tubule are associated with a compromised ability to excrete free water. Examples include true volume depletion and states of decreased effective arterial blood volume, such as congestive heart failure, cirrhosis, and nephrotic syndrome.

8. What pathologic states can affect functioning of the diluting segment?

Intrinsic disorders of function of the diluting segment are unusual. Endogenous prostaglandin E_2 and loop diuretics inhibit NaCl transport in this segment and can thereby limit formation of free water.

9. Explain the meaning of serum sodium concentration with respect to sodium balance and water balance.

Serum Na^+ concentration [Na^+], measured in mEq/L, reflects the concentration of this cation in extracellular fluid (ECF). Because its units are measured as mass per unit volume, [Na^+] indicates the relationship between Na^+ and water in the body. It is not indicative of total body Na^+ content but is more an indication of the water status (hydration) of the body. [Na^+] may be low, normal, or increased with any given perturbation of total body Na^+ content. Alterations of the [Na^+] reflect alterations in free-water balance. Therefore, a true low [Na^+] indicates a free-water excess compared to Na^+ content, and a high [Na^+] indicates a relative free-water deficit.

10. What is meant by a state of decreased effective arterial blood volume?

The extracellular space is dynamic, with an ongoing balance between its capacity and its actual volume. Both parameters are biologically monitored and normally coordinated to maintain optimal tissue perfusion. A state of decreased effective arterial blood volume occurs when a large capacity is combined with a smaller volume, as seen most commonly with congestive heart failure, cirrhosis, and nephrotic syndrome. Isotonic fluid losses, such as hemorrhage, cause a decrease in ECF volume with no change in [Na^+]. If, however, these losses are replaced with hypotonic fluids, dilutional hyponatremia results.

11. Why does Na^+ have an effective distribution in total body water despite being confined largely to the extracellular space?
Na^+ is the major determinant of serum osmolality, and changes in its concentration lead to water shifts between the extracellular and intracellular compartments. This osmotic shift of water gives Na^+ an effective distribution greater than its chemical distribution and equivalent to that for total body water.

12. What is the initial step in evaluating a patient with hyponatremia?
Determining the serum osmolality (both measured and calculated) (Fig. 8-1).

13. What is hyperosmolar hyponatremia?
Hyperosmolar hyponatremia is defined as serum osmolarity > 295 mOsm/kg H_2O. It usually results from administration of hypertonic solutions of dextrose or mannitol.

14. Define isotonic hyponatremia.
Isotonic hyponatremia is defined as serum osmolality of 280–295 mOsm/kg H_2O. It is seen with administration of isotonic solutions of dextrose and mannitol.

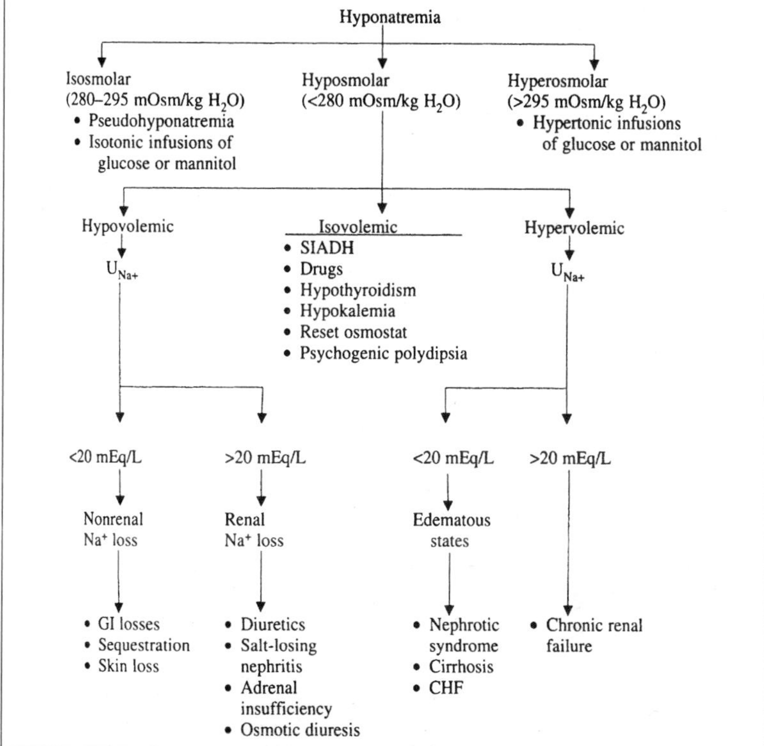

Figure 8-1. Classification of hyponatremia. SIADH = syndrome of inappropriate ADH secretion, GI = gastrointestinal, CHF = congestive heart failure.

15. **What is hyposmolar hyponatremia?**
Hyposmolar hyponatremia is defined as serum osmolality < 280 mOsm/kg H_2O). It can be associated with low, normal, or increased volume status and is seen with diuretic administration, salt-losing renal conditions, syndrome of inappropriate ADH secretion (SIADH), chronic renal failure, and a wide range of other causes.

16. **How can patients with hyposmolar hyponatremia be categorized according to history and physical findings?**
Patients with hyposmolar hyponatremia can be categorized as hypovolemic, hypervolemic, or euvolemic according to volume status as estimated from the physical exam and history.

17. **What findings suggest a hypovolemic state?**
Hypovolemia is supported by a history of volume loss or decreased intake and orthostatic blood pressure changes on examination.

18. **How is the hypovolemia treated?**
The lost volume must be replaced to turn off the factors that limit the kidney's ability to excrete free water.

19. **How do you recognize the hypervolemic patient?**
Hypervolemia is supported by a history of a condition with decreased effective arterial blood volume and an examination showing edema.

20. **Describe the treatment of the hypervolemia.**
Therapeutic attention must be directed to the underlying disorder. If the hyponatremia is mild and asymptomatic, free-water restriction, in addition to specific treatment of the underlying disorder, is the suggested initial therapeutic approach. If the hyponatremia is severe and symptomatic, more aggressive treatment with hypertonic saline and furosemide may be required.

21. **Summarize the approach to euvolemic hyposmolar hyponatremia.**
In patients with hyposmolar hyponatremia and apparently normal volume status or euvolemia, a wide variety of pathologic processes must be considered in the diagnostic evaluation, including SIADH and drugs that can limit free-water excretion (e.g., chlorpropamide).

22. **Define pseudohyponatremia.**
Pseudohyponatremia occurs when a quantitative serum Na^+ measurement is performed on a given volume of plasma that contains a greater-than-normal amount of water-excluding particles, such as lipid or protein. In this setting, plasma water (which contains the Na^+) composes a smaller fraction of the plasma volume, leading to a factitiously low serum Na^+ concentration (when expressed in mEq/L). The Na^+ concentration in plasma water is normal, and therefore patients are asymptomatic. Attention should be directed to hyperlipidemia or hyperproteinemia.

23. **How is spurious hyponatremia different from pseudohyponatremia?**
Spurious hyponatremia results from hyperosmolality of the serum (i.e., from hyperglycemia), resulting in movement of intracellular water to the extracellular space and subsequent dilution of the Na^+ in the ECF. These patients are not symptomatic from hyposmolality (unlike patients with true hyponatremia). If they are symptomatic at all, it is due to their hyperosmolar state. Attention should be directed to correcting the hyperosmolar state. It is important to distinguish these two categories of hyponatremia from true hyponatremia associated with hyposmolality because the diagnostic work-up and therapeutic management are different.

24. **How do you correct the serum Na^+ for a given level of hyperglycemia?**
Hyperglycemia, one of the causes of spurious hyponatremia, causes a decrease in the measured serum Na^+ concentration. For each increase in serum glucose of 100 mg/dL up to

600 mg/dL (an increase of 500, or 5×100 mg/dL), the serum Na^+ decreases by 8.0 mEq/L (5×1.6 mEq/L).

25. **Define essential hyponatremia.**
Essential hyponatremia, or "sick cell syndrome," denotes hyponatremia in the absence of a water diuresis defect. One hypothesis is that the osmoreceptor cells in the hypothalamus are reset so that they maintain a lower plasma osmolality. This is seen in several conditions, such as congestive heart failure, cirrhosis, and pulmonary tuberculosis, and is diagnosed by demonstrating normal urinary Na^+ concentration and dilution in the face of hyponatremia. Generally, this entity does not require treatment.

26. **What are the signs and symptoms of hyponatremia?**
The manifestations are mainly attributable to CNS edema, which is usually not seen until the serum Na^+ falls to 120 mEq/L or less. Symptoms range from mild lethargy to seizure, coma, and death. The signs and symptoms of hyponatremia are more a function of the rapidity of the drop in serum Na^+ than the absolute level. In patients with chronic hyponatremia, there has been time for solute equilibration, resulting in less CNS edema and less severe manifestations. In acute hyponatremia, there is no time for equilibration, and so smaller changes in serum Na^+ are accompanied by larger degrees of CNS edema and more severe manifestations.

27. **Why is hyponatremia often seen after transurethral resection of the prostate (TURP)?**
Often during the TURP procedure, large volumes of solutions containing mannitol, glycerol, or sorbitol are used to irrigate the prostate. A variable fraction of these fluids is absorbed into the systemic circulation, producing hyponatremia.

28. **How do you manage hyponatremia in edematous states?**
Treatment depends on the underlying etiology, any symptoms, and the rapidity of the drop in serum Na^+. In general, patients with edematous states such as the nephrotic syndrome, who have ECF expansion, have some degree of hyponatremia if they are not water-restricted. Generally, this condition is asymptomatic and requires no treatment. Treatment is required only if the hyponatremia is severe (< 125 mEq/L), and especially if there are symptoms such as lethargy, confusion, stupor, and coma.

29. **A 41-year-old black man is hospitalized with acute bacterial meningitis. His chemistry profile shows a BUN and creatinine of 11 and 1.2 mg/dL, respectively, but his serum Na^+ is 127 mEq/L. What is the likely cause of his hyponatremia?**
Hyponatremia in the setting of bacterial meningitis (or any pathologic CNS process) is usually due to SIADH. SIADH is a form of hyponatremia involving sustained or spiking levels of ADH that are inappropriate for the osmotic or volume stimuli that normally affect ADH secretion.

30. **List the essential points in the diagnosis of SIADH.**
- Presence of hypotonic hyponatremia
- Inappropriate antidiuresis (urine osmolality higher than expected for the degree of hyponatremia)
- Significant Na^+ excretion when the patient is normovolemic
- Normal renal, thyroid, and adrenal function
- Absence of other causes of hyponatremia, volume depletion, or edema

31. **Describe the work-up for the patient in question 29.**
The work-up includes measurement of serum and urine Na^+ concentration and osmolality. In most cases, urinary osmolality exceeds plasma osmolality, often by > 100 mOsm/L. Urinary Na^+ excretion exceeds 20 mEq/L unless the patient is wasting, and it improves with fluid restriction.

In most cases, restriction of fluids to 1000–1200 mL/day is all that is needed. Occasionally, patients with symptomatic and marked hyponatremia may require demeclocycline therapy and/or hypertonic saline.

32. **What is cerebral salt-wasting?**
Due to impaired renal water excretion, this condition is associated with hyposmolar hyponatremia in patients with cerebral trauma or disease. It mimics SIADH in all aspects including hypouricemia except that in this syndrome patients are volume-depleted, while in SIADH, patients are euvolemic. The high urinary Na^+ despite hypovolemia reflects renal salt-wasting. The etiology of this salt-wasting is unknown, although increased secretion of cerebral natriuretic factors is one likely explanation. A circulating factor that impairs renal tubular Na^+ reabsorption is another likely possibility.

Al-Mufti H, Arieff AI: Cerebral salt wasting syndrome: Combined cerebral and distal tubular lesion. Am J Med 77:740, 1984.

33. **How do you estimate the free-water deficit in a patient with hypernatremia?**
It can be assumed that the patient has lost free water without salt, and thus the patient has reduced total body water (TBW) but maintains the same total body Na^+ content. This change results in an increase in the serum Na^+ concentration that is proportional to the decrease in TBW. In other words, the ratio of the initial serum Na^+ (which is assumed to be normal) to the current serum Na^+ (which is higher than normal) is equal to the ratio of the present TBW (which is less than normal) to the initial TBW (which is assumed to have been normal).

$$\text{Current TBW} \div \text{Initial TBW} = \text{Initial } \{Na^+\} \div \text{Current } \{Na^+\}$$

This relationship can be used to calculate the current TBW. Subtracting this value from the initial (normal) TBW yields the estimated free-water deficit. This calculated free-water deficit must be replaced with fluids.

34. **What are the manifestations of hypernatremia?**
The manifestations of hypernatremia are basically those of hyperosmolality and are similar to the symptoms manifested by other causes of hyperosmolality, such as hyperglycemia. These are produced mainly by fluid shifts from the CNS and increased CNS osmolality, resulting in "shrinking" of the brain. The symptoms range from lethargy to seizures, coma, and death. The severity of the symptoms depends on the severity of the hyperosmolality and the speed with which it develops.

35. **What are some common causes of hypernatremia?**
Diabetes insipidus, severe dehydration due to extrarenal fluid losses (e.g., burns, excessive sweating), and hypothalamic disorders (e.g., tumors, granulomas, cerebrovascular accidents) leading to defective thirst and vasopressin regulation.

36. **How do you correct hypernatremia?**
Once the free-water deficit is calculated, hypernatremia is usually corrected by replacement of the water. In mild cases, this can be accomplished by simply having the patient drink or, if IV fluids are used, dextrose in water can be given. If salt-containing fluids are deemed necessary, the equivalent free-water volume must be given. For example, if half-normal saline is used (1 L of which contains 500 mL of normal saline and 500 mL of free water), then twice the amount of the estimated free-water deficit is needed to correct the free-water deficit. This volume deficit should be replaced slowly. The first half is given over 24 hours. If the patient is hemodynamically unstable, with signs of severe ECF volume depletion, therapy with 0.9% normal saline is warranted before dextrose infusion is started.

POTASSIUM BALANCE

37. How is potassium (K^+) distributed between the intracellular fluid (ICF) and ECF compartments?
A 70-kg man contains approximately 3500 mEq of K^+ (approximately 50 mEq/kg body weight). The vast majority of this (98%) is in the ICF space. Therefore, the amount in the ECF compartment (the portion that we routinely measure) represents only a small percentage of the total body K^+.

38. How is the large chemical gradient between intracellular and extracellular K^+ concentration maintained?
The Na^+-K^+ adenosine triphosphate (ATPase) pump actively extrudes Na^+ from the cell and pumps K^+ into the cell. This pump is present in all cells of the body. In addition, the cell is electrically negative compared to the exterior, which serves to keep K^+ inside the cell.

39. Given the relatively small extracellular compared to intracellular concentration of K^+, why are some electrical processes (cardiac conduction, skeletal and smooth muscle contraction) sensitive to changes in the ECF K^+ concentration?
It is the ratio of the ECF to ICF K^+ concentration more than the absolute level of either that determines the sensitivity of these electrical processes. Because the ECF concentration of K^+ is small compared to the ICF concentration, a small absolute change in ECF K^+ concentration results in a large change in the ECF to ICF K^+ ratio.

40. What factors commonly influence the movement of K^+ between the intracellular and extracellular compartments?

- **Acid-base changes:** Acidemia (increased concentration of H^+ in serum) leads to intracellular buffering of H^+, with subsequent extrusion of K^+ into the ECF, increasing the concentration of K^+ in this compartment. Similarly, alkalemia leads to hypokalemia.
- **Hormones:** Insulin, epinephrine, growth hormone, and androgens all promote net movement of K^+ into cells.
- **Cellular metabolism:** Synthesis of protein and glycogen is associated with intracellular K^+ binding.
- **Extracellular concentration:** All other things being equal, K^+ tends to enter the cell when its extracellular concentration is high and vice versa.

41. How is K^+ handled by the kidney?
Most of the filtered K^+ is reabsorbed in the proximal tubule, and there is net secretion or net resorption in the distal nephron, depending on the body's K^+ needs. Under most conditions, we are in K^+ excess, and the kidney must excrete K^+ to maintain whole-body K^+ balance. K^+ restriction leads to renal K^+ conservation, but this process is neither as rapid nor as efficient as the process for Na^+.

42. How does aldosterone influence K^+ metabolism?
Aldosterone is the main regulatory hormone for K^+ metabolism. It promotes Na^+ resorption and K^+ secretion in the distal nephron, gut, and sweat glands. Quantitatively, its greatest effect is in the kidney. Its secretion is increased by an increasing K^+ concentration in the ECF and is decreased by low K^+ concentrations.

43. How does hypoaldosteronism affect K^+ and Na^+ levels?
Asymptomatic hyperkalemia is a common presentation of patients with mineralocorticoid deficiency. Na^+ deficiency and volume depletion are not seen unless there is concomitant glucocorticoid deficiency. Na^+ balance is maintained by other factors, such as angiotensin II and catecholamines, although the ability to conserve Na^+ maximally is generally lost. Thus, urine $Na^+ < 10$ mEq/L is unusual in primary hypoaldosteronism.

44. How is hypoaldoteronism diagnosed?

To diagnose hypoaldosteronism, the first step is to exclude drug-induced hyperkalemia (such as angiotensin-converting enzyme (ACE) inhibitors, beta blockers, NSAIDs, heparin, or K^+-sparing diuretics). The next step is to obtain morning samples of plasma for renin, aldosterone, and cortisol measurements. Administration of furosemide (20–40 mg) at 6 PM and 6 AM before samples are drawn enhances the utility of the test by stimulating plasma renin activity in normal persons but not in those with hypoaldosteronism.

45. What is meant by transtubular K^+ gradient (TTKG)?

TTKG is an indirect method of evaluating the effect of aldosterone on the kidney. The principle is to measure K^+ at the end of the cortical collecting tube, after all the distal K^+ secretion has taken place:

$$TTKG = \frac{U_{K+}/(U_{osm}/P_{osm})}{P_{K+}}$$

It is assumed that urine osmolality (U_{osm}) at the end of the cortical collecting tube is the same as that of plasma (P_{osm}) because the interstitium here is iso-osmotic. It is also assumed that no further K^+ secretion or resorption takes place. But, since ADH-mediated water permeability continues in the medullary collecting tubule, the K^+ concentration in this duct rises. The above formula is applicable as long as the urine Na^+ concentration is 25 mEq/L, since Na^+ delivery should not be a limiting factor.

46. What is the TTKG value in normal and hyperkalemic subjects?

The TTKG in normal subjects is 8–10 on a normal diet. On a high K^+ diet, TTKG is > 11 because of increased K^+ secretion. Thus, in a hyperkalemic subject, a TTKG < 5 mEq/L indicates impaired tubular K^+ secretion and is highly suggestive of hypoaldosteronism.

Ethier JH, et al: The trans-tubular potassium gradient in patients with hypokalemia and hyperkalemia. Am J Kidney Dis 15:309, 1990.

47. List conditions that can lead to increased renal K^+ excretion.

- Increased dietary K^+ intake
- Increased aldosterone secretion (as in volume depletion)
- Alkalosis
- Increased flow rate in the distal tubule
- Increased Na^+ delivery to the distal nephron
- Decreased chloride concentration in tubular fluid in the distal nephron
- Natriuretic agents

48. How does increased sodium delivery promote renal excretion of K^+?

Increased Na^+ delivery to the distal nephron promotes Na^+ resorption in exchange for K^+ secretion. The process is accelerated in the presence of aldosterone.

49. Explain how decreased chloride concentration leads to an increase renal excretion of K^+.

Decreased chloride concentration in tubular fluid in the distal nephron allows Na^+ to be resorbed with a less permeable ion (e.g., bicarbonate or sulfate) that increases the negativity of the tubular lumen in the distal nephron. The increased negativity of the tubular lumen promotes K^+ secretion.

50. How do natriuretic agents increase renal excretion of K^+?

Natriuretic agents, such as loop diuretics, thiazides, and acetazolamide, lead to increased Na^+ delivery to the distal nephron, volume depletion with increased aldosterone secretion, and subsequent increased renal K^+ excretion.

51. **In addition to the kidney, what is the other major route of K^+ loss?**
The GI tract. Fluids in the lower GI tract, particularly those of the small bowel, are high in K^+. Therefore, diarrhea can result in significant losses of K^+. However, upper GI losses, such as vomiting or nasogastric suction, cause renal K^+ loss. This renal K^+ loss is multifactorial and includes the following:
- Alkalosis
- Volume depletion, which leads to increased aldosterone secretion
- Chloride depletion from the loss of HCl in gastric fluid, which leads to a high tubular concentration of HCO_3^-, a relatively nonresorbable anion

52. **What causes a spuriously elevated serum K^+ determination?**
- **Hemolysis**, with the release of intraerythrocytic K^+.
- **Pseudohyperkalemia**, seen in marked thrombocytosis or leukocytosis. It is due to the disproportionately increased amounts of the normally released K^+ that occurs with clotting. This condition can be corrected by inhibiting clotting and measuring the plasma K^+ concentration.

53. **List the four common mechanisms by which hyperkalemia develops.**
- Inadequate excretion
- Excessive intake
- Shift of potassium from tissues
- Pseudohyperkalemia (due to thrombocytosis, leukocytosis, poor venipuncture technique, in vitro hemolysis)

Singer GG, Brenner BM: Fluids and electrolytes. In Fauci A, et al (eds): Harrison's Principles of Internal Medicine, 14th ed. New York, McGraw-Hill, 1998.

54. **What factors lead to inadequate potassium excretion?**
- Renal disorders (acute renal failure, severe chronic renal failure, tubular disorders)
- Hypoaldosteronism
- Adrenal disorders
- Hyporeninemia (as with tubulointerstitial diseases, drugs such as NSAIDs, ACE inhibitosr, and beta blockers)
- Diuretics that inhibit potassium secretion (spironoloactone, triamterene, amiloride)

55. **What factors lead to a shift of potassium from tissues?**
- Tissue damage (muscle crush, hemolysis, internal bleeding)
- Drugs (succinylcholine, arginine, digitalis poisoning, beta blockers)
- Acidosis
- Hyperosmolality
- Insulin deficiency
- Hyperkalemic periodic paralysis

56. **What is the first step in the diagnostic approach to patients with disturbances in serum K^+ concentration?**
Determine whether the disturbance results from:
- Abnormal K^+ intake or metabolism (excessive catabolism or anabolism)
- Intra- and extracellular compartmental shifts
- Disturbances in renal excretion or extrarenal loss

57. **What should you do next?**
After the patient is placed in one of these three categories, it is possible to narrow the differential diagnosis, order appropriate diagnostic tests, and decide on the appropriate management. Disturbances of intake can be investigated by history and physical examination. The possibility of cellular shifts can be investigated by looking for any of the disturbances that result in

compartmental movement of this cation. Determination of the urinary K^+ concentration can help in distinguishing renal from nonrenal causes. High urinary K^+ excretion in the setting of hypokalemia is compatible with a renal cause for K^+ deficiency. In contrast, an appropriately low urinary K^+ excretion in the setting of hypokalemia suggests extrarenal (possibly GI) losses.

58. **How does hypokalemia present clinically?**
The major manifestations are seen in the neuromuscular system. When K^+ falls to 2.0–2.5 mEq/L, muscular weakness and lethargy are seen. With further decreases, the patient manifests paralysis with eventual respiratory muscle involvement and death. Hypokalemia also can cause rhabdomyolysis, myoglobinuria, and paralytic ileus. Prolonged hypokalemia can lead to renal tubular damage (called hypokalemic nephropathy).

59. **How do you manage a patient with hypokalemia?**
Management must be directed at the disturbance causing the abnormal K^+ concentration. If hypokalemia is associated with alkalosis, then the alkalosis should be corrected in addition to providing K^+ supplements. In general, patients with K^+ depletion should be given supplements slowly to replace the deficit. The oral route is preferred because of its safety as well as efficacy. Some instances require more rapid repletion with IV supplements, but this should not exceed 20 mEq/h. Cardiac monitoring should accompany infusions of > 10 mEq/h.

60. **What are the manifestations of hyperkalemia besides ECG changes?**
The most important manifestation is the increased excitability of cardiac muscle. With severe elevations in K^+, a patient can suffer diastolic cardiac arrest. Skeletal muscle paralysis also can be seen. Again, the symptoms produced by hyperkalemia are dependent on the rapidity of the change. Patients with chronically elevated serum K^+ levels can tolerate higher levels with fewer symptoms than patients with acute hyperkalemia.

61. **How is hyperkalemia generally managed?**
Treatment depends on the extent of the hyperkalemia and the clinical setting. Mild levels of hyperkalemia (5.0–5.5 mEq/L) associated with the hyporenin–hypoaldosterone syndrome are tolerated well and usually require no treatment. Higher levels not associated with ECG changes may require treatment with a synthetic mineralocorticoid.

62. **Describe the management of hyperkalemia as a medical emergency.**
Hyperkalemia occasionally presents as a medical emergency with very high levels (> 7.0 mEq/L) and cardiac conduction system abnormalities as determined by the ECG changes (see Chapter 3). In this emergent setting, management includes:
   - IV calcium must be administered to immediately counteract the effect of hyperkalemia on the conduction system.
   - Calcium administration must be followed by maneuvers to shift K^+ into cells, thereby decreasing the ratio of extra-to intracellular K^+. This goal can be accomplished by administering glucose with insulin and/or bicarbonate to increase serum pH.
   - Finally, a maneuver to remove K^+ from the body must be instituted, such as a cation-exchange resin (Kayexalate) and/or hemodialysis or peritoneal dialysis.

63. **A 61-year-old woman with end-stage renal disease missed her dialysis twice and presents to the emergency department with a serum K^+ of 6.4 mEq/L. How should you manage this patient?**
The severity of hyperkalemia is assessed by both the serum K^+ level and ECG changes. If the ECG shows only tall T waves and the serum K^+ is < 6.5 mEq/L, the hyperkalemia is mild, whereas K^+ levels of 6.5–8.0 mEq/L are associated with more severe ECG changes, including absent P waves and wide QRS complexes. At higher K^+ levels, ventricular arrhythmias tend to appear, and the prognosis is grave unless proper treatment is given.

64. If the ECG shows only tall T waves, which agents should you administer? Why?

- **Hypertonic glucose infusion**, along with 10 units of insulin (e.g., 10 units of insulin with 200–500 mL of 10% glucose in 30 min followed by 1 L of the same in the next 4–6 hours).
- **Sodium bicarbonate**, 50–150 mEq given by IV (if the patient is not in fluid overload).

Both of these agents shift K^+ into cells and start acting within an hour. Total body K^+ can be decreased by using cation-exchange resins, such as sodium polysterone sulfonate; usually, 20 gm with 20 mL of 70% sorbitol solution is started every 4–6 h.

65. If the ECG shows the more severe changes, what should you do?

The patient should first receive 10% calcium gluconate (10–30 mL IV) while being monitored. Arrangements must be made to dialyze the patient as soon as possible to correct the hyperkalemia.

66. A 71-year-old diabetic with a nonhealing foot ulcer is on tobramycin and piperacillin. This patient has a resistant hypokalemia. How do you approach this problem?

Aminoglycosides and penicillins are both known to deplete serum K^+. The former do this by defective proximal tubular K^+ resorption and the latter by increased renal K^+ excretion induced by the poorly resorbable anion (penicillin). With aminoglycosides, magnesium-wasting is another complication. Hence, in addition to K^+ repletion, correction of hypomagnesemia is important, since hypokalemia is often resistant to correction unless the magnesium deficit is also corrected.

67. A 67-year-old man with congestive heart failure treated with furosemide has a serum K^+ of 2.4 mEq/L. How would you correct his K^+ deficit?

Hypokalemia is an important complication of diuretic therapy (except with K^+-sparing diuretics). It is important to monitor serum K^+ periodically in these patients, especially those with cardiac illnesses who are likely to be on digoxin because hypokalemia can exacerbate digitalis toxicity. The K^+ deficit requires replacement (except in patients who are on minimal doses of diuretics), particularly if serum K^+ is < 3 mEq/L. The serum K^+ level is not an exact indicator of the total body deficit, but severe hypokalemia with serum K^+ of < 3 mEq/L is usually associated with a deficit of approximately 300 mEq. KCl elixir or tablets are the treatment of choice. Enteric-coated K^+ supplements are known to cause gastric ulceration.

68. What is the primary defect in Bartter's syndrome?

The primary defect in Bartter's syndrome seems to be impaired NaCl reabsorption in the thick ascending loop of Henle or distal tubule. Recent genetic studies indicate the defect involves a mutation of Na^+-K^+-2Cl cotransporter or K^+ channel in the thick ascending limb of Henle. The diagnosis is often made by exclusion. Surreptitious use of diuretics and vomiting (urine Cl^- is often low!) can mimic most of the findings of this syndrome.

69. Describe the treatment of Bartter's syndrome.

Treatment consists of a K^+-sparing diuretic (such as amiloride in doses of 10–40 mg) and NSAIDs to raise the plasma K^+ by reversing the physiologic abnormalities.

Wingo C: Disorders of potassium balance. In Brenner B, Rector CR (eds): The Kidney, 6th ed. Philadelphia, W.B. Saunders, 2000.

70. A 55-year-old man with a history of congestive heart failure and chronic obstructive pulmonary disease (COPD) presents with extreme weakness and fatigue. His medications include digoxin 0.25 mg/day, hydrochlorothiazide 50 mg/day, and albuterol inhalations for his asthma. The patient reports a few days

of exacerbation of COPD symptoms, forcing him to use the inhaler more frequently. What is the likely cause of his weakness?
The most likely cause of weakness in this patient is severe hypokalemia resulting from overuse of beta agonists such as albuterol especially in the presence of potassium losing diuretics, since both effects could be additive. The hypokalemic effects of inhaled beta agonists are often so potent that they are used to treat patients with hyperkalemia acutely.

ACID-BASE REGULATION

71. **What is the Henderson-Hasselbalch equation?**
An acid-base disorder is suspected on clinical grounds and confirmed by arterial blood gas (ABG) analysis of the pH, $PaCO_2$, or HCO_3^- concentration. The Henderson-Hasselbalch equation is used to test if a given set of parameters is mutually compatible:

$$pH = pKa + \log \frac{\{HCO_3^-\}}{\alpha CO_2 \times PaCO_2} = 6.1 + \log \frac{\{HCO_3^-\}}{0.03 \times PaCO_2}$$

The value of pK_a, the negative log of the equilibrium constant K, and the CO_2 solubility coefficient (αCO_2) are constant at any given set of temperature and osmolality. In plasma, at 37°C, the $pK_a = 6.1$ and $\alpha CO_2 = 0.03$.

72. **Explain the significance of the Henderson-Hasselbalch equation.**
The Henderson-Hasselbalch equation shows that pH is dependent on the ratio of $[HCO_3^-]$ to $PaCO_2$ and not on the absolute individual values alone. A primary change in one of the values usually leads to a compensatory change in the other value. This serves to limit the degree of the resulting acidosis or alkalosis.

73. **The integrated action of which three organs is involved in acid-base homeostasis?**
The **liver**, **lungs**, and **kidneys** cooperate to maintain acid-base balance. The liver metabolizes proteins contained in the standard American diet such that net acid (protons) is produced. Hepatic metabolism of organic acids (lactate) can consume acid, which is the equivalent of producing bicarbonate. Acid released into the ECF titrates HCO_3^- to H_2O and CO_2. The lungs excrete this CO_2 and the CO_2 produced from cellular metabolism. The kidney reclaims the filtered HCO_3^- and excretes the accumulated net acid.

74. **What is the fate of a load of nonvolatile acid administered to the body?**
The acid load is initially buffered by extracellular (40%) and intracellular (60%) buffers. These buffers minimize the decrease in pH that otherwise would occur. The major ECF buffer is the HCO_3^- system, and most intracellular buffering is provided by histidine-containing proteins. The administered acid reduces ECF HCO_3^-, and new HCO_3^- is then regenerated by the kidney during the process of proton (acid) secretion. So the administered acid is initially buffered and eventually excreted by the kidney.

75. **How does the kidney excrete acid to maintain the acid-base balance?**
The kidney must **reclaim** the filtered HCO_3^- and **regenerate** the HCO_3^- lost by acid titration. This latter process is equivalent to acid excretion. Reclamation of HCO_3^- is quantitatively a more important process than regeneration (4500 mEq/day versus 70 mEq/day). Nevertheless, without regeneration of new HCO_3^- (excretion of acid), the plasma HCO_3^- concentration could not be maintained, and net acid retention would result. Two principal urinary buffers allow net acid excretion (new HCO_3^- regeneration) Dibasic phosphate and ammonia. By accepting a proton,

they become monobasic phosphate and ammonium ions, respectively, and are excreted in the urine. The phosphate is measured as titratable acid, and the ammonium is measured directly. Urinary excretion of these two substances minus urinary HCO_3^- excretion constitutes net acid excretion.

76. List the four primary acid-base disturbances.

- Metabolic acidosis
- Metabolic alkalosis
- Respiratory acidosis
- Respiratory alkalosis

77. Explain what is meant by acidosis and alkalosis.

In the steady-state maintenance of normal acid-base balance, the addition of H^+ to the body fluids is balanced by their excretion, such that the H^+ concentration of the ECF remains relatively constant at 40 nM (40×10^{-9} M, or pH = 7.40). **Acidosis** refers to an imbalance in this process that leads to a net increase in $[H^+]$. **Alkalosis** refers to an imbalance that leads to a net decrease in $[H^+]$.

78. What is meant by *metabolic* and *respiratory* in referring to acid-base disturbances?

Metabolic and *respiratory* are terms used to describe how the imbalance occurred. Describing a disorder as **metabolic** infers that the imbalance leading to the change in H^+ occurred either because of addition of nonvolatile acid or base or because of a gain or loss of available buffer (HCO_3^-). HCO_3^- as a buffer reduces the concentration of free H^+ in solution. Referring to an acid-base disorder as **respiratory** infers that the net change in $[H^+]$ occurred secondary to a disturbance in ventilation that resulted in either a net increase or decrease in CO_2 gas in the ECF.

79. Define metabolic acidosis.

Metabolic acidosis means a net increase in $[H^+]$ as a result of a net gain in nonvolatile acid or from a net loss of HCO_3^- buffer.

80. Define respiratory acidosis.

Respiratory acidosis means a net increase in $[H^+]$ as a result of decreased ventilation, leading to CO_2 retention.

81. Define metabolic alkalosis.

Metabolic alkalosis means a net decrease in $[H^+]$ as a result of gain of HCO_3^- or loss of acid.

82. Define respiratory alkalosis

Respiratory alkalosis means a net decrease in $[H^+]$ because of increased ventilation leading to decreased CO_2.

83. What important points should be kept in mind about these four disorders?

These disorders refer to the imbalance that leads to the directional change in $[H^+]$ and do not denote what the final $[H^+]$, PCO_2, and $[HCO_3^-]$ will be. Two important facts should be kept in mind:

1. Compensatory changes occur in response to these disorders.
2. More than one acid-base disturbance may occur simultaneously; the final parameters measured depend not only on the algebraic sum of the different disorders but also on their respective compensatory responses.

84. How are the four primary acid-base disorders diagnosed?
See Table 8-2.

TABLE 8-2. RELATIONSHIPS BETWEEN HCO_3^- AND $PaCO_2$ IN SIMPLE ACID-BASE DISORDERS

Condition	Primary Disturbance	Predicted Response
Metabolic acidosis	$\downarrow HCO_3^-$	$\Delta PaCO_2 (\downarrow) = 1–1.4\ \Delta HCO_3^-$*
Metabolic alkalosis	$\uparrow HCO_3^-$	$\Delta PaCO_2 (\uparrow) = 0.4–0.9\ \Delta HCO_3^-$*
Respiratory acidosis	$\uparrow PaCO_2$	Acute: $\Delta HCO_3^- (\uparrow) = 0.1\ \Delta PaCO_2$ Chronic: $\Delta\ HCO_3^- (\uparrow) = 0.25–0.55\ PaCO_2$
Respiratory alkalosis	$\downarrow PaCO_2$	Acute: $\Delta HCO_3^- (\downarrow) = 0.2–0.25\ \Delta PaCO_2$ Chronic: $\Delta HCO_3^- (\downarrow) = 0.4–0.5\ \Delta PaCO_2$

*After at least 12–24 hours.
From Hamm L: Mixed acid-base disorders. In Kokko JP, Tannen KL (eds): Fluids and Electrolytes, 3rd ed. Philadelphia, W.B. Saunders, 1996, p 487.

85. What are secondary acid-base disturbances?
The phrase *secondary acid-base disturbance* is actually a misnomer. More correctly stated, these are compensatory physiologic responses to the cardinal acid-base disturbances. They usually alleviate the change in H^+ concentration and therefore the pH that otherwise would occur.

86. What equation helps explain the compensatory physiologic responses to acid-base disturbances?
The mass-action equation, derived from the more familiar Henderson-Hasselbalch equation, definies the relationship of H^+, HCO_3^-, and the $PaCO_2$:

$$[H^+] = \frac{PaCO_2}{\{HCO_3^-\}} \times 24$$

One can see that in the setting of metabolic acidosis, with a primary decrease in $[HCO_3^-]$, the $[H^+]$ increases. It is also evident that the increase in $[H^+]$ in this setting can be alleviated by concomitantly decreasing the $PaCO_2$, which is exactly what occurs as a result of a **physiologic** increase in ventilation. This situation is properly described as metabolic acidosis with a directionally appropriate respiratory response. It is incorrect to describe the condition as primary metabolic acidosis with secondary respiratory alkalosis; to say that a patient has respiratory alkalosis is to say that a patient has **pathologic** hypoventilation, which is not the case in this situation. Tables and formulas can be used to calculate the expected respiratory response to a given degree of metabolic acidosis.

87. What is a mixed acid-base disorder?
If the decrease in $PaCO_2$ in response to the degree of metabolic acidosis is exactly what we would have predicted from the formulas, the patient is said to have one acid-base disorder: metabolic acidosis. In contrast, if the measured decrease in $PaCO_2$ is more than that predicted for the degree of metabolic acidosis, then the patient has an *additional* (not secondary) acid-

base disorder: respiratory alkalosis in addition to metabolic acidosis. In other words, the patient has a mixed disorder, which is actually very common. If the measured $PaCO_2$ is higher than predicted, then the patient has an additional respiratory acidosis.

88. **What causes respiratory acidosis?**
Respiratory acidosis is a drop in the pH (acidosis) caused by alveolar hypoventilation. The alveolar hypoventilation leads to a rate of excretion of CO_2 that is less than its metabolic production. This net gain in CO_2 causes a rise in the $PaCO_2$. The lungs may be subject to diffuse hypoventilation (global alveolar hypoventilation), or only parts of the lungs may be involved (regional alveolar hypoventilation). As can be seen in the Henderson-Hasselbalch equation, any increase in the $PaCO_2$, if not accompanied by an increase in $[HCO_3^-]$, leads to a measurable drop in the pH.

89. **Describe the treatment of respiratory acidosis.**
Treatment is aimed at the correction of the cause of the hypoventilation. This goal may involve the treatment of airway obstruction or, in respiratory failure, even mechanical ventilation.

90. **What causes respiratory alkalosis?**
Respiratory alkalosis, the opposite of respiratory acidosis, is a rise in pH (alkalosis). It is due to alveolar hyperventilation, which in turn leads to an increase in the excretion of CO_2 and a drop in the $PaCO_2$. The causes of respiratory alkalosis include:
- CNS stimulation of ventilation: physiologic (voluntary, anxiety, fear, fever, pregnancy) or pathologic (intracranial hemorrhage, stroke, tumors, brainstem lesions, salicylates)
- Peripheral stimulation of ventilation: reflex hyperventilation due to abnormal lung or chest wall mechanics (pulmonary emboli, myopathies, interstitial lung diseases), arterial hypoxemia, high altitudes, pain, congestive heart failure, shock of any etiology, hypothermia
- Hyperventilation with mechanical ventilation
- Others: severe liver disease, uremia

91. **Are the plasma electrolytes alone (Na^+, K^+, Cl^-, and HCO_3^-) sufficient to determine a patient's acid-base status?**
No. Remember that the regulatory systems of the body work to maintain the pH (or $[H^+]$), and that pH is a function of the ratio of $PaCO_2$ and $[HCO_3^-]$. The pH is not determined by the absolute value of $PaCO_2$ or $[HCO_3^-]$ alone. Thus, a set of plasma electrolytes demonstrating a normal $[HCO_3^-]$ does not necessarily indicate a normal acid-base status.

92. **Give two interpretations of a low $[HCO_3^-]$ and high $[Cl^-]$.**
A low $[HCO_3^-]$ and high $[Cl^-]$ may represent either a metabolic acidosis (probably a nonanion gap acidosis) or a chronic respiratory alkalosis with an appropriate metabolic response (renal lowering of $[HCO_3^-]$ as a response to the chronically low $PaCO_2$). This is an attempt to maintain a more normal pH.

93. **Give two interpretations of a high $[HCO_3^-]$ and low $[Cl^-]$.**
Likewise, a high $[HCO_3^-]$ with low $[Cl^-]$ may represent a metabolic alkalosis or a chronic respiratory acidosis with an appropriate metabolic response (renal increase in $[HCO_3^-]$ in response to chronically high $PaCO_2$) in an attempt to maintain a more normal pH. Note that without an accompanying pH and $PaCO_2$, one cannot tell if an abnormal $[HCO_3^-]$ is due to a metabolic cause (a metabolic acidosis or alkalosis) or to a metabolic response to a primary respiratory disorder. This illustrates the importance of obtaining ABGs (with a pH and $PaCO_2$) in addition to a $[HCO_3^-]$ to properly assess a patient's acid-base status.

94. What is meant by the anion gap?
The anion gap (AG) represents the difference between the routinely measured cations and anions in the plasma. It is usually calculated as follows:

$$\text{Anion gap} = [Na^+] - [Cl^- + HCO_3^-]$$

95. Is the anion gap really a "gap"?
Since electroneutrality is always maintained in solution, there is no actual anion "gap." This gap is composed predominantly of negatively charged proteins in plasma and averages 12 ± 3 mEq/L. An increase is most commonly caused by addition of an acid salt (H^+A^-), which reduces plasma HCO_3^- concentration by titration. Electroneutrality is maintained in the face of the reduced plasma HCO_3^- concentration by the accompanying anion. Since the anion is not measured routinely in the electrolyte profile, the routine measurement would reveal only decreased HCO_3^- concentration. With plasma Na^+ and Cl^- remaining unchanged, this reduced HCO_3^- concentration leads to an increased anion gap. Note that the AG would not change if the added acid were HCl. Other circumstances that can increase the AG include increased protein concentration and alkalemia, which increase the net negative charge on plasma proteins. The presence of a large quantity of cationic (positively charged) proteins, as with multiple myeloma, can reduce the AG.

96. What is the conceptual difference between an anion-gap and a non–anion-gap metabolic acidosis?
An AG acidosis is caused by the addition of a nonvolatile acid to the ECF. Examples include diabetic ketoacidosis, lactic acidosis, and uremic acidosis. A non–anion-gap acidosis commonly (but not exclusively) represents a loss of HCO_3^-. Examples include lower GI losses from diarrhea and urinary losses due to renal tubular acidosis. Therefore, when approaching a patient with an anion-gap acidosis, one should look for the source and identity of the acid gained. By contrast, when evaluating a patient with a non–anion-gap acidosis, one should begin by looking for the source of the HCO_3^- loss.

97. What are the causes of anion-gap metabolic acidosis?
The mnemonic **KUSMAL** can be used to remember the differential diagnosis of AG metabolic acidosis.
K = **K**etones (diabetic, alcohol, starvation)
U = **U**remia
S = **S**alicylates
M = **M**ethyl alcohol
A = **A**cid poisoning (ethylene glycol, paraldehyde)
L = **L**actate (circulatory/respiratory failure, sepsis, liver disease, tumors, toxins)
Morganroth ML: An analytical approach in the diagnosis of acid-base disorders. J Crit Illness 5:138–150, 1990.

98. What is the significance of plasma osmolal gap? How does it help in the evaluation of a patient with metabolic acidosis?
The plasma osmolal gap is the difference between the measured and calculated plasma osmolality. Plasma osmolal gap of 0.25 mOsm/kg suggests, in a patient with AG metabolic acidosis, the possibility of ingestion of methanol or ethylene glycol. Isopropyl alcohol and ethanol increase the osmolal gap but not the anion gap, since acetone is not an anion.

99. What are the common causes of a non–anion-gap metabolic acidosis?

Associated with K^+ loss	**Drugs**
Diarrhea	Acetazolamide
Renal tubular acidosis (proximal or distal)	Amphotericin B

Associated with K^+ loss
Interstitial nephritis
Early renal failure
Urinary tract obstruction
Post-hypocapnia
Infusions of HCl (HCl, arginine HCl, lysine HCl)

Drugs
Amiloride
Spironolactone
Toluene ingestion

Urethral diversions
Ureterosigmoidostomy
Dual bladder
Ileal ureter

Toto RD: Metabolic acid-base disorders. In Kokko JP, Tannen RL (eds): Fluids and Electrolytes, 3rd ed. Philadelphia, W.B. Saunders, 1996.

100. How does the serum protein level affect the interpretation of AG?

The AG is significantly influenced by serum albumin level. If the concentration of serum albumin falls to 2 gm/dL (which is approximately half the normal), the expected normal AG should be reduced to half.

The paraproteins that accumulate in multiple myeloma are usually positively charged since they are rich in lysine and arginine. If there is a significant accumulation of these positively charged particles, the measured cations remain in the normal range. But, since these "unmeasured" cations are associated with Cl^- (which is measured), the calculated AG will be reduced proportionately and may even become negative.

101. Why is ammoniagenesis reduced in renal failure?

Renal ammoniagenesis is an important mechanism for removal of acid and H^+ from the body. Ammonia then combines with H^+ to form ammonium, which is then excreted in the urine. In renal failure, with reduction in the renal mass, there is a decrease in the ATP stores. Consequently, less ATP can be used to oxidize glutamine to ammonia. This is an important mechanism for defective acidification in chronic renal failure.

102. How is the urine anion gap useful in the evaluation of metabolic acidosis?

Measuring urine electrolytes and calculating the urine anion gap are useful diagnostically in the evaluation of some cases of hyperchloremic metabolic acidosis.

$$\text{Urine anion gap} = \text{Unmeasured cations} - \text{unmeasured anions} = (Na^+ + K^+) - Cl^-$$

In normal subjects excreting 20–40 mEq of NH_4^+/L, the urine anion gap is positive or near zero. On the other hand, in metabolic acidosis, the NH_4^+ excretion increases if the renal acidification mechanisms are intact. Consequently, urinary Cl^- excretion also increases to maintain electroneutrality. Urinary Cl^- therefore exceeds cation ($K^+ + Na^+$) excretion, and the urine anion gap is negative (often –20 to > –50 mEq/L. On the other hand, in acidosis where the renal acidification mechanisms are impaired (as in renal failure and renal tubular acidosis), the urine anion gap remains positive, as in normal subjects.

Battle DC, et al: The use of the urine anion gap in the diagnosis of hyperchloremic metabolic acidosis. N Engl J Med 318:594, 1988.

103. In which two clinical situations should the urine anion gap not be used?

- In **ketoacidosis**, the excretion of ketoacids neutralize the increased excretion of NH_4^+ cations, decreasing the negativity of anion gap.
- In **hypovolemia**, the avid proximal Na^+ reabsorption causes decreased distal Na^+ delivery resulting in a defect in acidification. The Cl^- reabsorption that accompanies Na^+ prevents NH_4Cl excretion, and the urine anion gap remains positive.

104. What causes a decreased anion gap?

Certain disorders are associated with an AG that is lower than normal. The lower AG may be due to an increase in **unmeasured cations** like (K^+, Ca^{++}, or Mg^{++}), the addition of **abnormal** cations

KEY POINTS: RENAL TUBULAR ACIDOSIS 

1. Type IV is the most common type of RTA in clinical practice.
2. It is often secondary to diabetic or nondiabetic renal disease (e.g., obstructive uropathy, aldosterone deficiency).
3. Drugs (e.g., triamterene and trimethoprim) are another common cause of RTA.

(lithium), or an increase in **cationic immunoglobulins** (plasma cell dyscrasias). AG also can be decreased by loss of unmeasured anions such as albumin (serum hypoalbuminemia) or if the effective negative charge on albumin is decreased by acidosis.

105. What is renal tubular acidosis (RTA)?

RTA refers to a disorder of tubular function in which the kidney has a compromised ability to excrete acid and/or recover filtered HCO_3^- in the setting of higher than normal $[H^+]$ in the ECF. The laboratory presentation is that of a non–anion-gap metabolic acidosis. There are four types of RTA.

106. Describe type I RTA.

Type I RTA (distal or classic RTA) is characterized by reduced net proton secretion by the distal nephron in the setting of systemic acidemia. Since the distal nephron is largely responsible for net acid excretion, patients with this disorder have continuous net acid retention (less net acid excretion than net acid production) and are therefore not in net acid balance. The diagnosis is made by demonstrating an inappropriately alkaline urine ($pH > 5.5$) in the setting of an acidemic serum ($pH < 7.36$) and by excluding the presence of drugs that alkalinize the urine (acetazolamide) or urea-splitting bacteria in the urine that can increase the urinary pH.

107. Describe type II RTA.

Type II RTA (proximal RTA) is characterized by a reduced capacity for HCO_3^- recovery by the proximal tubule but intact distal nephron function. These patients waste HCO_3^- in the urine until the ECF concentration of HCO_3^- is reduced to a level such that the reduced filtered load of HCO_3^- (GFR x plasma HCO_3^-) can now be more completely resorbed and the urine becomes nearly bicarbonate free. The reduction in plasma HCO_3^- concentration results in an increase in $[H^+]$. However, in the steady-state condition of low plasma HCO_3^-, these patients can excrete an appropriately acid urine ($pH < 5.5$) because distal nephron function is intact, and they are thus in acid balance (amount of acid excreted equals amount of acid produced), unlike the situation described for type I.

108. What is type III RTA?

Type III RTA represents a variant of type I, and the term is rarely used.

109. Describe type IV RTA.

Type IV RTA is characterized by reduced aldosterone effect on the renal tubules, which may result in insufficient secretion of acid necessary to maintain normal acid-base status. These patients nevertheless can excrete an appropriately acidic urine in the face of acidemic stress. Unlike the other types of RTA, type IV RTA is commonly associated with hyperkalemia due to a coexisting reduction in K^+ secretion. This disorder is commonly seen in patients with hyporenin-hypoaldosteronism but also is seen in isolated aldosterone deficiency and resistance.

110. How is type I (distal) RTA managed?
Alkali is given in amounts necessary (usually 1–2 mEq/kg/day) to correct the acidosis and to buffer the acid being retained. K^+ supplements are commonly required at the initiation of treatment but usually not in the steady-state treatment once the acidosis has been corrected.

111. How is type II (proximal) RTA managed?
Alkali is not usually required in adults because they do not have net acid retention and have only mild acidemia. But because the chronic acidemia inhibits bone growth in children, they must be treated with large amounts of alkali (10–20 mEq/kg/day) as well as large K^+ supplements (the increased urinary HCO_3^- losses are accompanied by accelerated urinary K^+ losses).

112. How is type IV RTA managed?
The clinically mild degrees of acidemia rarely require alkali treatment. Hyperkalemia is more commonly a clinical concern and dictates whether mineralocorticoid replacements with synthetic steroids are required.

113. What is lactic acidosis?
Lactic acidosis is due to the accumulation of lactic acid, the end product of glycolysis. This accumulation leads to a depletion of the body's buffers and a drop in pH. Lactate, being an unmeasured anion, is one of the causes of an increased anion-gap acidosis.

114. List the causes of lactic acidosis.
- Cellular hypoxia
- Decreased hepatic utilization of lactic acid (seen in advanced hepatocellular insufficiency of any cause)
- Cyanide poisoning
- Alcohol consumption
- Neoplasms with a large tumor burden
- Diabetic ketoacidosis (even in the absence of shock or other etiologies)
- Lactic acidosis X (severe lactic acidosis without obvious cause)
- Factitious lactic acidosis

115. How does cellular hypoxia cause lactic acidosis?
Oxygen is required for the oxidative phosphorylation of the lactic acid produced by glycolysis. Anything interfering with the available cellular supply of O_2 or its utilization will lead to the accumulation of lactic acid. This category includes respiratory failure, circulatory failure, and CO poisoning. This also can be seen in thiamine deficiency and has been reported in patients on long-term total parenteral nutrition without supplementation with thiamine.

KEY POINTS: LACTIC ACIDOSIS

1. In patients with lactic acidosis, bicarbonate administration is useful only when the pH is below 7.15.
2. Alkali may cause paradoxical increase in lactate production in patients with milder acidois.
3. The most common causes of lactic acidosis are cellular hypoxia, decreased hepatic utilization of lactic acid, alcohol consumption, neoplasms with a large tumor burden, and diabetic ketoacidosis.
4. Lactic acidosis X refers to severe lactic acidosis without obvious cause.

116. How does cyanide poisoning cause lactic acidosis?

CN causes increased lactic acid production because it blocks oxidative phosphorylation, leading to increased glycolysis, decreased utilization of lactic acid, and therefore lactic acid accumulation.

117. Explain how alcohol consumption may lead to lactic acidosis.

Alcohol causes a modest increase in lactic acid production. In association with caloric depletion, the lactic acidosis can be severe.

118. How does large tumor burden lead to lactic acidosis?

Neoplasms can lead to increased production of lactic acid, even with sufficient O_2, since the tumor cells can have higher rates of glycolysis than normal cells.

119. What causes factitious lactic acidosis?

When blood is stored for prolonged periods of time, the red and white cells generate lactic acid in the tube as it is stored. It is most commonly seen in patients with high WBC counts.

120. What causes metabolic alkalosis?

Metabolic alkalosis results from addition of excess HCO_3^- or alkali or loss of acid. Note that a low Cl^- and a high HCO_3^- concentration can result from both metabolic alkalosis as well as from a metabolic response to a respiratory acidosis. However, the pH and $PaCO_2$ help to differentiate these two disorders.

121. What are the two categories of metabolic alkalosis?

Chloride-responsive (urine $Cl^- < 10$ mEq/L) and chloride-resistant (urine $Cl^- > 20$ mEq/L). Forms of alkalosis responsive to chloride salt administration are generally associated with ECF fluid volume depletion and low urinary Cl^- concentration in spot urine tests, whereas the Cl^- unresponsive alkaloses are associated with ECF volume expansion and urine $Cl^- > 20$ mEq/L.

122. What conditions are associated with chloride-responsive metabolic alkalosis?

- Gastric fluid loss
- Postdiuretic therapy
- Posthypercapnia
- Congenital chloride diarrhea

123. List the conditions associated with chloride-resistant metabolic alkalosis.

- Primary aldosteronism
- Primary reninism
- Hyperglucocorticoidism
- Hypercalcemia
- Potassium depletion
- Liddle's syndrome
- Bartter's syndrome
- Chloruretic diuretics

Toto RD: Metabolic acid-base disorders. In Kokko JP, Tannen RL (eds): Fluids and Electrolytes, 2nd ed. Philadelphia, W.B. Saunders, 1990, p 356.

124. Which is the most common acid-base disturbance seen in cirrhosis?

Primary respiratory alkalosis due to centrally mediated hyperventilation is the most common acid-base disturbance in patients with severe hepatic disease, especially with superimposed encephalopathy. The exact etiology is unclear but may be related to the hormonal imbalance associated with liver failure. Estrogens and progesterone have been implicated, a situation somewhat similar to that seen in pregnancy.

125. How do you diagnose a mixed acid-base disorder?

1. Define the primary disturbance and the compensatory process involved. The primary disturbance is identified by the direction of the changes in pH, HCO_3^-, and $PaCO_2$ levels.
2. Determine whether the pulmonary or renal compensation is appropriate (see question 91). Two facts must be kept in mind while making these interpretations. First, adequate compensation takes 12–24 h to occur, and second, "overcompensation" never occurs in primary acid-base disturbances.
3. Consider the patient's history and clinical presentation to formulate a differential diagnosis. In general, the underlying clinical condition gives clues to the possible mixed acid-base disturbance, which are then defined using the nomograms of expected compensation.

Narins R, Emmett M: Simple and mixed acid-base disorders: A practical approach. Medicine 59:161–187, 1980.

126. What findings suggest a combined metabolic and respiratory acidosis?

In combined metabolic and respiratory acidosis, even though the HCO_3^- and $PaCO_2$ may not be changed, pH is distinctly lower.

127. What findings suggest combined metabolic acidosis and metabolic alkalosis?

In combined metabolic acidosis and metabolic alkalosis, the pH and HCO_3^- can be lower, normal, or higher, but an elevated anion gap with a high or normal HCO_3^- suggests the diagnosis.

128. What findings suggest combined metabolic alkalosis and respiratory acidosis?

Combined metabolic alkalosis and respiratory acidosis (which can be seen in patients with ARDS or COPD who are vomiting) causes HCO_3^- levels of higher-than-predicted compensation for a given high $PaCO_2$.

129. A 34-year-old woman is admitted to the hospital because of nausea and vomiting for the last 2 days. She admits to having taken several aspirin pills to alleviate her joint pains before she noticed epigastric pain and vomiting. Her arterial blood gas analysis reveals the following: pH 7.64, Pco_2 32, and plasma bicarbonate 33 mEq/L. What kind of acid-base disorder is present in this patient?

The patient has an alkalotic state since the pH is higher than normal range. Since the patient presented with significant emesis, it is logical to think that the primary disturbance is metabolic alkalosis, which is supported by the fact that plasma bicarbonate is significantly elevated. The expected respiratory compensatory response is to increase Pco_2 by 6–7 mmHg for every 10 mEq/L increase in plasma bicarbonate. However, in this patient the Pco_2 is actually lower than normal, indicating a primary respiratory alkalosis. Thus, this patient has a mixed acid-base disorder. The combined metabolic and respiratory alkalosis explains why the pH is so disproportionately high.

130. In what situations are potentially fatal mixed acid-base disorders encountered?

In general, combined respiratory and metabolic acidosis or metabolic and respiratory alkalosis can result in pH changes that are fatal. Common examples include:

- An alcoholic with ketoacidosis (metabolic acidosis) may have superimposed vomiting from gastritis (metabolic alkalosis) and hyperventilation associated with withdrawal (respiratory alkalosis).
- A combination of metabolic acidosis and respiratory alkalosis is seen typically in patients with sepsis, salicylate intoxication, and severe liver disease.
- Metabolic acidosis can coexist with metabolic alkalosis in patients with renal failure or with alcoholic or diabetic ketoacidosis (acidosis) who are vomiting or having gastric suction (alkalosis).

- Vomiting in a pregnant woman or a patient with liver failure causes a mixture of respiratory and metabolic alkalosis.

CALCIUM, PHOSPHATE, AND MAGNESIUM METABOLISM

131. **How is calcium distributed in the body and in the serum?**
A 70-kg man has approximately 1000 gm of calcium in his body. Of this amount, bone contains 99%, whereas the ECF and ICF contain only 1%. Furthermore, only about 1% of skeletal calcium is freely exchangeable with ECF calcium. The routine measurement for serum calcium (normal = 9–10 mg/mL = 4.5–5.0 mEq/L = 2.25–2.5 mM/L) measures total calcium. Approximately 40% is protein-bound, 5–10% is complexed to other substances (e.g., phosphate, sulfate), and 50% is ionized.

132. **Explain the significance of the ionized fraction of calcium.**
The ionized fraction determines the activity of calcium in cellular and membrane function. It is possible to vary the concentration of total calcium without changing the ionized fraction by changing the protein concentration. It is also possible to vary the ionized fraction without changing the total calcium by changing serum pH. Increasing serum pH decreases the ionized fraction of calcium and vice versa.

133. **What are the major sites of calcium resorption in the nephron?**
About 50% of the filtered calcium is reabsorbed in the proximal tubule, and most of the remainder (about 40% of the total) is reabsorbed in the loop of Henle, primarily the ascending limb of the loop of Henle. A small amount of calcium is reabsorbed in the distal convoluted tubule and an even smaller amount in the collecting tubule.

134. **What are the major hormones involved in calcium metabolism?**
Parathyroid hormone (PTH), vitamin D, and calcitonin.

KEY POINTS: ELECTROLYTE DISTURBANCES 

1. It is crucial to exclude magnesium deficiency in patients with resistant hypokalemia.
2. Hyperglycemia is the most common cause of nonhypotonic hyponatremia.
3. Although hypoalbuminemia results in reduction of total serum calcium, ionized calcium remains unchanged (physiologically more important fraction).

135. **Summarize the roles of these hormones in calcium metabolism.**
PTH is secreted in response to a decrease in serum calcium and promotes calcium resorption from bone because it enhances renal resorption of calcium and excretion of phosphate. Low serum calcium concentration stimulates 1-hydroxylation of 25-hydroxyvitamin D by the kidney to form 1,25-dihydroxyvitamin D (the active form of **vitamin D**). This hormone promotes calcium resorption from the gut and mineralization of bone. Increases in serum calcium lead to increased secretion of **calcitonin**. This hormone inhibits bone reabsorption and 1-hydroxylation of 25-hydroxyvitamin D and thereby ameliorates hypercalcemia.

136. What factors affect renal calcium excretion?

With some exceptions, renal calcium handling varies directly with renal Na^+ handling. Therefore, renal calcium excretion is increased by saline diuresis, loop diuretics, and volume expansion. In contrast, renal calcium excretion is decreased in volume depletion and other states associated with renal salt retention. One notable exception to this general rule is that the natriuresis associated with thiazide diuretics is accompanied by decreased, rather than increased, urinary calcium excretion.

137. Define pseudohypocalcemia and pseudohypercalcemia.

These terms refer to an alteration of the total calcium concentration in the setting of a normal ionized fraction. Since the ionized fraction is normal, such patients are asymptomatic. Abnormalities in the concentration of serum proteins are a common cause of these disorders. Hypoalbuminemia causes a decrease in the total serum calcium level without a change in the level of ionized calcium. For each decrease of 1.0 g/dL in serum albumin, one should expect a drop in the total serum calcium of approximately 0.8 mg/dL.

138. List the common causes of true hypocalcemia.

- Hypoparathyroidism (usually following thyroid or parathyroid surgery)
- Vitamin D deficiency
- Magnesium depletion (usually at levels < 0.8 mEq/L)
- Liver disease (decreased synthesis of 25-hydroxyvitamin D)
- CRF (hyperphosphatemia and decreased synthesis of 1,25-dihydroxyvitamin D)
- Acute pancreatitis
- Tumor lysis syndrome
- Rhabdomyolysis

139. What are the signs and symptoms of hypocalcemia?

The symptoms depend on the magnitude of the decrease in serum calcium, the rate of the drop, and its duration. The symptoms of hypocalcemia are due to the resultant decrease in the excitation threshold of neural tissue, which causes an increase in excitability, repetitive responses to a single stimulus, reduced accommodation, or even continuous activity of neural tissue. Specific signs and symptoms include:

- Tetany and paresthesia
- Altered mental status (lethargy to coma)
- Seizures
- QT interval prolongation on the ECG
- Increased intracranial pressure
- Lenticular cataracts

140. What are Trousseau's and Chvostek's signs?

Both are indications of the latent tetany caused by hypocalcemia. Of the two signs, Trousseau's is more specific and reliable.

- **Trousseau's sign:** A sphygmomanometer is placed on the arm and inflated to greater than systolic blood pressure and left in place for at least 2 minutes. A positive response is carpal spasm of the ipsilateral arm. Relaxation takes 5–10 seconds after the pressure is released.
- **Chvostek's sign:** Tapping the facial nerve between the corner of the mouth and the zygomatic arch produces twitching of the ipsilateral facial muscle, especially the angle of the mouth. This sign may be seen in 10–25% of normal adult patients.

141. What causes hypercalcemia?

The common causes of hypercalcemia include primary hyperparathyroidism (approximately 50% of cases), malignancy, use of thiazide diuretics, vitamin D excess, hyper-and hypothyroidism, granulomatous disorders, immobilization, and milk-alkali syndrome.

142. What are the signs and symptoms of hypercalcemia?
Symptoms include weakness, constipation, nausea, anorexia, polyuria, polydipsia, and pruritus. Severe hypercalcemia may present with progressive CNS symptoms of lethargy, depression, obtundation, coma, and seizures. Rapid onset is more likely to be symptomatic than a slowly progressive level, regardless of the ultimate level at presentation.

143. Describe the appropriate treatment for hypercalcemia.
Treatment depends on the calcium level and symptoms of the patient. Acute, symptomatic hypercalcemia should be treated aggressively, first with saline infusion to expedite calcium excretion. Most patients with hypercalcemia are significantly volume-depleted as a result of the osmotic diuresis related to the hypercalciuria.

144. How is normal saline infused?
Normal saline should be given at a rapid rate, 300 mL/h or more, with KCl and possibly magnesium added to the solution depending on measured blood values. After the patient is volume-repleted, furosemide may be given to promote calciuresis. Care must be taken to keep input equal to or greater than output to avoid making the patient hypovolemic again.

145. Explain the role of mithramycin in the treatment of hypercalcemia.
Mithramycin is effective when the patient cannot tolerate large fluid loads due to congestive heart failure or third-space losses or if there is an inadequate response to IV volume replacement. It should be given at a dose of 15 mg/kg (i.e., 1–2 mg) IVSS for one dose. The dose can be repeated if necessary, but doses more frequent than every 3–7 days have been associated with renal and hepatic toxicity. Mithramycin also can cause a coagulopathy, which can lead to serious bleeding complications.

146. How is calcitonin used in the treatment of hypercalcemia?
Calcitonin is useful for decreasing serum calcium and has the added advantage of rapid onset of action. It may be given in the presence of renal insufficiency, thrombocytopenia, or when mithramycin is contraindicated. Its disadvantage is that rapid resistance often develops, probably related to the development of antibodies. This resistance can sometimes be delayed by concomitant administration of prednisone.

147. Describe the role of bisphosphonates in the treatment of hypercalcemia.
Bisphosphonates inhibit osteoclast activity and are effective with those cancers in which this mechanism is present. They are given via IV infusion over 5 days or as oral tablets.

148. What other agents are useful for treatment of less significant levels of hypercalcemia?
Less significant levels of hypercalcemia can be treated with other agents, such as glucocorticoids (prednisone, 20–40 mg/day), phosphates (1–6 g/day), prostaglandin inhibitors (aspirin and NSAIDs), or oral bisphosphonates. All of these agents are less effective but may suffice for chronic maintenance.

Bilizekian JP: Management of acute hypercalcemia. N Engl J Med 326:1196–1203, 1992.

149. What factors regulate phosphate metabolism in the body?
Serum phosphate is lowered by insulin, glucose (by stimulating insulin secretion), and alkalosis, which cause transcellular translocation of phosphate from plasma. Phosphate is resorbed predominantly in the proximal tubule, with small amounts being absorbed in the distal tubule. Renal phosphate excretion is increased by PTH, alkalosis, saline diuresis, ketoacidosis, and increased dietary phosphate intake

150. In which clinical situations can hypophosphatemia develop?

- Decreased intake of phosphorus
- Shifts of phosphorus from serum into cells
- Increased excretion of phosphorus into urine
- Spurious hypophosphatemia (mannitol infusion)

151. What factors may lead to decreased intake of phosphorus?

- Decreased dietary intake
- Alcoholism
- Decreased intestinal absorption due to vitamin D deficiency, malabsorption, steatorrhea, secretory diarrhea, vomiting, or phosphate binders

152. What factors may cause shifts of phosphorus from serum into cells?

- Respiratory alkalosis (e.g., sepsis, heat stroke, hepatic coma, salicylate poisoning, gout)
- Recovery from hypothermia
- Hormonal effects (e.g., insulin, glucagon, androgens)
- Recovery from diabetic ketoacidosis
- Carbohydrate administration (hyperalimentation, fructose or glucose infusions)

153. List the factors that may lead to incresed excretion of phosphorus in urine.

- Hyperparathyroidism
- Renal tubule defects (as in aldosteronism, SIADH, mineralocorticoid administration, diuretics, corticosteroids)
- Hypomagnesemia

154. What electrolyte disturbances are commonly seen in progressive renal disease?

Patients with progressive renal disease develop hyperphosphatemia, hypocalcemia, and secondary hyperparathyroidism. They are also at risk of developing at least two kinds of bone disease.

155. What are the main disturbances thought to be responsible for the abnormalities of calcium and phosphate metabolism in progressive renal disease?

1. A rise in inorganic phosphate concentration in the serum due to poor renal excretion. This rise leads to a decrease in serum calcium concentration and stimulation of PTH secretion. The increased PTH secretion leads to increased bone resorption and osteitis fibrosa cystica.
2. Resistance to the action of vitamin D. One function of this hormone is to promote calcium resorption from the gut. Decreased gut resorption of calcium exacerbates the hypocalcemia and reduces available calcium for bone mineralization.
3. Defective synthesis of 1,25-dihydroxyvitamin D (the active form of this hormone). Reduced levels of 1,25-dihydroxyvitamin D result in defective bone mineralization (osteomalacia in adults, rickets in children).

156. How does magnesium depletion affect calcium and phosphate metabolism?

Magnesium depletion results in decreased secretion and end-organ responsiveness of PTH. This leads to functional hypoparathyroidism and the resultant effects on the serum level and urinary excretion of calcium and phosphate. This disorder can be corrected with magnesium repletion.

157. What are some common causes of magnesium deficiency?

Causes include dietary insufficiency (decreased intake, protein-calorie malnutrition, prolonged IV feeding), intestinal malabsorption, chronic loss of GI fluids, loop diuretics (Mg^{++} is reabsorbed predominantly in the thick ascending limb of the loop of Henle), other drugs (gentamicin, cisplatin, pentamidine, cyclosporine), alcoholism, hyper-parathyroidism, and lactation.

158. What is the milk-alkali syndrome?

The presence of hypercalcemia, increased BUN and creatinine, increased serum phosphate, and metabolic alkalosis in a patient ingesting large quantities of milk and calcium carbonate-containing antacids. The patient usually presents with nausea, vomiting, anorexia, weakness, polydipsia, and polyuria. If it continues, metastatic calcification can occur, leading to mental status changes, nephrocalcinosis, band keratopathy, pruritus, and myalgias. The treatment is withdrawal of the milk and antacid.

159. What electrolyte abnormalities are seen in HIV infection?

Apart from the main proteinuric syndrome caused by focal sclerosis (so-called HIV nephropathy), a variety of electrolyte disorders are commonly seen in patients with HIV. Asymptomatic **hyperkalemia** is a common manifestation. The hyperkalemia may be due to many possible causes, including hyporenin-hypoaldosteronism, adrenal insufficiency, drugs such as pentamidine and trimethoprim-sulfamethoxazole, and even isolated hypoaldosteronism. **Hyponatremia** is frequently caused by hypovolemia, adrenal insufficiency, and SIADH due to associated pulmonary or cerebral diseases. Other electrolyte abnormalities include hypocalcemia, hypomagnesemia, and hypouricemia. Hypercalcemia is seen in association with lymphomas and cytomegalovirus infection.

Klotman PE: AIDS and the kidney. Semin Nephrol 18:4, 1998.

160. List the electrolyte disturbances associated with alcoholism.

- Hypokalemia
- Hypophosphatemia
- Hypomagnesemia
- Hyponatremia

161. How common is hypokalemia in alcoholics? Explain.

Hypokalemia is seen in one-half of hospitalized, withdrawing alcoholics. This does not necessarily mean a total body K^+ deficit. Respiratory alkalosis, inadequate dietary intake, and GI losses (vomiting, diarrhea) are the common etiologic factors for hypokalemia. Withdrawal as well as severe liver failure causes respiratory alkalosis.

162. How common is hypophosphatemia in alcoholics? Explain.

Hypophosphatemia (< 2.5 mg/dL) is a common finding in hospitalized severe alcoholics, noted in more than half (50%) of patients in some series. The common predisposing factors are respiratory alkalosis, decreased dietary intake, transcellular shifts due to glucose administration, and, rarely, associated proximal tubular injury leading to phosphate wasting.

163. Explain the relationship between chronic alcoholism and hypomagnesemia.

Chronic alcoholism is the most common cause of hypomagnesemia in the U.S. It is seen in alcoholics who are withdrawing and more commonly in those who had withdrawal seizures. GI losses, cellular uptake, dietary deficiencies, and possibly lipolysis leading to fatty acid-magnesium precipitation are the possible causes.

164. How may beer contribute to hyponatremia?

Hyponatremia sometimes is seen in beer-drinkers who ingest large quantities of beer, which is virtually solute-free. When this free-water volume exceeds the excretory capacity of the kidney, hyponatremia results.

BIBLIOGRAPHY

1. Brenner RM (ed): Brenner & Rector's The Kidney, 7th ed. Philadelphia, W.B. Saunders, 2004.
2. Goldman L, Ausiello D (eds): Cecil Textbook of Medicine, 22nd ed. Philadelphia, W.B. Saunders, 2004.
3. Rose BD, Post T (eds): Clinical Physiology of Acid-Base and Electrolyte Disorders, 5th ed. New York, McGraw-Hill, 2001.
4. Schrier RW (ed): Renal and Electrolyte Disorders, 6th ed. Philadelphia, Lippincott Williams & Wilkins, 2003.

CHAPTER 9

HEMATOLOGY

Mark M. Udden, M.D., and Martha P. Mims, M.D., Ph.D.

Blood is the originating cause of all men's diseases.
The Talmud, *Baba Nathra, III.58a*

The blood is the life.
The Bible, *Deuteronomy 12:23*

HYPOPROLIFERATIVE ANEMIAS

1. What are the two most helpful laboratory tests in the initial evaluation of anemia?

Reticulocyte count and peripheral blood film. The peripheral blood film demonstrates important abnormalities of red blood cell (RBC) shape, size, or hemoglobinization. In addition, an impression of the white blood cell (WBC) count and platelet count can be obtained. RBCs also must be examined for the presence of inclusions (such as Howell-Jolly bodies).

2. What are reticulocytes? Why count them?

Reticulocytes are young RBCs newly released from the marrow. They can be detected by their lacy network of RNA. If the reticulocyte count is high, blood loss or hemolysis is likely to be the cause of anemia. Other possible causes include response to treatment of iron, folate, or vitamin B_{12} deficiency. If the reticulocyte count is low, a primary marrow disorder (hypoproliferative anemia) should be considered.

Cavill I: The rejected reticulocyte. Br J Haematol 84:563–565, 1992.

3. What methods are used to determine reticulocyte count?

The old method of determining the reticulocyte count relied on a manual count of 1000 cells stained with new methylene blue. Currently the reticulocyte count usually is determined by flow cytometric analysis of thiazole orange-stained cells or other automated analysis, which leads to greater reproducibility and allows discrimination between mature and immature reticulocytes. The release of immature reticulocytes is often a sign of early marrow recovery after bone marrow transplantation or response to treatment in deficiency states.

4. How are mean cell volume (MCV) and red cell distribution width (RDW) used in the evaluation of anemias?

The complete blood count (CBC) now includes the MCV, and many clinical laboratories also determine an index of the heterogeneity of cell size (RDW). In iron-deficiency anemia, for example, RBCs have been produced during periods of iron sufficiency and varying degrees of deficiency. Thus, cell size in iron-deficiency anemia is more heterogeneous than in thalassemia minor, in which all of the cells are small. This difference results in a larger RDW for iron-deficiency anemia and a normal RDW for thalassemia (Table 9-1).

5. What is the significance of the mean cellular hemoglobin content?

Current automated devices for determining the CBC can also determine the mean cellular hemoglobin content of reticulocytes. A decrease in reticulocyte cellular hemoglobin content is an

TABLE 9-1. CLASSIFICATION OF ANEMIAS BASED ON MCV AND RDW

MCV Low		MCV Normal		MCV High	
RDW Normal	*RDW High*	*RDW Normal*	*RDW High*	*RDW Normal*	*RDW High*
Chronic disease Nonanemic heterozygous thalassemia Children	Iron deficiency HbS-α or β thalassemia	Normal Chronic disease Nonanemic or enzyme abnormality Splenectomy CLL (except extreme high lymphocyte number) Acute blood loss	Early or mixed nutritional deficiency Anemic abnormal hemoglobin Myelofibrosis Sideroblastic anemia Myelodysplasia	Aplastic anemia	Folate or vitamin B_{12} deficiency Sickle cell anemia (one third of cases) Immune hemolytic anemia Cold agglutinins Preleukemia Newborn

Note: Chronic liver disease, chronic myelogenous leukemia, and cytotoxic chemotherapy may be associated with high or normal MCV and high or normal RDW. CLL = chronic lymphocytic leukemia.
From Bessman JD: Automated Blood Counts and Differentials: A Practical Guide. Baltimore, Johns Hopkins University Press, 1986, p 11, with permission.

early indicator of iron deficient erythropoiesis that can occur during treatment with erythropoietin and indicates a need for iron supplementation.

6. **Summarize the symptoms and signs of iron deficiency.**
Patients may have the symptoms of **anemia**: fatigue, dyspnea on exertion, and, in certain cases in which underlying cardiac disease exists, signs of congestive heart failure or angina. In many cases, however, the anemia develops insidiously and is well tolerated. Iron deficiency is associated with **pica**. Adults may crave ice, starch, or even dirt. Iron-deficient children in older neighborhoods may eat lead-containing paint chips, leading to the association of iron deficiency and plumbism. Iron deficiency is also associated with **esophageal webs** (sometimes causing dysphagia), painless stomatitis, and spooning of the fingernails (**koilonychia**). There also may be a connection between iron deficiency and restless leg syndrome.
Moore DF Jr, Sears DA: Pica, iron deficiency, and the medical history. Am J Med 97:390–393, 1994.

7. **In the treatment of iron-deficiency anemia, how much iron should be administered, in what form, and for how long?**
Iron is best given as ferrous sulfate in a formulation that does not include enteric coating. Typically, patients take 325 mg orally 3 times/day until the anemia corrects and for several months thereafter. This regimen provides 60 mg of elemental iron per tablet, or 180 mg/day. Of this, 18–36 mg can be absorbed and utilized by an otherwise unimpaired marrow. Intravenous iron therapy (as

ferrous gluconate or iron dextran) has been used in patients undergoing renal dialysis to optimize the response to erythropoietin therapy. Certain patients with ongoing blood loss (e.g., inflammatory bowel disease or Osler-Weber-Rendu syndrome) who cannot tolerate iron orally or who cannot absorb enough iron from the gut also benefit from iron dextran replacement.

8. Summarize the role of the serum ferritin value.

When a low serum ferritin value is used to make the diagnosis of iron deficiency, the ferritin can be checked to verify that iron stores have increased with therapy. In some instances, patients improve, but the anemia does not fully correct. If the ferritin has normalized, another cause of anemia (i.e., coexistent thalassemia minor) should be sought. A useful guide to success is the occurrence of reticulocytosis about 10 days after initiation of iron therapy.

Weiss, MJ: New insights into erythropoietin and epoetin alfa: Mechanisms of action, target tissues, and clinical applications. Oncologist 8 Suppl 3:18–29, 2003.

9. What are the common causes of iron deficiency?

- Dietary deficiency (particularly in infants)
- Malabsorption (sprue, postgastrecotmy patients)
- Chronic blood loss
- Chronic intravascular hemolysis
- Idiopathic pulmonary hemosiderosis
- Repetitive phlebotomy

10. List the most common causes of chronic blood loss.

- Gastritis
- Peptic ulcer disease/*Helicobacter pylori*
- GI varices
- GI malignancy
- GI polyps
- Diverticulosis
- Telangiectasia (Osler-Weber-Rendu disease, scleroderma)
- Angiodysplasia
- Long-distance running
- Menstrual loss and pregnancy

11. What is chronic intravascular hemolysis?

Chronic intravascular hemolysis is a disorder usually seen in paroxysmal nocturnal hemoglobinuria, a rare stem cell disorder, or in patients with malfunctioning cardiac valves. Examination of urine sediment stained for iron discloses iron-laden tubular cells (hemosiderosis).

12. What causes iron overload?

Iron overload results from chronic administration of iron to non–iron-deficient persons, chronic transfusion therapy, and disorders associated with increased absorption of dietary iron (hemochromatosis, thalassemia intermedia or major, and certain refractory anemias, such as sideroblastic anemia).

13. Summarize the consequences of iron overload.

Iron overload has many effects, including:

- Cardiomyopathy, arrhythmias
- Hepatic dysfunction and cirrhosis
- Hepatoma
- Endocrine dysfunction (hypothyroidism, hypogonadotrophic hypogonadism, hyperpigmentation, diabetes mellitus)

- Arthropathy (chondrocalcinosis, synovial fluid containing calcium pyrophosphate or hydroxyapatite crystals)
- Osteopenia and subcortical cysts

14. What test is frequently used to screen for hemochromatosis?
The serum transferrin saturation (serum iron divided by the total iron-binding capacity) is frequently used to screen for hemochromatosis. Because of the diurnal variation in serum iron, a fasting morning sample is best. A serum transferrin saturation > 50% for women and > 60% for men suggests the possibility of iron overload.

15. Summarize the genetic link to hemochromatosis.
Mutations in the HFE gene may account for most cases in white patients, who appear to have genetic hemochromatosis. Homozygosity for C282Y or the combination of C282Y and another mutation H63D in the HFE can be detected by the polymerase chain reaction (PCR) assay. Use of this genetic method in population studies shows that not all patients who appear to have the hemochromatosis genotype develop clinical iron overloading. Similarly, some white patients and most black patients with clinical iron overloading have a normal HFE genotype.

16. What other tests are used to screen for hemochromatosis?
Measurement of serum ferritin and assessment of hepatic iron (usually on liver biopsy) and/or a PCR study of HFE should be considered next in the evaluation of suspected hemochromatosis. Elevated serum ferritin levels, however, can occur in a number of inflammatory conditions without iron overload.

Beutler E, Hoffbrand AV, Cook JD: Iron deficiency and overload. Hematology (Am Soc Hematol Educ Program) 2003, pp 40–61.

17. How is hemochromatosis treated?
Treatment of hemochromatosis is simple: patients are recommended for phlebotomy with assessment of serum ferritin to determine success of therapy.

18. When is it appropriate to order hemoglobin electrophoresis to evaluate hypochromic microcytic anemia?
When iron stores are established as normal. The microcytic disorders that may be detected are beta-thalassemia minor and the so-called thalassemic hemoglobinopathies (including hemoglobin [Hb] E in Asians). Beta thalassemia minor is marked by an increased Hb A_2 and sometimes increased fetal Hb. Iron deficiency results in a decreased pool of alpha chains, for which the beta chain of Hb A and the delta chain of Hb A_2 must compete. Beta chains are more successful, resulting in diminished Hb A_2 during iron deficiency. For this reason, a search for beta-thalassemia may be thwarted when patients are also iron deficient.

Beutler E: The common anemias. JAMA 259:2433–2437, 1988.

19. Which diseases are usually associated with the anemia of chronic disease (ACD)?
ACD is typified by a low serum iron, low total iron-binding capacity, and low percent saturation but increased iron stores, as evidenced by an increased ferritin. Traditionally, ACD is associated with inflammatory states, including malignancy, rheumatologic disease, and infection. However, a study of hospitalized patients showed that the laboratory pattern of ACD occurs in a significant number of anemic patients who do not have inflammatory conditions. These patients were severely ill with complications of diabetes, renal failure, and hypertension.

Cash JM, Sears DA: The anemia of chronic disease: Spectrum of associated disease in a series of unselected hospitalized patients. Am J Med 87:638, 1989.

20. What causes macrocytosis?

Macrocytosis, or a large MCV, is not always associated with folate or vitamin B_{12} deficiency. Anemia with macro-ovalocytic RBCs (megaloblastic) is much more specific for folate or vitamin B_{12} deficiency. Causes of macrocytosis are listed in Table 9-2.

TABLE 9-2. CAUSES OF MACROCYTOSIS

Megaloblastic anemia (macro-ovalocytosis)	Sideroblastic anemia*
Alcoholism	Chronic obstructive pulmonary disease
Malignancy	Artifacts and idiopathic
Hemolysis (usually poorly compensated)	Pregnancy
Aplastic anemia	Liver disease
Hypothyroidism	Drugs (AZT, azathioprine, anticonvulsants)
Refractory anemias (myelodysplasia)	

*Often marked by dual populations of RBCs—one hypochromic microcytic and the other macrocytic.
From Colon-Otero G, et al: A practical approach to the differential diagnosis and evaluation of the adult patient with macrocytic anemia. Med Clin North Am 76:581–596, 1992; and Savage DG, et al: Etiology and diagnostic evaluation of macrocytosis. Am J Med Sci 319:343–352, 2000.

21. How are folate and vitamin B_{12} deficiency states recognized?

Common features of B_{12} and folate deficiency are those of megaloblastic anemia:

- **Marrow:** hyperplastic marrow demonstrating a markedly ineffective erythropoiesis; megaloblastic RBCs with open, granular nuclei, and mature cytoplasm or nuclear-cytoplasmic asynchrony; giant metamyelocytes.
- **Peripheral blood:** macro-ovalocytosis with occasional Howell-Jolly bodies and basophilic stippling; hypersegmented neutrophils; variable degree of neutropenia and thrombocytopenia.
- **Megaloblastic changes:** affect rapidly proliferative cells of mouth, gut, small intestine, and cervix, showing immature-looking nuclei (indeed, some cervical Pap smears are mistakenly read as atypical or malignant).
- **Homocystine levels:** elevated in both deficiency states.

22. What lab tests help distinguish folate and vitamin B_{12} deficiencies?

- Serum folate levels are normal in B_{12} deficiency but low in folate deficiency.
- RBC folate levels may be normal or low in B_{12} deficiency but are always low in folate deficiency.
- Folate deficiency responds to the physiologic dose of folate (200 mcg/day); B_{12} deficiency does not. Pharmacologic dose of folate (1 mg/day) can correct anemia but may exacerbate neurologic symptoms.
- Urine formiminoglutamic acid is increased in folate deficiency but absent in B_{12} deficiency.
- Serum methylmalonic acid is normal in folate in deficiency but increased in B_{12} deficiency.

23. How do diet and neurologic disease differ in vitamin B_{12} and folate deficiencies?

Diet may be normal in vitamin B_{12} deficiency, but patients with folate deficiency may be alcoholics or have a diet consisting mainly of junk food and "tea and toast," with no green vegetables.

Neurologic disease in vitamin B_{12} deficiency is subacute and involves combined systems; in folate deficiency it is absent or associated with alcohol.

Babior BM: The megaloblastic anemias. In Williams WJ, et al (eds): Hematology, 5th ed. New York, McGraw-Hill, 1995.

24. What processes may interrupt B_{12} absorption?

- Pernicious anemia associated with gastric atrophy and loss of intrinsic factor due to an autoimmune-mediated attack on the gastric mucosa.
- Gastrectomy: megaloblastic anemia develops 5–6 years after total gastrectomy.
- Disorders of the small intestine: ileal resection, Crohn's disease, sprue.
- Competition with intestinal flora: blind-loop syndrome, fish tapeworm *(Diphyllobothrium latum).*
- Pancreatic disease: deficiency of R-binders with chronic pancreatitis.
- Dietary: strict vegetarians (no meat, eggs, or milk), breastfed infants of strict vegetarians.

Carmel R, Green R, Rosenblatt DS, Watkins D: Update on Cobalamin, Folate, and Homocysteine. Hematology (Am Soc Hematol Educ Program). 2003, pp 62–81.

25. Describe the pattern of neurologic disease associated with B_{12} deficiency.

B_{12} deficiency is associated with the findings of combined-system disease:

- Posterior column: paresthesia, disturbed vibratory sense, loss of proprioception
- Pyramidal: spastic weakness, hyperactive reflexes
- Cerebral: dementia, psychosis (megaloblastic madness), optic atrophy

26. Is the severity of anemia a good predictor of neurologic involvement?

Of interest is the lack of correlation between severity of anemia and neurologic manifestations of B_{12} deficiency. A recent study suggests that a significant minority of patients with peripheral neuropathy or other neurologic manifestations of B_{12} deficiency have a normal hematocrit and MCV, but low or low-normal B_{12} levels. It is possible that serum methylmalonic acidemia and homocystinemia are better indicators.

Lindebaum J, et al: Neuropsychiatric disorders caused by cobalamin deficiency in the absence of anemia or macrocytosis. N Engl J Med 318:1720, 1988.

27. How much folate is required in pregnant women? Why?

Developmental anomalies of the fetal neural tube have been associated with poor folate intake early in pregnancy. For this reason, it has been recommended that women of child-bearing age consume 400 mcg/day of folate. This recommendation is controversial because folate supplementation may mask symptoms of vitamin B_{12} deficiency. However, cereals are now fortified with folate, and folate deficiency as a cause of anemia is less common.

Cziezel AE, Dudas I: Prevention of the first occurrence of neural-tube defects by periconceptional vitamin supplementation. N Engl J Med 327:1832–1835, 1992.

28. When are bone marrow biopsy and aspiration indicated?

Bone marrow biopsy and aspiration are safe and easily performed for the following indications:

- Pancytopenia: myelodysplasia, aplastic anemia, myelophthisic states, hypersplenism, megaloblastic anemia
- Anemia: sideroblastic anemia, refractory anemia, pure red cell aplasia
- Staging of malignancy: Hodgkin's disease, leukemias, non-Hodgkin's lymphoma, small cell carcinoma of the lung, multiple myeloma
- Thrombocytopenia: evaluation of idiopathic thrombocytopenic purpura
- Neutropenia
- Infectious diseases: typhoid, tuberculosis, pancytopenia seen in AIDS, brucellosis
- Lipid-storage diseases (such as Gaucher's disease)

29. **Why is bone marrow biopsy not always required for the diagnosis of hypoproliferative anemia?**
Because of the high prevalence of iron-deficiency anemia and anemia of chronic disease, a hypoproliferative (low reticulocyte count) anemia does not always require bone marrow biopsy if iron studies are consistent.

30. **Why is bone marrow biopsy essential to the diagnosis of sideroblastic anemia?**
The diagnosis of a sideroblastic anemia requires a bone marrow study to demonstrate the presence of ringed sideroblasts.

KEY POINTS: HYPOPROLIFERATIVE ANEMIA

1. The approach to anemia requires a good history and physical exam, careful examination of the peripheral blood smear, and reticulocyte count.
2. In microcytic anemias, the first step is to evaluate patients for iron deficiency via tests for serum iron, total iron-binding capacity, and ferritin levels.
3. Thalassemia is best evaluated after iron deficiency is ruled out or corrected.
4. In macrocytic anemias, vitamin B_{12} and folate deficiencies should be considered.
5. In a patient with normochromic normocytic anemia, anemia of chronic disease (which may also be microcytic) is the major consideration.
6. Renal insufficiency also should be considered, particularly in patients with long-standing diabetes mellitus.

31. **What are the diagnostic criteria for severe aplastic anemia?**
Aplastic anemia is marked by peripheral pancytopenia and a hypocellular bone marrow aspirate. Commonly used criteria for severe aplastic anemia are as follows:
- Marrow biopsy cellularity < 25%
- Neutrophil counts < 0.5×10^9/L
- Platelet counts < 20×10^9/L
- Corrected reticulocyte count < 1%

32. **Summarize survival rates for patients with severe aplastic anemia.**
Patients meeting the diagnostic criteria in question 31 have a median survival of < 6 months; only 20% survive 1 year.

33. **What is the best therapy for aplastic anemia in a young person?**
For patients who are under age 40, bone marrow transplantation (BMT) from a histocompatibility leukocyte antigen (HLA)–identical sibling is the current standard of care. HLA-identical but nonrelated donors may be used for such patients.

34. **How does BMT affect survival rates?**
For nontransfused patients, 80% long-term survival rates have been achieved with BMT, although survival may be accompanied by disabling graft-versus-host disease (GvHD) in 10–20%.

35. What other treatments are available for aplastic anemia? How effective are they?

Patients who do not have donors or who are otherwise unsuitable candidates for BMT have been successfully treated with immunosuppressive regimens. The most effective has been antithymocyte globulin, usually in combination with cyclosporine. This regimen produces remission rates of 40–60%. Severe serum sickness and thrombocytopenia are consequences. Patients frequently have partial responses, freeing them from infections or the need for transfusions. Unfortunately, relapses occur in 10%, and some patients, although clinically improved at first, develop myelodysplastic syndromes later.

Young NS: Acquired aplastic anemia. Ann Intern Med 136:534–546, 2002.

36. What is the principal indication for erythropoietin (EPO) therapy in the treatment of anemia?

EPO deficiency regularly accompanies end-stage renal disease, and the resultant anemia is the principal indication for use of EPO.

37. Summarize the other indications for EPO therapy in patients with anemia.

Recent studies suggest a role for EPO in patients with AIDS-related anemia, particularly when they receive zidovudine in high doses. The anemia of chronic disease is associated with inappropriately low EPO levels in some people with rheumatoid arthritis. Chemotherapy-related anemia and cancer-related anemia improve with EPO therapy. EPO has also been used with success to improve the ability of patients to undergo autologous blood donation before surgery. It also has been beneficial in the treatment of anemia of prematurity and myelodysplasia.

38. What is the novel quality of darbepoietin alfa?

Darbepoietin alfa, a recently developed EPO, has a long half-life, allowing weekly or every-other-week dosing regimens.

Smith R: Applications of darbepoietin-alpha, a novel erythropoiesis-stimulating protein, in oncology. Curr Opin Hematol 9:228–233, 2002.

HEMOLYTIC ANEMIAS

39. Patients with hemolytic anemia have shortened RBC survival. What are the laboratory features of hemolysis?

During hemolysis, the bone marrow responds to the premature destruction of RBCs by increasing its production of RBCs seven- to eight-fold. This expansion is marked by reticulocytosis. Other clues to accelerated RBC destruction are:

- Indirect hyperbilirubinemia-acholuric jaundice (unconjugated bilirubin is not secreted in urine)
- Hemoglobinuria
- Fall of hemoglobin > 1 gm/7 days in the absence of bleeding or massive hematoma

40. How is intravascular hemolysis distinguished from extravascular hemolysis?

See Table 9-3.

41. Give examples of intravascular hemolytic disorders.

Examples of intravascular hemolytic disorders include hemolytic transfusion reactions, paroxysmal nocturnal hemoglobinuria, march hemoglobinuria, and RBC fragmentation syndromes.

TABLE 9-3. LABORATORY STUDIES IN HEMOLYSIS

Intravascular	Extravascular and Intravascular
Hemoglobinemia	Increased reticulocyte count
Hemoglobinuria	Increased indirect, unconjugated bilirubin
Hemosiderinuria	Increased urobilinogen
Low serum haptoglobin	
Methemalbumin	
Low serum hemopexin	
Increased lactate dehydrogenase	

From Udden MM: Hemolytic anemias: Intravascular. In Goldman L, Bennett JC (eds): Cecil Textbook of Medicine. Philadelphia, W.B. Saunders, 2000, pp 882–884.

KEY POINTS: HEMOLYSIS

1. Review of the peripheral blood film for abnormal red cell morphology is required.
2. Uncomplicated patients have an elevated reticulocyte count.
3. If renal failure or inflammation is present, the reticulocyte count may be low; a drop in hemoglobin of 1 g/wk is an indication of hemolysis.
4. Blood loss or the presence of a large hematoma may be confused with hemolysis.
5. Ineffective erythropoiesis may have laboratory features resembling hemolysis, such as increased unconjugated bilirubin and LDH.

42. Name the three basic types of RBC defects that lead to hemolysis in the hereditary hemolytic anemias. Give examples of each.

Membrane disorders	Hemoglobin abnormalities	Enzymatic defects
Spherocytosis	Sickle cell anemia	G6PD deficiency
Elliptocytosis	Unstable hemoglobins	Pyruvate kinase
Stomatocytosis	Thalassemia	5′-Nucleotidase
Xerocytosis		

43. What is extraordinary about the normal RBC?

The RBC is extraordinarily adapted to a circulatory system that requires resistance to shear stresses in the arterioles and suppleness to negotiate small orifices in the spleen and capillaries.

44. Name the major acquired hemolytic disorders.

Whereas hereditary disorders are examples of intracorpuscular defects, acquired hemolytic disorders typically result from extracorpuscular defects. Examples include autoimmune hemolytic anemia, fragmentation syndromes, malaria, hypersplenism, and physical agents such as heat, copper, and certain oxidants.

45. List the complications of hereditary spherocytosis (HS).

- Aplastic crises (associated with parvovirus B19)
- Hemolytic crises

- Megaloblastic crises (increased demand for folate)
- Pigment gallstones
- Splenomegaly
- Stasis ulcers

46. Describe the underlying protein deficiency associated with HS.

HS is marked by decreased amounts of spectrin, the principal membrane protein found in erythrocytes. Spectrin has self-associative properties and forms a lattice with other RBC membrane proteins and actin. This supportive lattice on the inner aspect of the lipid bilayer gives the RBC its unique properties of strength and suppleness. Deficiency of spectrin correlates with the degree of hemolysis, changes in osmotic fragility, and response to splenectomy.

47. Describe the molecular mechanisms underlying HS.

The molecular mechanisms underlying HS include structural changes in spectrin itself, loss of ankyrin (a protein that links spectrin to the transmembrane protein band 3), and structural abnormalities of band 3. Most of these defects occur in what investigators call the "vertical interaction" in the RBC membrane cytoskeleton between band 3, ankyrin, and spectrin. Two mutations are associated with additional morphologic changes. A spectrin beta-chain mutation is associated with acanthocytic spherocytes that are accentuated by splenectomy.

A truncated band-3 protein is associated with so-called pincered RBCs. A deficiency of spectrin, for whatever reason, accounts for the decreased membrane surface area and spherocytosis.

Delaunay J: Molecular basis of red cell membrane disorders. Acta Haematol 108:210–218, 2002.

48. What is hereditary elliptocytosis (HE)?

HE includes a broad spectrum of disorders that result in an elliptical RBC shape and hemolysis. In general, HE results from genetic defects that arise in the horizontal interaction of the RBC membrane cytoskeleton that depends on alpha spectrin–beta spectrin association and interaction of spectrin with band 4.1 protein to form a high-molecular-weight oligomeric structure. Most patients with HE and its variants have a structural abnormality of the spectrin protein that results in failure of the protein to self-associate into higher-order tetramers and oligomers.

49. List the most important subsets of HE.

- **Mild common HE** (normal hematocrit and mild reticulocytosis).
- **Common HE with chronic hemolysis** (more striking degree of hemolysis, anemia, and more bizarre RBC morphology).
- **Infantile poikilocytosis** (present at birth; later associated with striking hemolysis, bizarre RBCs, and jaundice).
- **Homozygous HE** (rare subset accompanied by severe anemia).
- **Hereditary pyropoikilocytosis** (rare subset in which the spectrin is abnormally sensitive to heat. The peripheral blood picture resembles that seen in hemolysis associated with severe burns.)
- **Spherocytic elliptocytosis** (unusual autosomal dominant disorder in which the elliptocytes are rounded. Spherocytes and increased osmotic fragility are also found.)
- **Southeast Asian ovalocytosis**

50. Explain the unusual feature of Southeast Asian ovalocytosis.

This subset of HE is accompanied by resistance to malarial infection. The central pallor in RBCs is separated by a transverse ridge. The disorder is associated with an abnormal band-3 protein that leads to membrane rigidity but only mild hemolysis.

51. What is the most common enzymatic defect in RBCs leading to hemolysis? How is it diagnosed?
Glucose-6-phosphate dehydrogenase (G6PD) deficiency. Hundreds of variants of this X-linked enzyme have been characterized.

52. Summarize the consequences of G6PD deficiency.
Because G6PD is the first enzyme in the hexose monophosphate pathway, its deficiency compromises the RBC's ability to regenerate NADPH from NADP+. NADPH is necessary for the reduction of glutathione-containing disulfides (GSSG to GSH). The RBC as a carrier of oxygen is highly vulnerable to oxidative attack when GSH is depleted. Oxidation results in precipitation of hemoglobin, which can be detected as Heinz bodies by supravital staining with crystal violet.

53. How is G6PD deficiency diagnosed?
The diagnosis is established by measuring the enzymatic activity of G6PD.

54. Many abnormal hemoglobins with single amino acid changes are known. Of these, which sickle or participate in the sickling process during deoxygenation?
Sickle hemoglobin coexists with other beta-chain variants to produce a spectrum of disorders from clinically insignificant conditions such as sickle cell trait (AS and S-herediatry persistence of fetal hemoglobin) to severe disease represented by homozygous sickle syndrome (SS). Other forms of sickle cell disease include S-beta-thalassemia, SC, SD Punjab, SO Arab, S Lepore Boston, and S Antilles.

55. What is the incidence of sickle hemoglobinopathies in births among African-Americans?

AS	8.0% (1 of 12)	AC	3.00%	SBo	0.03%
SS	0.16%	SC	0.12%		

Note that the incidence of SBo and SC is approximately that of SS. In adults, as many patients with sickle beta-thalassemia or SC will be seen as homozygous S patients. Although SBo is clinically similar to SS disease, SB+ and SC patients are more likely to have palpable spleens and may experience splenic sequestration/infarctive crises as adults rather than in early childhood, as is the case with SS disease. SC patients also tend to have higher hematocrits. They may present with blindness due to retinopathy or aseptic necrosis of the hip.

56. Where else is the hemoglobin S gene found?
The hemoglobin S gene also can be found in Sicily, Northern Greece, Turkey, the eastern province of Saudi Arabia, and central India.

Serjeant GR: Sickle Cell Disease, 3rd ed. New York, Oxford University Press, 2001.

57. Is any morbidity truly associated with sickle trait?
Because 8% of African Americans are heterozygous for sickle trait, this is an important question. The following abnormalities have been associated with sickle trait:

Splenic infarction at high altitude	Pulmonary embolism
Hyposthenuria	Glaucoma, anterior chamber bleeds
Hematuria	Sudden death following exertion
Bacteriuria and pyelonephritis in pregnancy	Bacteremia in women

Sears DA: Sickle cell trait. In Embury SH, et al (eds): Sickle Cell Disease: Basic Principles and Clinical Practice. New York, Raven Press, 1994.

58. What are sickle crises?
Patients with sickle cell disease are susceptible to sudden, unheralded vaso-occlusive events that are called crises. The most common event is a simple pain crisis affecting the limbs, low

back, chest, or abdomen. Sometimes specific organs are affected by definite infarcts, including the bone and spleen (if splenic tissue has been preserved).

59. **Describe chest syndrome.**
The chest syndrome is marked by episodes of dyspnea, fever, pain, and sudden appearance of an infiltrate on chest x-ray consistent with pneumonia. As often as not, no infection exists; instead, there is probably a sickle vaso-occlusion. Recent studies of chest syndrome have emphasized the role of fat embolism from bone marrow infarcts and rib infarcts. Splinting while the patient is suffering a rib infarct may lead to hypoventilation and pulmonary vaso-occlusion. Incentive spirometry has been advocated to reduce the risk of chest syndrome in patients hospitalized with sickle crises and chest pain.

60. **Is acute chest syndrome associated with hospitalization for other disorders?**
Yes. In a recent multicenter study, acute chest syndrome often occurred as a complication in patients admitted for other reasons. Thirteen percent of patients who developed chest syndrome required mechanical ventilation, and 3% died. Half of the deaths involved infections. Thus, antibiotics, along with transfusion therapy, have an important place in management.

Vichinsky EP, et al: Causes and outcomes of the acute chest syndrome in sickle cell disease. N Engl J Med 342:1855–1865, 2000.

61. **How are patients in a sickle crisis managed? How often do crises occur?**
Patients with chest syndrome often receive antibiotics and require oxygen. When hypoxemia continues despite oxygen therapy, exchange transfusions are helpful. The pathophysiology of the pain crisis is not well understood.

62. **How often do crises occur?**
Of note, most patients experience pain relatively infrequently—once every year or two. About 20% of patients, however, are troubled by more frequent crises and may visit the emergency department or hospital monthly. Why some homozygotes do poorly while others do relatively well is one of the mysteries of sickle cell disease. Similarly, it is not known what initiates crises or what mechanisms of spontaneous recovery terminate crises while patients are receiving only supportive care. The severity and duration of crises are variable. Stays for patients requiring hospitalization vary from 3 to 10 days.

Platt OS, et al: Pain in sickle cell disease: Rates and risk factors. N Engl J Med 325:11–16, 1991.

63. **What routine health maintenance measures are used in children with sickle cell anemia?**
Now that many states routinely screen all births for hemoglobin S, practice guidelines for follow-up of parents and identified infants have been developed. Parents are taught to bring in their child when he or she is febrile and to examine the child for splenic enlargement. Penicillin prophylaxis is emphasized. Children should receive the polyvalent pneumococcal vaccine at age 2 years, *Haemophilus influenzae* type B and meningococcal vaccine, and hepatitis B immunization.

64. **Summarize routine health maintenance for adults with sickle cell anemia.**
For adults, routine health maintenance includes genetic counseling about the risk of sickle cell disease in relatives or children. Patients are given folate supplementation and periodic ophthalmoscopic exams. All adults should receive pneumococcal vaccine if they have not already been vaccinated. As patients get older, periodic review of renal function seems prudent.

65. **Is RBC transfusion recommended for the treatment of typical pain crises?**
No.

66. Under what circumstances should RBC transfusion be considered in the treatment of sickle cell disease?

Strong indications	Relative indications
Aplastic crises	Before general anesthesia
Hypoxemia and chest syndrome	During pregnancy
Heart failure	Baseline anemia
CNS events, stroke	Simple surgery
Sequestration crises	Priapism
	Before arteriography

67. What protocol is recommended for RBC transfuion in sickle cell disease?
A national cooperative study found that simple transfusions to an arbitrary level of hemoglobin seemed to enable patients to undergo general anesthesia with no worse outcome than patients who had exchange transfusions. Because less blood was used, the conservative transfusion protocol was complicated less often by alloimmunization.

Claster S, Vichinsky EP: Managing sickle cell disease. BMJ 327:1151–1155, 2003.

68. A patient with sickle cell disease presents with a history of a viral syndrome, followed by dramatic worsening of the anemia. What entity needs to be strongly considered?
Aplastic crisis. Typically, patients have a flulike illness, with or without an evanescent rash, fever, and myalgias, followed 5–10 days later by weakness and dyspnea. The patient presents with a sharply reduced hematocrit. A key finding is the nearly absolute absence of reticulocytes. This disorder is in fact a transient pure red cell aplasia. The platelet and WBC counts are usually unaffected. Bone marrow shows the absence of erythroid progenitors, except for a few "giant pronormoblasts."

69. What is the most common cause of aplastic syndrome?
Parvovirus B19, which seems to have a unique tropism for erythroid progenitors.

KEY POINTS: SICKLE CELL DISEASE

1. Patients should have hemoglobin electrophoresis and or HPLC to determine which sickling disorder is present.
2. All patients with sickle hemoglobinopathies should receive pneumococcal vaccine. Vaccination for HIB and meningococcus is also recommended.
3. Treatment with hydroxyurea should be considered in adult patients with SS Hb who have more than three severe pain crises/year.
4. Transfusions in sickle cell patients carry risk and should be avoided unless the patient has a severe complication (chest syndrome, stroke, aplastic crises).
5. Chest syndrome is a frequent cause of death in hospitalized patients with sickle cell disease. Treatment with transfusions/exchange transfusion, antibiotics, and oxygen is essential.

70. Explain the physiologic and clinical significance of parvovirus-induced aplasia.
In patients with hemolysis, parvovirus-induced aplasia is significant because the duration of aplasia (5–10 days) coincides with the half-life of RBCs. Thus, cessation of RBC production for 10 days in a patient with a hematocrit of 22% and RBC lifespan of 9 days spells trouble.

Transfusions of packed RBCs are life-saving. The 10-day cessation of erythropoiesis caused by the parvovirus goes unnoticed in a normal person with a hematocrit of 40% and an RBC life-span of 120 days. The parvovirus may be the cause of fifth disease, arthritis, and spontaneous abortions.

Saarinen UM, et al: Human parvovirus B19-induced epidemic acute red cell aplasia in patients with hereditary hemolytic anemia. Blood 67:1411, 1986.

71. **Discuss the role of hydroxyurea in the treatment of patients with severe (> three crises/year) sickle cell anemia.**

Perhaps the greatest therapeutic advance in sickle hemoglobinopathy was the recognition that certain chemotherapeutic agents can reverse the developmental "switch" from fetal to adult hemoglobin (Hb) synthesis. The rise in Hb F in each RBC suppresses sickling and offers the promise of reduced hemolysis and vaso-occlusive phenomena. A double-blinded trial of hydroxyurea was halted early when it was shown to reduce the rate of crises by about 40% and also to reduce the incidence of chest syndrome and frequency of transfusions and, in a follow-up study, prolonged survival.

Charache S, et al: Effect of hydroxyurea on the frequency of painful crises in sickle cell anemia. N Engl J Med 332:317–322, 1995.

72. **Summarize the disadvantages of hydroxyurea therapy.**

Issues related to compliance with daily medications, frequent follow-up, need in contraception, and the potential for leukemogenesis, all of which have spurred the search for alternative agents that increase Hb F production.

73. **Discuss the role of bone marrow transplantation in the treatment of severe sickle cell anemia.**

BMT has been used in the treatment of severe sickle cell disease with good results. It is controversial because of the morbidity and mortality associated with allogeneic BMT and GVHD. The longevity enjoyed by most patients and the promise of regimens such as hydroxyurea cast doubt on the usefulness of BMT except for the sickest patients.

Steinberg MH: Management of sickle cell disease. N Engl J Med 340:1021–1030, 1999.

74. **What is thalassemia minor?**

Thalassemia minor is a frequent cause of microcytic hypochromic anemia. It is due to an imbalance of alpha- and beta-chain production.

75. **What causes thalassemia minor?**

The genetic information for the alpha-chain of hemoglobin is organized as two adjacent genes on chromosome 16. Thus, normal people have four copies of the gene for alpha hemoglobin. In alpha-thalassemias, deletions of one or more of these genes result in a deficiency of alpha-chains and an excess of beta-chains. Deletion of a single gene is silent, but deletion of two genes is noticed as a microcytic mild anemia, with a normal hemoglobin electrophoresis. People with only one functional alpha-gene have a mild hemolytic anemia (Hb H disease). Hemolysis results from oxidative attack by the $beta_4$ tetramers present in the RBCs of affected people.

76. **How common is thalassemia minor in African Americans?**

About 30% of African-Americans are heterozygous for a single-gene deletion; thus, alpha-thalassemia is found in about 2.0%.

77. **How common is thalassemia minor in Asians?**

Asians have a much higher incidence of a chromosome 16 with two deleted alpha-genes and therefore are at risk for bearing children with only one or no functional alpha-genes. A study of

Chinese patients with Hb H disease found that adult patients had significant disability due to iron overload despite the absence of a need for chronic transfusion therapy.

78. Define hydrops fetalis.
Hydrops fetalis in association with a tetramer of gamma-chains (hemoglobin Bart's) is the cause of death at birth of a fetus with four alpha-gene deletions.

79. What is beta-thalassemia major?
In beta-thalassemia major, the absence of beta-chains results in the presence of $alpha_4$, a tetrameric alpha-chain protein that is highly toxic to the RBC membrane. Developing RBCs perish in the marrow or limp out to live a short, withered existence in the circulation. Erythropoiesis is highly ineffective. Patients have tremendous expansion of the bone marrow and extramedullary hematopoiesis. Affected children are transfusion-dependent; if not transfused aggressively, they develop pathologic fractures and significant growth retardation.

Oliveri N: The beta-thalassemias. N Engl J Med 341:99–109, 1999.

80. Is there an effective treatment for children with beta-thalassemia major?
Aggressive transfusion therapy has greatly improved the outlook for these children. Iron overload is the price for this therapy. Chelation with deferoxamine by continuous subcutaneous infusion with a pump has been effective in reducing iron burden and prevents the onset of cardiomyopathy. However, the expense and inconvenience of chelation therapy are burdensome to patients when they reach young adulthood. Noncompliance with subcutaneus chelation has led to the pursuit of an effective oral agent.

81. Discuss the role of BMT in the treatment of beta-thalassemia.
Children with thalassemia major have been successfully treated with BMT. In the very young, GVHD is less frequent, and mortality and morbidity rates seem to be acceptable. After restoration of normal hematopoiesis, iron overload can be aggressively treated by phlebotomy.

Lucarelli G, et al: Marrow transplantation in patients with thalassemia responsive to iron chelation therapy. N Engl J Med 329:840, 1993.

82. A 20-year-old woman with a history of two previous laparotomies for abdominal pain presents with confusion, fever, tachycardia, abdominal pain, and peripheral neuropathy. Her mother had a similar history and died at a young age. What disorder do you suspect? How do you make a diagnosis?
The history is strongly suggestive of porphyria, acute intermittent type (AIP), which results from a deficiency of porphobilinogen deaminase. AIP is inherited in an autosomal dominant pattern. Physicians must be aware of two unfortunate facts about porphyria: (1) many people carry a diagnosis that is not based on adequate testing, and (2) many others with the disease are unrecognized. Hence, before embarking on specific therapy, laboratory studies must be obtained to confirm the diagnosis. Urine tests positive for delta-aminolevulinic acid, porphobilinogen, and uroporphyrin.

83. Summarize the symptoms and signs of AIP.
- Abdominal pain: fever, leukocytosis, vomiting, constipation
- Neurologic manifestations: peripheral neuropathy, paraplegia, Guillain-Barré syndrome, respiratory arrest, cranial nerve findings, psychosis, seizure, coma
- Other: hyponatremia, hypertension, tachycardia

84. How is AIP treated?
Treatment includes carbohydrate infusions, hematin, beta blockers, and observation for respiratory compromise while appropriate lab studies are obtained to confirm the diagnosis. The patient should avoid barbiturates, anticonvulsants, estrogens, oral contraceptives, and alcohol.

Tefferi A, et al: Acute porphyrias: Diagnosis and management. Mayo Clin Proc 69:991–995, 1994.

85. A young man presents with asymptomatic cyanosis. What are the most likely hematologic causes?
Congenital methemoglobinemia and methemoglobin reductase (cytochrome b_5 reductase) deficiency.

86. What causes congenital methemoglobinemia?
Congenital methemoglobinemia is due to abnormal hemoglobin (M-hemoglobinopathy). Congenital cyanosis is transmitted as an autosomal dominant disorder. The M-hemoglobins are among the 400 or more human hemoglobin variants that have been reported in various parts of the world and are generally known by place names of first discovery, such as M-Boston, Saskatoon, Milwaukee, and Kochikuro. M-hemoglobins have been identified only rarely in black people. These hemoglobins stabilize iron in its oxidized (Fe^{+3}) state and have a muddy brown appearance.

Jaffe E: Methemoglobinemia in the differential diagnosis of cyanosis. Hosp Pract 20(12):92–110, 1985.

87. Explain methemoglobin reductase deficiency.
Methemoglobin reductase (cytochrome b_5 reductase) deficiency is an autosomal recessive disorder. Cyanosis caused by hypoxemia requires at least 5 gm/dL of deoxyhemoglobin to be noticeable, whereas only 1.5 gm/dL of methemoglobin will be recognized.

Dinneen SF, Mohr DN, Fairbanks VF: Methemoglobinemia from topically applied anesthetic spray. Mayo Clin Proc 69:886–888, 1994.

88. What disorder is associated with chronic intravascular hemolysis, anemia, iron deficiency, and dark urine after waking from sleep?
Paroxysmal nocturnal hemoglobinuria (PNH), an acquired clonal or oligoclonal disorder that results in increased sensitivity to complement. Most patients have chronic hemolysis, hemoglobinuria, and hemosiderinuria without the paroxysmal nocturnal component. The sucrose hemolysis test is a useful screen. An old but favorite "pimp question" is to ask for the two disorders that result in a low leukocyte alkaline phosphatase score—chronic myelogenous leukemia and PNH.

89. Explain the relationship between PNH and aplastic anemia.
PNH also has a close relationship to aplastic anemia. Some patients with aplastic anemia have a typical PNH defect but produce few cells. PNH may arise after a hypoplastic event. The hemolytic disorder is complicated by unusual thrombi, including Budd-Chiari syndrome.

90. What is the cause of PNH on the molecular level?
The biochemical defect leading to increased complement lysis has been a hot topic for decades. New research has focused on abnormalities of the many proteins that are linked to the cellular membrane by a glycosylphosphatidylinositol anchor. These proteins usually are reduced or absent in PNH. Japanese investigators have identified abnormalities in an X-linked gene PIG-A (phosphatidylinositol glycan class A) that apparently are responsible for PNH in the patients studied to date.

Hillmen P, et al: Natural history of paroxysmal nocturnal hemoglobinuria. N Engl J Med 333:1253–1258, 1995.

91. Compare the laboratory and clinical features of warm and cold antibody-mediated immune hemolytic anemias.
See Table 9-4.

TABLE 9-4. COMPARISON OF WARM AND COLD ANTIBODY-MEDIATED IMMUNE HEMOLYTIC ANEMIAS

	Warm	Cold
Antibody	IgG	IgM
Complement	±	+
Spontaneous agglutination	-	+++
Active temperature	37°C	4°C
Antigen	Rh(pan)	I,i
Response to therapy with:		
Steroids	Good	Poor
Splenectomy	Good	Poor
Gloves, warmth	None	Good

92. **With which disorders are warm and cold antibody-mediated immune hemolytic anemias associated?**
Cold agglutinin disease may be a self-limited disorder brought on by mycoplasmal infection (usually anti-I) or infectious mononucleosis (usually anti-i). Chronic cold agglutination disease may be an idiopathic syndrome or associated with a lymphoproliferative disorder. In contrast, warm autoimmune hemolytic anemia is associated with lupus, chronic lymphocytic leukemia, Hodgkin's disease, non-Hodgkin's lymphomas, and certain drugs.

93. **Explain the direct Coombs' test used to evaluate autoimmune hemolytic anemia.**
The Coombs' test is used to detect antibodies on RBCs (direct Coombs' or direct antiglobulin test positive) or in plasma. In the direct test, the RBCs are washed and incubated with an antiglobulin serum (rabbit or other species) and then examined for agglutination.

94. **Explain the indirect test.**
In the indirect test, the serum is reacted with a panel of RBCs bearing antigens of interest. Antibodies, if present in the sera, bind to the RBCs bearing the relevant antigen. The panel cells are washed to reduce nonspecific binding, then incubated with an antiglobulin serum to detect agglutination. The antiglobulin reagent is necessary because antibodies attached to RBCs are usually IgG in low numbers and cannot ordinarily cross-link to agglutinate. The antiglobulin serum bridges these antibodies, favoring agglutination.

95. **How is the Coombs' test used to evaluate autoimmune hemolytic anemia?**
In autoimmune hemolytic anemia, the direct test is usually positive, indicating the presence of an autoantibody on the RBCs. The indirect test, indicating the presence of the same antibody in serum, also may be positive. Persons who have been exposed to blood or have had a miscarriage or abortion may develop antibodies to certain antigens on the transfused RBCs that do not exist on native RBCs. Later, they have a positive indirect Coombs' test and negative direct Coombs' test.

96. **What is fragmentation hemolysis?**
Fragmentation hemolysis (fragmented RBCs) on a periperhal smear from a patient with hemolytic anemia is characterized by the appearance of schistocytes, helmet cells, burr cells (echinocytes), and spherocytes. The hemolysis is intravascular and can be associated with a wide variety of conditions.

97. List the macroangiopathic causes of fragmentation hemolysis.

- Valve hemolysis
- Endocardial cushion defect repair
- Extracorporeal circulation

98. List the microangiopathic causes of fragmentation hemolysis.

Thrombocytopenia is often present with the following disorders:

- Cavernous hemangiomas
- Thrombotic thrombocytopenic purpura (TTP)
- Hemolytic uremic syndrome (HUS)
- Eclampsia/preeclampsia
- Malignant hypertension
- Scleoderma
- Disseminated carcinomatosis
- Disseminated intravascular coagulation (DIC)

99. How does HUS differ from TTP?

In HUS, renal failure is the predominant organ syndrome associated with thrombocytopenia and fragmentation hemolysis. Metalloprotease activity, absent in TTP, is present in HUS, indicating a different pathogenesis. HUS has been observed after infection with *Escherichia coli* O157:H7, a newly arising contaminant of undercooked meat. This *E. coli* serotype elaborates a shiga-like toxin that may participate in the genesis of HUS. In some families a deficiency in plasma factor H, a complement control factor, is associated with recurrent HUS.

LEUKOCYTES

100. What is the lower limit for the absolute neutrophil count?

For adults, the level below which neutropenia is a consideration is 1.8×10^9/L (1800/mm^3). African Americans have a lower mean neutrophil count, which may be encountered during routine exams. However, they do not have an increased incidence of infections, nor do they have increased severity of infectious diseases. When the neutrophil count is $< 0.5 \times 10^9$/L (500/mm^3), neutropenia is severe, and there is a greater propensity for compromised response to infection.

101. What three mechanisms may lead to neutropenia?

- Decreased production
- Peripheral destruction
- Peripheral pooling (transient neutropenia)

102. What disorders cause decreased production of neutrophils?

- Drug-induced disorders
- Hematologic diseases (idiopathic disease, cyclic neutropenia, Chediak-Higashi syndrome, aplastic anemia, infantile genetic disorders)
- Tumor invasion, myelofibrosis
- Nutritional deficiencies (vitamin B_{12}, folate, especially in alcoholics)
- Infections (tuberculosis, typhoid fever, brucellosis, tularemia, measles, dengue fever, mononucleosis, malaria, viral hepatitis, leishmaniasis, AIDS)

103. Which drugs commonly cause neutropenia?

The cytotoxic chemotherapeutic agents (including alkylating agents and antimetabolites) as well as immunosuppressive drugs are obvious choices, but other drugs such as phenothiazines, antithyroid drugs, or chloramphenicol may cause neutropenia in a dose-dependent fashion by inhibiting cell replication. Immune-related neutropenia may be seen with penicillins, cephalosporins, and other agents. The more common agents associated with idiosyncratic neutropenia are listed in Table 9-5.

Young NS: Agranulocytosis. JAMA 271: 935–938, 1994.

TABLE 9-5. DRUGS THAT COMMONLY CAUSE NEUTROPENIA

Analgesics/anti-inflammatory agents	**Antibiotics**	**Others**
Indomethacin	Chloramphenicol	Phenytoin
Para-aminophenol derivatives	Penicillins	Cimetidine
Acetaminophen	Sulfonamides	Captopril
Phenacetin	Cephalosporins	Chlorpropamide
Pyrazolone derivatives	**Phenothiazines**	
Aminopyrine	Clozapine	
Dipyrone	Antithyroid drugs	
Oxyphenbutazone		
Phenylbutazone		

104. Which disorders may lead to peripheral destruction of neutrophils?

- Antineutrophil antibodies and/or splenic or lung (alveolar macrophage) trapping
- Autoimmune disorders (Felty's syndrome, rheumatoid arthritis, systemic lupus erythematosus)
- Drugs as haptens (aminopyrine, α-methyl dopa, phenylbutazone, mercurial diuretics, some phenothiazines)
- Wegener's granulomatosis

105. Which disorders may cause peripheral pooling of neutrophils?

- Overwhelming bacterial infection (gram-negative septicemia)
- Hemodialysis
- Cardiopulmonary bypass

Stock W, Hoffman R: White blood cells. 1: Non-malignant disorders. Lancet 355:1351–1357, 2000.

106. What is the significance of finding myelocytes, metamyelocytes, and nucleated RBCs in the peripheral blood?

Leukoerythroblastosis, or the presence of immature WBCs and nucleated RBCs, often is associated with a malignancy (prostate, breast, or GI tumors, lymphoma, myelofibrosis, leukemia, preleukemia) that has metastasized to the bone marrow. Numerous other, less serious conditions also affect leukoerythroblastosis, sometimes transiently:

- Hemolysis, including sickle cell disease
- Thrombocytopenic purpura
- GI bleeding
- Renal transplants
- Septicemia
- Chronic lung disease
- Myocardial infarction
- Liver disease

107. Describe the features of lymphocytosis caused by infections.

When infections (usually viral) cause lymphocytosis, the lymphocyte morphology is unusual or atypical. Thus, infection with Epstein-Barr virus (EBV) or cytomegalovirus (CMV) can cause an infectious mononucleosis syndrome of fever, sore throat, lymphadenopathy, hepatosplenomegaly, and, in the case of EBV, an increased titer of the heterophile antibody. In EBV infection, B cells are penetrated by the virus, eliciting a polyclonal T-cell response manifested in the peripheral blood as atypical lymphocytosis. Cold agglutinin disease also may occur in EBV disease. The IgM antibodies are usually directed against the i antigen. An acute lymphocytosis may be associated with primary infection with HIV-1, adenovirus, rubella, or herpes simplex II. These disorders are usually self-limited.

108. Is lymphocytosis dangerous to the fetus in pregnant women?

CMV, toxoplasmosis, and, less commonly, EBV infection during the first trimester of pregnancy have been associated with serious developmental defects in the newborn.

MYELOPROLIFERATIVE DISORDERS

109. Polycythemia is frequently encountered by internists. Before you embark on a long and expensive work-up, what two steps are necessary?

There is no point in pursuing a work-up of polycythemia without demonstrating that (1) the RBC mass is increased and (2) hypoxemia is not present as a cause of secondary erythrocytosis. Many patients who take diuretics have an increased hematocrit, but typically they also have decreased plasma volume and normal RBC mass. Some patients who are not taking diuretics (usually smokers) have so-called stress erythrocytosis, with normal RBC mass and reduced plasma volume. Patients with chronic lung disease or congenital heart disease resulting in significant left-to-right shunts are also polycythemic.

Djulbegovic B, et al: A new algorithm for the diagnosis of polycythemia. Am Fam Physician 44:113–120, 1991.

110. List the major and minor criteria widely used to diagnose polycythemia vera (PCV).

The Polycythemia Study Group originally developed guidelines to establish a diagnosis of PCV; recently these guidelines have been amended to include modern laboratory tests :

Category A (major criteria)

1. Increased red blood cell mass (> 25% above normal mean for sex)
2. Absence of causes for secondary polycythemia (see below)
3. Palpable splenomegaly
4. Clonality marker

Category B (minor criteria)

1. Thrombocytosis: platelets > 400 × 10^9/L
2. Leukocytosis: WBC > 10 ▽ 10^9/L
3. Splenomegaly based on imaging studies
4. Growth of erythroid colonies in the absence of erythropoietin or low serum erythropoietin level

111. How are these criteria used to reach a diagnosis of PCV?

A diagnosis of PCV is supported by finding (1) A1 + A2 and either A3 or A4 or (2) A1 + A2 and any two B criteria (see question 110 for list of criteria).

112. What secondary causes of polycythemia must be considered?

Carboxyhemoglobin should be measured if the patient is a heavy smoker, and in certain families a high-affinity hemoglobin may be identified by determining the P_{50} (oxygen half-saturation pressure). Several kindreds have alterations in the gene for the erythropoietin receptor, resulting in familial erythrocytosis. Mutations in hypoxia inducing factor alpha have also been identified in a hereditary condition known as Chuvash polycythemia. A neoplasm-producing ectopic erythropoietin also may result in erythrocytosis.

113. **How are secondary causes of polycythemia differentiated from PCV?**
Typically, secondary causes are obvious, but CT scans or liver scans may be necessary to evaluate the possibility of an occult neoplasm of the kidney or liver. In PCV the erythropoietin level is usually low or normal, whereas in secondary conditions, erythropoietin levels are increased.
Pearson TC: Evaluation of diagnostic criteria in polycythemia vera. Semin Hematol 38:21–24, 2001.

114. **Once the diagnosis of PCV is established, how are patients treated?**
Treatment of PCV is important because untreated patients are uncomfortable and at risk for life-threatening thrombotic events. Initially, phlebotomy of 500 mL of blood every other day as tolerated is undertaken until the hematocrit is reduced to a normal range. Phlebotomy alone usually suffices for younger patients, but some conditions are not well-controlled and require myelosuppressive therapy with hydroxyurea.
Tefferi A, Solberg LA, Silverstein MN: A clinical update in polycythemia vera and essential thrombocythemia. Am J Med 109:141–149, 2000.

115. **What is the major complication of phlebotomy?**
As phlebotomy proceeds, patients develop iron deficiency, which reduces the rate at which phlebotomy is necessary for control of the disease.

116. **Do other drugs have a role in the treatment of PCV?**
An important study by the Polycythemia Vera Study Group compared treatment with phlebotomy, 32P, or chlorambucil. Phlebotomy alone was associated with an increased incidence of stroke and other thrombotic events, whereas treatment with chlorambucil or 32P was associated with a high incidence of transformation into acute leukemia. Therefore, patients who are over age 70 or those who have had previous thrombotic events may do better with hydroxyurea and occasional phlebotomy. A recent publication from Europe suggests that low-dose aspirin (100 mg/day) may prevent thrombotic complications in PCV patients with no contraindications.
Landolfi R. et al: Efficacy and safety of low-dose aspirin in polycythemia vera. N Engl J Med 351:114–124, 2004.

117. **What was the prognosis of chronic myelogenous leukemia (CML) with traditional treatment?**
Before the introduction of imatinib in 2001, symptoms of CML were controlled with agents such as hydroxyurea. Despite these measures, CML uniformly transformed into an acute leukemia. Median survival of CML patients was 39–47 months with a risk of transformation into blast phase of about 20% per year.

118. **How has imatinib changed the prognosis of CML?**
Imatinib, a tyrosine kinase inhibitor, induces complete hematologic remissions in more than 95% of patients with chronic phase CML and complete cytogenetic remissions in more than 70%. Comparison of survival of imatinib-treated patients with historical controls suggests that imatinib-treated patients who achieve cytogenetic remission live longer than those treated with alternatives. Nevertheless, induction of remissions in patients who present in blast crisis is short-lived, and imatinib resistance develops in the majority of patients treated in advanced phase. Imatinib is now considered to be the first-line treatment for chronic-phase CML by most hematologists, but more time is needed to see whether imatinib will prolong survival compared with older treatments.

Goldman JM, Melo JV: Chronic myelogenous leukemia: Advances in biology and new approaches to treatment. N Engl J Med 349:1451–1464, 2003.

119. Describe the clinical features of acceleration of CML into blast phase.
Certain clinical events herald the transformation of CML from chronic to blast phase, including an enlarging spleen (with splenic infarcts), increased basophilia and eosinophilia, fever, fibrosis in the marrow, and resistance to hydroxyurea. In many instances, an accelerated phase (marked by an increased percentage of blasts and promyelocytes) occurs before frank leukemia.

120. What laboratory features herald the transformation of CML into acute leukemia?
In about two thirds of cases of transformation into acute leukemia, a new cytogenetic abnormality appears in addition to the Philadelphia chromosome. These new cytogenetic abnormalities suggest that the Ph^1 clone evolves into a more malignant cell. Four typical chromosomal changes are seen in the setting of transformation: (1) a second Ph^1 chromosome, (2) trisomy 8, (3) isochromosome 17, and (4) trisomy 19. Of interest, the phenotype of a leukemic cell in the blast crisis of CML is variable. Although most patients have blasts with the characteristics of myeloid cells, about one third have cells that are lymphoid in character. Less often, the cells have features of erythroblastic leukemia or megakaryocytic leukemia.

121. Compare the roles of imatinib and BMT in the treatment of CML.
BMT is the only current therapy that offers a hope of cure for CML. Although the peritransplant mortality rate is significant, the long-term outlook is better for young patients who have CML and an HLA-identical sibling. Patients should undergo BMT during the chronic phase, because once patients reach blast crises, the outlook is poorer. At this point it is unclear whether imatinib or transplant offer superior long-term outcome. Most hematologists offer a trial of imatinib to newly diagnosed patients with CML and reserve transplantation for those who fail to achieve a complete or near complete cytogenetic remission in the first 6–9 months of therapy and are good transplant candidates.

122. Patients presenting with large spleens, fibrotic marrows, and teardrop-shaped erythrocytes on the peripheral blood film have what myeloproliferative disorder?
Myelofibrosis, or agnogenic myeloid metaplasia. This myeloproliferative disease is marked by splenomegaly, tear-drop RBCs, fibrotic marrow, and immature erythroid and myeloid cells in peripheral blood (leukoerythroblastic blood picture). Extramedullary hematopoiesis is usually present in the liver and spleen. Patients may have neutrophilia, thrombocytosis, and anemia, but other patients, typically with massively enlarged spleens, may be cytopenic instead. Patients with enlarged spleens and neutrophilia resemble patients with CML. Determination of the presence of Ph^1 chromosome may distinguish the two.

123. Describe the fibroblast proliferation associated with myelofibrosis.
The fibroblast proliferation that is typically present in the marrows of such patients is polyclonal and appears to be fostered by fibroblast growth factors released by abnormal megakaryocytes. Patients may be troubled by bone pain and often have radiographic evidence of osteosclerosis. Massive splenomegaly may lead to portal hypertension and varices.

Tefferi A: Myelofibrosis with myeloid metaplasia. N Engl J Med 342:1255–1265, 2000.

124. How is myelofibrosis treated?
Treatment is largely supportive and ineffective. As in other myeloproliferative diseases, transformation into acute leukemia has been observed in some patients.

125. Patients without massive splenomegaly may have platelet counts above 1,000,000/mL ("platelet millionaires"). What myeloproliferative disease do they have?

Patients may become platelet millionaires for various reasons. Occasionally patients with severe **iron deficiency** and concurrent hemorrhage or inflammatory disease have platelet counts > 1,000,000/mL. Once iron deficiency is corrected or the inflammatory disorder resolves, platelet counts return to normal levels.

Another myeloproliferative disorder, **essential thrombocythemia**, should be considered when the platelet count rises above 600,000/mL, although a count > 1,000,000/mL is the rule.

126. What are the signs and symptoms of essential thrombocythemia?

Patients also have evidence of clonal proliferation. Physical exam may show modest splenic enlargement and purpura. Patients often are troubled by hemorrhage due to poorly functioning platelets. Purpura, epistaxis, and gingival bleeding are typical manifestations and may be exacerbated by aspirin. Erythromelalgia, characterized by a localized burning pain and warmth of the distal extremities, is commonly seen. Dramatic relief is obtained with small doses of aspirin. Also seen are neurologic manifestations such as dizziness, seizures, and transient ischemic attacks.

Schafer AI: Thrombocytosis. N Engl J Med 350:1211–1219, 2004.

127. List the causes of thrombocytosis.

Reactive disease	Myeloproliferative disorders
Malignancy	Essential thrombocythemia
Iron deficiency	PCV
Splenectomy	CML (Ph^1+)
Inflammatory bowel disease	Myelofibrosis
Infection	Myelodysplastic syndromes
Collagen-vascular diseases	

128. How are the potential causes of thrombocytosis differentiated?

Iron studies, collagen vascular screen, and cytogenetic studies of the bone marrow aspirate are helpful in differentiating these disorders. PCV may present as essential thrombocythemia and iron deficiency with chronic GI blood loss. When the iron deficiency is corrected, the erythrocytosis of PCV becomes evident.

Buss DH, et al: Occurrence, etiology, and clinical significance of extreme thrombocytosis: A study of 280 cases. Am J Med 96:247–253, 1994.

129. What is the most likely complication in a patient with a myeloproliferative disease who presents with a swollen, hot ankle?

Patients with myeloproliferative syndromes (PCV, CML, myelofibrosis, essential thrombocythemia) may develop hyperuricemia and gout. Thus, arthritis in such patients should be investigated thoroughly, including arthrocentesis and examination for intracellular, negatively birefringent crystals under polarized light.

ACUTE MYELOGENOUS LEUKEMIA

130. Which cytogenetic abnormalities have been described in acute myelogenous leukemia (AML)?

At least 90% of patients with AML have cytogenetic abnormalities. Some of these, when detected, indicate a relatively good prognosis, and others bode ill. Specific morphologic variants of AML have been linked to characteristic cytogenetic abnormalities, as shown in the Table 9-6.

TABLE 9-6. CYTOGENETIC ABNORMALITIES IN MORPHOLOGIC VARIANTS OF AML

Cytogenetic Abnormality	Leukemia Type	Prognosis
Trisomy 8	M2	Average
t(8;21)	M2 with splenomegaly, chloromas, Auer rods	Good
t(15;17)	M3, many promyelocytes, DIC	Good
inv 16	M4 with abnormal eosinophils	Good
t(9;11)	M5, monocytic leukemia	Average
t(6;9)	M2 with increased basophils	Average
(4;11)	Biphenotypic leukemia lymphoid and monocytic phenotype	Poor
5q-, 7-, 5-, 7-	Therapy-related leukemia	Poor

Löwenberg B, Downing JR, Burnett A: Acute myeloid leukemia. N Engl J Med 341:1051–1062, 1999.

131. **How is AML diagnosed?**
The diagnosis of AML M1–M5 requires a cellular bone marrow aspirate with blasts representing > 20% of all nucleated WBCs. If erythroblasts comprise > 50% of the nucleated bone marrow cells, erythroleukemia (M6) is present. If the marrow is cellular but blasts account for < 20% of the nucleated RBCs, myelodysplasia is present. Peroxidase stain is important in the definition of AML; in practice, the blasts are peroxidase (or Sudan black)-positive in AML and peroxidase-negative in acute lymphoblastic leukemia (ALL).

132. **How is AML classified? How do the subtypes differ in natural history and complications?**
See Table 9-7.

133. **How does the presentation and treatment of acute promyelocytic leukemia (APL) differ from other AML subtypes?**
Patients with APL present with lower WBC counts and may have a normal count when first examined. Careful attention to the morphology of the circulating WBCs discloses the presence of the hypergranular blasts or blasts with multiple Auer rods. Less frequently the blasts are hypogranular. A significant hemorrhagic diathesis may complicate either the presentation or the treatment of APL with standard AML chemotherapy. A picture resembling DIC is characteristic and may be accompanied by CNS bleeding, which is sometimes fatal. Patients may require intensive support with platelets, fresh frozen plasma, and cryoprecipitate. In the past, heparin has been used to abrogate the consumptive coagulopathy.

134. **Why are patients more susceptible to infections during induction chemotherapy?**
Patients receiving induction chemotherapy usually endure a period of absolute granulocytopenia (leukocyte nadir) at a time when there have been breakdowns of important barriers to infection. These breakdowns include mucositis throughout the GI tract and the presence of chronic indwelling venous catheters.

TABLE 9-7. FRENCH-AMERICAN-BRITISH (FAB) CLASSIFICATION OF AML		
Type	**Description**	**Criteria**
M1	Myeloblastic leukemia without maturation	> 3% of blasts are peroxidase-positive. A few granules, Auer rods, or both; one or more distinct nucleoli; no further maturation
M2	Myeloblastic leukemia with maturation	> 50% of marrow cells are myeloblasts and promyelocytes. Myelocytes, metamyelocytes, and mature granulocytes are seen; eosinophilia may predominate in some cases
M3	Hypergranular promyelocytic leukemia	Majority of cells are abnormal promyelocytes, reniform (kidney-shaped) nuclei, bundles of Auer rods; also some have closely packed bright pink or purple granules
M4	Myelomonocytic leukemia	> 20% of bone marrow, peripheral blood nucleated cells, or both are promonocytes and monocytes; an eosinophilic variant is also recognized
M5	Monocytic leukemia (M5a = poorly differentiated) (M5b = differentiated)	Granulocyte component, 10% of marrow cells, monocytoid cells have a fluoride-sensitive esterase reaction cytochemically
M6	Erythroleukemia	> 50% of cells are erythroblasts; myeloblasts represent > 30% of nonerythroid nucleated cells
M7	Megakaryoblastic	> 30% of marrow cells are blasts; platelets peroxidase-positive on electron microscopy, or blasts react with antiplatelet monoclonal antibodies; marrow fibrosis is prominent; cytoplasmic budding is also a feature

From Bennett JM, et al: Proposal for the classification of the acute leukemias. Br J Hematol 33:451, 1976.

135. Which organisms most frequently cause infection during induction chemotherapy-induced bone marrow aplasia?

Bacteria

Pseudomonas aeruginosa
E. coli
Staphylococcus aureus
Klebsiella aerobacter
Proteus vulgaris
Bacteroides spp.
Alpha-hemolytic streptococci
Staphylococcus epidermidis

Fungi

Candida spp.
Aspergillus spp.
Phycomycetes spp.

136. How are chemotherapy-induced infections treated?

Antibiotic therapy usually is designed to cover the bacterial pathogens listed in the previous question. If after a period of adequate treatment the patient remains febrile, antifungal therapy is usually begun. Recent meta-analyses support the use of liposomal amphotericin B and itraconazole in empirical antifungal therapy. Controversy still rages over the need for reverse isolation, enteric sterilization with antibiotics, or other prophylactic measures that may be taken to reduce infection.

Gotzsche PC, Johansen HK. Routine versus selective antifungal administration for control of fungal infections in patients with cancer. Cochrane Database of Systematic Reviews. 2002:CD000026.

137. What are the most important causes of death in patients undergoing BMT?

BMT is a challenging mode of therapy. After conditioning, patients become pancytopenic during the 3 weeks or so required for engraftment. During that time, they are prone to **infectious complications** similar to those experienced by patients undergoing remission-induction chemotherapy for AML. These patients are treated prophylactically with antibiotics and transfusions of RBCs and platelets. Blood products must be irradiated to prevent **GvHD** from lymphocytes in the donor units. After engraftment, **interstitial pneumonitis** is a frequent complication, with a high mortality rate. Some of these deaths are due to infectious agents such as CMV. Recently, a severe form of **veno-occlusive disease** of the liver has emerged as a cause of morbidity and mortality after BMT.

138. Describe the clinical findings in GvHD.

One consequence of engraftment is the potential for GvHD, which is caused by T cells from the donor. GvHD may be either acute or chronic.

139. Characterize acute GvHD.

Acute GvHD arises during the first 100 days after transplant, with donor T cells targeting the host's skin, liver, and GI tract. Patients may have mild skin rashes or more severe disease resulting in toxic epidermal necrolysis. Diarrhea and transient elevation of liver enzymes may occur and, in some patients, are more severe, resulting in massive diarrhea and liver failure. Immunologic competence is also delayed by GvHD, so that patients are susceptible to new infections, including those mediated by encapsulated organisms such as pneumococci.

140. Characterize chronic GvHD.

Chronic GvHD results in the same organ involvement, with additional features of a scleroderma-like illness. Dry eyes, dry mouth, myasthenia, bronchiolitis, and infections are also observed.

ACUTE LYMPHOBLASTIC LEUKEMIA

141. Can acute lymphoblastic leukemia (ALL) be reliably differentiated from AML (M1) by examination of the peripheral blood smear only?

No. Although hematologists can sometimes distinguish between the two entities by looking at the morphology of the blasts, there is a high rate of discordance with the results of special studies. Flow cytometry is frequently used to show typical lymphoid markers in ALL and myeloid markers in AML. Some patients with leukemia show evidence of both types of markers and are called biphenotypic. AML can be differentiated from ALL by using sensitive markers such as CD19 and CD7 for B- and T-cell lineages, respectively, and CD13 or CD33 for AML.

142. Summarize the distinguishing cytologic features of ALL and AML.

See Table 9-8.

TABLE 9-8. DISTINGUISHING CYTOLOGIC FEATURES OF ALL AND AML

	AML	ALL
Wright's stain morphology		
Cytoplasm	More abundant	Scanty
Granules	Sometimes present	Absent
Nucleoli	3–5 distinct	1–3, often indistinct
Auer rods	May be present	Absent
Staining characteristics		
Peroxidase or Sudan black	+	–
Periodic acid–Schiff	+/–	+

From Pui C-H, Evans WE: Acute lymphoblastic leukemia. N Engl J Med 339:605–615, 1998.

143. What are the indicators of a poor prognosis in adults with ALL?

ALL has an 80% cure rate in young children with good prognostic features, but in adults the outlook is much worse. Certain features at presentation of ALL in adults confer a poorer prognosis and may suggest the need for highly aggressive therapy. Adults are more likely than children to show:

- Unfavorable chromosomal abnormalities, such as Ph^1 and 8:14 translocation
- Biphenotypic disease and other than early pre-B immunophenotype
- Leukocytosis at presentation
- Multidrug resistance
- Mediastinal mass

Copelan EA, McGuire EA: The biology and treatment of acute lymphoblastic leukemia in adults. Blood 85:1151–1168, 1995.

LYMPHOPROLIFERATIVE DISEASE

144. What is the most common leukemia of adults?

Chronic lymphocytic leukemia (CLL), which is a neoplastic growth of lymphocytes, most often B lymphocytes. Patients are often elderly, and CLL is detected during examination for other problems. Lymphadenopathy and splenomegaly are also relatively common. Some patients present only with an elevated WBC count, composed of lymphocytes with a normal morphology.

145. List the diagnostic criteria for CLL.

1. Sustained lymphocyte count $> 10 \times 10^9$/L. Morphology should be "typical."
2. Bone marrow involvement (> 30% lymphocytes)
3. B-cell immunophenotypes (typically weak expression of membrane immunoglobulin, CD 20, expression of the T-cell antigen CD5)

To make a diagnosis of CLL, criterion 1 should be satisfied along with either criterion 2 or 3. If criterion 1 is not satisfied (lymphocyte count $< 10 \times 10^9$/L), criteria 2 and 3 must be present.

International Workshop on Chronic Lymphocytic Leukemia: Chronic lymphocytic leukemia: Recommendations for diagnosis, staging, and response criteria. Ann Intern Med 110:236–238, 1989.

146. Why is staging of CLL important?

Patients with CLL are typically staged to determine prognosis and therapy. Many patients with CLL present with limited disease and live without problems from leukemia. Because most are elderly, death from other causes is most likely. Patients with more advanced disease, however, do less well; unfortunately, chemotherapy has not improved survival. Treatment is usually given to patients who have anemia, thrombocytopenia, or bulky lymphadenopathy.

147. What are the two currently used staging systems for CLL?

The Rai Staging System (Table 9-9) and the Binet Staging System (Table 9-10).

TABLE 9-9. RAI STAGING SYSTEM FOR CLL

Stage	Clinical Features	Survival (mo)*
0	Lymphocytosis in blood and bone marrow only	> 120
I	Lymphocytosis and enlarged lymph nodes	95
II	Lymphocytosis plus hepatomegaly, splenomegaly, or both	72
III	Lymphocytosis and anemia (hemoglobin < 110 gm/L)	30
IV	Lymphocytosis and thrombocytopenia (platelets $<100 \times 10^9$/L)	30

*Weighted median survival was derived from eight series that involved a total of 952 patients.

TABLE 9-10. BINET STAGING SYSTEM FOR CHRONIC LYMPHOCYTIC LEUKEMIA

Stage	Clinical Features	Survival (mo)*
A	Hemoglobin > 100 gm/L; platelets $> 100 \times 10^9$/L and < 3 areas involved†	> 120
B	Hemoglobin > 100 gm/L; platelets $> 100 \times 10^9$/L and > 3 areas involved	61
C	Hemoglobin < 100 gm/L or platelets $< 100 \times 10^9$/L or both (independent of the areas involved)	32

*Weighted median survival was derived from eight series that involved a total of 1117 patients.
†Cervical, axillary, and inguinal lymph nodes (whether unilateral or bilateral); spleen; and liver.
From International Workshop on Chronic Lymphocytic Leukemia: Chronic lymphocytic leukemia: Recommendations for diagnosis, staging, and response criteria. Ann Intern Med 110:236–238, 1989.

Recently it has been recognized that patients with CLL cells that express a “germinal center” phenotype as defined by absence of mutation of the immunoglobulin heavy chain variable region genes (IgV_H genes) have a worse prognosis and more rapid disease course than patients with a post germinal center phenotype and presence of IgV_H gene mutation. Two markers, Zap-70 and CD 38, correlate relatively well the the germinal center phenotype and are finding their way into clinical practice as a way of determining who will need early or more aggressive treatment.

Shanafelt TD, Geyer SM, Kay NE: Prognosis at diagnosis: integrating molecular biologic insights into clinical practice for patients with CLL. Blood 103:1202–1210, 2004.

148. What are the complications of CLL?

- Autoimmune phenomena (warm antibody autoimmune hemolytic anemia, immune thrombocytopenia, neutropenia)
- Pure red blood cell aplasia
- Hypogammaglobulinemia
- Transformation into a large cell lymphoma with poor prognosis (Richter's syndrome)

Rozman C, Montserrat E: Chronic lymphocytic leukemia. N Engl J Med 333:1052–1057, 1995.

149. Which lymphoproliferative disorder is associated with pancytopenia, splenomegaly, absence of lymphadenopathy, and circulating lymphoid cells with multiple projections?

Hairy cell leukemia (HCL). Although an uncommon malignancy (2% of all leukemias), HCL receives a great deal of attention because of advances in treatment and the unusual infections observed in the course of the disease. HCL is an important consideration in the work-up of patients who present with pancytopenia. Some patients have presented with aplastic anemia.

150. How is HCL diagnosed?

Although the bone marrow aspirate is often scanty, characteristic "hairy" lymphs may be observed. The biopsy may show a diffusely involved marrow with mononuclear cells situated in a network of fibrosis. Although hairy cells may be present in the marrow, the biopsy picture is one of profound hypocellularity. The hairy cell is a B lymphocyte with an immunophenotype consistent with a cell between a CLL-lymphocyte and a plasma cell. Hairy cells also possess the Tac antigen (CD25), a receptor for interleukin-2, usually seen on activated T cells. The distinctive cytochemical feature of the hairy cell is a tartrate-resistant acid phosphatase activity.

151. What is the differential diagnosis of HCL?

The differential diagnosis of a patient with splenomegaly and circulating abnormal but relatively mature lymphocytes includes HCL, CLL, leukemic phase of non-Hodgkin's lymphoma, and splenic lymphoma with villous lymphocytes (SLVL). SLVL shows many features of HCL, including lymphocytes with projections or villi. However, the lymphocyte in SLVL has usually just one or two polar projections. SLVL is considered to be the leukemic counterpart of marginal zone lymphoma. SLVL has an epidemiologic association with hepatitis C infection; in such patients, treatment with interferon can lead to regression of the lymphoma.

Catovsky D: Chronic lymphoproliferative disorders. Curr Opin Oncol 7:3–11, 1995.

152. How is HCL treated?

In the past many patients improved after splenectomy. Interferon has been used successfully in alleviating this disorder, but recent trials show that the most effective agent is the purine analog 2-chlorodeoxyadenosine.

153. What infectious complications are seen in HCL?

The course of HCL is marked by an increased incidence of infections with atypical mycobacteria or fungi, such as *Histoplasma* and *Cryptococcus* spp. There also may be an increased incidence of bacterial infections and perhaps legionellosis. Factors contributing to the occurrence of atypical mycobacterial and fungal infections may include decreased neutrophils, absolute monocytopenia, and inability to form granuloma normally.

Westbrook CA, Golde DW: Clinical problems in hairy cell leukemia: Diagnosis and management. Semin Oncol 11:514, 1984.

HODGKIN'S AND NON-HODGKIN'S LYMPHOMAS

154. What are the common presentations of Hodgkin's disease?
Most patients often present with lymphadenopathy in the neck or axilla; lymph nodes are non-tender, rubbery, and discrete. Sometimes the nodes wax and wane in size until attention is sought. Important symptoms in the staging of Hodgkin's disease are fever, weight loss (> 10% of body weight), and night sweats. Some patients are troubled by pruritus. Hodgkin's disease tends to originate in central lymph nodes, so that some patients present with mediastinal lymphadenopathy.

155. How does Hodgkin's disease spread?
Hodgkin's disease is thought to spread from a unifocal site to contiguous lymph nodes. There may be early hematogenous dissemination to the spleen, with subsequent spread to the splenic hilar and retroperitoneal nodes as well as the liver. If large tumor masses develop, there may be extension into adjacent organs. Often the spleen is significantly involved in the absence of palpable splenomegaly. Hence, some centers recommend staging laparotomy to avoid missing splenic and hepatic disease. The importance of staging in Hodgkin's disease is to determine the extent of disease and thereby decide on therapy.

156. How is Hodgkin's disease staged?
See Table 9-11.

TABLE 9-11. ANN ARBOR STAGING OF HODGKIN'S DISEASE

Stage	Substage	Involvement
I	I	Single lymph node
	IE	Single extralymphatic organ
II	II	Lymph nodes on same side of diaphragm
	IIE	With localized extralymphatic site
III	III	Lymph nodes above and below diaphragm
	IIIE	With localized extralymphatic site
	IIIS	With isolated splenic site
	IIISE	With both extralymphatic and splenic sites
IV	IV	Disseminated or diffuse involvement of one or more extralymphatic sites
	IVA	Asymptomatic
	IVB	Fever, sweats, weight loss > 10% body weight

From Aisenberg A: The staging and treatment of Hodgkin's disease. N Engl J Med 299:1228, 1978.

157. What are the histologic subtypes of Hodgkin's disease?
- Nodular sclerosis (35%)
- Mixed cellularity (33%)
- Lymphocyte predominant (16%)
- Lymphocyte depletion (16%)

158. Summarize the gender distribution of the histologic subtypes.
Nodular sclerosis more frequently affects women, whereas the other three types more often affect men.

159. Which subtypes carry the worst prognosis?
Although staging generally determines the outlook, histologic subtype is also important. Nodular-sclerosing and lymphocyte-predominant subtypes tend to present with limited disease. Lymphocyte depletion is associated with more advanced disease, retroperitoneal involvement, and presentation in older adults.

160. What should be done before patients with Hodgkin's disease undergo staging laparotomy?
Patients first must undergo a comprehensive clinical staging evaluation before surgical staging is contemplated. The key elements in the clinical staging are as follows:

- Detailed history
- Detailed physical exam, with attention to lymph node areas, spleen, and liver
- Laboratory tests: CBC, erythrocyte sedimentation rate, alkaline phosphatase, renal and liver function tests
- Radiology: posteroanterior and lateral views of chest, abdominal and chest CT scans, bilateral lower-extremity lymphangiogram
- Bone marrow aspirate and biopsy

161. When is staging laparotomy needed?
There is no need for staging laparotomy if disseminated or diffuse extralymphatic involvement is found, unless the results would change therapy. In centers where treatment includes chemotherapy for limited disease, the need for laparotomy is less apparent. Unfortunately, staging laparotomy carries a high morbidity due to pulmonary emboli, subphrenic abscesses, stress ulcers, and wound infections.

Urba WJ, Longo DL: Hodgkin's disease. N Engl J Med 326:678–687, 1992.

162. In patients cured of Hodgkin's disease, what are the late sequelae of therapy?
The most important of the late sequelae are myelodysplasia, leukemia, and non-Hodgkin's lymphoma (3–10 years after therapy). Certain complications of the high-dose irradiation are also evident: acute radiation pneumonitis with fever, cough, and shortness of breath. Cardiac effects of irradiation include pericarditis, pericardial effusions, and pericardial fibrosis. Coronary artery disease may be accelerated. Neurologic effects of irradiation include Lhermitte's syndrome (paresthesia produced by flexion of the neck). Hypothyroidism is also a frequent sequelae of radiation therapy.

Bookman MA, Longo DI: Concomitant illness in patients treated for Hodgkin's disease. Cancer Treat Rev 13:77, 1986.

163. How does the pattern of lymph node involvement in non-Hodgkin's lymphoma (diffuse versus nodular) correlate with the pace of disease progression?
In nodular lymphomas, the neoplastic lymphocytes congregate into aggregates that superficially resemble germinal centers. Lymphomas of this type generally pursue an indolent course. Diffuse lymphomas tend to behave in a more aggressive manner. Other adverse prognostic factors include older age, elevated lactate dehydrogenase, two or more extranodal sites, T-cell phenotype, and masses > 10 cm.

164. How often do patients with lymphoma have bone marrow involvement?
Bone marrow involvement is extremely common in non-Hodgkin's lymphoma, whereas it is relatively uncommon in Hodgkin's disease. Diffuse well-differentiated lymphocytic lymphoma is associated with bone marrow involvement in 100% of cases. Small, cleaved-cell lymphomas, follicular and diffuse types, are associated with bone marrow involvement in 40–50% of cases.

Large-cell lymphomas are less likely to spread to the marrow (15% incidence). When bone marrow involvement occurs in large cell lymphoma, there is a greater risk for CNS disease.

165. **In Africa, Denis P. Burkitt described an aggressive neoplasm that bears his name. What are the salient clinical features of this lymphoma?**
Burkitt's lymphoma results from a proliferation of B lymphocytes with a striking appearance. They present as round or oval cells with abundant basophilic cytoplasm-containing vacuoles that stain positively for fat. The tissue is replaced with a monotonous infiltrate of cells with interspersed macrophages, giving a "starry sky" appearance. When it presents as a leukemia, it is classified as L3 in the FAB scheme. These cells proliferate rapidly and have a potential doubling time of 24 hours.

166. **Distinguish the African and American forms of Burkitt's lymphoma.**
In African Burkitt's lymphoma, patients present with large extranodal tumors of the jaws, abdominal viscera (including kidney), and ovaries and retroperitoneum. In the American form of Burkitt's lymphoma, patients present with intra-abdominal tumors arising from the ileocecal region or mesenteric lymph nodes. In Africa, the disease is associated with EBV, but this association is less common in American cases.

167. **What characteristic cytogenetic abnormalities are seen in Burkitt's lymphoma?**
A t(8:14) translocation is recognized in most cases. The proto-oncogene *c-myc* is located on chromosome 8 and usually becomes translocated to the locus of the heavy-chain immunoglobulin gene although translocations to the light-chain loci on chromosomes 2 and 22 are also seen. This results in the activation of *c-myc*. Burkitt's is now classified as a subset of small noncleaved cell lymphoma (SNCL). SNCL is a frequent neoplasm diagnosed in association with HIV infection and has a predilection for CNS and bone marrow involvement.

Mashal RD, Canellos GP: Small non-cleaved cell lymphoma in adults. Am J Hematol 38:40–47, 1991.

168. **When should patients with non-Hodgkin's lymphoma receive chemo-or radiotherapy?**
In an evaluation of patients with favorable histology and stage III or IV disease, it was found that deferral of treatment until patients became symptomatic did not adversely affect survival. In fact, during the course of nontreatment, spontaneous regression was frequently observed. The median time to treatment was 31 months. Thus, in the absence of curative chemotherapy for indolent lymphomas, deferral of treatment is a reasonable course, provided patients are followed closely.

PLASMA CELL DYSCRASIAS

169. **How do you differentiate multiple myeloma (MM) from benign monoclonal gammopathy (BMG)?**
Table 9-12 summarizes the distinguishing features. The discovery of a monoclonal protein on serum protein electrophoresis should be followed by a careful work-up for MM. Patients who have a small serum spike, normal CBC, no proteinuria, and no lytic lesions, hypercalcemia, or renal dysfunction usually are followed with periodic serum protein electrophoresis. Patients meeting some of the criteria for MM but showing no progression with follow-up are described as having indolent MM. Such patients generally do not have anemia or lytic bone lesions.

170. **What are the renal manifestations of multiple myeloma?**
Myeloma kidney
Dense tubular casts and progressive azotemia
Glomerulonephritis
Urate nephropathy
Pyelonephritis

TABLE 9-12. MULTIPLE MYELOMA VERSUS BENIGN MONOCLONAL GAMMOPATHY

	MM	BMG
M-protein	> 3.5 gm/dL	< 3.5 gm/dL
IgG IgA	> 2.0 gm/dL	< 2.0 gm/dL
Anemia or other cytopenia	Usually present	Absent
Urine protein	> 500 mg/24 h	< 500 mg/24 h
Bones	Lytic lesions or osteoporosis	Normal
Marrow plasma cells	> 10%	< 10%
Serum beta$_2$-microglobulin	> 3.0 mg/L	< 3.0 mg/L
Calcium	Elevated in 30%	Normal
Creatinine	± Elevation	Normal
Change in monoclonal protein with time	Increases	No change

Hyperviscosity
Renal tubular dysfunction
Isosthenuria
Renal tubular acidosis
Adult Fanconi syndrome
Dye-nephropathy
Hypercalcemia renal damage
Plasma cell infiltration
Amyloid kidney
Nephrotic syndrome

171. Describe the clinical manifestations of Waldenström's macroglobulinemia.
Waldenström's macroglobulinemia is a B-cell disorder of proliferating plasmacytoid lymphs that produce an IgM monoclonal protein. Patients frequently have hepatosplenomegaly, lymphadenopathy, and bone marrow involvement. The elderly are affected most often. Neurologic disease, including peripheral neuropathy and cerebellar dysfunction, is also seen. A prominent feature is retinopathy with large sausage-shaped, dilated retinal veins. Bleeding and purpura are also common. Of particular importance is the recognition of hyperviscosity syndrome, which also may occur in MM.

Dimopoulos MA, Alexanian R: Waldenstrom's macroglobulinemia. Blood 83:1452–1459, 1994.

172. How is Waldenström's macroglobulinemia treated?
This syndrome can respond dramatically to plasmapheresis because IgM does not have a large extravascular distribution.

173. List the manifestations of the hyperviscosity syndrome.
Global CNS dysfunction and stupor
Retinopathy
Retinal hemorrhages
Papilledema
Hypervolemia, congestive heart failure
Headache, vertigo, ataxia
Stroke
Coagulopathy

174. Patients with the lambda-light-chain type of MM are prone to develop amyloidosis. What are the laboratory clues to the presence of this systemic disorder?
Amyloid is a lardaceous substance that accumulates in the tissues of patients with various disorders, including MM. The amyloid in MM is composed of light chains, most often of the lambda type, arranged in a beta-pleated sheet. When stained with Congo red and viewed under polarized light, amyloid shows an apple-green birefringence.

KEY POINTS: THROMBOCYTOPENIA

1. A good history includes careful questioning about prescription and nonprescription and herbal medication use.
2. Patients also should be asked about high-risk behavior for HIV infection.
3. A good physical exam gives careful attention to temperature, blood pressure, assessment for bleeding sites, lymphadenopathy, and hepatosplenomegaly.
4. The peripheral blood smear must be reviewed carefully to look for platelet clumping (spurious thrombocytopenia), schizocytes and other fragmented RBCs, macro-ovalocytes (megaloblastic anemia), and atypical WBCs (viral syndrome, leukemia, lymphoma).

175. How do patients with amyloidosis present?

Patients may develop purpura from skin involvement, hepatosplenomegaly, macroglossia, orthostatic hypotension, congestive heart failure, malabsorption, nephrotic syndrome, peripheral neuropathy, and carpal tunnel syndrome. Of interest, the consequences of amyloid include an acquired factor X deficiency, resulting in a prolonged PT and PTT and functional hyposplenism. The latter results in the presence of Howell-Jolly bodies, even though the spleen is present.

Gertz MA, Kyle RA: Primary systemic amyloidosis—a diagnostic primer. Mayo Clin Proc 64:1505–1519, 1989.

HEMOSTASIS

176. Define the primary and secondary phases of hemostasis.

Hemostasis is a complicated process with several components, all of which must work well for normal hemostasis to occur. The two overlapping phases of the formation of a clot or hemostatic plug are (1) **primary hemostasis**, in which the ruptured vessel wall interacts with platelets that must adhere and aggregate to form the basis of the clot, and (2) **secondary hemostasis**, in which clotting factors circulating in the blood activate each other in a cascade that results in the activation of thrombin and the deposition of fibrin around the platelet plug.

177. How do disorders of primary and secondary hemostasis differ in clinical presentations?

See Table 9-13.

178. Describe idiopathic thrombocytopenic purpura (ITP).

In ITP, an autoantibody arises (usually IgG) that interacts with the patient's own platelets. Sometimes these antibodies interact with specific antigens related to functional proteins; platelets coated with the auto-IgG are then sequestered and removed by macrophages in the spleen, liver, and bone marrow. Production of megakaryocytes, as judged by a bone marrow aspirate, appears to be normal. However, recent studies indicate that megakaryocytopoiesis is, in fact, suboptimal for the degree of peripheral destruction. Thus, megakaryocytes may be affected by the autoantibody of ITP.

Cines DB, Blanchette VS: Immune thrombocytopenic purpura. N Engl J Med 346:995–1008, 2002.

TABLE 9-13. DISORDERS OF PRIMARY VERSUS SECONDARY HEMOSTASIS

	Primary	Secondary
Onset	Immediate	Delayed, hours after trauma
Sites, type of lesion	Mucosa, GI, GU, skin (purpura, petechiae) hematuria, hematomas	Joints, retroperitoneum, muscles
Components involved	Vessel wall, platelet adhesion	Generation of fibrin from fibrinogen
Typical disorder	von Willebrand disease	Hemophilia A (factor VIII deficiency)

From Schafer AI: Approach to bleeding. In Loscalzo J, Schafer AI (eds): Thrombosis and Hemorrhage, 3rd ed. Philadelphia, Lippincott Williams & Wilkins, 2003, p 315–329.

179. How is ITP diagnosed?

ITP implies no known cause and is a diagnosis of exclusion. ITP occurs early in HIV infection, often before typical AIDS-defining illness. Diagnosis does not always require a bone marrow aspirate and biopsy.

180. How is ITP treated?

Treatment remains empiric. Patients typically respond to prednisone. Refractory ITP or relapsed ITP may require splenectomy and/or additional immunosuppressive therapy. Treatment with intravenous IgG often produces a significant though transient increase in the platelet count.

George JN, et al: Idiopathic thrombocytopenic purpura: A practice guideline developed by explicit methods for the American Society of Hematology. Blood 88:3–40, 1996.

181. What disorders are associated with nonimmune destruction of platelets?

Thrombocytopenia occurs with a wide variety of disorders of hematopoiesis. Of most concern are situations that result in the increased peripheral destruction of platelets. Some of these conditions may have immune components. The following disorders are associated with increased platelet destruction:

Infections
Sepsis, gram-negative or gram-positive
Viral, rickettsial
Histoplasmosis
Malaria
Typhoid, brucellosis
Hypersplenism
Extracorporeal circulation, hypothermia

Microangiopathic disease
Disseminated intravascular coagulation
Thrombotic thrombocytopenic purpura
Eclampsia, preeclampsia
Burns
Cavernous hemangiomas
Kasabach-Merritt syndrome
Massive transfusion

182. Name the most common hereditary disorder resulting in a prolonged bleeding time.

Von Willebrand's disease, an autosomal dominant disorder, results from several abnormalities in the production of a large, multimeric adhesive protein, von Willebrand factor (vWF). Classic VWF (type 1) disease results from decreased release of VWF from the endothelial cell. vWF is also synthesized by megakaryocytes and is a constituent of the alpha-granules of platelets.

Decreased presence of vWF at the site of endothelial damage results in impairment of platelet adhesion and consequently poor primary hemostasis.

183. What are the signs and symptoms of von Willebrand's disease?
Patients with von Willebrand's disease have problems with epistaxis, hematuria, menorrhagia, GI bleeding, and bleeding after trauma. In classic type I disease, the platelet count is normal, but the bleeding time is prolonged. Factor VIII activity is also reduced in the plasma of patients with type 1 disease. The reduction of vWF seems to shorten the circulating life of factor VIII. Understanding of the pathophysiology of von Willebrand's disease has advanced rapidly so that now multiple types are recognized.

Sadler JE, Mannucci PM, Berntorp E, et al. Impact, diagnosis and treatment of von Willebrand disease. Thromb Haemost. 84:160–174, 2000.

184. What are the hereditary disorders of platelet function?
Because von Willebrand's disease is associated with platelet dysfunction, it is often considered with disorders resulting from congenital structural abnormalities of the platelet. These bleeding disorders are identified by a prolonged bleeding time and abnormal functional behavior in platelet aggregation tests. Three of these disorders are described in Table 9-14.

TABLE 9-14. HEREDITARY DISORDERS RESULTING IN PLATELET DYSFUNCTION

	Von Willebrand's Disease	Bernard-Soulier Syndrome	Glanzmann's Thrombasthenia
Defect	Reduced or abnormal factor VIII:vWF	Absence of platelet gp Ib, a receptor for vWF	Absence of platelet gp IIb, IIIa, a receptor for vWF and fibrinogen
Inheritance	Autosomal dominant	Autosomal recessive	Autosomal recessive
Platelet appearance	Normal	Macrothrombocytes	Normal
Aggregometry			
Ristocetin	Decreased	Decreased	Normal
ADP	Normal	Normal	Decreased
Collagen	Normal	Normal	Decreased

gp = glycoprotein, vWF = von Willebrand factor, ADP = adenosine diphosphate.

185. What drug results in an acquired platelet defect?
The biggest offender is aspirin. Platelet cyclooxygenase is irreversibly inhibited by low doses of aspirin. As a result, the platelet has lifelong impaired function. Aspirin exacerbates the bleeding tendencies associated with von Willebrand's disease and other platelet disorders and by itself can produce prolongation of the bleeding time. It is important to note that the bleeding time does not predict the risk of hemorrhage in an individual patient. The potential benefit of this aspirin effect is to reduce platelet activity in critical areas, such as a stenosed coronary artery. The typical finding in platelet aggregometry with aspirin-treated platelets is the absence of the secondary wave of aggregation produced by ADP.

186. Give another example of an acquired disorder of platelet function.
Another important acquired disorder of platelet function is that associated with uremia. Although the pathogenesis of this mild hemostatic defect is poorly understood, it appears that the administration of the vasopressin analog desmopressin increases vWF and shortens the bleeding time.

George JN, Shattil SJ: The clinical importance of acquired abnormalities of platelet function. N Engl J Med 324:27–39, 1991.

187. What two factor deficiencies result in hemophilia? What is their pattern of inheritance?
Hemophilia results from a deficiency of factor VIII (hemophilia A) or factor IX (hemophilia B). These are X-linked disorders, and the family history of an affected boy reveals affected maternal uncles and cousins. Patients may have mild or severe disease. Severe disease requires frequent administration of factor VIII or IX concentrates. In the past, hemophilia was a crippling disorder because of the frequency of hemarthroses and arthritis. Prophylactic administration of factor VIII concentrate after trauma has reduced the incidence of complications dramatically.

Bolton-Maggs PH, Pasi KJ: Haemophilias A and B. Lancet 361:1801–1809, 2003.

KEY POINTS: HEMOSTASIS

1. Obtaining a bleeding history and history of aspirin use, liver or kidney disease is as or more important than obtaining screening PT, PTT, or bleeding times prior to elective procedures.
2. Disorders of primary hemostasis (thrombocytopenia, von Willebrand disease) demonstrate purpura and mucosal bleeding.
3. Disorders of secondary hemostasis such as hemophilia are complicated by deep tissue bleeding and hemarthroses.
4. The first steps in working up a bleeding disorder include the PT, PTT (with mixing study if prolonged), and a CBC with platelet count.
5. Hereditary thrombophilia is more likely in patients with thrombosis who are young or who have a thrombosis in an unusual site. The most common such disorder in European patients is factor V Leiden.
6. Increased homocysteine, lupus anticoagulants, and the related antiphospholipid antibody syndrome are important causes of acquired thrombophilia.

188. What questions about bleeding problems need to be asked in the history?
The patient interview should include questions about personal or family history of bleeding problems, including prolonged bleeding after dental extraction, injury, or surgical procedure. Patients should be asked about frequent nosebleeds, menorrhagia, melena, and bruising. A history of liver disease, obvious malnutrition, or malabsorption syndrome also should be sought. Although irrelevant to PT and PTT, a recent history of aspirin ingestion needs to be sought. The physical exam should include inspection of the skin and mucosa for purpura or petechiae, hematomas, and ecchymotic lesions.

189. What hereditary disorders result in a prolonged PTT without bleeding?
When routine preoperative screening PT and PTT tests are obtained, patients occasionally have a dramatic, reproducible prolongation of the PTT but no historical or physical findings to suggest

a hemostatic disorder. Familial disorders causing this phenomenon are (1) hereditary deficiency of factor XII (Hageman factor) and (2) deficiency of factors in the contact activation system that activates XII, including Fletcher factor (prekallikrein) and Fitzgerald factor (high-MW kininogen). These disorders produce an interesting in vitro phenomenon that does not seem to result in any hemorrhagic tendency. In fact, Mr. Hageman, the first person recognized to be deficient in factor XII, died of pulmonary embolism.

190. What is the lupus anticoagulant (LA)?

LA is an autoantibody that binds to the phospholipid component required in the formation of the prothrombin activation complex. Its presence on the phospholipid disrupts the association between factor Xa, prothrombin, factor V, and calcium, leading to an abnormally long PTT (and sometimes PT). The name is truly a misnomer because in vivo it is not an anticoagulant, nor does it occur only in patients with lupus. There is a high but incomplete level of concordance with other known phospholipid antibodies, such as anticardiolipin antibodies.

191. Describe the relationship between LA and antiphospholipid antibody syndrome.

Antiphospholipid antibody syndrome (APS) refers to patients with antiphospholipid antibodies that react with cardiolipin or with beta$_2$-glycoprotein I. Some of these patients also may have typical LAs. APS and LA are associated with thrombosis (arterial and venous), recurrent pregnancy loss, and thrombocytopenia.

Levine JS, Branch DW, Rauch J: The antiphospholipid syndrome. N Engl J Med. 346: 752–63, 2002.

192. What are the causes of disseminated intravascular coagulation (DIC)?

See Table 9-15.

TABLE 9-15. CAUSES OF DISSEMINATED INTRAVASCULAR COAGULATION

Infections	Collagen-vascular disease
Viral (epidemic hemorrhagic fevers, herpes, rubella)	Vasculitis
Rickettsial (Rocky Mountain spotted fever)	Polyarteritis
Bacterial (gram-negative sepsis, meningococcemia)	Systemic lupus erythematosus
Fungal (histoplasmosis)	Obstetric complications
Protozoan (malaria)	Abruptio placentae
Neoplasms	Septic abortion
Carcinomas (prostate, pancreas, breast, lung, ovary)	Amniotic fluid embolism
Acute promyelocytic leukemia	Intrauterine fetal death
Vascular disease	Saline-, urea-induced abortions
Cavernous hemangiomas (Kasabach-Merritt syndrome)	Eclampsia
Aneurysms	Hemolytic transfusion reactions
	Hypothermia-rewarming
	Shock
	Cocaine-induced rhabdomyolysis
	Use of factor IX concentrates

193. When DIC is present, which coagulation tests are abnormal?
DIC occurs in patients with inappropriate activation of thrombin and disseminated clotting, which in turn is associated with increased fibrinolysis. During this process, multiple coagulation factors are consumed. Byproducts of thrombin and plasmin activity circulate as well. As endothelial cell damage occurs, there is consumption of platelets and, in some instances, fragmentation of RBCs, resulting in significant intravascular hemolysis. Laboratory findings are summarized in Table 9-16.

TABLE 9-16. LABORATORY FINDINGS IN DIC

Peripheral blood smear	
Platelets	↓
Red cell fragmentation	Present
PT, PTT	Both ↑
Fibrinogen	↓
Fibrin degradation products	↓
D-dimers	↓
Platelet count	↑

From Levi M, Ten Cate H: Disseminated intravascular coagulation. N Engl J Med 341:586–592, 1999.

194. How do patients with DIC present?
Although DIC is often a hemorrhagic condition, certain patients present with thrombotic complications: digital ischemia, decreased mentation, migrating thrombophlebitis, and renal involvement.

195. How does the bleeding diathesis associated with liver disease resemble DIC?
The liver may not be the seat of the soul, but it is definitely the site of production of all clotting factors (except vWF). Severe liver disease compromises hemostasis in a number of ways. Most readily detected is a decrease in the activity of the vitamin K–dependent factors II, VII, IX, and X. Patients with severe liver disease have a prolonged PT and PTT that does not improve after the administration of vitamin K.

196. Explain the significance of low fibrinogen levels.
Low fibrinogen levels elaborate a poorly functioning fibrinogen. Dysfibrinogenemia produces prolongation of the PT, PTT, and thrombin time.

197. How does the onset of cirrhosis and portal hypertension complicate the clinical picture?
With the onset of cirrhosis and portal hypertension, splenomegaly and a reduced platelet count occur. Because the liver is also an important organ of clearance of plasminogen activators, increased fibrin degradation products may be measured. Thus, the laboratory abnormalities in severe liver disease may mimic DIC.

198. What serious complication can occur with anticoagulation therapy in patients with congenital hypercoagulable states?
Proteins C and S are vitamin K–dependent anticoagulants. When patients are placed on warfarin for treatment of DVT, the goal of therapy is to reduce the activity of procoagulant factors (VII

included). This effect is monitored by following the PT, which detects early changes in the activity of factor VII. When warfarin therapy is initiated, particularly at high doses or in patients with a congenital deficiency, the levels of protein C may drop precipitously before the onset of anticoagulation because of decreased factor VII activity. One consequence of this drop is a serious disorder known as warfarin skin necrosis.

199. What are the acquired causes of hypercoagulability?
See Table 9-17.

TABLE 9-17. SECONDARY HYPERCOAGULABLE STATES

Abnormalities of coagulation and fibrinolysis	Abnormalities of blood vessels and rheology
Malignancy	Conditions promoting venous stasis (immobilization, obesity, advanced age, postoperative state)
Pregnancy	Artificial surfaces
Use of oral contraceptives	Vasculitis and chronic occlusive arterial disease
Infusion of prothrombin complex concentrates	Homocystinuria
Nephrotic syndrome	Hyperviscosity (polycythemia, leukemia, sickle cell disease, leukoagglutination, increased serum viscosity)
Disseminated intravascular coagulation	Thrombotic thrombocytopenic purpura
Antiphospholipid antibody syndrome, Lupus anticoagulant	
Abnormalities of platelets	
Myeloproliferative disorders	
Paroxysmal nocturnal hemoglobinuria	
Hyperlipidemia	
Diabetes mellitus	
Heparin-induced thrombocytopenia	

Adapted from Schafer AI: The hypercoagulable states. Ann Intern Med 102:818, 1985.

200. What is thrombopoietin?
Thrombopoietin acts in concert with other growth factors, such as IL-3, IL-6, and IL-11, to increase the number of megakaryocytic precursors. Thrombopoietin appears to be the predominant factor in megakaryocyte maturation. Thrombopoietin levels vary inversely with platelet counts in bone marrow failure syndromes. Mature platelets remove thrombopoietin from plasma so that levels are low when the platelet count is high. However, patients with clonal disorders associated with thrombocytosis, such as essential thrombocytosis, may have elevated thrombopoietin levels because of the decreased binding of thrombopoietin to presumably abnormal megakaryocytes and platelets.

Kaushansky K: Regulation of megakaryopoiesis. In Loscalzo J, Schafer AI, eds: Thrombosis and hemorrhage. 3rd ed: Philadelphia, Lippincott Williams & Wilkins, 120–139, 2003.

201. Why does the platelet count need to be monitored in patients receiving heparin?

Heparin-induced thrombocytopenia (HIT) occurs in 1–3 % of patients who receive heparin as prophylaxis or treatment for thrombosis or when heparin is used to flush catheters. Heparin-naive patients may develop thrombocytopenia 7–10 days after initiation of the drug. Unlike other causes of drug-induced thrombocytopenia, HIT is associated with thrombosis—venous and arterial. Heparin should be discontinued, and another form of anticoagulation (heparan, argatroban, or hirudin) should be substituted.

Warkentin TE, Kelton JG: A 14-year study of heparin-induced thrombocytopenia. Am J Med 101:502– 507, 1996.

WEB SITES

1. www.hematology.org
2. www.bloodline.net

BIBLIOGRAPHY

1. Greer JP, et al (eds): Wintrobe's Clinical Hematology, 11th ed. Philadelphia, Lippincott Williams & Wilkins, 2004.
2. Hoffbrand AV, Fantini B (eds): A Century of Hematology. Semin Hematol 36(Suppl 7), 1999.
3. Loscalzo J, Schafer AI (eds): Thrombosis and Hemorrhage, 3rd ed. Philadelphia, Lippincott Williams & Wilkins, 2003.

PULMONARY MEDICINE

Sheila Goodnight-White, MD

Medicine is the only world-wide profession, following everywhere the same methods, actuated by the same ambitions, and pursuing the same ends.

Sir William Osler (1849–1919)
Aequanimitas (1932)

The difference in sound during inspiration, expiration, and the retention of the breath is important in fixing our diagnosis.

Leopold Auenbrugger (1722–1809)
Inventum Novum (1761)

PHYSIOLOGY

1. Define hypoxemia.
Hypoxemia usually is defined as a partial arterial oxygen tension (PaO_2) < 60 mmHg.

2. List and explain the five basic pathophysiologic mechanisms that can cause hypoxemia.

- **Decreased inspired oxygen (P_IO_2):** high altitude, nonpressurized airplane cabin.
- **Hypoventilation:** decreased minute ventilation resulting in increased arterial carbon dioxide (CO_2) that leads to hypoxemia. (CNS impairment, respiratory muscle fatigue, or neuromuscular disease).
- **Diffusion abnormality:** diffuse interstitial pulmonary fibrosis.
- **Ventilation-perfusion (V/Q) abnormalities:** mismatching of ventilation and perfusion.
- **Shunt:** perfusion of nonventilated lung (pneumonia, pulmonary edema). Hypoxemia secondary to shunting is refractory to oxygen therapy.

3. Which is the most common cause of hypoxemia?
V/Q abnormalities, which are responsive to oxygen therapy.

4. How can the five basic mechanisms of hypoxemia be differentiated?
The values of PaO_2, $PaCO_2$, alveolar–arterial oxygen ($A–aO_2$) difference, and response to breathing 100% oxygen can be used to separate the basic causes of hypoxemia (Table 10-1).

5. What is the alveolar-arterial oxygen difference ($P_A\text{-}aO_2$)?
The $P_A\text{-}aO_2$ is the difference in the partial pressure of oxygen between alveolar air (P_AO_2) and arterial blood (PaO_2):

$$P_A\text{-}aO_2 = P_AO_2 - PaO_2$$

TABLE 10-1. DIFFERENTIATION OF THE CAUSES OF HYPOXEMIA

Machanism	PaO_2	$PaCO_2$	$A\text{–}aO_2$ Difference	Response to 100% O_2
P_IO_2	↓	↔ or ↓	↔	NA
Hypoventilation	↓	↑	↔	NA
Diffusion abnormality	↓	↔ or ↓	↑	Yes
V/Q mismatch	↓	↔ or ↓	↑	Yes
Shunt	↓	↔ or ↓	↑	No

↓ = decreased, ↔ = normal, ↑ = increased, NA = not applicable.

6. **What is a normal $P_A\text{-}aO_2$?**
   A normal $P_A\text{-}aO_2$ is usually < 10 mmHg in a patient breathing room air. In conditions that interfere with gas exchange between the alveoli and pulmonary capillaries, the $P_A\text{-}aO_2$ increases. In pure hypoventilation, when lung function is not impaired, the $P_A\text{-}aO_2$ is normal.

7. **How does aging affect $P_A\text{-}aO_2$?**
   Oxygenation normally decreases slightly with increasing age. An age-adjusted normal $P_A\text{-}aO_2$ can be estimated as follows: 2.5 + 0.21(age). Thus, a healthy 70-year-old is expected to have a $P_A\text{-}aO_2$ of approximately 17 mmHg. Of course, this equation yields only an approximation; there may be a great deal of individual variation.

8. **How do you calculate the $P_A\text{-}aO_2$?**
   The $P_A\text{-}aO_2$ can be calculated by using a simplified form of the alveolar gas equation:

$$P_AO_2 = FiO_2\,(P_{atm} - PH_2O) - (PaCO_2/RQ)$$

   where RQ is the respiratory quotient, FiO_2 is the fraction of the inspired gas that is oxygen (21% in room air), P_{atm} is the atmospheric pressure (760 mmHg at sea level), and PH_2O is the vapor pressure of water (assumed to be 47 mmHg).

9. **What value is used for RQ?**
   Usually a value of 0.8 can be used for RQ, which reflects the normal mixture of dietary substrates.

10. **Give an example of how to calculate the $P_A\text{-}aO_2$.**
    In a patient breathing room air with a P_AO_2 of 91 mmHg and $PaCO_2$ of 40 mmHg (measured by arterial blood gas), the P_AO_2 is calculated as follows:

$$\begin{aligned} P_AO_2 &= 0.21\,(760 - 47) - 40/0.8 \\ &= 150 - 50 \\ &= 100 \text{ mmHg} \\ P_A\text{-}aO_2 &= P_AO_2 - PaO_2 \\ &= 100 - 91 \\ &= 9 \text{ mmHg} \end{aligned}$$

    The calculated value is within normal limits.

11. **What is the oxyhemoglobin equilibrium curve? What does it demonstrate?**
The oxyhemoglobin equilibrium curve (or dissociation curve) is a plot of the hemoglobin percent saturation (SaO_2) against the PaO_2. It demonstrates the binding reaction of hemoglobin and oxygen.

12. **Explain what the dissociation curve shows about the relationship between hemoglobin and the binding or releasing of oxygen.**
The sigmoid-shaped curve shows that the binding (or releasing) of oxygen and hemoglobin is not a linear relationship (as is the case with dissolved oxygen). Oxygen is readily released at the lower range of PaO_2 values but very tightly held at the upper range of PaO_2 values—i.e., the affinity of hemoglobin for oxygen increases as more oxygen molecules bind to it. This enables the oxygen content of blood to remain high at high PaO_2 levels but still allows hemoglobin to release oxygen readily as the PaO_2 drops below 60 mmHg (the "steep" part of the curve).

13. **Clinicians refer to a shift of the oxyhemoglobin equilibrium curve to the left or right. What does this mean?**
Because the curve represents the affinity of hemoglobin for oxygen over the range of PaO_2, a shift in the curve in either direction represents a change in that affinity. A shift of the curve to the **left** represents an **increase** in the affinity of hemoglobin for oxygen; in other words, oxygen is taken up more readily and released less readily for any given PaO_2. Conversely, a shift to the **right** represents a **decrease** in affinity; in other words, oxygen is taken up less readily and released more readily (Fig. 10-1).

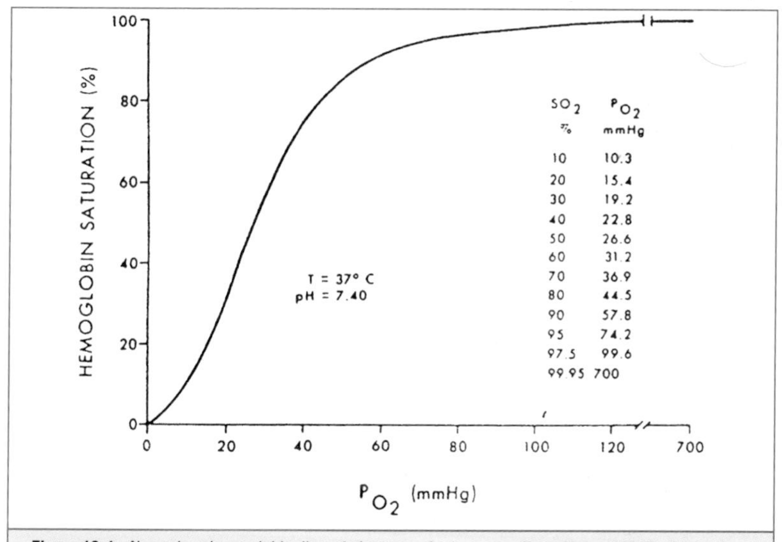

Figure 10-1. Normal oxyhemoglobin dissociation curve for humans. (From Murray JF: The Normal Lung, 2nd ed. Phildelphia, W.B. Saunders, 1986, p 174.)

14. **What factors can shift the oxyhemoglobin equilibrium curve?**
See Table 10-2.

15. **If the dissolved oxygen content of blood, measured by the PaO_2, is so small compared with the oxygen bound to hemoglobin, why do we measure and follow the PaO_2 as we treat patients?**
The PaO_2, although directly measuring only a tiny fraction of the total oxygen content of blood, is related to the total oxygen content through the dissociation curve. As the PaO_2 drops below

TABLE 10-2. FACTORS INFLUENCING THE OXYHEMOGLOBIN EQUILIBRIUM CURVE

Shift to the Left (↑ Hb/O_2 affinity)	Shift to the Right (↓ Hb/O_2 affinity)
Hypothermia	Hyperthermia/fever
Alkalosis	Acidosis
Hypocapnia	Hypercapnia
? 2,3DPG	↑2,3DPG
↑ Carboxyhemoglobin	↓ Carboxyhemoglobin
Hemoglobin F, Chesapeake Yakima, Ranier	Hemoglobin E, Seattle, Kansas

DGP = diphosphoglycerate

60 mmHg, the curve is very steep, whereas at a PaO_2 over 60 mmHg, the curve is flat. A drop of PaO_2 from 100 to 60 mmHg (drop of 40 mmHg) represents a drop of SaO_2 from 99% to 90%, a loss of only 9% of the blood's total oxygen content. However, a further drop of 40 mmHg (from a PaO_2 of 60 to 20 mmHg) represents a drop in SaO_2 from 90% to about 30%, or a loss of 60% of the blood's total oxygen content.

16. **What is the goal of oxygen therapy?**
The goal of oxygen therapy is to provide adequate supplemental oxygen to maintain tissue oxygenation, usually at a PaO_2 just over 60 mmHg. Below this level, small decreases in PaO_2 are accompanied by very large drops in the SaO_2 and therefore very large drops in the total oxygen content of blood. Attempts to increase the PaO_2 further do not result in significant increases in the oxygen content of blood but may increase the risk of oxygen toxicity. Because of potential oxygen toxicity, use of high concentrations of therapeutic oxygen (> 60%) should be limited to as short a duration as possible.

PHYSICAL EXAMINATION, SYMPTOMS, AND DIAGNOSTIC TECHNIQUES

17. **What is the most common cause of cough of short duration?**
Cough of short duration (< 3 weeks) is most commonly caused by acute upper respiratory tract infection (acute bronchitis).

18. **List the most common causes of chronic cough.**
- Post nasal drip
- Asthma
- Gastroesophageal reflux
- Sequelae of recent URI
- Medications (ACE inhibitor)
- Chronic bronchitis
- Lung cancer

19. **Since "all that wheezes is not asthma," what should be included in the differential diagnosis for wheezing?**
See Table 10-3.

20. **What is hemoptysis?**
Hemoptysis is defined as blood in the sputum and includes the full range of bloody sputum, from blood streaks to frank blood. In addition to history and physical examination, all patients should have a chest x-ray. Further diagnostic procedures should be guided by the findings of

TABLE 10-3. DIFFERENTIAL DIAGNOSIS OF WHEEZING

Laryngeal Obstruction	Peripheral Airway Obstruction	
Foreign body	Asthma and other reactive airway diseases	
Edema	Nonasthmatic causes	
Anaphylaxis	*Acute*	
Vocal cord dysfunction	Pulmonary embolism	
Epiglottitis and abscess	Pulmonary edema (cardiac asthma)	
Trauma	Aspiration of gastric contents or toxic liquids	
Enlarged thyroid	Inhalation injury (thermal or irritant)	
Tumors	Eosinophilic pneumonia	
Anomalous arteries	*Chronic*	
Aneurysm	COPD	Bronchiolitis
	Cystic fibrosis	Sarcoidosis
	Bronchiectasis	

these studies. The combined use of bronchoscopy and chest CT may be indicated, especially in smokers above the age of 40.

21. **Which neoplasms are most likely to cause hemoptysis?**
Bronchial carcinoma, metastatic lung cancer, and adenoma.

22. **List the vascular causes of hemoptysis.**
- Pulmonary infarct/embolism
- Mitral stenosis
- Bronchial-arterial fistula
- Ruptured thoracic aneurysm
- Arteriovenous malformation

23. **Which infections may cause hemoptysis?**
Mycobacteria (especially tuberculosis), fungal infections, lung abscess, necrotizing pneumonia, paragonimiasis, hydatid cyst.

24. **What are the two most common iatrogenic causes of hemoptysis?**
Rupture of pulmonary artery by balloon-tipped catheter and anticoagulant therapy.

25. **List the other causes of hemoptysis.**
Behçet's disease, Wegener's granulomatosis, Goodpasture's syndrome, coagulopathies, lymphangioleiomyomatosis, trauma/foreign body, cocaine use, and cryptogenic bleeding.

26. **What is massive hemoptysis?**
Massive hemoptysis implies copious bleeding and has been defined as the expectoration of > 600 mL of blood in a 24-hour period. The prognosis depends on the etiology and magnitude of the bleeding. This potentially lethal and alarming clinical situation requires expeditious evaluation, close observation, and possible arterial embolization or surgical intervention.

27. **What is clubbing?**
Clubbing is the distal enlargement of the digits at the nail bed secondary to an increase in soft tissue. The pathogenesis is unknown. It is usually bilateral and symmetrical and affects both fingers and toes. Clubbing is most often aquired but may be familial.

28. **List the disorders associated with clubbing.**
   - **Pulmonary:** lung cancer, pulmonary fibrosis, chronic infection (e.g., tuberculosis, cystic fibrosis), chronic obstructive pulmonary disease (COPD), arteriovenous malformations.
   - **Cardiac:** endocarditis, congenital heart disease
   - **Gastrointestinal:** cirrhosis, inflammatory bowel disease, malignancy, malabsorption
   - **Endocrine:** hyperthyroidism

29. **Define dyspnea.**
Dyspnea is a term used clinically to describe shortness of breath.

30. **List the causes of acute and chronic dyspnea.**

Acute	**Chronic**
Asthma	COPD
Pulmonary edema	Interstitial lung disease
Pneumothorax	Anemia
Pulmonary embolism	Chronic LV dysfunction
Pneumonia	Pulmonary vascular diseases
Pleural effusion	Psychogenic

Diagnostic evaluation of dyspnea. Available at: http://www.aafp.org/afp/ 980215ap/morgan.html

KEY POINTS: DIAGNOSTIC USES OF BRONCHOSCOPY 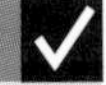

1. Evaluation of an abnormal chest film
2. Unexplained symptoms (wheezing, cough, hemoptysis, stridor) or unexplained findings (recurrent laryngeal nerve paralysis, recent diaphragmatic paralysis)
3. Preoperative staging of cancer
4. Bronchoalveolar lavage for interstitial lung disease or infection
5. Evaluation for lung transplant rejection
6. Diagnosis of pneumonia or infiltrate (specimen collection)
7. Chest trauma or inhalation injury

31. **What are the contraindications to fiberoptic bronchoscopy?**
Although there are no *absolute* contraindications to bronchoscopy, sound clinical judgment should guide any decision concerning an invasive procedure with potential risk for morbidity and mortality. Well-trained and experienced bronchoscopists, careful supervision, and consideration of potentially high-risk conditions (e.g., uremia, thrombocytopenia, pulmonary hypertension, bleeding diathesis) reduce morbidity and mortality risks.

32. **List the major and minor complications of bronchoscopy.**
Major complications: significant hemorrhage, pneumothorax, respiratory failure.
Minor complications: syncope, epistaxis, bronchospasm.

33. **Give the mortality and overall complication rates for bronchoscopy.**
The mortality rate is < 0.05%, and the overall complication rate is < 0.1%.
Virtual Hospital: Bronchoscopy. Available at: http://www.vh.org/adult/provider/radiology/LungTumor/Diagnosis/Bronchoscopy/Text/Bronchoscopy.html

34. **What conditions place patients at increased risk during bronchoscopy?**
- Bleeding diathesis
- Hypoxia
- Unstable asthma
- Acute hypercapnia
- Hepatitis
- Lung abscess
- Superior vena cava syndrome
- Inability to cooperate with exam
- Cardiac arrhythmias
- Recent myocardial infarction
- Partial tracheal obstruction
- Uremia
- Immunosuppression
- Respiratory failure

35. **What is the most common clinical use of pulmonary function tests (PFTs)?**
PFTs help to identify and quantify abnormalities of the pulmonary system, categorized as obstructive or restrictive. The most common use of PFTs is the evaluation of obstructive airway disease. Obstruction is defined as a decrease in forced expiratory flow rates. FEV_1 (forced expiratory volume in 1 second) and FEV_1/FVC (forced vital capacity) are decreased.

KEY POINTS: THERAPEUTIC USES OF BRONCHOSCOPY 

1. Removal of mucous plugs/secretions and foreign bodies
2. Difficult endotracheal intubations
3. Local treatment of endobronchial neoplasm

36. **List the common cause of an obstructive ventilatory defect.**
- COPD (emphysema, chronic bronchitis)
- Asthma
- Cystic fibrosis
- Bronchiectasis
- Upper airway obstruction (tumors, foreign bodies, stenosis, and edema).

Virtual Hospital: Interpretation of Pulmonary Function Tests. Available at: http://www.vh.org/Providers/Simulations/Spirometry/SpirometryHome.html

37. **What lung volumes and capacities are measured with PFTs? (Fig. 10-2)**
- **Functional residual capacity (FRC):** volume of air remaining in the lungs at the end of a normal respiration
- **Tidal volume (TV):** volume drawn into the lungs during inspiration from the end-expiratory position
- **Expiratory reserve volume (ERV):** volume of air that can be forcibly exhaled after a quiet expiration has been completed (i.e., from the end-expiratory position)
- **Residual volume (RV):** volume that remains in the lungs after a maximal expiratory effort

- **Inspiratory capacity (IC):** maximal volume of air that can be inhaled from the end-expiratory position. It consists of two subdivisions: tidal volume and inspiratory reserve volume
- **Total lung capacity (TLC):** contained in the lungs at the end of a maximal inspiration
- **Vital capacity (VC):** volume of air exhaled by a maximal expiration after a maximal inspiration

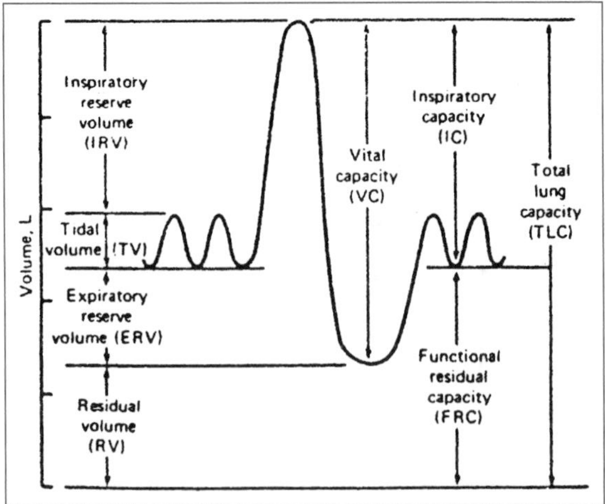

Figure 10-2. Summary of lung volumes and capacities measured with PFTs. (From Fishman AP: Pulmonary Diseases and Disorders. New York, McGraw-Hill, 1998, p 150, with permission.)

38. What PFT findings are suggestive of a restrictive ventilatory defect?

A restrictive defect implies that lung volumes are decreased with normal expiratory flow rates (decreased VC, normal expiratory flow rates, and normal maximal voluntary ventilation). Diagnosis of a restrictive process rests on a **decreased total lung capacity (TLC)**. Other supporting data may include decreased lung compliance and decreased diffusion of carbon monoxide (DL_{CO}).

39. What are the common causes of restrictive pulmonary disease?

- Interstitial lung disease (fibrosis, pneumoconiosis, edema)
- Chest wall disease (kyphoscoliosis, neuromuscular disease)
- Space-occupying lesions (tumors, cysts)
- Pleural disease (effusion, pneumothorax)
- Extrathoracic conditions (obesity, ascites, pregnancy)

40. What factors determine DL_{CO}?

The diffusing capacity of carbon monoxide (DL_{CO}) estimates the transfer of oxygen from the alveolus to the red blood cell. The diffusion is determined by the thickness of the alveolar-capillary membrane, the “driving pressure” or oxygen tension difference between the alveolus and capillary, and the area of the alveolar-capillary membrane.

41. What causes a reduced DL_{CO}?

DL_{CO} may be reduced due to decreased area for diffusion (emphysema, lung resection, anemia) or increased thickness of the membrane (pulmonary fibrosis, CHF).

42. **What patient factors suggest that preoperative PFTs may help to assess postoperative risk?**
    - Known pulmonary dysfunction
    - Current smoking, especially if > 1 pack/day
    - Chronic productive cough
    - Neuromuscular disease (amyotrophic lateral sclerosis, myasthenia)
    - Recent respiratory infection
    - Advanced age
    - Obesity
    - Thoracic cage deformity

43. **List the procedural factors that favor preoperative PFTS.**
    - Thoracic or upper abdominal operation
    - Pulmonary resection
    - Prolonged anesthesia

44. **What PFT parameters suggest increased postoperative risk?**
    - FVC < 50% predicted
    - FEV_1 < 2.0 L or M 50% predicted

45. **List the PFT paramters that indicate high postoperative risk.**
    - FVC < 1.5 L
    - FEV_1 < 1.0 L
    - MVV < 50% predicted
    - $PaCO_2$ > 45 mmHg

PLEURAL AND MEDIASTINAL DISEASE

46. **What causes pleural effusion?**
    A pleural effusion represents an increase in fluid in the pleural space, which may be due to increased hydrostatic pressure, decreased oncotic pressure, decreased pleural space pressure (lung collapse), obstruction of lymphatic drainage, or increased permeability.

47. **Explain the two basic categories of pleural effusion.**
    A **transudative** effusion classically is associated with volume overload states, such as CHF, nephrotic syndrome, and cirrhosis. An **exudative** effusion is a protein-rich effusion secondary to inflammation of the pleura or failure of lymphatic protein removal. Exudates occur in neoplasms, infection, and various collagen vascular diseases.

48. **What findings on physical examination are suggestive of a pleural effusion?**
    - Small effusions (< 500 mL) frequently have minimal findings.
    - Larger effusions: dullness to percussion, diminished breath sounds, and reduced tactile and vocal fremitus over the involved hemithorax.
    - Large effusions (> 1500 mL), with concomitant atelectasis: bronchial breath sounds, egophony, and inspiratory lag.
    - Pleural friction rubs may be noted in the early stages or near resolution.

49. **Which diagnostic tests are used to distinguish transudative from exudative pleural effusions?**
    Thoracentesis (percutaneous removal of pleural fluid) is used to obtain pleural fluid for analysis. Light's criteria are then used to distinguish transudative from exudative effusions. Other

tests that may be helpful include pleural fluid glucose, pH, cell count and WBC differential, amylase, cytology, Gram stain, special stains as clinically indicated, and culture.

50. **What are Light's criteria?**
An exudative pleural effusion meets one or more of Light's criteria, whereas a transudative meets none:
- Pleural fluid protein/serum protein ratio > 0.5
- Pleural fluid lactate dehydrogenase (LDH)/serum LDH ratio > 0.6
- Pleural fluid LDH > two thirds the upper limit of normal for serum

51. **Define pleural fluid acidodsis.**
Pleural fluid acidosis has a pH < 7.30 and a glucose level < 60 mg/dL.

KEY POINTS: CAUSES OF PLEURAL FLUID ACIDOSIS 

1. Rheumatoid effusion
2. Lupus pleuritis
3. Empyema
4. Malignancy
5. Esophageal rupture
6. TB empyema

52. **Which radiologic test should be performed in patients with suspected pleural effusion?**
A small amount of pleural fluid can be detected as the obliteration of the posterior part of the diaphragm on lateral chest x-ray. When a larger amount of fluid is present, the lateral costophrenic angle on the posteroanterior radiograph is blunted. When pleural fluid is suspected, **lateral decubitus films** should be obtained to detect free fluid gravitating to the dependent side and accumulating between the chest wall and lung.

53. **How is the amount of pleural fluid estimated?**
The amount of fluid present can be roughly quantified by measuring the distance between the inner border of the chest wall and the outer border of the lung. When this distance is < 10 mm, the amount of fluid present is small, and usually a diagnostic thoracentesis should be performed under ultrasonographic guidance.

54. **What is an empyema?**
Empyema describes the presence of infected liquid or frank pus in the pleural space. It may result from infection of a contiguous structure, instrumentation of the pleural space, or hematogenous spread of infection.

55. **What is the significance of a parapneumonic effusion?**
A parapneumonic effusion is any effusion associated with pneumonia. Up to 40% of all pneumonias may be associated with a pleural effusion. Morbidity and mortality rates are higher in pneumonias with effusion than in pneumonia alone.

56. **How is a parapneumonic effusion treated?**
Most effusions resolve without specific intervention. However, the effusion may be complicated and require tube thoracotomy (chest tube) or surgical decortication. In addition to protein and LDH analysis, pleural fluid pH, Gram stain/culture, and glucose may help to classify parapneumonic effusions and determine an appropriate treatment plan.

57. **In how many patients with exudative effusion is a definitive diagnosis never made?**
20%.

58. **What is the next step if routine pleural fluid analysis is nondiagnostic?**
Closed-needle biopsy of the parietal pleura in patients with a suspected neoplasm or TB pleural effusion may establish the diagnosis. Although the overall yield from pleural fluid cytology is slightly higher, needle biopsy of the pleura is positive in 40% of patients with malignant pleural disease. When TB is suspected, a portion of the biopsy should be cultured. The initial biopsy is positive for granuloma in 50–80% of patients. The combined results of pleural fluid culture and biopsy are diagnostic in 90% for TB.

59. **What other diagnostic procedures are available?**
- **Bronchoscopy,** if the patient has a parenchymal abnormality on chest x-ray or CT scan.
- **Thoracoscopy,** which allows direct visualization of the pleural surface, and guided or open pleural biopsy.

60. **Which population of patients is most likely to experience a primary spontaneous pneumothorax?**
Primary spontaneous pneumothorax, occurring in patients with no history of pulmonary disease, likely results from spontaneous rupture of a subpleural emphysematous bleb. It has a peak incidence at 20–30 years of age, is more common in smokers and exsmokers, has a 4:1 male-to-female ratio, and is seen most often in tall, thin people.

61. **In which patients is a secondary spontaneous pneumothorax most often seen?**
Secondary spontaneous pneumothorax, occurring in patients with underlying pulmonary disease, is most often seen with COPD.

62. **Summarize the treatment for both primary and secondary spontaneous pneumothorax.**
Recurrence rates for both primary and secondary spontaneous pneumothorax range are common. Therefore, repeated spontaneous pneumothorax should be treated by pleurodesis or surgical intervention (including parietal pleurectomy).

63. **In which patients should spontaneous pneumothorax be included in the differential diagnosis?**
Spontaneous pneumothorax, although not common, should be considered in any patient with underlying lung disease and unexplained clinical decompensation.

64. **What underlying lung diseases may cause pneumothorax?**
Causes of pneumothorax secondary to underlying lung disease include COPD, asthma, lung abscess, adult respiratory distress syndrome (ARDS), AIDS/*Pneumocystis carinii* pneumonia (PCP), neoplasm, Marfan's syndrome, sarcoidosis, cystic fibrosis, tuberculosis, and eosinophilic granuloma.

65. **Summarize the other possible causes of pneumothorax.**
Pneumothorax may be iatrogenic (after thoracentesis or transbronchial biopsy or secondary to barotrauma) or traumatic. Catamenial pneumothorax is rare and occurs in women at the time of menstruation.

66. **How does pneumothorax present clinically?**
Spontaneous pneumothorax usually occurs at rest. Ipsilateral pleuritic chest pain and acute dyspnea are the most common complaints. Findings on physical exam (which may be subtle with small pneumothoraces) include:

- Sinus tachycardia
- Reduced breath sounds
- Reduced tactile fremitus
- Hyperresonance
- Reduced chest wall excursion on the ipsilateral side

Pneumothorax and Pneumomediastinum. Available at: http://www.sbu.ac.uk~dirt/museum/p6–73.html.

67. **What is a tension pneumothorax?**
Tension pneumothorax is due to unidirectional flow of air into the pleural space from which it cannot escape. It develops when intrapleural pressure > atmospheric pressure during expiration, causing collapse of the involved lung, shift of the mediastinum, and potentially acute deterioration in cardiopulmonary status requiring prompt relief of the positive pleural pressure.

KEY POINTS: TENSION PNEUMOTHORAX

1. Tension pneumothorax is a medical emergency.
2. It should be suspected in any patient with sudden, unexplained deterioration in cardiopulmonary status or a history of pneumothorax.
3. It also should be suspected after a procedure known to cause pneumothorax and in patients receiving mechanical ventilation
4. Tension pneumothorax also may occur during CPR, if it is difficult to ventilate the patient or if electromechanical dissociation is present.

68. **List the physical findings that suggest tension pneumothorax.**
    - Signs of a significant pneumothorax (no tactile fremitus, markedly decreased or absent breath sounds, and hyperresonance)
    - Cardiopulmonary compromise (rapid pulse, hypotension, cyanosis, electromechanical dissociation)
    - Possibly a shift of the trachea away from the involved side

69. **Name the most common masses found in each compartment of the mediastinum.**
    - **Anterior mediastinum:** thymoma, germ cell tumors (teratoma), lymphoma, thyroid or parathyroid tumors.
    - **Middle mediastinum:** lymphoma, granulomatous disease, development cysts, vascular masses and enlargements, diaphragmatic hernia.
    - **Posterior mediastinum:** neurogenic tumors, esophageal lesions, diaphragmatic hernia (Fig. 10-3).

70. **What is Hamman's sign?**
Mediastinal emphysema or pneumomediastinum can be detected on auscultation by the presence of a mediastinal "crunch" coinciding with cardiac systole and diastole. It is named after American physician Louis Hamman (1877–1946).

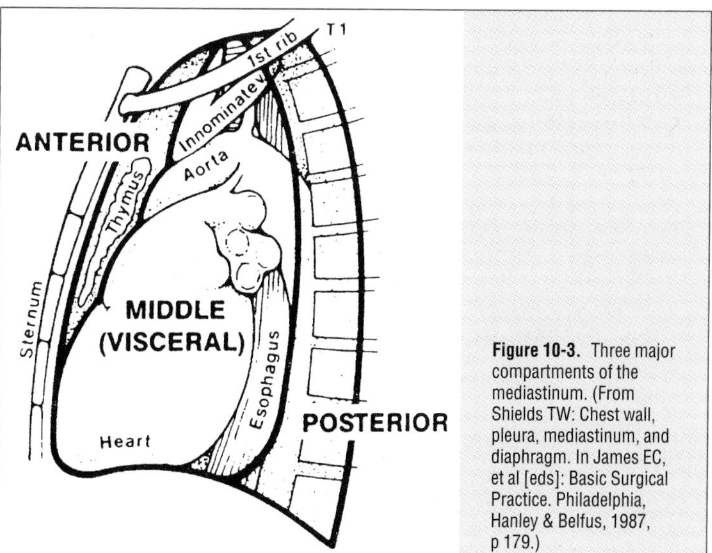

Figure 10-3. Three major compartments of the mediastinum. (From Shields TW: Chest wall, pleura, mediastinum, and diaphragm. In James EC, et al [eds]: Basic Surgical Practice. Philadelphia, Hanley & Belfus, 1987, p 179.)

PULMONARY INFECTIONS

71. Define community-acquired pneumonia (CAP).
CAP is defined as pneumonia contracted in the community rather than in the hospital setting.

72. What is the most common cause of CAP?
The most common cause of CAP is *Pneumococcus* spp., which account for up to 55% of cases requiring hospitalization. Other causes include *Mycoplasma* and *Legionella* spp., *Haemophilus influenzae*, atypical organisms, and viruses. However, the cause and incidence of CAP vary depending on the community, patient age, and comorbidities.

MEDLINEplus: Pneumonia. Available at: http://www.nlm.nih.gov/medlineplus/pneumonia.html.

73. What clinical manifestations may help to diagnose pneumonia?
- **History:** Fever, cough (productive versus nonproductive), dyspnea, pleuritic pain, abdominal pain, malaise
- **Physical examination:** Fever, tachycardia, cyanosis (with severe pneumonia), tachypnea
- **Auscultation:** Crackles (rales), pectoriloquy, egophony, dullness to percussion (pleural effusion)

74. What laboratory tests and imaging modalities may help to diagnose pneumonia?
- **Laboratory tests:** sputum Gram stain and culture, WBC count (elevated, normal, low)
- **Chest x-ray** showing consolidation/infiltrate (bilateral?) and/or pleural effusion
- **Other evaluations:** oxygen saturation, possibly arterial blood gas

75. What factors predispose to the development of pneumococcal pneumonia?
- Severe underlying illness such as multiple myeloma, lymphoma, and leukemia
- Cirrhosis and renal failure

- Poorly controlled diabetes mellitus
- Sickle cell anemia
- Splenectomy
- Advanced age

Community-Acquired Pneumonia. Interactive Guidelines. Available at: www.vh.org/Providers/ClinGuide/CAP/CapHome.html.

76. Give the mortality rate associated with pneumococcal pneumonia.

The mortality rate associated with pneumococcal pneumonia ranges from 6% to 19% in hospitalized patients without complications. For patients with bacteremic disease the mortality rate approaches 25%.

77. List the factors that may help identify patients at risk for adverse outcome or complications secondary to pneumococcal pneumonia.

- Bacteremia
- Older age
- Immunodeficiency or AIDS
- Preexisting lung disease
- Nosocomial infection
- Initial body temperature < 38°

78. List the possible complications of pneumococcal pneumonia.

- Bacteremic seeding of other sites
- Parapneumonic effusion or empyema
- Necrotizing pneumonia
- Lung abcess

Marfin AA, Sporrer J, Moore PS, Siefkin AD: Risk factors for the adverse outcome in persons with pneumococcal pneumonia. Chest 107(20):457–462, 1995.

79. Who should receive the pneumococcal vaccine, and is revaccination necessary?

- People older than 65 years.
- People aged 2–64 years with cardiopulmonary disease, diabetes, alcoholism, chronic liver disease, CSF leaks, cochlear implant, or residence in special environments or chronic care facility.
- Immunocompromised people older than 2 years: HIV, malignancy, splenectomy, immunosuppressive treatment, transplant.

Centers for Disease Control and Prevention: MMWR 51:931, 2002.

80. For which groups is revaccination necessary?

- People older than 65 years: revaccinate if first vaccine was given 5 or more years ago and the person was younger than 65 at the time.
- People aged 2–64 years: no revaccination recommended.
- Immunocompromised people older than 2 years: revaccinate if 5 or more years have elapsed; if the person was 10 years old or younger when the initial vaccine was given, consider revaccination at 3 years.

81. Which risk factors predispose to the development of nosocomial pneumonia?

- Increased severity of underlying illness
- Previous hospitalization
- Indwelling urethral catheters
- Presence of intravascular catheters or nasogastric tube
- Intubation (especially prolonged intubation, reintubation)

- Recent thoracic or upper abdominal surgery
- Use of broad-spectrum antibiotics (increased risk of superinfection)
- H_2 blocker or antacids (?)
- Age > 70 years

82. Define nosocomial pneumonia. How serious a problem is it?
Nosocomial pneumonia is acquired > 48 hours after admission to the hospital. It is the number one cause of nosocomial mortality. The mortality rate remains at 30–50% despite antimicrobial therapy. The incidence of infections caused by resistant organisms is increasing.

83. Which organisms most commonly cause nosocomial pneumonia?
Nosocomial pneumonia is caused most commonly by gram-negative organisms, including *Pseudomonas aeruginosa, Klebsiella pneumoniae, Escherichia coli,* and *Enterobacter* spp. *Staphylococcus aureus*, including methicillin-resistant organisms, *Streptococcus pneumoniae*, anaerobes, *Candida* spp., enterococci, and polymicrobial infections are also common. Overall, *Pseudomonas* and *S. aureus* are most common.

84. Describe the radiologic manifestations of PCP.
PCP is the most common AIDS-defining illness and should be suspected in the appropriate clinical setting. The most common radiologic manifestation of PCP is bilateral interstitial or alveolar infiltrates. Other presentations include pneumothorax, cysts, nodules, lobar infiltrates, or pleural effusion.

85. What symptoms are associated with tuberculosis (TB)?
The symptoms associated with TB are often nonspecific. Common complaints include productive cough, weight loss, weakness, anorexia, night sweats, and generalized malaise. These nonspecific symptoms are most often subacute or chronic (> 8 wk) in duration. Both fever, present in one-third to one half of the patients, and hemoptysis correlate with cavitary disease and positive sputum smears.

86. Describe the common anatomic distribution of chest x-ray changes in postprimary (reactivation) TB.
- Apical and posterior segments of the upper lobes (85%). A lesion found only in the anterior segment suggests a diagnosis other than TB (e.g., malignancy).
- Superior segments of the lower lobe (10%).
- Remainder of the lower lobe (< 7%).
- The right lung is more often affected than the left.

87. Which diseases may be associated with infiltrates in the upper lobes?
The differential diagnosis of upper lobe infiltrates with or without cavitation includes atypical mycobacterial infections, silicosis, pneumonia, malignancy, pulmonary infarct, ankylosing spondylitis, actinomycosis, fungal infections, and nocardial infection.

88. What specific factors are associated with an increased risk for developing TB?
Increased risk for developing TB is related to increased susceptibility to acquire the disease (silicosis, chronic renal failure, alcoholism, malignancy, diabetes mellitus, weight loss, immunosuppressive therapy, HIV infection, gastrectomy) or high risk for exposure (foreign birth, IV drug users, low socioeconomic status, prisoners, elderly patients in nursing home, hospital employees/physicians).

Joint Statement of the American Thoracic Society and the Centers for Disease Control and Prevention: Targeted tuberculin testing and treatment of latent tuberculosis infection. Am J Respir Crit Care Med 161(4 Pt 2):S221–S247, 2000.

89. What clinical problems are associated with the treatment of TB?

- **Drug resistance:** Primary resistance (resistant organisms in the initial infection), most common for isoniazid (INH), is increasing in the U.S. Resistance to both INH and rifampin may be seen. Resistance varies by location, ethnic background, and origin of birth. Secondary drug resistance develops during treatment.
- **Noncompliance:** Multiple drug regimens given over an extended period (≥ 6 months) may lead to noncompliance. Therefore, directly observed therapy (DOT) is highly recommended.
- **Medication side effects:** Hepatotoxicity, the most important side effect, is seen in 2–5% of patients, most frequently occurring with INH therapy. All patients should be fully informed of potential complications of therapy.

90. How do you monitor for adverse drug reactions during TB therapy?

Before therapy is started, the following tests should be performed: baseline liver function tests (INH, rifampin, PZA); CBC with platelets (ethambutol), blood urea nitrogen, creatinine, and calcium (INH, rifampin); uric acid (PZA, ethambutol); and visual acuity (retrobulbar optic neuritis, ethambutol). Patients receiving INH should be questioned monthly about potential symptoms, including peripheral neuropathy.

91. What special consideration applies to patients with liver disease or alcoholism?

For persons with liver disease/alcoholism or age > 35 years, liver function tests should be performed periodically and symptoms monitored.

92. Why is multidrug therapy used in the treatment of TB?

Early work established the large numbers of organisms found in tuberculous cavities, with spontaneous resistance developing in 1 in 100,000–1,000,000 organisms. Therefore, single-drug therapy leads to the selection of resistant organisms and treatment failure.

93. What are the guidelines for determining a positive tuberculin skin test reaction?

See Table 10-4.

94. Which infectious agents can mimic TB?

Fungal infections, especially histoplasmosis and coccidioidomycosis, and *Nocardia* spp. (gram-positive, aerobic, partially acid-fast organisms).

95. With what is nocardiosis associated? How is it treated?

Nocardiosis is most commonly associated with underlying disease, such as pulmonary alveolar proteinosis. Most strains are susceptible to sulfonamides.

96. What are the mechanisms of hemorrhage from the site of previous pulmonary TB?

- Reactivation of TB
- Bronchiectasis
- "Scar carcinoma"
- Vessel erosion by a broncholith (calcified lymph node)
- Fungal infection (usually aspergillosis) in the cavity
- Rasmussen's aneurysm (terminal pulmonary artery)

TABLE 10-4. GUIDELINES FOR DETERMINING A POSITIVE TUBERCULIN SKIN TEST REACTION

Induration ≥ 5 mm	Induration ≥ 10 mm	Induration ≥ 15 mm
HIV-positive Recent contacts of TB case Chest x-ray changes consistent with old TB Organ transplant or immunosuppressed	Recent arrivals (< 5 yr) from high-prevalence countries IV drug users Residents/employees of high-risk congregate settings: prisons, jails, nursing homes, homeless shelters Mycobacteriology lab personnel High-risk clinical conditions: silicosis, diabetes, chronic renal failure, some hematologic malignancies (leukemia, lymphoma), specific malignancies (lung, head and neck), weight loss 10% ideal weight	No risk

From American Thoracic Society: Diagnostic standards and classification of tuberculosis in adults and children. Am J Respir Crit Care Med 161:1376–1395, 2000, with permission.

KEY POINTS: PRINCIPLES FOR PHARMACOLOGIC MANAGEMENT OF TB

1. Provide the safest, most effective therapy in the shortest time.
2. Use two or more drugs to which the organism is susceptible.
3. Never add a single drug to a failing regimen.
4. Consider directly observed therapy for all patients or monitor compliance closely.
5. Children should be treated in the same way as adults, with appropriate dosage adjustments.
6. Extrapulmonary TB should be treated according to the principles and drug regimens for pulmonary TB.
7. The major determinant of outcome is patient compliance.

NEOPLASTIC DISEASE

97. **How does lung cancer rank in cancer-related deaths?**
Lung cancer is the leading cause of cancer deaths for both men and women in the United States, with over 170,00 deaths per year. Lung cancer now exceeds breast cancer in women,

who develop lung cancer at an earlier age and with fewer years of smoking. From 1950 to 1995, there was a 500% increase in women. In 1999, over 60,000 women died of lung cancer.

98. **What is the survival rate for patients with lung cancer?**
Fewer than 15% of patients survive for 5 years and over 85% present with advanced disease.

99. **What are the major risk factors for lung cancer?**
Cigarette smoking accounts for over 80% of risk, with environmental exposures and genetic factors contributing to the rest. All major cell types have been associated with cigarette smoking.

100. **Which chest x-ray and clinical criteria can help distinguish between a benign and malignant pulmonary nodule?**
A pulmonary nodule can be described as a rounded lesion measuring < 3 cm at maximal diameter on a chest x-ray. Although no single characteristic or group of characteristics definitely predicts the nature of a solitary pulmonary nodule, the following factors favor a malignant process:
- Age > 40 years
- History of smoking
- Progressive growth
- Absence of calcification
- Size > 3 cm
- Irregular borders

Lung Tumors: A Multiidisciplinary Data Base: Risk of Malignancy in a Solitary Pulmonary Nodule. Available at: http://www.vh.org/cgi-bin/noduletool.cgi.

101. **What are the most common histologic types of lung cancer?**
- Non-small cell cancer (70%)
- Squamous cell (25–30%)
- Adenocarcinoma (30–35%)
- Bronchoalveolar cell (10–15%)
- Large cell undifferentiated (10–15%)
- Small cell lung cancer (20–25%)

102. **Where is lung cancer most likely to develop?**
Lung cancer occurs lightly more frequently in the right lung, upper lobes, and anterior segment. Squamous and small cell carcinomas occur more commonly in a central location, whereas adenocarcinoma usually develops more peripherally.

103. **What complications are associated with lung cancer?**
- Pancoast's tumor (squamous cell), commonly associated with Horner's syndrome
- Superior vena cava syndrome (non-small cell), associated with facial swelling, dilated neck and chest wall veins, confusion
- Central airway obstruction (sqaumous cell), associated with flattened limbs of the flow-volume on PFTs

104. **Which paraneoplastic syndromes are associated with lung cancer?**
- Syndrome of inappropriate antidiuretic hormone (SIADH), associated with small cell cancer and hyponatremia
- Hypercalcemia, associated with squamous cell cancer, lethargy, and confusion
- Eaton-Lambert syndrome (ELS), associated with small cell cancer and fatigability
- Increased adrenocorticotropic hormone (ACTH), associated with small cell cancer and Cushing's syndrome
- Digital clubbing, associated with non-small cell cancer, pain, and swelling

105. **Describe the symptoms and location of a Pancoast tumor.**
First described in 1932 by Henry Khunrath Pancoast, a Philadelphia radiologist, this tumor is located in the extreme apex of the upper lobe of the lung and represents approximately 4% of all

lung cancers. Although the tumor may be of various cell types, the most common is squamous cell carcinoma. Pancoast's original criteria: arm/shoulder pain, Horner's syndrome, destruction of bone, and atrophy of the hand muscles.

106. List the most common *pulmonary* complications of lung cancer.
Atelectasis, postobstructive pneumonia secondary to endobronchial obstruction, hemoptysis, pleural effusion, and respiratory failure are most frequent. Symptoms may include cough, wheezing, stridor, chest pain, and hemoptysis.

107. What is Eaton-Lambert syndrome (ELS)?
ELS is a paraneoplastic myopathy; that is, it is associated with malignancy but not secondary to the direct effects of the tumor or its metastases. ELS is most often seen with small cell carcinoma.

108. How is ELS differentiated from myasthenia gravis (MG)?
Clinically, ELS resembles MG, but careful neurologic and electromyographic (EMG) examination can distinguish between the two. Unlike MG:

- ELS involves proximal muscle groups
- ELS has little response to neostigmine challenge
- ELS demonstrates increased muscular response/strength to repetitive stimulation

109. Is hypertrophic pulmonary osteoarthropathy (HPO), a well-recognized paraneoplastic syndrome, a contraindication to surgical resection of lung cancer?
No. Removal of lung cancer or treatment results in regression in the clinical manifestations of HPO. The cause is unknown. HPO is seen more often in squamous cell and adenocarcinoma.

110. Describe the symptoms and signs of HPO.
Patients complain of a deep burning pain, usually in the distal extremity. Other symptoms usually include clubbing of the fingers and/or toes, periostitis of the long bones, and occasionally polyarthritis. The most commonly involved bones are the tibia, fibula, humerus, radius, and ulna. The x-ray of the extremity reveals subperiosteal new bone formation.

111. Which tumors commonly metastasize to the lung?

- Lung cancer
- Colorectal cancer
- Thyroid cancer
- Ovarian cancer
- Pancreatic/hepatic
- Head and neck
- Genitourinary (renal, prostate, bladder)
- Breast cancer
- Testicular cancer
- Melanoma
- Gastric
- Sarcoma

112. With which cancers are endobronchial metastases most common?
Renal cell carcinoma, melanoma, and breast carcinoma.

PULMONARY VASCULAR DISEASE

113. What are the predisposing factors for the development of venous thromboembolism (VTE)?
Risk factors for the development of VTE include age > 40, prior VTE, prolonged anesthesia (> 30 min), prolonged immobilization, CVA, CHF, cancer, fracture of the pelvis, hip, or tibia, pregancy and postpartum, estrogen-containing medications, obesity, inflammatory bowel disease, and genetic or aquired thrombophilia (lupus anticoagulant, factor V Leiden,

anticardiolipin antibody syndrome, protein S or C deficiency, antithrombin III deficiency, prothrombin G20210A mutation).

Fedullo PF, Tapson VF: Clinical practice. The evaluation of suspected pulmonary embolism. N Engl J Med 349:1247–1256, 2003.

114. What is the mortality rate for pulmonary embolism (PE)?
PEs occur in over 600,000 people per year, resulting in over 100,000–200,000 deaths. Thirty percent are diagnosed antemortem.

115. Summarize the chest x-ray findings associated with PE.
Often the interpretation of the chest x-ray of patients with acute PE is "normal," although subtle nonspecific abnormalities are generally found. Examples include differences in diameters of vessels that should be similar in size, abrupt cut-off of a vessel followed distally, increased radiolucency in some areas, regional oligemia (Westermark's sign), a peripheral wedge-shaped density over the diaphragm (Hampton's hump), or an enlarged right descending pulmonary artery (Palla's sign).

116. How common is pulmonary infarction?
Approximately 1 in 10 PEs results in pulmonary infarction.

117. What findings are associated with pulmonary infarction?
Pleuritic chest pain, hemoptysis, and low-grade fever are present when infarction has occurred. Pulmonary infarction is classically described as a wedge-shaped infiltrate that abuts the pleura (Hampton's hump). It often is associated with a small pleural effusion that is usually exudative and may be hemorrhagic.

118. What is the starting point for the diagnosis of PE?
It is impossible to diagnose PE on clinical grounds alone; therefore, further testing is needed. The V/Q scan is often the starting point of the evaluation. Although highly sensitive, it is nonspecific, and interpretation may be difficult in patients with underlying pulmonary disease.

119. What other tests help to establish the diagnosis of PE?
Helical CT, although with fairly wide ranges of sensitivity and specificity, when coupled with other less invasive testing, may prove to be a safe strategy. Pulmonary angiography is still the gold standard to demonstrate PE, but the procedure is not without risk and is usually reserved for unstable patients, when thrombolysis is considered, or when less invasive tests (guided by the clinical situation) are nondiagnostic. The role of D-dimers is currently being evaluated.

120. What major complications may be associated with pulmonary angiography?
Complications may include death (< 0.5%), cardiac perforation, arrhythmias, contrast reaction, renal insufficiency secondary to dye, and bleeding. Overall, the risk of major complications is 4% and appears to be the highest in the most critically ill patients.

American Thoracic Society: The diagnostic approach to acute venous thromboembolism. Am J Respir Crit Care Med 160:1043–1066, 1999.

121. Discuss the role of D-dimers in the evaluation of suspected PE.
The enzyme-linked immunosorbent assay (ELISA) has a high negative predictive value and is sensitive for thrombosis, but lacks specificity. Recent data for the use of rapid D-dimer assays as an exclusionary test, in combination with a low pretest probability/low-probability VQ or helical CT, are encouraging.

Kelly J, Rudd A, Lewis RG, Hunt BJ: Plasma D-dimers in the diagnosis of venous thromboembolism. Arch Intern Med 162:747–756, 2002.

122. Discuss the causes of nonthrombotic PE.
The pulmonary vasculature filters the venous circulation and is exposed to nonthrombotic emboli. Fat embolism usually follows bone trauma or fracture, and symptoms begin 12–36 hours after the event. Amniotic fluid embolism results from entrance of amniotic fluid into the venous circulation, with consequent shock and disseminated intravascular coagulation (DIC). Other causes include air, tumor, and trophoblast.

123. What are the clinical manifestations of fat emoblism?
Clinical manifestations include altered mental status, respiratory decompensation, anemia, thrombocytopenia, and petechiae.

124. List the potential risk factors for the development of primary pulmonary hypertension (PPH)?
Although most cases are sporadic, PPH may be associated with: familial factors (<10%, autosomal dominant with incomplete penetration), anorectic drug use, chronic illicit drug use (cocaine, amphetamines), portal hypertension, and HIV.

OBSTRUCTIVE LUNG DISEASE

125. What causes chronic obstructive pulmonary disease (COPD)?
Cigarette smoking has a primary role in most cases of COPD. Not all smokers develop COPD, however, even those with a high-dose history. Pulmonary function declines normally with aging, and patients who experience a rate of loss that significantly exceeds the norm are classified as having COPD.

126. How serious a problem is COPD?
COPD is the fourth leading cause of death in the United States and is the only major chronic disease for which the mortality is increasing.

American Lung Association. COPD Fact Sheet. Available at: http://www.lungusa.org/diease/copd_factsheet.html.

127. Define chronic bronchitis.
Chronic bronchitis is defined clinically by symptoms, which include a productive cough on most mornings for ≥ 3 consecutive months for ≥ 2 or consecutive years.

128. How does emphysema differ from chronic bronchitis?
Unlike chronic bronchitis, which is described in terms of symptoms, emphysema is an anatomic/structural term. Emphysema is an abnormal enlargement of air-containing space distal to the terminal bronchioles accompanied by destruction of alveolar tissue. Most patients with COPD have some characteristics of both processes.

129. Describe the radiographic changes are associated with COPD.
The chest x-ray findings are secondary to overdistention of the lungs. Examples include a low, flat diaphragm; increased retrosternal airspace (on lateral x-ray); and an elongated, narrow heart shadow (Fig. 10-4). Bullae, which appear as rounded radiolucent areas, are occasionally seen and reflect emphysematous changes.

130. What is the prognosis of severe COPD? How is the severity staged?
Prognosis is based on age, severity of hypoxemia, presence of hypercapnia, and severity of airflow obstruction (FEV_1). Of these, the most relevant is the FEV_1. The severity of COPD is staged on the basis of airflow obstruction:

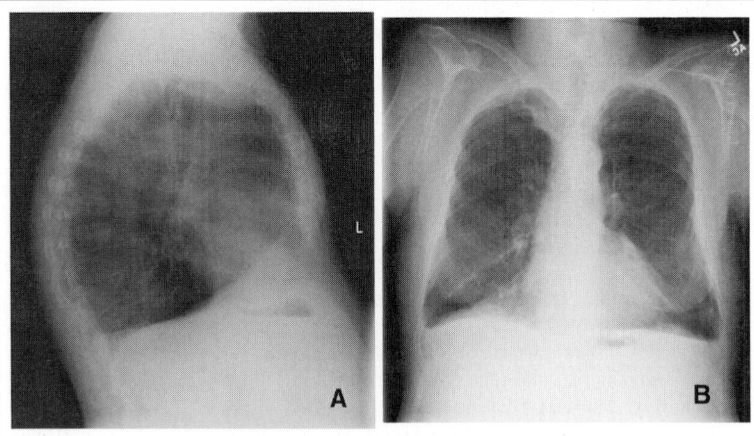

Figure 10-4. Lateral (A) and posteroanterior (B) radiographs of a patient with COPD.

Stage	**Characteristics**
0: At risk	Normal spirometry Chronic symptoms (cough, sputum)
I: Mild	$FEV_1 \geq 80\%$ predicted, with or without symptoms
II: Moderate	FEV_1 50–80% predicted; with or without symptoms
III: Severe	FEV_1 30–50% predicted, with or without symptoms
IV: Very severe	$FEV_1/FVC < 70\%$; FEV1 < 30% predicted or $FEV_1 < 50\%$ plus respiratory failure ($PaO_2 < 60$) or signs of right heart failure

Fabbri LM: GOLD Guidelines, Executive Summary. Eur Respir J 22:1–2, 2003.
Global Initiative for Obstructive Lung Disease (GOLD): http://www.goldcopd.com.
Global Initiative For Obstructive Lung Disease (GOLD): www.goldcopd.com.

131. When should antibiotics be given to patients with an acute exacerbation of COPD?

Antibiotics are recommended if two or three of the following are present: increasing dyspnea, increased sputum production, and/or purulent sputum.

132. Summarize the three types of acute exacerbations in patients with COPD.

- **Type 1:** increases in dyspnea, sputum volume, and sputum purulence (severe)
- **Type 2:** two of the above three symptoms (moderate)
- **Type 3:** one of the above three symptoms (mild) and at least one of the following: URI within 5 days, fever without other cause, increased wheezing, increased cough, and increased respiratory rate or heart rate increased by 20% or more.

Anthonisen NR, Manfreda J, Warren CP, et al: Antibiotic therapy in exacerbations of chronic obstructive pulmonary disease. Ann Intern Med 106:196–204, 1987.

133. What are the poor prognostic signs in an acute exacerbation of asthma?

- Pulse rate > 100/min
- Pulsus paradoxus > 10 mmHg
- PEFR < 16% of predicted
- $PaCO_2 > 45$ mmHg

- Retraction of sternocleidomastoid muscles
- FEV_1 < 600 mL before treatment or FEV_1 < 1600 mL after treatment

American Lung Association (ALA): Asthma Information Center. Available at: http:// www. lungusa.org/asthma

134. What is Samter's syndrome?
Approximately 4–20% of asthmatics are sensitive to aspirin. Of aspirin-sensitive patients, 90% have associated nasal polyposis and rhinosinusitis. This triad is known as Samter's syndrome.

135. What is bronchiectasis?
It is a fixed dilatation of bronchi due to destructive changes in the elastic and muscular layers of the bronchial wall. The hallmark of bronchiectasis is overproduction of sputum. It was a more common disease before the advent of appropriate antibiotic therapy for pulmonary infection.

136. What conditions predispose to bronchiectasis?
Conditions predisposing to bronchiectasis include severe inflammation (including infections), congenital syndromes (e.g., cystic fibrosis [CF], Kartagener's syndrome, Young's syndrome), airway obstruction, traction of the airways (e.g., fibrosis, TB, radiation), immune deficiencies, and anatomic malformations.

137. Describe the presentation of bronchiectasis.
Patients usually present with a chronic cough productive of large quantities of foul, often blood-tinged sputum. High-resolution CT scan has replaced bronchography as the gold standard for diagnosis.

Barker AF. Bronchiectasis.N Engl J Med 346: 1383–1393, 2002.

138. How common is CF?
CF is the most common genetic disease in the US. Its incidence is 2000–3000 annually.

139. What causes CF?
The CF gene is located on the long arm of chromosome 7 and encodes for a protein that acts as a regulated chloride channel. This abnormal ion transport leads to thick secretions in many organs, resulting in the clinical findings of CF, as well as the elevated sweat choride used in diagnosis.

140. How is CF diagnosed?
Most simply, CF is diagnosed based on clinical history and an abnormal sweat chloride test (> 60 mEq/dL) on at least two occasions.

INTERSTITIAL LUNG DISEASE

141. Which interstitial lung diseases (ILDs) are most likely associated with pneumothorax?
Eosinophilic granuloma, neurofibromatosis, lymphangioleiomyomatosis, and tuberous sclerosis.

142. Which pulmonary syndromes are associated with rheumatoid arthritis (RA)?
RA may be associated with ILD. The condition is more common in men, rarely precedes joint disease, and may be associated with cutaneous nodules. The most common pulmonary complication is pleural effusion. Other conditions include pulmonary vasculitis, parenchymal nodules, and bronchiolitis obliterans.

143. What is Caplan's syndrome?
Caplan's syndrome (rheumatoid pneumoconiosis) refers to the association of RA and nodules on chest x-ray in patients with coalworker's pneumoconiosis. This syndrome has been associated with the risk for pneumothorax.

144. How prevalent is sarcoidosis?
Sarcoidosis is a multisystem disorder of unknown etiology that has a prevalence of approximately 20 cases/100,000 population. Although it may occur at any age, patients are usually 20–40 years of age. Women have a slightly higher prevalence, and in the U.S. sarcoidosis is more common in blacks than whites (10:1 ratio).

145. Which organs are involved in sarcoidosis?
Many organs may be involved, but the lung is involved most frequently (> 90% of cases).

146. How is sarcoidosis diagnosed?
Sarcoidosis is a diagnosis of exclusion. The diagnosis rests on the combination of history, radiographic, and histologic findings. The typical pathologic finding is noncaseating granuloma.

KEY POINTS: CONDITIONS THAT MAY BE ASSOCIATED WITH NONCASEATING GRANULOMAS

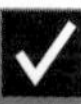

1. Sarcoidosis
2. Mycobacterial and fungal disease
3. Extrinsic allergic alveolitis
4. GI diseases (celiac disease, Crohn's disease, Whipple's disease)
5. Pneumoconiosis
6. Drug reaction
7. Foreign body reaction
8. Syphilis
9. Berylliosis

147. What is Goodpasture's syndrome?
Goodpasture's syndrome usually refers to a combination of glomerulonephritis and diffuse pulmonary hemorrhage associated with development of antiglomerular basement membrane (anti-GBM) antibodies and, less frequently, antipulmonary basement membrane antibodies. Immunofluorescent staining of tissue reveals a linear pattern of deposition of IgG.

148. Who gets Goodpasture's syndrome?
Goodpasture's syndrome is predominantly a disease of young adults (mean age, 21 years) and is more common in males.

149. Summarize the differential diagnosis of Goodpasture's syndrome.
The differential diagnosis includes other pulmonary-renal syndromes, including vasculitis, Wegener's granulomatosis, polyarteritis nodosa, uremia with pulmonary edema, and immune complex disease (e.g., systemic lupus erythematosus).

ACUTE RESPIRATORY FAILURE

150. **Can cardiogenic pulmonary edema be distinguished from noncardiogenic pulmonary edema based on clinical and radiographic findings?**
No. The two conditions can be differentiated by measurement of the pulmonary capillary wedge pressure (PCWP), which reflects left ventricular (LV) filling pressures (normally 6–12 mmHg). The PCWP is elevated in cardiogenic pulmonary edema, reflecting the elevated LV filling pressures, but it is normal in acute respiratory distress syndrome (ARDS), because LV filing pressures are normal (the defect resulting in increased interstitial fluid is at the alveolar-capillary membrane). The most common causes are sepsis, trauma, aspiration, and pneumonia.

151. **List the indications for initiation of mechanical ventilation.**
The need for ventilatory support should be based on a bedside assessment of impairment. Indications include:
- Loss of ventilatory reserve: increased respiratory rate (> 35), increased CO_2 (>10 mmHg), decreased tidal volume (< 5 mL/kg), decreased vital capacity (< 10 mL/kg), decreased (< 10 L/min), decreased negative inspiratory force (<–25 cmH_2O)
- Refractory hypoxemia

Slutsky AS: Mechanical ventilation. American College of Chest Physicians' Consensus Conference. Chest 104:1833, 1993.

ENVIRONMENTAL LUNG DISEASE

152. **Define pneumoconiosis.**
The term is derived from the Greek words *pneumo* (lung) and *konis* (dust). It currently refers to an accumulation of inorganic dust in the lungs and the consequences of the tissue's response to the presence of the dust. The most common pneumoconioses are silicosis, asbestosis, and coalworker's pneumoconiosis (black lung).

153. **What clinical manifestations are associated with asbestos exposure?**
Asbestosis (bibasilar-predominant fibrosis), pleural plaques, pleural effusions, mesothelioma, and malignancies (marked increase risk for lung cancer in smokers).

APNEA SYNDROMES

154. **How do you differentiate central apnea and obstructive sleep apnea?**
Apnea refers to a pause in respiration for more than 10 seconds and is seen in both central sleep apnea (CSA) and obstructive sleep apnea (OSA). They are differentiated by a lack of respiratory effort in CSA versus continued but ineffective respiratory effort in OSA. Hypopnea is defined as a reduction in airflow of at least 50% that results in a decrease in arterial saturation of 4% or more (due to partial airway obstruction).

155. **What is the respiratory distress index (RDI)?**
The number of apneas and hypopneas/hour is termed the respiratory distress index. RDI helps to determine the severity of OSA.

156. **List the clinical characteristics of a patient with OSA.**

Obesity (common)	Sexual dysfunction
Daytime hypersomnia	Morning headache

Rarely awaken during sleep	Nocturnal enuresis
Loud snoring	Intellectual deterioration

BIBLIOGRAPHY

1. Baum GL, Wolinsky E (eds): Textbook of Pulmonary Diseases, 7th ed. Boston, Little, Brown, 2001.
2. Bone RC, et al (eds): Pulmonary and Critical Care Medicine. St. Louis, Mosby, 1997.
3. Fishman AP: Pulmonary Diseases and Disorders, 4th ed. New York, McGraw-Hill, 2002.
4. Muray JF, Nadel JA (eds): Textbook of Respiratory Medicine, 3rd ed. Philadelphia, W.B. Saunders, 2003.
5. Parsons PE, Heffner JR (eds): Pulmonary/Respiratory Therapy Secrets. Philadelphia, Hanley & Belfus, 1997.

RHEUMATOLOGY

Richard A. Rubin, M.D.

CHAPTER 11

The wolf, I'm afraid, is inside tearing up the place.
Flannery O'Connor (1925–1964)
Novelist, sufferer from lupus erythematosus (letter)

Screw up the vise as tightly as possible—you have rheumatism; give it another turn, and that is gout.
Anonymous

1. **Give an operational definition for rheumatic diseases.**
Rheumatic diseases are syndromes of pain and/or inflammation in articular or periarticular tissues.

2. **What is undifferentiated connective tissue disease (UCTD)?**
An exact diagnosis of a rheumatic disease is not always possible at initial presentation. All of the clinical manifestations of a given rheumatic disease may not develop at once but may unfold over time, and many features are shared among different rheumatic diseases. Myositis, for example, can be found as a primary condition (polymyositis) or as part of other systemic diseases (dermatomyositis, systemic sclerosis, and even systemic lupus erythematosus [SLE]). In addition to shared clinical features, these illnesses may have shared serologic features. The most obvious example is antinuclear antibody (ANA), which may be found in various diseases, including SLE, systemic sclerosis, Sjögren's syndrome, inflammatory myopathies, Hashimoto's thyroiditis, and inflammatory bowel disease. When clinical and laboratory features suggest an autoimmune or inflammatory etiology but clinical and serologic heterogeneity make an exact diagnosis impossible, the designation UCTD has been used.

3. **How is UCTD different from mixed connective tissue disease (MCTD)?**
MCTD was first described as a separate entity in 1972 and is a more specific designation than UCTD. It is not the mixture or overlap of any rheumatic diseases; rather, MCTD is used specifically when features of SLE and systemic sclerosis are present with high titers of antibody to U_1RNP.

4. **What is a "joint mouse"?**
Osteocartilaginous bodies within a joint are often termed *joint mice* or *loose bodies* and occur commonly in osteoarthritis. They are believed to arise when bits of articular cartilage and subchondral bone break from the surface and enter the joint. There may be proliferation and deposition of new bone on these fragments.

5. **What is chondromalacia patella?**
Chondromalacia is a softening and degeneration of articular cartilage. In the patella, it is often associated with meniscal disease, knee laxity, or recurrent trauma. Typically, pain is associated with activity, often with descending stairs.

Moskowitz RW: Clinical and laboratory findings in osteoarthritis. In McCarty DJ, Koopman WJ (eds): Arthritis and Allied Conditions, 12th ed. Philadelphia, Lea & Febiger, 1993, pp 1735–1760.

6. **How do bunions occur?**
A bunion (hallux valgus) is a deviation of the proximal phalanx of the great toe toward the fibular side of the foot. It can be caused by biomechanical factors (tight and pointy-toed shoes that push the proximal phalanx across the other toes), inflammatory disease (gout or rheumatoid arthritis), or abnormal alignment (usually congenital) at the first metatarsal-cuneiform joint. If the cuneiform is abnormal, the first metatarsal may deviate excessively toward the midline (a primary varus deformity), which leads to a valgus deformity (lateral deviation) of the great toe when the abnormal foot is placed into standard shoes.

7. **What conditions are associated with avascular necrosis of bone?**

Trauma (femoral head fractures)	Gaucher's disease
Hemoglobinopathies	Pregnancy
Exogenous or endogenous overproduction of glucocorticoids	SLE
	Kidney transplantation
Alcoholism	Lymphoproliferative diseases
HIV A	Anticardiolipin antibody syndrome

8. **What mechanisms contribute to bone loss with the use of glucocorticoids?**
Use of glucocorticoids is a cornerstone of treatment of many rheumatic diseases, but one of its most concerning toxicities is accelerated bone loss. The severity parallels the dose and duration of treatment. It occurs to some degree in almost all patients at doses of greater than 7½ mg/day. Trabecular bone is most affected. Glucocorticoid effects include decrease in synthesis of bone matrix constituents and altered production of various cytokines and growth factors important for bone. Corticosteroids have also been shown to decrease intestinal absorption of calcium and increase urinary calcium excretion. The calcium loss stimulates parathyroid hormone (PTH) production and PTH levels are often elevated. It should also be remembered that patients taking corticosteroids are not spared the factors influencing osteoporosis in the general population (smoking, low calcium intake, lack of weight-bearing exercises, among others.

Sambrook PN, et al: Corticosteroid osteoporosis. Br J Rheum 34:8–12, 1995.

9. **What is Behçet's syndrome?**
Behçet's syndrome is an inflammatory disease manifested principally by ocular inflammation and oral, nasal, and genital ulcerations. Other features include arthritis, thrombophlebitis, and vasculitis.

10. **Describe Buerger's disease.**
Buerger's disease (also called thromboangiitis obliterans) is a vasculopathy in which acute inflammatory lesions produce occlusive thrombosis of arteries and veins. It has been associated overwhelmingly with tobacco use.

11. **Define Caplan's syndrome and Cogan's syndrome.**
Caplan's syndrome: rheumatoid arthritis (RA) with pneumoconiosis.
Cogan's syndrome: an unusual vasculopathy associated with interstitial keratitis, sensorineural hearing loss, tinnitus, and vertigo. Systemic features such as fever, weight loss, and fatigue are present in about one-half of patients.

12. **What are deQuervain's tenosynovitis and Dupuytren's contacture?**
DeQuervain's tenosynovitis: inflammation of the synovial lining and subsequent narrowing of the membrane (stenosing tenosynovitis) of the abductor pollicis longus and extensor pollicis brevis tendons at the radial styloid.
Dupuytren's contracture: nodular fibrosis of the palmar fascia and flexion contractures of the digits.

13. What is Ehlers-Danlos syndrome?
Ehlers-Danlos syndrome refers to a group of disorders characterized by hyperextensibility of skin and hypermobility of joints, predisposing to early development of osteoarthritis.

14. Describe Kawasaki's disease.
Kawasaki's disease (also called mucocutaneous lymph node syndrome) is an acute febrile disease, usually in children under 5 years of age, associated with conjunctivitis, fissuring of the lips, strawberry tongue, painful lymphadenopathy, and vasculitis, especially of the coronary arteries.

15. Distinguish between Legg-Calvé-Perthes disease and Osgood-Schlatter disease.
Legg-Calvé-Perthes disease: idiopathic osteonecrosis of the femoral capital epiphysis usually in boys ages 3–8 that may result in a large flat femoral head.
Osgood-Schlatter disease (also called tibial tubercle apophysitis): inflammation at the site where the patellar tendon inserts onto the tibial tubercle. It is probably a repetitive motion injury, usually occurring in adolescents, and presents as knee pain.

16. What is Saint Vitus' dance?
Saint Vitus' dance (also called Sydenham's chorea or chorea minor) is a neurologic disorder consisting of abrupt, purposeless involuntary movements that disappear during sleep. It is found in patients with rheumatic fever.

17. Describe SAPHO syndrome.
SAPHO syndrome (synovitis, acne, pustulosism hyperostosis) is a representative example of a group of syndromes that produce seronegative asymmetric arthritis usually with chest wall pain (sternoclavicular hyperostosis), chronic aseptic osteomyelitis, and severe acne. Sacroiliac joint involvement can occur and is usually unilateral. There is no HLA B27 association.

18. Define Still's disease.
Still's disease is a subset of juvenile RA that has systemic features (fever, lymphadenopathy, pleuropericarditis, hepatosplenomegaly, and leukocytosis) as major manifestations.

19. What is Sudek's atrophy?
Sudek's atrophy (also called reflex sympathetic dystrophy) is characterized by severe pain, edema, vasomotor abnormalities, and atrophy of bone, muscle, and skin.

20. Define Tietze's syndrome.
Tietze's syndrome (also called osteochondritis) is painful enlargement of the upper costal cartilages.

21. Distinguish between Bouchard's nodes and Heberden's nodes.
Bouchard's nodes: one of the most common manifestations of osteoarthritis with bony enlargement of the proximal interphalangeal (PIP) joints.
Heberden's nodes: one of the most common manifestations of osteoarthritis with bony enlargement of the distal interphalangeal (DIP) joints. Women are affected more frequently than men (10:1 ratio). Heredity plays a particularly strong role in mothers, daughters, and sisters.

22. Distinguish between Charcot joint and Charcot-Leyden crystals.
Charcot joint: progressive degenerative arthropathy associated with a neuropathic joint; historically, it was associated most commonly with tabes dorsalis, but now it is seen most frequently with syrinx or diabetic neuropathy.

Charcot-Leyden crystals: crystals formed in the cytoplasm of disrupted eosinophils found in the sputum of asthmatics and in the synovial fluid of patients with eosinophilic synovitis.

23. **Define the following disorders named after occupations.**
Housemaid's knee: prepatellar bursitis.
Tailor's seat (also called weaver's bottom): inflammation of the ischial bursa (the bursa that separates the gluteus maximus from the ischial tuberosity).

24. **Define the following disorders named after specific sports.**
Little leaguer's shoulder: separation of the proximal humeral epiphysis, probably secondary to the repetitive motion associated with pitching.
Tennis elbow: lateral epicondylitis.

25. **What is trigger finger?**
Trigger finger is the sticking or locking of a finger in flexion as a result of stenosing tenosynovitis. The finger can be extended manually, often with discomfort.

26. **What is Finkelstein's test?**
Finkelstein's test is a maneuver to demonstrate de Quervain's tenosynovitis. A fist is made around the thumb, and ulnar motion of the wrist is produced. In patients with de Quervain's tenosynovitis, this maneuver reproduces the typical sharp, exquisite pain.

27. **Describe Phalen's sign.**
Phalen's sign is a test of diagnostic usefulness in carpal tunnel syndrome. By raising both arms, opposing the dorsum of the hands, and then slightly dropping the elbows (maximally flexing the wrist), one can reproduce the discomfort of carpal tunnel syndrome.

28. **What is the Shober test?**
The Shober test is a test for spinal flexion. Two points on the patient's lumbar spine (usually the lumbar sacral junction and a point 10 cm above) are marked while the patient is standing. The distance is remeasured after the patient bends to touch the toes (maximal forward flexion). An elongation < 5 cm suggests spine stiffness.

29. **Define Tinel's sign.**
Tinel's sign is defined as focal pain and electrical sensations elicited by tapping on a nerve at the site of entrapment.

30. **What is POEMS syndrome?**
POEMS syndrome is a plasma cell dyscrasia characterized by **p**olyneuropathy, **o**rganomegaly, **e**ndocrinopathy, **m**onoclonal protein, and **s**kin changes, which may resemble scleroderma.

31. **What are rice bodies?**
Aggregates of fibrin frequently found in the synovial fluid of patients with RA.

32. **Which clinical syndromes are associated with complement deficiencies?**
See Table 11-1.

33. **What is "en coup de sabre"?**
Smaller areas of skin fibrosis (localized scleroderma) can take several forms. Morphea can be present as a single patch of involved skin or appear in multiple lesions (generalized morphea). In linear scleroderma, the lesion is band-like and may expand across dermatomes. Fibrosis may be so deep that it disrupts growth and can cause distortion and contracture. "En coup de sabre" refers to the specific curvilinear band (resembling a dueling scar) that occurs across the face.

TABLE 11-1. COMPLEMENT DEFICIENCIES ASSOCIATED WITH SPECIFIC DISEASES

Complement Deficiency	Disease(s)
C1q	Glomerulonephritis and poikiloderma congenita
C1r	Glomerulonephritis, lupus-like syndrome
C1s	Lupus-like syndrome
C1INH	Discoid lupus, SLE, lupus-like syndrome
C4	SLE, Sjögren's syndrome
C2	SLE, discoid lupus, polymyositis, Henoch-Schönlein purpura, Hodgkin's disease, vasculitis, glomerulonephritis, common variable hypogammaglobulinemia
C3	Vasculitis, lupus-like syndrome, glomerulonephritis
C5	SLE, neisserial infection
C6	Neisserial infection
C7	SLE, rheumatoid arthritis, Raynaud's phenomenon and sclerodactyly, vasculitis, neisserial infection
C8	SLE, neisserial infection
C9	Neisserial infection

From Ruddy S: Complement deficiencies and rheumatic diseases. In Kelly WN, et al (eds): Textbook of Rheumatology, 4th ed. Philadelphia, W.B. Saunders, 1993, pp 1283–1289.

DIAGNOSIS

34. Which studies should generally be performed on synovial fluid after arthrocentesis?

Gram stain and bacterial culture may confirm the presence of an infective agent. In the right clinical setting, similar procedures for mycobacteria or fungi are important. A white blood cell (WBC) count with differential is one of the best indicators of the degree of inflammation. Evaluation for crystals by polarized light microscopy may confirm the diagnosis. Although a good deal has been written about various other tests (e.g., glucose, complement, rheumatoid factor, ANA, lactate dehydrogenase, protein), they add little diagnostic information.

35. What are the "string" and "mucin clot" tests?

The primary component of joint fluid is hyaluronic acid. It is quite viscous and makes a "string" when expressed from a syringe as a single drop. Dilute acetic acid causes hyaluronate and protein to clump and fall to the bottom of a test tube (producing the famous "mucin clot"). Inflammatory mediators cause fragmentation of the hyaluronate–protein complex, rendering it unable to form a good mucin clot.

36. Are the "string" and "mucin clot" tests still of clinical value?

Basically, these tests provide a crude bedside estimate of the level of synovial inflammation. Because the wet prep and total synovial fluid WBC count give more objective data, the mucin clot and string tests are primarily of historic interest. It is also probably true that when done in the traditional manner at the bedside, these tests violate regulations for the handling of bodily fluids established by the Occupational Safety and Health Administration and Clinical Laboratories Improvement Act.

Schumacher HR Jr: Synovial fluid analysis and synovial biopsy. In Kelly WN, et al (eds): Textbook of Rheumatology, 4th ed. Philadelphia, W.B. Saunders, 1993, pp 562–578.

37. Straight leg raising is a useful diagnostic maneuver in what common condition?

The straight leg raising test is designed to reproduce back pain secondary to nerve root compression. The leg is lifted by the calcaneus with the knee remaining straight. Bringing the heel across the other leg (called cross-table straight leg raising) may increase the sensitivity of this maneuver.

38. What is onychodystrophy? With which diseases is it associated?

Separation of the nail plate, usually beginning at the free margin and progressing proximally, is called onychodystrophy. Both systemic and local processes are associated with this finding, including hypo- and hyperthyroidism, pregnancy, syphilis, trauma (particularly clawing), psoriasis, SLE, atopic dermatitis, eczema, use of solvents (including nail hardeners), and mycotic, pyogenic, or viral infections.

Domonkos AN, et al: Diseases of the skin appendages. In Andrews' Diseases of the Skin: Clinical Dermatology, 7th ed. Philadelphia, W.B. Saunders, 1982, pp 930–984.

39. Which rheumatic syndromes have been associated with uveitis?

Ankylosing spondylitis	Juvenile RA
Reactive arthritis	Sjögren's syndrome
Psoriasis	Sarcoidosis
Inflammatory bowel disease	Behçet's disease
Kawasaki disease	Relapsing polychondritis

Rosenbaum JT: Uveitis. In McCarty DJ (ed): Arthritis and Allied Conditions, 11th ed. Philadelphia, Lea & Febiger, 1989, pp 1563–1568.

40. Which diseases are associated with soft tissue calcification?

Soft tissue calcification detected by plain roentgenograms can be an important clue in the diagnosis of rheumatic conditions. A partial list includes:

Calcific tendinitis	Neuropathic arthropathy
Chondrocalcinosis	Parathyroid disease
Dermatomyositis	Renal osteodystrophy
Diabetes	Sarcoidosis
Ehlers-Danlos syndrome	Scleroderma
Neoplasia	Trauma

Resnick D, Niwayama G: Soft tissues. In Resnick D, Niwayama G (eds): Diagnosis of Bone and Joint Disorders, 2nd ed. Philadelphia, W.B. Saunders, 1988, pp 4171–4294.

41. Which conditions commonly mimic systemic vasculitis?

Bacterial endocarditis, atrial myxoma, and multiple cholesterol embolization syndrome have many of the same presenting signs and symptoms as systemic vasculitis. Thrombotic states, including hypercoagulability (as occurs with phospholipid antibodies), cryoglobulinemia, hemoglobinopathies, thrombotic thrombocytopenic purpura, or hemolytic uremic syndrome, may be confused with vasculitis. Drugs that induce vasospasm (cocaine, ergots, and other sympathomimetics) sometimes produce the arteriographic appearance of vasculitis. Finally, processes that produce vascular malformation, such as fibromuscular disease and moyamoya, may be included in the differential diagnosis of vasculitis.

Sack KE: Mimickers of vasculitis. In Koopman WJ (ed): Arthritis and Allied Conditions, 13th ed. Baltimore, Williams & Wilkins, 1997, pp 1525–1546.

42. **What are Gottron's papules?**
Patches of erythematous scaly plaques on knuckles in patients with dermatomyositis.

KEY POINTS: SIGNIFICANCE OF LAB VALUES IN RHEUMATOLOGIC DISEASE

1. ANA titers are not associated with intensity of disease.
2. Measurement of single-stranded DNA antibodies are of absolutely no clinical value.
3. The HLA B27 association with arthritis is highest in AS and reactive arthritis but lower with the spondylitis associated with psoriasis and inflammatory bowel disease.
4. A patient with low positive RF and arthralgia should be checked for hepatitis C, which can produce a low-grade synovitis and cryoglobulins (which, in turn, can produce a falsely positive RF).
5. Serum transaminases (ALT, AST) are found in muscle. Therefore, elevated LFTs, especially when no concomitant gamma-glutamyl transferase is available, may reflect muscle inflammation in a patient with rheumatic disease. Check the creatine phosphokinase level.

43. **What is the difference between scleroderma and sclerodactyly?**
Both scleroderma and sclerodactyly refer to the fibrotic changes in skin occurring in systemic sclerosing conditions. The term *scleroderma* is used when these changes occur diffusely over the body: arms, torso, and face for example. *Sclerodactyly* is usually reserved to describe the skin tightening when it occurs in the fingers and hand (distal to the wrist).

RHEUMATOID ARTHRITIS

44. **What are the American College of Rheumatology (ACR) criteria for RA?**
Patients can be said to have RA if they satisfy at least four of the seven criteria in Table 11-2. Criteria 1–4 must be present for at least 6 weeks.

45. **Discuss the HLA association of RA.**
Upward of 90% of patients meeting the ACR criteria for RA have been found to have the HLA class II genes DR4 or DR1. Closer review shows that the specific alleles of these otherwise disparate genes have a common sequence (often called the shared epitope) at loci 70–74 of the third hypervariable region of DRβ_1 chains, which code for one side of the peptide-binding groove. The estimated prevalence of the susceptibility alleles in the general population (5–15%) makes it clear that most people with these alleles do not develop RA; therefore, genetic testing is not a useful tool in the clinical practice. Other genes are likely associated and include those coding for galactosylation of immunoglobulins, and cytokines including TNF and IL-1a.
Nepom GT, Byers P, et al. HLA gene association with RA: Identification of susceptibility alleles using specific oligopeptide probes. Arthr Rheum 32:15, 1989.

46. **Who gets RA?**
RA affects about 1% of the general adult population. It occurs two to three times more frequently in women than in men. It can develop as early as infancy or in the geriatric population, but its peak onset is the fifth decade of life. Worldwide, the prevalence is fairly stable. Exceptions include several Native American tribes, including the Chippewa, Pima, and Yakima

TABLE 11-2. ACR CRITERIA FOR RHEUMATOID ARTHRITIS

1. Morning stiffness around the joints, lasting at least 1 hour before maximal improvement.
2. Arthritis of three or more joints. A physician has observed simultaneous soft tissue swelling or fluid (not bony overgrowth alone) in at least three joint areas. The 14 possible joint areas include PIP, metacarpophalangeal (MCP), wrist, elbow, knee, ankle, and metatarsophalangeal (MTP) joints.
3. Arthritis of hand joints. At least one joint area is swollen, as above, in the wrist, MCP, or PIP joint.
4. Symmetric arthritis: simultaneous involvement of the same joint areas on both sides of the body.
5. Rheumatoid nodules: subcutaneous nodules over bony prominences or extensor surfaces or in juxta-articular regions, observed by a physician.
6. Serum rheumatoid factor (RF): demonstration of abnormal amounts of serum RF by any method that has been positive in < 5% of normal control subjects.
7. Radiographic changes typical of RA on posteroanterior hand and wrist x-rays, which must include erosions or unequivocal bony decalcification localized to or most marked adjacent to the involved joints (osteoarthritis changes alone do not qualify).

From Arnett FC, et al: The American Rheumatism Association 1987 revised criteria for the classification of rheumatoid arthritis. Arthritis Rheum 31:315–324, 1988.

tribes. Conversely members of the Blackfeet and Haida tribes as well as rural African Blacks seem to be protected. Socioeconomic factors may influence the severity of established disease, but there are few compelling data to support a role in disease susceptibility.

47. **Summarize the genetic predispostion to RA.**
The genetic predisposition based on HLA DR4 and the "shared epitope" is well described. Twin studies suggest that 30–50% of risk for disease development comes from genetic factors.

48. **What factors may be noted in women with RA?**
Hormonal status even beyond the female preponderance may play a role. Some studies have shown that nulliparity may increase the risk of disease. Pregnancy certainly influences the disease with upwards of 70% of pregnant women developing remission (with most suffering postpartum relapse). Another study suggested a role for breast-feeding in raising the risk of developing RA. Finally, one study in the U.K. suggested that use of oral contraceptives reduced the risk of developing RA significantly.

49. **What is "gelling"?**
Gelling describes the achiness and stiffness that occurs in patients with RA after a period of inactivity (such as getting up from the dinner table or rising from a seat after a movie). The stiffness that occurs on rising from bed in the morning is also a form of gelling.

50. **Which joints are most commonly involved in RA?**
RA is a symmetric polyarthropathy that can involve almost any diarthrodial joint. The hands and wrists are involved in over 90% of patients. About one half of patients with RA develop

x-ray evidence of hip involvement. Foot and ankle disease can have a major impact on function, although ankle involvement is rare in the absence of MTP involvement. Palpable swelling at the radiohumeral joint, along with incomplete extension, marks elbow involvement. Nodules and concomitant swelling of the olecranon bursae also may suggest elbow disease. Knee involvement is common. Other joints involved include the shoulders, temporomandibular joints, cricoarytenoid joints (sometimes explaining why patients commonly have "sore throats" without signs of pharyngitis), and ossicles of the ears (which may be in part responsible for some hearing loss).

51. How does RA commonly affect the spine?

The thoracic and lumbar spines are rarely if ever involved with RA. The cervical spine is commonly involved and deserves special mention. Cervical spine involvement usually is heralded by pain with motion and occipital headache. Significant laxity at the alantoaxial joint with subluxation makes patients prone to slowly progressive, spastic quadriparesis. If this laxity is present, the hyperextension of the neck that occurs during intubation for general anesthesia can produce quadriplegia. Thus patients with neck pain or long-standing disease should undergo cervical spine evaluation before any surgical procedure.

52. What is Baker's cyst? How does it form?

Swelling of the knee capsule extending posteriorly to the popliteal fossa (hence the synonym popliteal cyst). Baker's cyst is thought to develop as the knee is flexed, producing a significant rise in intra-articular pressure and an outpouching of the synovium posteriorly. The cruciate ligaments may act as a one-way valve, making it hard for the fluid to resorb. Posterior rupture may lead to swelling of the leg below the knee. When rupture occurs, a crescentic hematoma may form beneath one of the malleoli.

Kraag G, et al: The hemorrhagic crescent sign of acute synovial rupture [letter]. Ann Intern Med 85:477, 1976.

53. What is the major differential diagnosis of Baker's cyst?

The major differential diagonsis is thrombophlebitis. Although a ruptured popliteal cyst may mimic thrombophlebitis, the increased pressure in the calf from the fluid may compress venous return and predispose to clot as well.

54. What are the two layers of normal synovium?

The **synovial lining** is a thin, delicate structure (only one or two cells thick) and contains two types of synoviocytes: type A (macrophage-like cells probably derived from bone marrow) and type B (fibroblast-like cells that are probably of mesenchymal origin). The **subsynovium** constitutes the second layer of normal synovium.

55. How does RA affect the synovium?

The synovium is a primary target for the inflammatory process in RA. Both layers are radically affected quite early (perhaps within weeks) in the course of the disease. Type A synoviocytes thicken the synovial lining probably by local proliferation. The subsynovium also thickens by infiltration of lymphocytes and macrophages. Although B cells are present, the majority of infiltrating cells are T lymphocytes with a phenotype characteristic of memory T cells. Suppressor T cells are notably scarce. Multinucleate giant cells and hemosiderin-laden macrophages are also seen. Angiogenesis is a prominent and early change as well. Later, fibronectin is deposited on articular cartilage. In contrast to the synovial tissue, synovial fluid has a predominance of polymorphonuclear leukocytes, and of the T cells present in the fluid, most are CD_8^+.

56. What is pannus?

Pannus is the term used to describe the area of proliferating synovium that meets the articular cartilage. It is believed to be the source of erosive damage in RA.

57. **How does pannus lead to articular destruction in RA?**
Although the source of stimulation for the synovial swelling and development of pannus that occurs in RA has not been entirely elucidated, concepts are emerging. The presence of specific adhesion molecules may support the attachment of pannus to articular cartilage since normal cartilage does not support the adhesion of pannus. There is also a preponderance of proinflammatory cytokines within the synovium and synovial fluid—mainly TNF-alpha, IFN-alpha, and IL-15. These in turn lead to cellular activation and production of metalloproteinases, cathepsins, and other destructive enzymes. RANK-L production leads to osteoclast activation, almost certainly the principle source of bone loss in RA. Although the exact mechanism remains a mystery, it appears that articular damage in RA results from cartilage destruction that is a direct consequence of a relentless inflammatory attack that includes both pannus formation and soluble inflammatory mediators.

58. **What mechanisms underlie the classic swan neck deformitiy?**
The swan neck deformity describes flexion at the MCP and DIP joints with extension at the PIP joints. This deformity results from inflammation and subsequent contraction of interosseous and flexor muscles and tendons. Other contributing factors include tenosynovitis and destruction leading to MCP subluxation. Flexion at the MCP leads to exaggerated pull on the extensor tendon of the PIP. The flexion at the DIP is caused because the pull of the flexor tendon overcomes the pull of the extensor tendon.

59. **What mechanisms underlie the classic boutonnière deformity?**
Flexion contracture at the PIP with extension of the DIP is referred to as the *boutonnière deformity*. The pathogenesis of this deformity is thought to be related to injury of the extensor tendon. If it becomes lengthened or torn, the flexor tendons are unopposed. The altered mechanics and location of the joint lead to functional shortening of the lateral tendons and hyperextension of the DIP joint.

60. **Decribe the mechanism for the development of cocked-up toes in RA.**
Inflammation of the MTP joints in RA often leads to subluxation of the metatarsal heads and collapse of the arch of the foot. A claw-like or cocking-up appearance of the toes follows.

McCarty DJ: Clinical picture of RA. In McCarty DJ, Koopman WJ (eds): Arthritis and Allied Conditions, 12th ed. Philadelphia, Lea & Febiger, 1993, pp 781–809.

61. **What are rheumatoid factors (RFs)?**
RFs are antibodies directed at the Fc portion of the IgG molecule. Although IgM RFs are the most common, all isotypes have been reported. (IgG RFs are associated with a greater likelihood of vasculitis.)

62. **Which conditions are associated with their presence in the circulation?**
The presence of RF is not specific for RA. Patients with other conditions that have rheumatic features, including sarcoidosis, interstitial lung disease, cryoglobulinemia, SLE, and Sjögren's syndrome, may have circulating RFs. Viral, parasitic, and other infectious diseases, including mononucleosis, hepatitis, malaria, tuberculosis, and bacterial endocarditis, may be associated with RFs. Up to 70% of patients with active hepatitis C infection have RFs in the circulation, probably because of the cross-reactivity between cryoglobulins (produced commonly in hepatitis C) and RF. Since chronic hepatitis can also produce achiness and occasionally a mild synovitis, careful attention should be paid to excluding hepatitis C (even if the patient has normal serum transaminase levels) before establishing a diagnosis of RA. Finally, human parvovirus B19 infection (fifth disease or slapped-cheek syndrome) may produce a symmetric polyarthropathy that can mimic RA, at times with modest titers of RFs in the circulation.

63. **Do all patients with RA have circulating RF?**
Up to 25% of patients with clinical RA have no circulating RF. In addition, it may take as long as 2 years for the RF to become detectable. Thus, just when it would be most helpful diagnostically,

RF is least likely to be present. The titer has little prognostic value in an individual patient, and remeasurements provide little added information.

64. What are anti-CCP antibodies?

Antibodies directed against the citrullinated portion of certain molecules (filaggrin and fibrin among others) have been found in the sera of patients with RA and are called anti-cyclic citrullinated peptide antibodies. They are present in about 66% of RA patients and in fewer than 5% of control subjects making them quite specific for RA. Their clinical usefulness seems to be in helping to distinguish true RA in patients who are otherwise seronegative, or if the exact diagnosis of an inflammatory arthropathy is otherwise unclear.

65. Why is early treatment of RA so important?

RA is now recognized to be profoundly disabling in most patients. The disability is related to the structural damage to the joint that can come very early in the course of the disease. This structural damage produces mechanical derangements in the joint leading inexorably to deformity and thus to profoundly reduced joint function.

66. What evidence confirms the fact that reduced function rapidly follows the mechanical derangement of the joint?

One study revealed that patients treated conservatively (putting off disease-modifying antirheumatic drugs [DMARDs] until trials of NSAIDs, low-dose steroids, physical therapy, splinting, and other modalities had failed) suffered a moderate loss of function with 2 years, a severe loss of function with 6 years, and a very severe loss by 10 years. If ability to maintain work status is used as a measure of function, statistics are even grimmer. Fifty percent of patients were disabled after 10 years and 60% after 15 years. An increased mortality rate (see previous question) has been recognized in patients treated in this way. Therefore, in an attempt to improve outcome, most rheumatologists now recommend earlier initiation of DMARDs and a more aggressive approach to management.

67. How is the functional capacity of RA patients classified?

Class I	No restrictions, able to perform normal activities
Class II	Moderate restriction, but able to perform normal activities
Class III	Marked restriction, inability to perform most duties of the patient's usual occupation or self-care
Class IV	Incapacitation or confinement to a wheelchair

68. Why is functional capacity so important in patients with RA?

Functional status may be one of the best predictors of premature mortality in patients with RA.

69. What classification scheme is used to describe the progression of RA?

See Table 11-3.

70. Which factors suggest an aggressive disease course in RA?

Explosive onset of disease with involvement of multiple joints, high titers of RF, positive ANA, nodules, lower socioeconomic status, and fewer years of formal education.

71. How does pregnancy affect RA?

Signs and symptoms of RA subside in approximately 70% of women during pregnancy. No data suggest that RA has a detrimental effect on the fetus. However, arthritis should be assessed before pregnancy, if possible, because anesthesia and intubation can be problematic and even dangerous when cervical spine disease is present. Delivery also can be difficult if arthritis limits hip motion. Postpartum flares of disease occur in approximately 90% of women who experience improvement.

TABLE 11-3. CLASSIFICATION OF PROGRESSION OF RA

Stage I: early
- No destructive changes on x-ray.
- X-ray evidence of osteoporosis is acceptable.

Stage II: moderate
- X-ray evidence of osteoporosis with or without slight subchondral bone destruction; slight cartilage destruction may be present.
- No joint deformities, although joint mobility may be limited.
- Adjacent muscle atrophy.
- Extra-articular soft tissue lesions such as nodules or tenosynovitis may be present.

Stage III: severe
- X-ray evidence of cartilage and bone destruction in addition to osteoporosis.
- Joint deformity, such as subluxation, ulnar deviation, or hyperextension, without fibrosis or bony ankylosis.
- Extra-articular soft tissue lesions such as nodules or tenosynovitis may be present.

Stage IV: terminal
- Criteria of stage III.
- Bony or fibrous ankylosis.

Griffin J: Rheumatoid arthritis: Biological effects and management. In Scott JS, Bird HA (eds): Pregnancy, Autoimmunity and Connective Tissue Disorders. Oxford, Oxford University Press, 1990, pp 140–162.

72. List the major extra-articular manifestations of RA.
- Nodules
- Vasculitis
- Pulmonary involvement
- Cardiac disease
- Eye involvement
- Felty's syndrome

73. What are rheumatoid nodules? Where are they found?
The classic rheumatoid nodule has a central area of necrosis surrounded by a rim of palisading fibroblasts that, in turn, is surrounded by a collagenous capsule with perivascular collections of chronic inflammatory cells. Rheumatoid nodules occur in 20–35% of patients with RA and can be found at the elbow, wrist, soles, Achilles tendon, head, or sacrum. RF is usually present. Accelerated nodule formation has been described in patients receiving methotrexate treatment for RA, even when methotrexate shows efficacy at calming the arthritis and the patient has had no previous nodule formation. Nodulosis goes away when methotrexate is discontinued.

74. Does Still's disease occur in adults? How is it diagnosed?
Still's disease is the eponym assigned to systemic-onset juvenile arthritis. It has been reported in adults as a seronegative polyarthropathy associated with sudden-onset high fever and chills, with evanescent rash on the trunk and extremities. Bony erosions are uncommon, although fusion of the carpal bones may occur.

Reginato AJ: Adult onset Still's disease. In Schumacher HR Jr, et al (eds): Primer on the Rheumatic Diseases, 10th ed. Atlanta, Arthritis Foundation, 1993, pp 182–183.

75. Describe the basic mechanism of action of NSAIDs.
All NSAIDs work by inhibiting cyclooxygenase (COX). This enzyme forms an important step in the production of many proinflammatory mediators, including prostaglandins. Without COX

there are fewer circulating prostaglandins and therefore less inflammation and pain. As with most mediators in the body, prostaglandins do not have a unique function. They are important in regulating blood flow to the kidney, producing protective mucus in the stomach among many others. In fact, the toxicities of NSAIDs are related primarily to inhibition of all prostaglandins, whether they produce useful or harmful effects.

76. **What are COX-2 anti-inflammatory drugs?**
Recently two subtypes of COX have been described. The traditionally recognized enzyme, designated COX-1, seems to be most involved with normal cellular processes, often described as housekeeping functions. COX-2 seems to be involved more specifically in the synthesis of inflammatory mediators. It is normally not easily detectable in tissue and is thought to be "upregulated" under inflammatory conditions.

77. **How do COX-2 anti-inflammatory drugs differ from older NSAIDs?**
By preferentially inhibiting COX-2, newer NSAIDs are able to reduce inflammation with less impact on the remaining prostaglandins and therefore fewer side effects. Two points should be emphasized. The side effects of NSAIDs remain by and large toxicities for the entire class of compounds. COX-2 NSAIDs may preferentially inhibit COX-2, but there is much individual variation. So although it is much less likely for a patient to develop an ulcer with a COX-2 inhibiting NSAID, it remains possible. Finally, although there is a clear and measurable improvement in safety, there is no real improvement in efficacy; COX-2 NSAIDs are less likely to cause trouble, but no more likely to control pain than older NSAIDs.

78. **How do the effects of aspirin on platelets differ from those of other NSAIDs?**
NSAIDs, including aspirin, decrease platelet aggregation by inhibiting the COX. Acetylated salicylates (such as aspirin) irreversibly destroy this enzyme, whereas other NSAIDs (including nonacetylated salicylates) allow the return of normal enzyme function once the drug level has dropped. Because COX-2 does not regulate platelet aggregation, newer COX-2 NSAIDs have little effect on platelet function.

79. **What are DMARDs and how are they used in the treatment of RA?**
DMARDs are medications thought to alter the natural history of RA, lessening the likelihood of joint destruction and deformity.

80. **Which agents were first used as DMARDs?**
Gold (oral or parenteral) and **D-penicillamine,** which are rarely used now because of their limited efficacy and significant toxicities compared with newer agents.

81. **Are antimalarial agents useful as DMARDs?**
Hydroxychloroquine (Plaquenil) is pretty well the uniquely used antimalarial medication in the U.S. (over **chloroquine** [Aralen] and **quinacrine** [Atabrine]). Antimalarial medications are believed to be weak, have a slow onset of action, and are generally used in mild disease or in combination with other DMARDs.

82. **Which DMARD is the cornerstone of treatment for RA in the U.S.?**
In the U.S, **methotrexate** remains the cornerstone of treatment for RA. Its exact mechanism of action is unclear, but its anti-folate effect contributes to its effect as a potent anti-inflammatory agent. It has a more rapid onset of action than many of the older DMARDs. Although it has many potential toxicities, most are reversible when the drug is stopped. These include bone marrow suppression, stomatitis, nausea, alopecia and hepatic toxicity. Idiopathic pulmonary hypersensitivity is perhaps the most dangerous side effect and must be dealt with promptly to avoid serious impairments. Because of these toxicities, methotrexate must be monitored carefully.

83. **How effective are sulfasalazine and leflunomide?**
Sulfasalazine is an easy to use and well-tolerated medication. Some studies have shown it to be as effective as methotrexate as a DMARD. It is used more frequently in Europe than in the U.S.
Leflunomide (Arava) has been available for a number of years. It is known to inhibit pyrimidine synthesis and thereby alter T-cell function. Studies show it to be about as effective as methotrexate. It must be monitored as closely as methotrexate since its toxicities are remarkably similar. The rate of diarrhea and hair loss may be a bit higher with leflunomide, but it does not have the risk of pulmonary reaction.

84. **Which immunosuppressive drugs are effective as DMARDs?**
Immunosuppressive drugs have been shown to be effective DMARDs in RA. To a large degree their use is restricted by their toxicities. **Chlorambucil** and **cyclophosphamide** are generally reserved for severe disease including the development of extra-articular features such as vasculitis. **Azathioprine** has been studied in RA, but its greater toxicity risk and lack of efficacy advantage over **methotrexate** make it a less common therapeutic choice. **Cyclosporine** has been used in the treatment of RA with good effect. Unfortunately, when used as a single agent, the doses required confer a high risk of hypertension and renal insufficiency. It has been used synergistically in combination with **methotrexate**, allowing lower doses of each drug.

85. **What are the newest options for treatment of RA?**
The newest options for the treatment of RA are anti-cytokine regimens. Three preparations (**etanercept** [Enbrel], **infliximab** [Remicade], and **adalimunmab** [Humira]) target TNF-α and one targets IL-1R (**anakinra** [Kineret]). All of these options are given parenterally and are fairly expensive. **Anakinra**, although proven efficacious, requires daily injections and has a slower onset of action and is therefore used less frequently.

86. **How effective are the TNF inhibitors in the treatment of RA?**
The TNF inhibitors have shown dramatic efficacy in the treatment of RA. Careful studies have shown significant improvements in function, lessening the number of swollen and tender joints and a slowing of the radiographic progression of disease. These medications have been used safely and effectively with more traditional DMARDs as well. The most common toxicities are injection site reactions, but they are also associated with increased infection risk, including TB and other opportunistic organisms and drug-induced lupus.

87. **Summarize the role of more traditional agents in the treatment of RA.**
Although NSAIDs, low-dose steroids, and narcotics may lessen symptoms (such as pain and swelling), they do not alter the long-term course of the disease. Basically, they produce less pain on the way to the wheelchair rather than allowing the patient to avoid the wheelchair altogether.

SJÖGREN'S SYNDROME

88. **What is Sjögren's syndrome?**
Sjögren's syndrome is an inflammatory disease of exocrine glands manifested primarily by dryness of the eyes and mouth. It can occur as an isolated entity (primary Sjögren's syndrome) or in association with another rheumatic disease, commonly RA or SLE (secondary Sjögren's syndrome).

89. **How does one document keratoconjunctivitis sicca?**
Many believe that Sjögren's syndrome is underdiagnosed. The first step is to ask the appropriate historical questions. Inquiries about eye grittiness or the ability to eat crackers without water have been suggested as nonleading ways to ask about dryness. Schirmer's test can document diminished output of the lacrimal glands. Likewise, biopsy of the salivary glands (usually in the lower lip), showing the presence of infiltrating lymphocytes, establishes the diagnosis.

Talal N: Sjögren's syndrome and connective tissue diseases association with other immunologic disorders. In McCarty DJ, Koopman WJ (eds): Arthritis and Allied Conditions, 12th ed. Philadelphia, Lea & Febiger, 1993, pp 1343–1356.

90. What percent of patients with primary Sjögren's syndrome subsequently develop a connective tissue syndrome?
If symptoms of an underlying connective tissue disease do not appear within 12 months of the keratoconjunctivitis sicca, the chances are approximately 10% that it will appear later in life.

91. Are patients with Sjögren's syndrome at increased risk for certain malignancies?
Yes—non-Hodgkin's lymphoma. The lymphomas are usually B cell–derived, and some patients also have serum protein spikes. The diagnosis of tumor may be difficult, given that the nonmalignant lymphoid infiltration of lymphocytes often simulates neoplasm (pseudolymphoma).

SYSTEMIC LUPUS ERYTHEMATOSUS

92. What are the most common clinical and laboratory features of SLE?
See Table 11-4.

TABLE 11-4. LABORATORY AND CLINICAL FEATURES OF SLE

Feature	Frequency (%)	Feature	Frequency (%)
Positive ANA	97	Leukopenia	46
Arthritis/arthralgia	80	Anemia	42
Fever	48	Myalgia	60
Skin involvement	71	Nephritis	42
Low complement	51	Pleurisy	44
Elevated anti-dsDNA	46	CNS symptoms	32

Adapted from Wallace DJ: The clinical presentation in SLE. In Wallace DJ, et al (eds): Dubois' Lupus Erythematosus, 4th ed. Baltimore, Williams & Wilkins, 1993, pp 317–321.

93. What are the ACR criteria for the classification of SLE, and how should they be used?
The ACR criteria for the classification of SLE were revised in 1997 (see Table 11-5) and are intended to allow comparison among patients with different manifestations of SLE and to help distinguish patients with SLE from those with other connective tissue diseases. They should not be thought of as diagnostic criteria as in "two from column A, one from column B and you get the lunch special."

94. Describe the common skin manifestations of acute SLE.
The skin is a frequent target organ in SLE. The classic lesion of acute lupus is the malar (butterfly) rash, which consists of an area of redness across the cheeks, usually involving the bridge of the nose, and often is exacerbated by ultraviolet light (artificial or sunlight). Atrophic dermal scarring does not develop with clearing of the rash.

TABLE 11-5.	ACR CRITERIA FOR CLASSIFICATION OF SLE
Malar rash	Fixed erythema, flat or raised, over the malar eminences, sparing the nasolabial folds
Discoid rash	Erythematous raised patches with adherent keratotic scaling and follicular plugging: atrophic scarring may occur in older lesions
Photosensitivity	Skin rash as a result of unusual reaction to sunlight, by patient history or physician observation
Oral ulcers	Oral or nasopharyngeal ulceration usually painless, observed by physician
Nonerosive arthritis	Involving two or more peripheral joints, characterized by tenderness, swelling or effusion
Pleuritis or pericarditis	(a) Pleuritis: convincing history of pleuritic pain or rub heard by physician or evidence of pleural effusion *or* (b) Pericarditis: documented by electrocardiogram or rub or evidence of pericardial effusion
Renal disorder	(a) Persistent proteinuria > 0.5 gm/day or > 3+ if quantitative not performed *or* (b) Cellular casts: may be red cell, hemoglobin, granular, tubular or mixed
Seizures or psychosis	(a) Seizures: in the absence of offending drugs or known metabolic derangement (e.g., uremia, ketoacidosis, electrolyte imbalance) (b) Psychosis: in the absence of offending drugs or known metabolic derangement (e.g., uremia, ketoacidosis, electrolyte imbalance)
Hematologic disorder	(a) Hemolytic anemia with reticulocytosis *or* (b) Leukopenia: < 4000/mm^3 on two occasions *or* (c) Lymphopenia: < 1500/mm^3 on two occasions *or* (d) Thrombocytopenia: < 100,000/mm^3 in the absence of offending drugs
Immunologic disorder	(a) Anti-DNA: antibody to native DNA in abnormal titer *or* (b) Anti-Sm: presence of antibody to Sm nuclear antigen *or* (c) Positive findings of antiphospholipid antibodies based on: (1) An abnormal serum concentration of IgG or IgM anticardiolipin antibodies (2) A positive test for lupus anticoagulant using standard method *or* (3) A false-positive test for at least 6 months and confirmed by *Treponema palladium* immobilization fluorescent treponemal antibody absorption test.

TABLE 11-5. ACR CRITERIA FOR CLASSIFICATION OF SLE *(continued)*

Positive ANA	An abnormal titer of ANA by immunofluorescence or an equivalent assay at any point in time in the absence of drug

Adapted from Hochberg MC: Updating the American College of Rheumatology revised criteria for the classification of systemic lupus erythematosus [letter]. Arthritis Rheum 40:1725, 1997.

95. **Describe the common skin manifestations of subacute cutaneous lupus.**
Symmetric, superficial, nonscarring annular lesions of the shoulders, upper arms, and back are the classic lesions of subacute cutaneous lupus. Nonscarring alopecia often occurs concurrently. Patients may or may not have circulating anti-Ro antibodies. Lesions are highly photosensitive.

96. **Describe the common skin manifestations of discoid lupus.**
The skin lesions of discoid lupus (chronic cutaneous lupus erythematosus) most commonly occur over the face and neck. They eventually become hypopigmented and atrophic.

97. **List the less common skin lesions of lupus.**
Less common skin lesions include urticaria, periungual erythema, bullae, livedo reticularis petechiae, purpura, and ecchymoses.
Sontheirmer RD: Clinical manifestations of cutaneous lupus erythematosus. In Wallace DJ, et al (eds): Dubois' Lupus Erythematosus, 4th ed. Philadelphia, Lea & Febiger, 1993, pp 285–301.

98. **What is subacute cutaneous lupus (SCLE)?**
Some consider this cutaneous eruption on a spectrum between chronic discoid lupus and acute cutaneous lupus. The lesions generally occur on the shoulders, upper chest, and neck and are symmetric and nonscarring. They can be annular and resemble psoriasis. Between 25% and 50% of patients have constitutional symptoms, and they may have circulating antibodies to Ro antigen. SCLE is associated with HLA-DRW3.
McCauliffe DP, Sontheimer RD: Subacute cutaneous lupus erythematosus. In Wallace DJ, et al (eds): Dubois' Lupus Erythematosus, 4th ed. Philadelphia, Lea & Febiger, 1993, pp 302–309.

99. **Describe the relationship between discoid lupus and systemic lupus.**
This area is somewhat controversial. Approximately 25% of patients with classic discoid lesions may have constitutional symptoms but do not meet the ARA criteria for SLE. Approximately 10% of patients with discoid lupus eventually develop SLE. These data are inexact, because early epidemiologic studies lumped SCLE and discoid lupus together in assessing risk for the development of systemic disease.

100. **How commonly does SLE affect the GI tract?**
GI manifestations may be present in up to 50% of patients with SLE. Anorexia, nausea, and vomiting are among the most common. Oral ulcerations (most commonly buccal erosions) were identified in 40% of one group of patients. Esophageal involvement, as esophagitis, esophageal ulceration, or esophageal dysmotility, seems to correlate with the presence of Raynaud's phenomenon. Intestinal involvement results in abdominal pain, diarrhea, and occasionally hemorrhage. Intestinal ischemia may be present and may progress to infarction and perforation. Pneumatosis intestinalis in SLE is usually benign and transient but may represent an irreversible necrotizing enterocolitis. In addition, pancreatitis and abdominal serositis are

well-recognized. Abnormal liver functions also occur. A vasculitic process has been implicated in the pathogenesis of GI manifestations.

Wallace DJ: Gastrointestinal manifestations and related liver and biliary disorders. In Wallace DJ, et al (eds): Dubois' Lupus Erythematosus, 4th ed. Philadelphia, Lea & Febiger, 1993, pp 410–417.

101. What is the most common pathologic abnormality in patients with lupus CNS disease?

Small infarcts and hemorrhages are more commonly the source for the neuropsychiatric features of lupus than vasculitis. In fact, vasculitis, as suggested by such commonly used designations as "lupus cerebritis," occur in < 15% of patients.

Johnson RT, Richardson EP: The neurological manifestations of systemic lupus erythematosus. Medicine 47:337–369, 1968.

KEY POINTS: SPECIFIC RHEUMATOLOGIC DISEASES

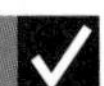

1. RA increases mortality.
2. Mixed connective tissue disease is a specific diagnosis with features of SLE and scleroderma in association with anti-RNP antibodies.
3. Undifferentiated connective tissue disease is a description commonly applied to a patient with signs and symptoms definitive enough to be clearly autoimmune and inflammatory in nature, but not sufficient to render a more exact diagnosis.
4. True articular hip pain is usually experienced as pain in the buttocks or groin. Pain at the outside of the hips is usually greater trochanteric bursitis.
5. Claudication can be either neurogenic or vascular in origin. Whereas arterial lower limb claudication often eases when the activity stops, even if there is no change in posture, neurogenic claudication may even intensify in a similar circumstance.

102. What are the neuropsychiatric manifestations of SLE?

Because of the difficulty in establishing an unequivocal diagnosis, rates of CNS features cross a broad range. Neuropsychiatric manifestations of lupus may occur in around 70% of patients. Examples include psychosis (5%); cranial, autonomic, and peripheral neuropathies; migraine headaches; seizure; aseptic meningitis; pseudotumor cerebri; chorea; and cerebral infarction. Rarely, transverse myelitis has been observed. Organic brain syndromes are easier to recognize in lupus when they are profound (delirium) but now are recognized more frequently as changes in mentation, such as mild memory loss and impaired concentration. The more subtle features of cognitive dysfunction may be the most common CNS syndrome in SLE. Abnormal SPECT or PET scanning and decreasing intellectual function, as measured by a standard battery of neurocognitive function tests, are present. The cause for this problem is not known, but cytokines are believed to play an important role.

Wallace DJ, Metzger AL: Systemic lupus erythematosus: Clinical aspects and treatment. In Koopman WJ (ed): Arthritis and Allied Conditions: A Textbook of Rheumatology, 13th ed. Baltimore, Williams & Wilkins, 1997, pp 1319–1345.

103. Describe the pulmonary manifestations of lupus.

Pulmonary involvement is fairly common in lupus and usually takes the form of pleurisy or pleural effusion. Up to 60% of patients may have pleuritic pain over the course of their illness.

Effusions can be either transudative or exudative and in rare cases are the presenting feature. The so-called shrinking lung syndrome describes dyspnea associated with diaphragmatic dysfunction, probably secondary to chronic pleural scarring. Pulmonary parenchymal involvement or lupus pneumonitis has been described, as have pulmonary hemorrhage, pulmonary emboli, and pulmonary hypertension. Emboli and hypertension are more common when phospholipid antibodies are also present.

104. List some conditions associated with a positive ANA.

- Lupus
- Drug-induced lupus
- Rheumatoid arthritis
- Systemic sclerosis
- CREST syndrome
- Polymyositis
- Dermatomyositis
- Mixed connective tissue disease
- Chronic hepatitis
- Infectious mononucleosis

105. Summarize the mortality rate associated with SLE.

Death rates from SLE have declined significantly over the last half of the 20th century. The 5-year survival rate in the 1950s was only 50%, whereas it is now > 90%. Survival in those with late-onset disease seems to be reduced compared with survival among those patients afflicted at an earlier age.

106. What are the common causes for death in patients with SLE?

Cause of death may be related to active disease, toxicity of medications, or other causes. Death early in the course of disease is usually related to the disease itself. Nephritis and CNS disease are the most ominous prognostic factors. Of the causes of death not directly related to active disease, infection is singly most common followed by myocardial infarction, stroke, and other atherosclerotic complications. Two recent studies have shown the presence of accelerated atherosclerosis in SLE.

Gladman DD, Urowitz MB: Prognostic subsets and mortality in systemic lupus erythematosus. In Wallace DJ, Hahn BH (eds): Dubois' Lupus Erythematosus, 5th ed. Baltimore, Williams & Wilkins, 1997.

Roman MJ, Shanker BA, et al: Prevalence and correlates of accelerated atherosclerosis in systemic lupus erythematosus. N Engl J Med 349:2399–2340, 2003.

Asanuma Y, Oeser A, et al: Premature coronary-artery atherosclerosis in systemic lupus erythematosus. N Engl J Med 349:2407, 2003.

107. Is ANA one antibody?

No. The detection of the LE cell initiated the study of autoantibodies. With the development of immunofluorescent techniques, different staining patterns were discovered, and it became clear that many different nuclear antigens can elicit an antibody response. Thus, many antibodies can be classified as ANA (see Table 11-6). Detecting the specific antibody reaction requires more refined techniques.

108. Do ANA staining patterns detect specific ANAs? What is their clinical relevance?

The fluorescence test for ANA is performed by incubating the patient's serum with a fixed monolayer of human larynx epithelioma cancer (HEp-2) cell lines. If ANAs are present in the serum, they bind to the nuclear component of the substrate. Next, fluorescent anti-Ig is added, which binds to antibodies (if present) in the test serum. With the fluorescent tag, the ANA can be directly visualized under fluorescent light. Different patterns of staining occur, and although they may provide some information, they do not identify the specific antibody present, nor are they specific for a disease entity. For example, the rim or peripheral pattern (usually associated with antibodies directed against nuclear membrane proteins) may be obscured if another autoantibody (staining a homogeneous pattern) is present.

TABLE 11-6. ANTINUCLEAR ANTIBODIES

Antigen	Antibody
Deoxyribose phosphate backbone of DNA	Anti-DNA (double-stranded or native)
Purine and pyrimidine bases	Anti–single-stranded DNA
H1, H2A, H2B, H3, H2A/H2B complex, H3/H4 complex	Antihistones
DNA topoisomerase I	Anti–SCL-70
Histidyl tRNA transferase	Anti–Jo-1
Kinetochore	Anticentromere
RNA polymerase I	Antinucleolar
Y1–Y5 RNA and protein	Anti-Ro
U1–6 RNA and protein	Anti-RNP (includes anti-Sm)

Adapted from von Mühlen CA, et al: Autoantibodies in the diagnosis of systemic rheumatic diseases. Semin Arthritis Rheum 24:323–358, 1995.

109. Why is it helpful to know which specific ANA is present in a given patient?
Although no laboratory test is absolutely diagnostic for a rheumatic disease, the presence of certain autoantibodies in the appropriate clinical setting can be helpful. Some common disease associations include:

Ro/SSA	SLE, neonatal lupus syndrome, subacute lupus, Sjögren's syndrome, RA
DS DNA	SLE
Sm	SLE
Jo-1	Polymyositis with pulmonary involvement
Centromere	CREST syndrome
SCL-70	Systemic sclerosis

Craft J, et al: Antinuclear antibodies. In Kelly WN, et al (eds): Textbook of Rheumatology, 4th ed. Philadelphia, W.B. Saunders, 1993, pp 164–187.

110. Which drugs are commonly associated with the development of a clinical syndrome of lupus and a positive ANA?
Historically, a clinical syndrome of arthritis, fever, rash, and positive ANA was seen in some patients after initiating antihypertensive treatment with hydralazine. Since then, the development of circulating ANA or clinical symptoms has been demonstrated with many drugs, including procainamide, diphenylhydantoin, isoniazid, chlorpromazine, d-penicillamine, sulfasalazine, methyldopa, and quinidine. So-called slow acetylators more commonly develop clinical symptoms. The clinical features usually regress fairly promptly, although the laboratory abnormality may persist (sometimes indefinitely) when the drug is discontinued. The clinical features commonly present in drug-induced lupus rarely, if ever, include CNS disease or nephritis.

Fritzler MJ, Rubin RL: Drug-induced-lupus. In Wallace DJ, et al (eds): Dubois' Lupus Erythematosus, 4th ed. Philadelphia, Lea & Febiger, 1993, pp 442–453.

111. What antibody is often touted to be diagnostic for drug-induced lupus?
Although often touted to be diagnostic for drug-induced lupus, an antihistone antibody is not particularly helpful when a patient taking one of the above medications has features of lupus and a positive ANA. Although antihistone antibody is present in the syndrome of drug-induced

lupus (perhaps as many as 90% of cases), it is also true that nearly 75% of patients with idiopathic disease may produce this antibody, making it of little diagnostic usefulness.

112. Does lupus nephritis recur in a transplanted kidney?

Disease activity in SLE often quiets with the onset of uremia and dialysis. Several studies note the ability to discontinue glucocorticoids without a return of extrarenal manifestations once dialysis has been initiated. Although there are reports of subsequent disease exacerbations, disease activity usually does not recur in transplanted kidneys.

113. Discuss the interaction of pregnancy and SLE.

1. Fertility is unaffected by the disease (i.e., patients become pregnant just as readily as women without lupus).
2. Although recent data suggest that pregnant patients with lupus do not have disease flares more frequently than nonpregnant patients, disease exacerbations during pregnancy do occur. Because such flares can be severe, patients with SLE should be considered at high risk. Active disease during the antecedent 3–6 months may increase the risk of a flare.
3. Preeclampsia occurs more frequently in pregnant patients with lupus. There is also increased risk of miscarriage, abortion, intrauterine growth delay, and prematurity in patients with SLE compared with controls.
4. The Ro antibody crosses the placenta and is responsible for most of the neonatal lupus syndromes, including skin manifestations and congenital heart block.

Lochshin MD: Pregnancy does not cause systemic lupus erythematosus to worsen. Arthritis Rheum 32:665–670, 1989.

114. Describe the role of cytotoxic therapy in the treatment of lupus-associated nephritis.

Cytotoxic agents, such as cyclophosphamide and chlorambucil, are useful in the management of life-threatening rheumatic diseases. Because of their toxicity, they should be used only in situations in which careful clinical trials point to significant advantages. Clinical trials of cytotoxic agents have shown an advantage in patients with lupus nephritis. Patients with inflammatory renal lesions avoided or had a slower progression to end-stage renal disease and diminished mortality rates when the treatment regimen included cyclophosphamide.

115. What is the antiphospholipid antibody (APA) syndrome?

APA syndrome consists of one or more of the following: multiple miscarriages, arterial or venous thrombosis, and thrombocytopenia in association with a laboratory finding of antibodies directed against phospholipids. These antibodies can be specific (such as anticardiolipin antibodies), or they may be identified by their effect on the clotting cascade (lupus anticoagulant). Common laboratory tests indicating the presence of antibodies to various phospholipids include prolonged partial thromboplastin time, false-positive VDRL test for syphilis, or positive anticardiolipin antibodies. A less common example is the dilute Russell viper venom clotting time. APA syndrome may occur by itself (primary APA syndrome) or in association with an underlying connective tissue syndrome, primarily lupus (secondary APA syndrome).

116. What is catastrophic APA syndrome?

Catastrophic APA syndrome is described as the sudden overwhelming vascular occlusion mediated by APAs. Clinical features result from widespread thrombosis of small vessels and the systemic inflammatory response which may include ischemic bowel, pulmonary emboli, ARDS, infarctive skin lesions, encephalopathy with altered consciousness, seizure MI and cardiac valvular lesions. Renal involvement is present in the majority of cases.

117. With what factors is catastrophic APA syndrome associated?
Up to 50% of patients may have previously known (and even treated) diseases including SLE, APA syndrome, and Behçet's disease, among others. Other clinical events may coincide with onset, including infections, vaccination, flare of underlying disease and even withdrawal of anticoagulation.

118. Summarize the prognosis of patients with catastrophic APA syndrome.
Mortality is high, even with prompt intervention.

119. How is catastrophic APA syndrome treated?
Treatment begins with anticoagulation with heparin, use of glucocorticoid, and treatment of any associated conditions. IVIg, plasma exchange, and cytotoxic agents have been used if patients fail to respond promptly.

Petri M. Management of thrombosis in antiphospholipid antibody syndrome. Rheum Dis Clin NA 27(3):633–641, 2001.

120. Describe Raynaud's phenomenon.
Raynaud's phenomenon is the eponym given to the color change (usually white, blue, then red) in the hands (or any distal part of the body) that is incited by intense emotion or exposure to cold. When one inquires about Raynaud's, it is sometimes difficult not to suggest a positive answer. Thus, one may ask, "While grocery shopping, do you notice any problems in the frozen food section?" or "If you look at your hands when you get cold, do they look any different to you?"

121. Distinguish between primary and secondary Raynaud's phenomenon.
When Raynaud's occurs without a disease association it can be called *primary Raynaud's phenomenon* or *Raynaud's disease.* Raynaud's occurring in association with another condition is usually termed *Raynaud's syndrome* or *secondary Raynaud's phenomenon.* The primary/secondary designation seems much easier to remember.

122. Which rheumatic conditions are typically associated with Raynaud's phenomenon?

- SLE
- APA syndrome
- CREST syndrome
- Drug-induced lupus
- Reflex sympathetic dystrophy
- Systemic sclerosis
- Idiopathic Raynaud's phenomenon
- Carcinoid syndrome
- Carpal tunnel syndrome
- Polymyositis
- Sjögren's syndrome
- Cold agglutinin disease
- Cryoglobulinemia (primary or associated with active hepatitis C)
- Systemic vasculopathies
- Cholesterol emboli
- Drug-induced (especially beta blockers)

123. What factors predict the development of a systemic autoimmune disease in a patient presenting with Raynaud's phenomenon?
One study showed that 12.6% of patients presenting with Raynaud's phenomenon went on to develop a rheumatic disease. Positive ANA (positive predictive value 30%), abnormal nail bed capillaries (positive predictive value 47%), or abnormal pulmonary function studies suggest an increased risk for developing systemic disease.

Spenser-Green G: Outcomes in primary Raynaud's phenomenon: With metaanalysis of frequency rates and predictions of transformation to secondary diseases. Arch Intern Med 158:595, 1998.

124. **What is meant by systemic sclerosing conditions?**
Systemic sclerosing conditions are a group of illnesses producing fibrosis of skin and other tissues. They can be systemic (scleroderma, CREST) or localized (morphea, linear scleroderma). Although a systemic form of the disease, CREST (**c**alcinosis, **R**aynaud's, **e**sophageal dysmotility, **s**clerodactyly, **t**elangiectasias) is less likely to involve internal organs and therefore has a lower mortality than scleroderma.

125. **Summarize the epidemiology of CREST.**
There is a significantly higher prevalence in the U.S. population than worldwide. Women are more commonly affected then men. African Americans more commonly suffer with scleroderma while Caucasians are more commonly afflicted with CREST.

126. **Summarize the genetic component of scleroderma.**
There is clearly a genetic component, with family members having a significant increased risk of developing scleroderma compared with an individual with no family history. One likely culprit is an abnormality in the fibrillin gene. This has been elegantly shown in a population study of Choctaw Indians, in whom a genetic defect has been traced to a single common ancestor.
Tan FK, Arnett FC: Genetic factors in the etiology of systemic sclerosis and Raynaud's phenomenon. Curr Opin Rheum 12:511, 2000.

127. **List the noncutaneous features of scleroderma.**
Arthritis, inflammatory muscle disease, GI dysmotility with resulting malabsorption, pulmonary interstitial pulmonary fibrosis with or without pulmonary hypertension, and scleroderma renal crisis.

128. **Do specific autoantibodies help predict the form of scleroderma a patient may develop?**
Yes. Although > 80% of patients with scleroderma have a positive ANA, this test adds little specificity. Anti-topoisomerase 1 (anti–Scl-70) has a positive predictive value of 70% of developing scleroderma. Centromere antibodies have a positive predictive value of 88% for the development of CREST.
Spencer-Green G: Tests preformed in systemic sclerosis: Anticentromere antibody and anti Scl-70 antibody. Am J Med 103:242, 1997.

129. **What is scleroderma renal crisis?**
Scleroderma renal crisis is a life-threatening aspect of scleroderma manifested by sudden onset of malignant hypertension, hemolytic anemia, hyperreninemia, and renal failure. Angiotensin-converting enzyme inhibitors have been life saving.

130. **What further evaluation for an occult malignancy should be undertaken in an adult diagnosed with dermatomyositis?**
The risk of malignancy is increased in patients with myositis. The data are strongest for patients with dermatomyositis, and the risk increases with age. Studies should include chest x-ray, mammography, stool guaiac, prostate-specific antigen, and full gynecologic examination. Depending on the results, follow-up evaluation may include endoscopy, colonoscopy, and biopsy.

131. **What is Jaccoud's deformity?**
Deformities of the hands secondary to chronic inflammation of the joint capsule, ligaments, and tendons. The changes may mimic those of RA (ulnar deviation of the fingers, MCP joint subluxation). Erosions are not present, although after several recurrences, notches may be seen in x-rays on the ulnar side of the metacarpal heads. Early in the course, patients can correct these changes voluntarily. Although originally described in rheumatic fever, this disorder has been extended to include the arthropathy in other conditions, most commonly SLE.

132. What is inclusion body myositis? How is it different from other inflammatory myopathies?
There are many significant differences between inclusion body myositis and inflammatory myopathy. Inclusion body myositis more often affects older people. Its onset is rarely sudden. The patient may notice both proximal and distal muscle involvement that may be focal, diffuse, or asymmetrical. It occurs more frequently men than in women. CPK levels are rarely as elevated in inclusion body myositis as they are in polymyositis and may be normal in as many as 25% of patients. Biopsy may show inflammation quite similar to that seen in polymyositis. Ragged red fibers and atrophic fibers are present in inclusion body myositis and intracellular lined vacuoles is a classical finding. Finally, EM reveals intracytoplasmic, intranuclear tubular or filamentous inclusions.

SPONDYLOARTHROPATHIES

133. What is a spondyloarthropathy? Which diseases are usually so classified?
Spondyloarthropathies are a group of inflammatory diseases of uncertain etiology that affect the spine and sacroiliac joints. In addition, they are characterized by the absence of RF or other autoantibodies and a high association with HLA B27. Other unifying features include peripheral oligoarthropathy, enthesopathy, and extra-articular foci of inflammation. Diseases classified as spondyloarthropathies include:

Ankylosing spondylitis	Arthropathy of psoriasis
Reactive arthritis	Enteropathic arthritis
Juvenile spondyloarthropathy	

Arnett FC: Seronegative spondyloarthropathies. In Scientific American Medicine Sect 15, 2002.

134. What mechanisms may explain the association of HLA-B27 with arthropathy?
The mechanism by which HLA B27 predisposes to arthritis is unknown. The observation that transgenic rats expressing B27 spontaneously develop features of spondyloarthritis strongly suggests that it is the B27 gene itself (and not a closely linked gene) that confers risk. The B27 may act as a receptor for a microorganism, or it may be modified by an infecting microorganism to elicit an immune reaction against the new antigen. Alternatively, B27 may resemble the microbial epitopes; thus antibodies directed against the microorganism cross-react with host antigens (molecular mimicry).

135. Describe the principal clinical features of ankylosing spondylitis.
Ankylosing spondylitis is one of the few inflammatory arthropathies that occurs more commonly in men than in women. The disease begins in late adolescence, usually with gradually worsening low back pain and stiffness. The pain typically improves with activity and worsens with rest, leading to the commonly experienced symptom of night-time awakening with pain and stiffness that require getting out of bed to stretch. Peripheral joints may be involved early in the course of the disease, mostly in the lower limbs. The disease is generally progressive, and extra-articular features may develop. The peripheral arthropathy occurs in both sexes, although sacroiliac and spinal involvement is more prominent in men.

Gran JT: An epidemiological survey of the signs and symptoms of ankylosing spondylitis. Clin Rheum Dis 4:161, 1985.

136. Name the extra-articular features of ankylosing spondylitis.
Anterior uveitis (occurring in ~25% of patients), aortitis (often progressing to aortic valve insufficiency), cardiac conduction defects, and pulmonary fibrosis (occurring in < 1% of patients).

137. What is the difference between a syndesmophyte and an osteophyte?
Syndesmophytes are thin, vertical outgrowths that represent calcifications of the annulus fibrosus. As syndesmophytes enlarge, ossification can involve adjacent anterior longitudinal and paravertebral connective tissue. Syndesmophytes predominate on the anterior and lateral aspects of the spine, particularly near the thoracolumbar junction, eventually bridging the disc space and connecting one vertebral body with its neighbor. **Osteophytes** are triangular and arise several millimeters from the discovertebral junction.

138. Describe the mucocutaneous manifestations of reactive arthritis.
Skin and mucous membranes are commonly involved in reactive arthritis. Small painless areas of desquamation on the tongue may not even be noticed by the patient. Circinate balanitis, conversely, is rarely missed. It primarily affects the glans penis and can range from small erythematous macules to larger areas of dry, flaking skin. Keratoderma blennorrhagica is a thickening and keratinization of the skin that generally involves the feet, hands, and nails. The lesions resemble psoriasis both clinically and pathologically.

Fan PT, Yu TY: Reiter's syndrome. In Kelly WN, et al (eds): Textbook of Rheumatology, 4th ed. Philadelphia, W.B. Saunders, 1993, pp 961–973.

139. List the five patterns of arthritis associated with psoriasis and their relative frequencies.

1. DIP joints of hands and/or feet	8%
2. Peripheral asymmetric oligoarthropathy	48%
3. Symmetric polyarthritis resembling RA	18%
4. Arthritis mutilans ("opera glass hands")	2%
5. Sacroiliitis with or without higher levels of spinal involvement	24%

Arnett FC: Sero-negative spondyloarthropathies. Bull Rheum Dis 37:1–12, 1987.

140. What is pyoderma gangrenosum?
Pyoderma gangrenosum consists of skin lesions that begin as pustules or erythematous nodules and break down to form spreading ulcers with necrotic, undermined edges. It is associated with IBD but also occurs in chronic active hepatitis, seropositive RA (without evidence of vasculopathy), leukemia, and polycythemia vera. Differential diagnosis of the lesions includes necrotizing vasculitis, bacterial infection, and spider bites.

KEY POINTS: TREATMENT OF RHEUMATOLOGIC DISEASE 

1. COX_2 NSAIDs are no more efficacious then older standard NSAIDs but are significantly less toxic.
2. Unless death or irreversible organ damage is imminent (e.g., likely to occur before cyclophosphamide and steroids can have sufficient therapeutic effect), plasma exchange adds little to the long-term outcome in patients with lupus with CNS disease or nephritis.

CRYSTAL ARTHROPATHY

141. What three principal crystals are associated with joint inflammation?
1. Urate (gout)
2. Calcium pyrophosphate (CPP; "pseudogout")
3. Hydroxyapatite

Dieppe P, Calvert P: Crystals and Joint Disease. London, Chapman & Hall, 1983.

142. What conditions have been associated with CPPD disease?

Hemochromatosis	Hypothyroidism	Neuropathic joint
Hyperparathyroidism	Hemosiderosis	Amyloidosis
Hypophosphatasia	Gout	Trauma, including surgery
Hypomagnesemia		

143. Why is the polarizing microscope important in the diagnosis of rheumatic diseases?

Use of a polarizing microscope allows the identification of specific etiologies in certain clinical syndromes. Its function is based on the relatively simple observation that crystals rotate light (i.e., they are birefringent). Polarized light passing through a crystal is no longer parallel to light not passing through the crystal. If a second polarizer is added so that its axis is rotated 90° (extinction) to the light as it emerges from the first polarizer but before it reaches the crystal, the only light reaching the observer's eye is the light that the crystal has rotated.

144. Where is chondrocalcinosis commonly demonstrated roentgenographically?

Chondrocalcinosis describes the radiographic appearance of CPP crystals in the joint cartilages. The prevalence in the general population (as assessed by multiple radiologic studies) is 10–15% in people aged 65–75 years but rises above 40% in people over 80 years old. They are generally punctate and linear densities in the articular cartilages: menisci of the knees, radiocarpal joints, annulus fibrosus of intervertebral discs, and symphysis pubis.

145. What are the four stages of gout?

Stage 1: asymptomatic hyperuricemia.
Stage 2: the first attack of acute articular disease.
Stage 3: the period between attacks, described as intercritical gout.
Stage 4: chronic tophaceous gout.

146. Describe stage 1 of gout.

Serum urate levels are elevated without articular disease or nephrolithiasis. Not all patients with asymptomatic hyperuricemia develop gout, but the higher the serum level, the greater the likelihood of developing articular disease. In most cases, 20–30 years of sustained hyperuricemia pass before an attack of nephrolithiasis or arthropathy.

147. Characterize the first attack of acute articular disease.

It is exquisitely painful and usually occurs in a single joint. Fever, swelling, erythema, and skin sloughing may be associated findings. Fifty percent of initial attacks occur as podagra, and 90% of patients with gout have podagra at some stage of disease without treatment.

148. Characterize stage 3 of gout.

During the intercritical period, most patients are completely asymptomatic. However, 62% of patients have a second attack of articular disease within 1 year of the first attack, 16% within 1–2 years, 11% within 2–5 years, 4% after 5–10 years, and 7% after > 10 years.

149. What is chronic tophaceous gout?

Chronic tophaceous gout occurs with the development of chronic arthritis and tissue deposition of urate. The principal determinant of the rate of urate deposition is the serum urate concentration.

Gutman AB: The past four decades of progress in the knowledge of gout with an assessment of present status. Arthritis Rheum 16:431, 1973.

OSTEOARTHRITIS

150. Is osteoarthritis (OA) a genetic disease?

The role of genetic factors in rheumatic disease is an area of vigorous research. OA clearly has a hereditary component. Perhaps the most recognized feature is the presence of Heberden's nodes in mothers and sisters. Recent studies have uncovered a mutation in a type II collagen gene (Arg519 to Cys) that predisposes to early OA.

Pun YL, et al: Clinical correlations of osteoarthritis associated with a single-base mutation (arginine 519 to cysteine) in type II procollagen gene: A newly defined pathogenesis. Arthritis Rheum 37:264–269, 1994.

151. Compare the biochemical changes of the aged joint with the osteoarthritic joint.

Although age is the single most significant epidemiologic factor associated with OA, there are biochemical differences between an old joint and an osteoarthritic joint (Table 11-7). The major components of the joint are bone and cartilage. The major components of the cartilage include the chondrocytes and matrix (which in turn is composed of collagen, water, and proteoglycans).

TABLE 11-7. BIOCHEMICAL DIFFERENCES BETWEEN THE AGING JOINT AND OSTEOARTHRITIS

	Aging	Osteoarthritis
Bone	Osteoporosis	Thickened cortices, osteophytes, subchondral cysts, remodeling
Chondrocyte activity	Normal	Increased
Collagen	Increased cross-linking of fibrils	Irregular weave Smaller fibrils
Water	Slight decrease	Significant increase
Proteoglycan	Normal total content	Decreased total proteoglycan component
	Decreased chondroitins	Increased chondroitins
	Increased keratin	Decreased keratin
	Normal aggregation	Decreased aggregation

From Brandt KD, Fife RS: Aging in relation to the pathogenesis of osteoarthritis. Clin Rheum Dis 12:117–130, 1986.

152. Describe the syndrome of spinal stenosis.

Progressive narrowing of the spinal canal leads to the syndrome of spinal stenosis, which results most commonly from OA of the lumbar or cervical spine. With cervical disease, patients typically present with pain and limitation of motion. Hyperreflexia is common. Other signs may include muscle weakness, spastic gait, and Babinski's sign. In the lumbar region, the clinical manifestations are mostly those of compression of the cauda equina (commonly claudication).

153. What is the difference between spondylolysis and spondylolisthesis?

Spondylolysis is an interruption of the pars interarticularis of the vertebra. **Spondylolisthesis** refers to displacement of one vertebra on another. The most common cause of spondylolisthesis is bilateral spondylolysis. Severe OA of the apophyseal joints can produce spondylolisthesis without spondylolysis.

154. What is the vacuum sign?
A radiographic sign of intervertebral osteochondrosis. Radiolucencies represent gas (nitrogen) that appears at the site of negative pressure produced by abnormal spaces or clefts. Clefts are produced by degeneration of intervertebral disc, especially the nucleus pulposus.

155. What is DISH?
Diffuse idiopathic skeletal hyperostosis (DISH) is a syndrome characterized by extensive ossification of tendinous and ligamentous attachments to bone. Involvement of the spine with flowing calcification over the anterior longitudinal ligament is among the most common findings. Extraspinal manifestations also are reported. Clinical symptoms are often mild and consist of morning stiffness and deep achiness of the affected portion.

156. What radiographic features help to distinguish DISH from ankylosing spondylitis, degenerative spine disease, and spondylosis deformans?
1. Flowing calcification along the anterolateral aspect of at least four contiguous vertebral bodies.
2. Relative preservation of intervertebral disc height in the involved vertebral segment and absence of extensive radiographic changes of "degenerative" disc disease (vacuum phenomena, vertebral body marginal sclerosis).
3. Absence of apophyseal joint ankylosis and sacroiliac joint erosion, sclerosis, and intra-articular osseous fusion.

157. List five classic radiographic findings of OA.
1. Subchondral cyst formation
2. New bone formation (osteophytes)
3. Sclerosis of bone
4. Joint space narrowing
5. Lack of osteoporosis

INFECTIOUS ARTHRITIS

158. Describe the mechanism for acute rheumatic fever.
Rheumatic fever occurs after group A streptococcal pharyngitis (which may be asymptomatic). Data indicate that the immune response initiated against the bacteria plays an important role. Antibodies cross-react with human antigens, leading to a persistent autoimmune reaction and tissue destruction (molecular mimicry). Development of immune complexes also has been documented.

159. What viral illnesses may be associated with arthropathy?
Common viruses associated with arthropathy include hepatitis B and C, parvovirus B19, rubella, and HIV. Some rare viral infections strongly associated with arthropathy include the group A arboviruses (Ross River virus, chikungunya, o'ynong-nyong, sindbis, Mayaro). Common viral infections that occasionally produce arthropathy include mumps, smallpox (vaccinia), Epstein-Barr virus, cytomegalovirus, and enteroviruses (ECHO and coxsackievirus).

Naides SJ: Viral arthritis including HIV. Curr Opin Rheumatol 7:337–342, 1995.

160. Summarize the association of hepatitis B and hepatitis C with arthropathy.
Chronic hepatitis B with persistent circulating B antigen has been associated with polyarteritis nodosa. Hepatitis C has a dramatically high rate of occurrence in patients with mixed cryoglobulinemia; this virus also has been documented in several cases of otherwise unexplained inflammatory polyarthropathy.

161. How is parvovrius associated with arthropathy?
Active infection with parvovirus has been associated with a nondestructive RA-like picture, with RFs documented in the circulation. Of interest, the arthropathy clears with no chronic or destructive sequelae.

162. Summarize the association of rubella infection with arthropathy.
Rubella infection is associated with arthralgia and arthritis, especially in adult women. Joint symptoms usually begin within 1 week of the onset of the rash of German measles. In the past, arthritis and arthralgias often were seen after rubella vaccination, but they are less common since a less arthrogenic strain of virus is used for the vaccine.

163. Summarize the common articular problems experienced by patients infected with HIV.
Patients infected with HIV suffer a variety of joint problems, the most common of which is arthralgia. Reactive arthritis is also well described in HIV-infected patients. The syndrome can have many of the classical features of reactive arthritis, including an association with HLA B27. Still, axial disease is uncommon and sacroiliac involvement is rare. Therefore, it has been suggested that HIV-infected patients should be described as having an undifferentiated spondyloarthropathy. Arthritis associated with psoriasis is also seen in patients with HIV infection. Its course may be more severe than in non–HIV-infected sufferers. It tends to follow an asymmetric polyarticular pattern in most patients. The "painful articular syndrome" has been used to describe an exquisitely painful asymmetrical minimally inflammatory arthritis, usually of the large joints of the lower extremities. Finally, septic arthritis is also well documented in patients with HIV infection. As in non–HIV-infected patients, the most common pathogen is *Staphylococcus aureus*. Also documented are cases of septic arthritis due to *Streptococcus*, *Salmonella*, atypical *Mycobacteria*, and other opportunistic organisms.

Solomon G, Brancato L, Winchester R. An approach to the human immunodeficiency virus-positive patient with a spondyloarthropathic disease. Rheum Dis Clin North Am 17:43–58, 1991.

164. What are the specific muscle problems encountered by patients infected with HIV?
Muscle involvement in patients with HIV takes several well-described forms. Simple arthralgias are common in all patients with viremia and, although uncomfortable, are rarely debilitating or dangerous. Inflammatory muscle disease clinically identical with polymyositis and dermatomyositis has also been well described. When present with evidence of peripheral neuropathy, a systemic vasculopathy should be considered. Nemaline rod myopathy has been described; its presence is noted pathologically without much inflammatory change in the muscle. Severe wasting in HIV-inflected patients is associated with a non-inflammatory myopathy. Pyomyositis, or direct muscle infection in the form of small muscle abscesses, is also reported. The most common infectious agents is *S. aureus*, but *Mycobacterium avium*, cryptococci, and *Microsporidia,* among others, have been reported. Finally, treatment itself has been associated with producing myopathy. Most cases have been reported with AZT, but other antiviral medications have been implicated.

165. What is DILS? Is it the same as Sjögren's syndrome?
DILS (diffuse infiltrative lymphocytosis syndrome) is a condition occurring in between 3% and 8% of HIV-infected patients. Although it produces profound salivary gland enlargement and symptoms of dryness (sicca), it is a distinct entity with different immunogenetics and pathophysiology from Sjögren's syndrome. African American DILS sufferers show a high incidence of HLA-DR8, while DR6 and DR7 are more prevalent in Caucasians. By contrast, in patients with Sjögren's syndrome, HLA DR2 and DR3 predominate.

166. What other organs may be involved in DILS?
In addition to salivary glands, other organs can become infiltrated with lymphocytes (CD8 cells in contrast to the CD4 cells characteristic of Sjögren's syndrome). Clinical features sometimes seen include neuropathy, interstitial pneumonitis, interstitial nephritis, and hepatitis.

167. Which bacterial pathogens are most commonly responsible for septic arthritis?
Septic arthritis is usually classified as gonococcal or nongonococcal. Of the nongonococcal bacteria causing joint infections, staphylococci remain the most common. Species of streptococci are the next most common cause when grouped together. Finally, gram-negative bacilli may cause 20–30% of septic joints.

168. Describe the common clinical manifestations of gonococcal arthritis.
Gonococcal arthritis occurs in approximately 0.1–0.5% of patients with gonorrhea. Clinical manifestations may differ from those of other bacterial arthropathies. Even under optimal conditions, joint fluids are culture positive in < 50% of cases. The arthropathy is commonly migratory and often accompanied by tenosynovitis. Skin lesions are often present, usually as a small macule or papule on a distal extremity.

169. What are the clinical manifestations of Lyme disease? When do they occur in the natural course of untreated disease?
The earliest manifestations of Lyme disease are erythema chronicum migrans and a flulike illness. In subsequent weeks, neurologic features may develop, including meningitis, cranial neuropathies (most commonly Bell's palsy), and peripheral neuropathy. Up to 8% of untreated patients may develop cardiac involvement including an AV block and myopericarditis. Anywhere from weeks to years after infection, an inflammatory arthritis can develop with knees being the most commonly afflicted.

170. Describe the classic skin manifestation of Lyme disease.
Erythema chronicum migrans (ECM) is an expanding erythematous ring (often asymptomatic) with central clearing beginning at the sight of the tick bite. The *Borrelia* organism can be cultured from the margin of the lesion. The rash occasionally is accompanied by flu-like symptoms (arthralgia, myalgia, and fever). In endemic regions ECM is the most common presenting feature of early Lyme disease. Other skin manifestations include benign lymphocytoma and acrodermatitis chronica atrophicans.

171. What other infections can accompany Lyme disease?
The tick that transmits *Borrelia burgdorferi*, usually *Ixodes scapularis* in the U.S., can also transmit *Babesia microtii* and *Anaplama phagocytophila. B. microtii* is often asymptomatic but can be responsible for a mild flu-like illness or in the immunosuppressed a severe malaria-like illness. *A. phagocytophila* produces ehrlichiosis. Studies have shown a coinfection rate with *B. microtii* of 11% and with *A. phagocytophila* of 4%. It appears that the resulting illness is more severe when coinfection occurs.

172. Is chronic arthritis of Lyme disease produced by active joint infection?
About 70% of untreated patients with Lyme disease in the U.S. develop arthritis. It may take the form of arthralgia, intermittent episodes of arthritis, or, in about 10% of patients, a chronic inflammatory synovitis. Treatment failure is associated with HLA DR4. It seems unlikely that chronic Lyme arthritis is due to persistent live infection since live spirochetes have rarely been documented. In addition, spirochetal DNA has not been reliably discovered after amplification with PCR technology.

MISCELLANEOUS RHEUMATIC CONDITIONS

173. What are the muscles of the rotator cuff?
The muscles of the rotator cuff include the supraspinatus, infraspinatus, teres minor, and subscapularis.

174. **What syndromes are associated with malfunction of the rotator cuff muscles?**
Disease of the rotator cuff is a common cause of shoulder pain. Impingement syndrome occurs when the supraspinatus tendon is caught between the head of the humerus and the acromion, resulting in pain. The activity most likely to bring these structures into proximity (and thus cause pain) is overhead movement and internal rotation of the arm. Night pain is characteristic. If the tendon ruptures (rotator cuff tear), significant weakness may result. Impingement syndrome usually results from injury to the supraspinatus during repetitious elevation and forward motion of the arm. Rotator cuff tendinitis is often an acute problem and may be associated with calcification.

175. **What are the most common causes of neuropathic joints in the upper extremity?**
Without sensation and proprioception as regulators of joint function, gradual relaxation of supporting structure, abnormal mechanics, and ultimately joint destruction develop. Many diseases, including congenital pain insensitivity, amyloidosis, diabetes mellitus, alcoholism, and tabes dorsalis, can lead to neuroarthropathy. In the upper extremities, particularly the elbow, syringomyelia is a common cause of sensory abnormalities leading to arthropathy.

176. **What is sarcoidosis?**
Sarcoidosis is a systemic disease characterized by a noncaseating granulomatous reaction of unknown origin. Besides the lungs, involvement of the eyes, skin, and joints is not uncommon. Skin involvement, including erythema nodosum, occurs in approximately 30% of patients. Asymptomatic sarcoid granulomas have been found in muscle biopsy and may occur in bones, appearing radiographically as cysts. Osteolysis also has been described.

177. **Describe the rheumatic manifestations of sarcoidosis.**
Articular symptoms are present in most patients with acute sarcoidosis (hilar adenopathy, fever, erythema nodosum), often affecting the ankles and knees. This articular syndrome is usually self-limited, lasting up to 4 weeks. When the disease is less acute in onset, articular involvement is less common. It can, however, be recurring and protracted, although joint destruction is infrequent. The articular involvement may predate pulmonary involvement or occur after 10 years of disease.

178. **Which conditions are associated with Dupuytren's contracture?**
Fibrosis and thickening of the palmar fascia can lead to the flexion contracture first described by Dupuytren. Associated diseases include diabetes mellitus, chronic liver disease, epilepsy, plantar fasciitis, carpal tunnel syndrome, RA, trauma to the hand, pulmonary tuberculosis, and alcoholism, to name a few.

179. **Describe the characteristic features of Wegener's granulomatosis (WG).**
WG is one of the systemic necrotizing vasculopathies. The organs primarily affected are the respiratory tract (upper and/or lower) and kidneys. Respiratory tract involvement can manifest as recurrent sinusitis, otitis media, tracheobronchial inflammation and erosions, or pneumonitis with cavitation. With the inflammatory process unchecked, a saddle-nose deformity can occur. Additional symptoms, such as arthritis, neuropathies, and eye inflammation, may occur. Laboratory data are generally nonspecific, but recently an antibody to cytoplasmic components of the PMN leukocyte (c-ANCA) has been associated with active disease.

180. **Compare polyarteritis nodosa (PAN), microscopic polyangiitis (MPA), WG, and Churg-Strauss syndrome (CSS).**
See Table 11-8.

181. **What are antineutrophil cytoplasmic antibodies (ANCAs)?**
ANCAs are antibodies directed against enzymes (proteinase-3 [PR-3] and myeloperoxidase) found in primary granules of PMNs and lysosomes of monocytes. Immunofluorescence detects two principal staining patterns: a fine granular cytoplasmic staining (c-ANCA) and a perinuclear

TABLE 11-8. COMPARISION OF PAN, MPA, WG, AND CSS

	Vessels Affected	Target Tissue	Laboratory Data
PAN	Predominantly medium-sized venules	Uniformly: peripheral nerve, sparing arterioles, capillaries, and GI tract. No glomerulonephritis or pulmonary involvement.	No ANCA; possible hepatitis B or C
MPA	Small to medium-sized vessels, including capillaries, venules, and arterioles	Uniformly: glomerulonephritis, skin. Commonly: pulmonary + alveolar hemorrhage. Less commonly: nerve, CNS, upper airway.	Usually p-ANCA (anti-MPO)
WG	Small to medium-sized vessels including capillaries, venules, and arterioles	Uniformly: glomerulonephritis, upper airway and pulmonary eye. Commonly: alveolar hemorrhage, peripheral nerve. Less commonly: skin, CNS.	Usually c-ANCA (anti-PR3)
CSS	Small to medium-sized vessels including capillaries, venules, and arterioles	Uniformly: pulmonary and peripheral nerve. Commonly: upper airway, skin, CNS, glomerulonephritis. Less commonly: alveolar hemorrhage.	Eosinophilia Usually p-ANCA (anti-MPO)

MPO = myeloperoxidase.

collection of antibody (p-ANCA). Despite the similar in vivo location of these enzymes, ethanol fixation produces an artifactual migration of the myeloperoxidase to a perinuclear location. There is no movement of the PR-3, which produces the cytoplasmic staining pattern. Although artifactual, the staining distinction is useful.

182. With which diseases are ANCAs associated?

The p-ANCA is most associated with a microscopic polyarteritis or a pauci-immune (meaning lack of immune complex deposition or complement consumption) crescentic glomerulonephritis. The PR-3 ANCA (usually staining as c-ANCA) is more sensitive and specific for WG. In fact, the antibody often allows earlier diagnosis and descriptions of what appear to be milder forms of the disease. There seems to be a correlation between disease activity and titers of c-ANCA in patients with WG. p-ANCA is found in higher titer than expected in ulcerative colitis, RA, and SLE.

Ball GV, Gay RM: Vasculitis. In Arthritis and Allied Conditions, 14th ed. Baltimore, Williams & Wilkins, 2001, pp 1645–1695.

183. What is fibromyalgia (FM)?

FM is a chronic nondestructive illness characterized by fatigue, generalized pain, sleep disturbance (sometimes termed "nonrestorative" sleep), and tender points in a characteristic distribution (see Fig. 11-1). FM replaced the term *fibrositis* because no inflammatory process has been objectively documented. Patients may have FM alone or concomitant diseases (e.g., RA, osteoarthritis, Lyme disease, sleep apnea). The disease is often mimicked by hypothyroidism.

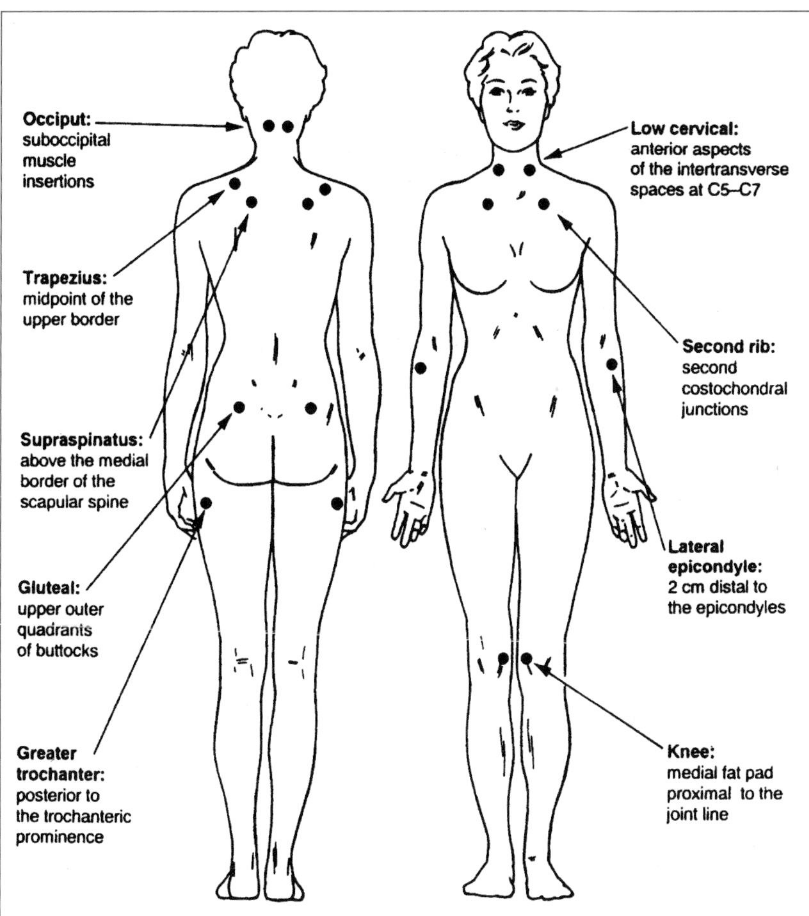

Figure 11-1. Location of tender points in fibromyalgia. (From Freundlich B, et al: The fibromyalgia syndrome. In Schumacher HR Jr, et al [eds]: Primer on Rheumatic Diseases, 10th ed. Atlanta, Arthritis Foundation, 1993, p 247, with permission.)

184. What other symptoms may be associated with FM?

In addition to the generalized achiness, patients may have associated irritable bowel syndrome, tension headaches, irritable bladder, and even a chronic cough. Sleep is disturbed by alpha intrusion into delta sleep as documented by EEG. Eighteen reproducible tender points have been established, and diagnosis of FM requires the presence of at least 11.

Wolfe F, et al: The American College of Rheumatology 1990 criteria for the classification of fibromyalgia: Report of the multicenter criteria committee. Arthritis Rheum 33:160–172, 1990.

185. How is FM treated?

Treatment is aimed at reconditioning muscles (slow but consistent physical training), restoration of more normal sleep patterns (tricyclic antidepressants in low doses are often helpful), and pain control (generally with nonnarcotic medications such as NSAIDs or acetaminophen and other techniques such as biofeedback).

BIBLIOGRAPHY

1. Harris ED, Budd RC, Firestein GS, et al (eds): Kelley's Textbook of Rheumatology, 7th ed. Philadelphia, W.B. Saunders, 2005.
2. Hochberg MC (ed). Rheumatology, 3rd ed. St. Louis, Mosby, 2003.
3. Klippel JH (ed): Primer on the Rheumatic Diseases, 12th ed. Atlanta, Arthritis Foundation, 2002.
4. Koopman WJ (ed): Arthritis and Allied Conditions: A Textbook of Rheumatology, 15th ed. Philadelphia, Lippincott Williams & Wilkins, 2005.
5. Resnick D (ed): Diagnosis of Bone and Joint Disorders, 4th ed. Philadelphia, W.B. Saunders, 2002.
6. Sheon RP, et al (eds): Soft Tissue Rheumatic Pain: Recognition, Management and Prevention, 3rd ed. Philadelphia, Lippincott Williams & Wilkins, 1996.

CHAPTER 12

ALLERGY AND IMMUNOLOGY

Roger D. Rossen, M.D., and Holly H. Birdsall, M.D., Ph.D.

Some men also have strange antipathies in their natures against that sort of food which others love and live upon. I have read of one that could not endure to eat either bread or flesh; of another that fell in a swooning fit at the smell of a rose . . . . there are some who, if a cat accidentally come into the room, though they neither see it, nor are told it, will presently be in a sweat, and ready to die away.

Increase Mather (1639–1723), *Remarkable Providence*

1. **Name the two major divisions of the immune system. Which is older?**
   The immune system can be considered to have two major divisions: the **innate immune system** and the **adaptive** or **cognitive immune system**. The innate immune system is phylogenetically older.

2. **Which is the first line of defense against infection?**
   Innate immunity is the first line of defense against infection because its elements are already present in the circulation and can respond immediately to microbial invasion. However, the innate system has no memory; on subsequent exposure to the same antigen, the response is no greater, no faster, and no more effective than it was on first exposure to antigen.

3. **What are the major components of the innate immune system?**
   Neutrophils, monocytes, macrophages, eosinophils, basophils, mast cells, natural killer (NK) cells, complement proteins, and acute-phase reactants. All of these elements have germline-encoded receptors that recognize motifs commonly present on microbes.

4. **What are the major components of the adaptive immune system? How do they work?**
   The adaptive immune system includes elements such as the B lymphocytes that make antibodies and T lymphocytes that provide the effector elements of antigen-specific cell-mediated immune responses. Elements of the adaptive immune system display a large repertoire (e.g., tens of millions) of specific antigen receptors that are generated by DNA rearrangements. Each lymphocyte and its clonal descendants express one of the millions of possible antigen receptors. Since numerically there are very few cells at any one time that can recognize newly introduced antigens, B cells and T cells must be appropriately stimulated and induced to divide and produce multiple copies of themselves.

5. **What is the major advantage of the adaptive immune system?**
   The distinct advantage of the adaptive immune system is its ability to select B cells and T cells that have high-affinity receptors for new antigens and to stimulate them to replicate and provide a specific, fine-tuned response to foreign invaders.

6. **What is the major disadvantage of the adaptive immune system?**
   The disadvantage of the adaptive immunes response is that the required expansion process takes time after the first encounter with antigen, in some cases more than 2 weeks. Many infectious agents can cause death or severe disability in less time than it takes the adaptive immune

system to mobilize a specific response. This disadvantage leaves a gap in the host defense system.

7. **Explain the role of vaccines in the adaptive immune system.**
The major reason that vaccines have been developed is to stimulate specific immune responses in advance of an encounter with a pathogenic microorganism so that an appropriate immune recognition system is in place before any real-life encounters take place.

8. **Explain immunologic memory.**
Although circulating antibodies and T cells produced during the initial response to a foreign substance may be lost with time, a second encounter with the same antigen typically induces a much more vigorous response that comes into play often within only a day or two following the second encounter. The innate and adaptive immune systems work together. For instance, T cells activate macrophages, allowing them to kill the organisms they ingest more effectively. Phagocytic cells ingest microbes coated by antibodies from the adaptive immune system. In order to mount an immune response, naive lymphocytes require costimulatory signals that are typically provided either by microbes or by cells of the innate system after encounter with microbial products.

9. **What are the major divisions of the adaptive immune system?**
The adaptive immune system may be divided into **humoral immunity** and **cell-mediated immunity**. The effector functions that they mediate often involve cells of the innate immune system.

10. **How does humoral immunity work?**
Humoral immunity involves antibodies, produced by B cells. Terminally differentiated B cells, called plasma cells, produce most of the antibodies. Humoral immune responses defend the host against extracellular bacteria and toxins. Blocking antibodies can prevent the adherence of bacteria, viruses, or toxins to host cells. Antibodies can activate complement through the classical pathway and lyse cells. Complement activation also generates chemotactic fragments that activate mast cells and phagocytes and chemotactically attract phagocytic cells into sites of inflammation. NK cells can bind to antibody-coated targets and lyse them in antibody-mediated cytotoxicity. Antibodies can also opsonize; in other words, their binding facilitates uptake of the antigen by phagocytic cells.

11. **How does cell-mediated immunity work?**
Cell-mediated immunity involves the action of T cells. $CD8^+$ cytolytic T cells can kill target cells directly. $CD4^+$ helper cells can activate macrophages to become more effective at killing the organisms they ingest. This process is also considered to be cell-mediated immunity, although, again, a cell of the innate system carries out the ultimate effector function. Cells of the innate system are also needed to initiate humoral and cell-mediated responses. Dendritic cells and macrophages ingest organisms, digest them into peptides, and present them to T cells and B cells in a way that causes antigen-specific lymphocytes to proliferate and differentiate into effector cells.

12. **What is the major histocompatibility complex (MHC)?**
The MHC is a cluster of genes (located on chromosome 6 in humans) that play a critical role in directing the activities of T cells.

13. **Name the two major classes of MHC molecules and their subtypes.**
MHC class I molecules, which are found on all somatic cells, and MHC class II molecules, which are found on a group of cells called antigen-presenting cells (e.g., dendritic cells, monocytes, macrophages, B cells). Humans have three major types of class I MHC molecules: HLA-A, HLA-B, and HLA-C. The class II MHC molecules include HLA-DR, HLA-DQ, and HLA-DP.

14. **How do MHC molecules function in the immune system?**
The antigen receptor of T cells can recognize only peptides displayed in MHC molecules. CD8-positive T cells (cytolytic T cells) bind only to antigenic peptides displayed within the antigen-presenting cleft of MHC class I molecules. CD4-positive T cells bind only to antigenic peptides displayed in MHC class II molecules.

15. **Describe the process by which antigens are displayed in MHC class I molecules.**
Under normal conditions, host proteins in the cytoplasm are broken down in an intracellular recycling process. Peptide fragments, generated by enzymes in an intracellular structure called a proteasome, are loaded into MHC class I molecules and displayed on the cell membrane. If an infecting virus has usurped the host synthetic machinery, some of the proteins displayed in MHC-I as a result of this process will be of viral origin. These proteins can be recognized by specific CD8 cells, which then lyse the infected host cell.

16. **Describe the process by which antigens are displayed in the MHC class II molecules.**
Extracellular antigens ingested by phagocytic cells and B cells are digested within endosomal vesicles by proteolytic enzymes; peptides generated here are loaded into MHC class II molecules. CD4 T cells recognize peptides displayed in MHC class II molecules on antigen-presenting cells. If the CD4 cells simultaneously receive additional signals from costimulatory molecules that are also displayed by these antigen-presenting cells, they become activated. Activated helper T cells produce messenger molecules called cytokines that further activate B cells to produce antibodies, CD8 T cells to become killer cells, and macrophages to produce molecules that can kill ingested microorganisms.

17. **What two signals are required to activate naive T cells?**
The first signal is provided by antigenic peptides displayed in MHC molecules. The second is provided by one or more costimulatory molecule produced by the antigen-presenting cell, in response to molecules displayed by pathogens. If these costimulatory signaling molecules are not present, the T cell–MHC interaction may alternatively cause the T cell to undergo programmed cell death, a process known as apoptosis.

18. **What are MCH class III genes?**
Included within the stretch of chromosome 6 that contains the genes for MHC class I and class II molecules are genes for complement components C2, C4, and factor B as well as other molecules with immunoregulatory properties, including the genes for tumor necrosis factor (TNF) alpha and TNF beta, also known as lymphotoxin. These additional genes within the MHC region of chromosome 6 are also known, in aggregate, as MHC class III genes.

19. **What are B lymphocytes (B cells)?**
B cells are derived from hematopoietic stem cells and are the precursors of plasma cells, the antibody- or immunoglobulin (Ig)-producing cells in the body. They differentiate from stem cells in the bone marrow, migrate through the blood, and eventually come to reside in the B cell areas of the spleen, lymph nodes, and submucosal tissues of the respiratory tree and the gut. The **B** designation comes from the discovery that antibody-producing cells develop in the **b**ursa of Fabricius, an anatomic structure located in the cloaca of **b**irds.

20. **Explain the basic structure of an antibody.**
An antibody or Ig molecule is a protein produced by B cells that binds to antigen. Ig molecules are composed of two identical heavy chains and two identical light chains. Each light and heavy chain combine to form an antigen-binding cleft at their amino terminus, and the two heavy chains associate with each other at their carboxy end. Overall, the structure resembles a lobster

with the claws representing the two antigen-binding sites. The tail of the lobster is composed only of heavy chains and is called the Fc piece. This end can bind to Fc receptors, structures that are largely found on phagocytes, and certain other effector cells of the immune system such as mast cells and eosinophils.

21. **Summarize the functions of the heavy chains and light chains.**
There are five classes of heavy chains (mu, gamma, alpha, epsilon and delta) that form the five isotypes or Ig classes: IgM, IgG, IgA, IgE, and IgD, respectively. There are two types of light chains, kappa and lamba, that are used by all Ig classes. IgA can polymerize into dimers and higher multimers. Secreted IgM is a pentamer of five basic subunits joined by a protein called J, the joining piece.

22. **What are the seven domains of the heavy chain constant region?**
The heavy chain constant region contains three domains in IgG, IgD, and IgA and four domains in IgE and IgM. These constant regions are responsible for the functional aspects of the Ig molecules (i.e., complement binding to the CH2 region, half-life in the circulation, ability to be transported across the placenta [IgG] or across mucous membranes [IgA]).

23. **Explain the heavy-chain variable region.**
The amino-terminal half is the variable region: V_L and V_H have three regions where the amino acid sequences are highly variable. It is the variation in sequence within these regions that determines the ability of antibodies to bind to one but not another antigen. That is, the variable regions confer specificity. A given B cell produces antibodies of a single specificity. However, during isotype switching, progeny of a given B cell may stop making IgM and begin producing IgG, IgA, or IgE. In that case the gene sequence encoding the V_H domain is transferred to genes encoding the C_H domains of the new Ig class. (See Fig. 12-1.)

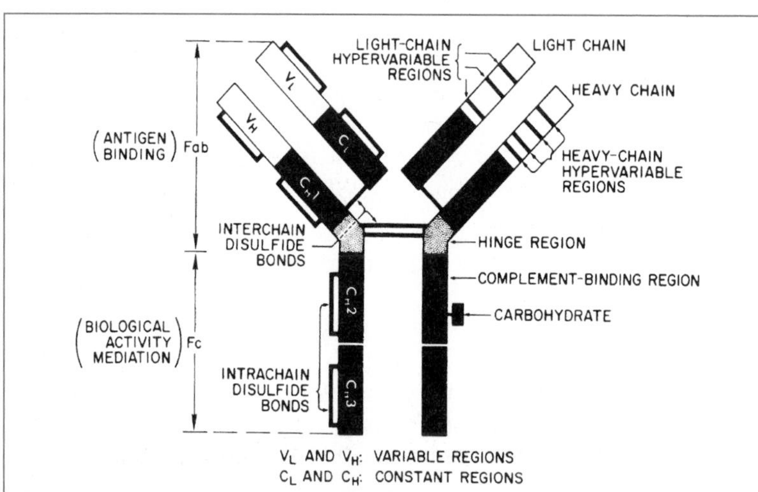

Figure 12-1. Chain and domain structure of an Ig molecule with hypervariable regions within variable regions of both H and L chains. Fab and Fc refer to fragments of the IgG molecule formed by protein cleavage. The former contains the V_H and C_H1 H chain regions and intact L chain; the latter consists of the C_H2 and C_H3 regions of two H chains linked to one another by disulfide bonds. (From Wasserman RL, Capra JD: Immunoglobulin. In Horowitz MI, Pigman W [eds]: The Glycoconjugates. New York, Academic Press, 1977, pp 323–348, with permission.)

24. **What are the features of primary and secondary antibody responses?**
A primary antibody response occurs following the first exposure to an antigen, while secondary antibody response occurs with the second and subsequent exposures. A secondary response is faster, bigger, and contains antibodies that bind with higher affinity to antigen and a greater diversity of T cells that react with the target antigens. In a secondary response, the antibody levels increase and new effector T cells enter the circulation within 1–2 days. In contrast, during a primary response the emergence of these elements of an adaptive response can take a week or more. During a secondary response the quantity of antibodies and the number of effector T cells is increased tenfold or higher. The average affinity of the antigen binding sites is also higher in a secondary response. Finally, during a secondary response more of the antibodies belong to the IgG class, whereas in a primary response most of the antibodies are IgM. Major features of these two responses are illustrated in Figures 12-2 and 12-3.

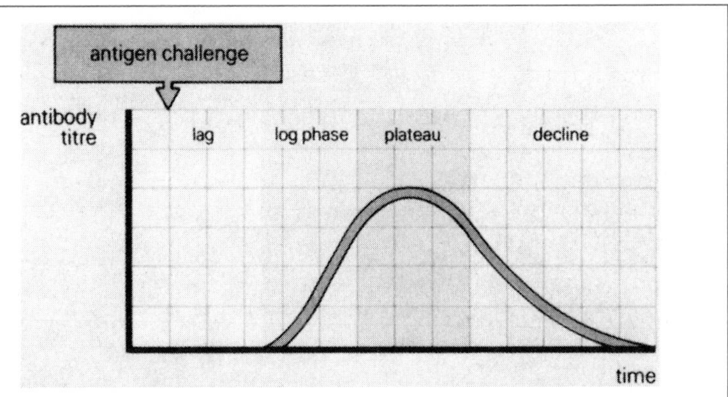

Figure 12-2. After antigen challenge, the primary antibody response proceeds in four phases: (1) a lag phase when no antibody is detected; (2) a log phase in which the antibody titer rises logarithmically; (3) a plateau phase during which the antibody titer stabilizes; and (4) a decline phase during which the antibody is cleared or catabolized. (From Roitt IM, et al: Immunology. New York, Gower Medical, 1989, p 8.1, with permission.)

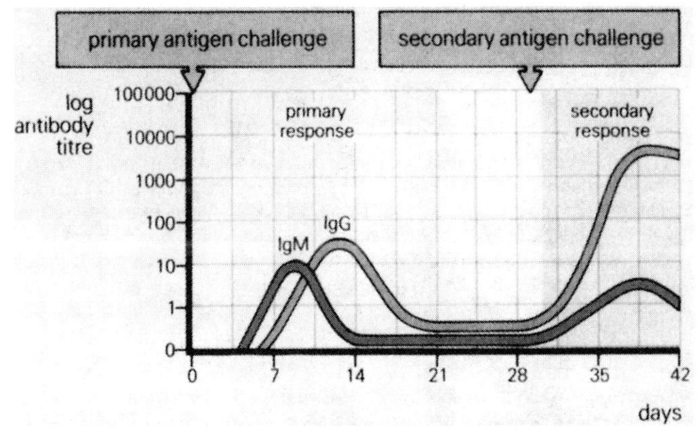

Figure 12-3. Primary and secondary antibody responses. In comparison with the antibody response to primary antigenic challenge, the antibody level after secondary antigenic challenge in a typical immune response (1) appears more quickly and persists for longer, (2) attains a high titer, and (3) consists predominantly of IgG. In the primary response the appearance of IgG is preceded by IgM. (From Roitt IM, et al: Immunology. New York, Gower Medical, 1989, p 8.1, with permission.)

25. Why are IgG antibodies "better" than IgM antibodies?
IgG antibodies can be considered "better" in that they enable neutrophils and monocyte/macrophages to phagocytose antibody-coated particles. This process is called opsonization. They can also direct the killing of infected cells, tumors, and parasites in a process called antibody-dependent cellular cytotoxicity. IgG molecules, because of their smaller size, can more readily enter interstitial fluids, and, in contrast to IgM molecules, they can be transported across the placenta.

26. What are the physical and biologic properties of the different classes of Ig?
See Table 12-1.

TABLE 12-1. PHYSICAL AND BIOLOGIC PROPERTIES OF HUMAN IMMUNOGLOBULINS*

Property	IgG	IgA	IgM	IgD	IgE
Molecular form	Monomer	Monomer, polymer	Pentamer	Monomer	Monomer
Subclasses	IgG 1,2,3,4	IgA 1,2	None	None	None
Molecular weight	150,000 for IgG 1,2,4 180,000 for IgG3	160,000 + polymers	950,000	175,000	190,000
Serum level (mg/cc)	9,3,1,0.5	2.1	1.5	4	0.03
Serum half-life (days)	23D for IgG 1,2,4 7D for IgG 3	6	5	3	3
Complement fixation	IgG 1,2,3+	(–)	+	(–)	(–)
Alt. Pathway activtn.	IgG4	+	(–)	+	?
Placental transfer	+	(–)	(–)	(–)	(–)
Other properties	Secondary response	Abundant in mucous secretions	Primary response, rheumatoid factor	–	Binds to mast cells

*The plus and minus signs indicate whether the molecules have or do not have the indicated property. Modified from Paul, WE, Fundamental Immunology, 2nd edition, Raven Press, New York, NY, 1989 and Samter M, et al (eds): Immunological Diseases, 4th ed. Boston, Little, Brown, 1988, p 44.

27. Summarize the functions of the complement system.
The complement system functions as the innate part of humoral immunity by promoting inflammatory reactions, and it facilitates the effector functions of antibodies, especially IgM and IgG antibodies. C3b, generated by the cleavage of C3, binds to the surface of antigens, including microbes, and facilitates their uptake by neutrophils and monocytes that express a C3b receptor. C5a and, to some extent, C3a are chemotactic for neutrophils and monocytes and serve to

recruit leukocytes into sites of inflammation. C3a and C5a are also known as anaphylatoxins because of their ability to induce mast cell degranulation. The terminal complement components, C6, C7, C8, and C9, form the membrane attack complex, a tubular structure that inserts through the plasma membrane of cells and microbes and kills them. Figure 12-4 summarizes specific functions of the complement system.

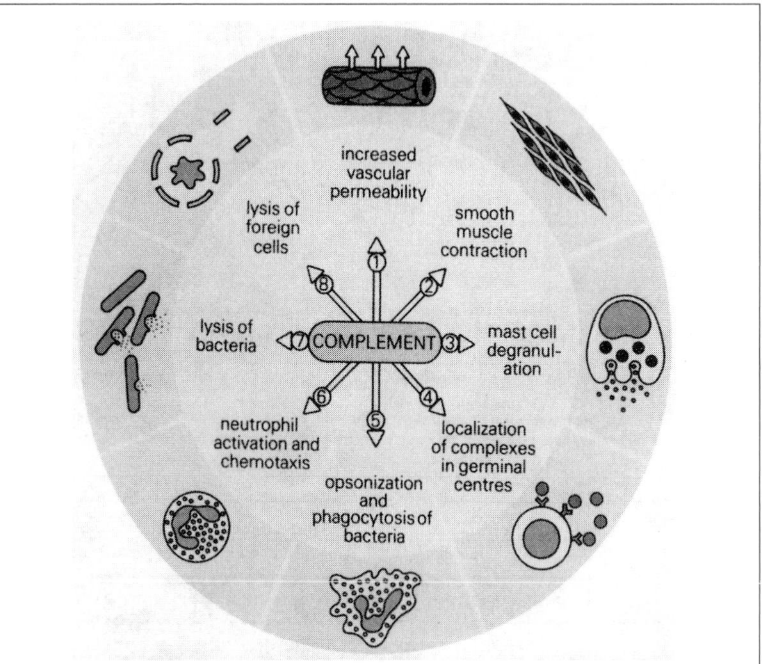

Figure 12-4. Summary of the actions of complement and its role in the acute inflammatory response. Note how the elements of the reaction are induced. Increased vascular permeability (1) due to the action of C3a and C5a on smooth muscle (2) and mast cells (3) allows exudation of plasma protein. C3 facilitates both the localization of complexes in germinal centers (4) and the opsonization and phagocytosis of bacteria (5). Neutrophils, which are attracted to the area of inflammation by chemotaxis (6), phagocytose the opsonized microorganisms. The membrane attack complex, C5–9, is responsible for lysis of bacteria (7) and other cells recognized as foreign (8). (From Roitt IM, et al: Immunology. New York, Gower Medical, 1989, p 13.11, with permission.)

28. **Summarize the activation sequences of the classical complement pathways.**
Initiation of classical complement pathway activation starts with binding of the C1 complex and proceeds through the activation cascade shown in Figure 12-5. C1 is composed of C1q, C1r, and C1s. To be activated, two of the five arms of C1q must interact with binding sites located near the hinge region of IgG and IgM molecules. Therefore, C1q activation requires two adjacent IgG molecules or a single IgM molecule.

29. **Summarize the activation sequences of the alternative complement pathways.**
Activation of the alternative pathway is initiated by binding of C3b to the surface of antigens, particularly microbial membranes. The alternative pathway bypasses C1, C2, and C4. Therefore, measurement of C3 and C4 can give some indication as to whether the activation has been via the classical (immune complex) or alternative (pathogen) pathways. The activation of C3 and

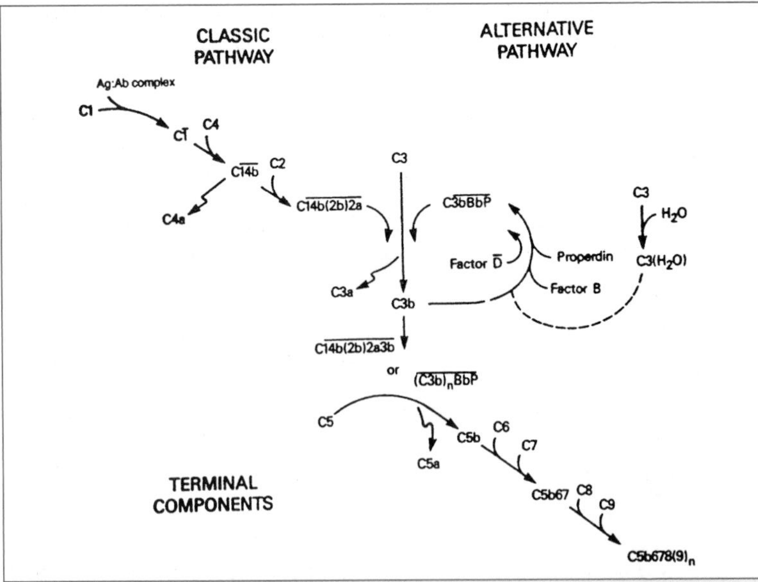

Figure 12-5. An overview of the complement cascade showing the classic and alternative pathways. The central position of C3 in both pathways is indicated. (From Samter M [ed]: Immunological Diseases, 4th ed. Boston, Little, Brown, 1998, p 205, with permission.)

the downstream participation of C5, C6, C7, C8, and C9 is the same for both pathways and the biologic activities of opsonization, recruitment of inflammatory cells, mast cell degranulation, and cell lysis are identical for both pathways. The alternative pathways are also diagrammed in Figure 12-5.

30. **What is mannose-binding protein?**
A third mechanism for activation of the complement cascade is mediated by a protein that is structurally similar to C1q of the classical pathway. This protein, called the mannose-binding lectin, reacts with repeating carbohydrate residues on bacterial surfaces that are commonly displayed by a wide array of microbes. Mannose-binding lectin employs C4 and C2 in an activation pathway that is closely homologous to that utilized by the classical complement activation pathway.

31. **What is the common purpose of all of these activation cascades?**
The purpose of all of these activation cascades is to assemble an enzyme that cleaves and activates C3 so that C3 can bind covalently to a microbial surface, and provide a template for the assembly of an enzyme that cleaves and activates C5 and the remaining elements of complement (C6–C9).

32. **What factors cause activation of the classical complement pathway?**
Antibody-antigen (immune) complexes activate the classical pathway. When bound to antigens, a single IgM or two IgG molecules (IgG doublet) of the IgG subclasses 1, 2, and 3, but not 4, can bind C1, and initiate complement activation. The binding site for C1q in the Ig molecule is not exposed until the antibody binds antigen. Therefore, soluble antibodies in the circulation do not activate complement. Certain viruses, urate crystals, DNA, and mitochondria that are released by damaged cells also activate the classical pathway by binding C1q, the ligand protein

of the C1 complex. Progression of the cascade through C3, 5, 6, 7, 8, and 9 requires assembly of these components on a planar surfaces, as are provided by target cell membranes.

33. **What factors protect the body cells against the complement cascade?**
Activation of the complement cascade does not proceed in fluids like blood plasma beyond C3 because enzymes in the blood promptly degrade activated C3 that is not covalently attached to a membrane structure or an antigen-antibody complex. In addition, mammalian somatic cells, but not red cells, are protected against injury by activated complement by three proteins, decay-accelerating factor, membrane cofactor protein, and CD59, also called protectin. These proteins interfere with the assembly of the enzymes that could otherwise complete the complement cascade and lyse the cell.

34. **What factors cause activation of the alternative complement pathway?**
Substances that activate the alternative pathway are mainly found on bacterial or yeast cell walls. Aggregates of Ig and cells whose surfaces are poor in sialic acid residues can also activate the alternative pathway. C3 has a highly reactive thioester bond that allows activated C3 to bind covalently to a wide variety of substrates. Most bacteria, some parasites, and virtually all plant cells display these residues.

35. **In evaluating patients, does it help to measure serum complement levels?**
Hospital clinical laboratories can usually measure serum C3 and C4. When the differential diagnosis includes sepsis, an active collagen vascular disease, or an allergic reaction, measurements of C3 and C4 are sometimes helpful. If the disease process is more than 24 hours old, one must realize that the complement proteins are among the acute-phase reactants and complement biosynthesis is stimulated by acute inflammation. Although complement may have been consumed in the first hours of the disease, new protein synthesis will cause a prompt rebound in plasma levels to normal or even supernormal levels. When interpreting serum complement levels (C3 and C4), one must realize that a normal level does not rule out either complement activation or complement-mediated tissue damage.

36. **How does liver disease affect complement levels?**
Since complement proteins are made in the liver, persistently low complement protein levels may be found only in patients with severe liver disease.

37. **What patterns of serum C3 and C4 levels are seen with activation of the classical and alternative complement pathways? Name at least one disease associated with each pattern.**
See Table 12-2.

TABLE 12-2. SERUM COMPLEMENT LEVELS IN DISEASE

Pathway	C4	C3	Disease
Classical	↓	↓	Systemic lupus erythematosus, serum sickness
Classical (fluid phase)	↓	N	Hereditary angioedema
Alternative	N	↓	Endotoxemia (gram-negative sepsis)
Alternative (fluid phase)	N	↓	Type II membranoproliferative glomerulonephritis (C3 nephritic factor)

↓ = Decreased, N = normal.

38. What are alpha, beta, and gamma interferons (IFNs)?
Interferons have been divided into three classes, IFN-alpha, IFN-beta, and IFN-gamma. IFN-alpha and IFN-beta were previously classified as type I and IFN-gamma as type II. IFN-beta is divided into two major subtypes: IFN-$beta_1$ and IFN-$beta_2$.

39. How are IFN-alpha, IFN-$beta_1$, and IFN-$beta_2$ produced? Explain the major function of each.
IFN-alpha is produced by leukocytes, fibroblasts (to a lesser degree), and other cells and is composed of 20 or more subtypes. IFN-$beta_1$ is produced by fibroblasts, leukocytes (to a lesser degree), and many other cells. IFN-$beta_2$ (IL-6) is produced by fibroblasts, T cells, monocytes, and endothelial cells.

40. Summarize the major functions of IFN-alpha, IFN-$beta_1$, and IFN-$beta_2$.
Both IFN-alpha and IFN-$beta_1$ modulate antibody production, graft rejection, and delayed-type hypersensitivity (DTH) reactions. They can induce autoimmune and inflammatory reactions, and they have important antiviral, antibacterial, antifungal, and antitumor activities. IFN-$beta_2$ has important immunomodulatory activity and poor antiviral activity. It has also been called "B-cell differentiation factor" because it stimulates mature B to differentiate into Ig-secreting plasma cells. It also plays a role in early hematopoiesis and may be an important autocrine growth factor for B cell malignancies

41. What produces IFN-gamma? Summarize its functions.
IFN-gamma is unrelated to the other IFNs in either structure or function. IFN-gamma is produced by activated T lymphocytes, natural killer (NK) cells, and lymphokine-activated killer (LAK) cells. Its biologic effects include enhancing cytotoxic T-cell and NK-cell activity, induction of class II antigen expression on B cells, and other antigen-presenting cells, and induction of IL-2 receptor expression on T cells. It down-regulates collagen synthesis and inhibits IL-4–induced IgE synthesis.

42. Outline B cell ontogeny from stem cell to plasma cell.
Stem cell → pre-B → immature B → mature B → activated B → secretory B → plasma cell. Immature B cells can be identified by the expression of IgM on their surface. Encounters with cognate antigen at this stage can lead to clonal deletion or anergy. Mature B cells have both IgM and IgD on their surface, and interaction with cognate antigen stimulates cell differentiation and survival.

43. What is the role of surface Ig on B cells?
Before active secretion of Ig begins, B cells produce Ig with an added polypeptide tail at the carboxy terminus. This tail anchors Ig in the B cell membrane. Cell surface Ig molecules provide antigen-binding sites. Binding of antigen to these cell surface Ig molecules activates the B cells. If the B cell receives additional costimulatory signals via specific cell surface molecules on T cells (e.g., from molecules called CD40 ligand or CD154), the B cell differentiates into an antibody-producing cell. In the absence of costimulatory signals, it does not differentiate further nor does it produce antibody.

44. Summarize the role of T cells. Where do they mature?
T cells function both as effectors and regulators of the immune response. Like B cells, they are derived from embryonic hematopoietic stem cells in the bone marrow. Unlike B cells, T cells mature in the thymus, hence their name. In the thymus, T cells are selected for their ability to interact weakly with either MHC class I or class II molecules (positive selection). However, cells that react strongly with these molecules are deleted (negative selection). Since antigenic peptides expressed in the thymus are from self proteins, negative selection removes potential autoreactive cells. Thymic epithelial cells have the ability to express many self proteins normally

produced only in specialized tissues (such as insulin), allowing the thymus to screen for T cells that might react with a wide diversity of host antigens.

45. **What are the major subtypes of T cells?**
CD4 T cells and CD8 T cells.

46. **Describe the principal function of CD4 T cells.**
CD4 cells function primarily as helper/inducer T cells that provide soluble and cognate signals to (a) B cells to stimulate antibody production, (b) CD8 cytolytic T cells, and (c) monocytes and macrophages to facilitate their ability to carry out cell-mediated immune responses. Recently it has been recognized that CD4 T cells can also act as killer cells or even as suppressor cells—that is, cells that can suppress cell-mediated responses carried out by other T cells. These immunomodulatory CD4 cells express high levels of the IL-2 receptor protein called CD25Y.
The incontrovertible fact about CD4 T cells is that they are stimulated to recognize and react against antigen presented by MHC class II molecules displayed on antigen-presenting cells.

47. **Describe the principal function of CD8 T cells.**
CD8 T cells classically are considered to carry out killer functions; for example, they kill virus-infected cells. As was noted with the CD4 T cell, many of functional restrictions no longer apply since numerous exceptions have been noted. What is important is that they recognize antigen only when presented by MHC class I molecules.

48. **What is the CD nomenclature for phenotyping cells?**
The CD (cluster designation) nomenclature is a system for the identification of cell surface antigens that have been defined by monoclonal antibodies. Development of a monoclonal antibody to a cell surface protein is one important step in its characterization. These antibodies allow identification of target proteins on cell surfaces. They can be used to help purify the proteins and illuminate their function. Over 200 CD antigens thus far have been recognized by international committees that assign these numbers. CD markers identify targets that can be used to remove whole classes of cells from the circulation by means of cytolytic monoclonal antibodies or by machines, called cell sorters, that recognize and segregate cells expressing specific molecules identified by monoclonal antibodies.

49. **How is the CD nomenclature used in clinical medicine?**
In clinical medicine, antibodies to CD3 and CD4 have been used to help control transplant rejection reactions by removing and inactivating the effector T cells. A few important CD markers are listed in Table 12-3.

TABLE 12-3. CD MARKERS, ISOFORMS, SITES OF EXPRESSION, AND FUNCTION

Surface Marker	Isoforms	Sites of Expression	Comments
CD2	50 kd protein	Thymocytes, T cells, NK cells (large granular lymphocytes)	Adhesion molecule that binds to LFA-3, a ligand on APC. Ligation with LFA-3 activates T cells.

(continued)

TABLE 12-3. CD MARKERS, ISOFORMS, SITES OF EXPRESSION, AND FUNCTION *(continued)*

Surface Marker	Isoforms	Sites of Expression	Comments
CD3	γ: 25 kD glycoprotein, δ: 20 kD glycoprotein, ε: 20 kD protein	Thymocytes, T cells	Associated with T-cell antigen receptor (TCR). Required for cell surface expression of TCR.
CD4	57 kD glycoprotein	Thymocytes, TH1 and TH2 T cells, monocytes, and some macrophages	Coreceptor for MHC class II, and for HIV-1 + HIV-2 gp120.
CD8	α: 32 kD glycoprotein β: 32–34 kD	Thymocytes, CD8 T cells	Coreceptor for MHC class I; anti-CD8 blocks cytotoxic T-cell responses.
CD16	50–80 kD	NK cells, granulocytes, macrophages	Low-affinity Fcγ receptor that plays a role in antibody-dependent cell mediated cytotoxicity and activation of NK cells.
CD19	95 kD	B cells	Coreceptor for B cells involved in B-cell activation.
CD28	44 kD homodimer	T-cell subsets Activated B cells	Binding to CD80 (on B cells) or CD86 (on macrophages or dendritic cells) sends costimulatory, differentiation-inducing signal.
CD45RO	180 kD glycoprotein	Memory T cells, B-cell subsets, monocytes	See CD45RA.
CD45RA	205–220 kD glycoprotein	Naive T cells, B cells, monocytes	Role in signal transduction, tyrosine phosphatase.
CD56	135–220 kD heterodimer	NK cells	Promotes adhesion of NK cells.
CD80	60 kD protein	B-cell subset Ligand for CD28 on T cells	Costimulator involved in antigen presentation.
CD86	80 kD protein	Activated B cells Monocytes, dendritic cells	Costimulatory ligand for CD28 on T cells, during antigen presentation.

From David J: Immunology. In Dale DC, Federman DD (eds): Scientific American Medicine. New York, Scientific American, Inc., 1996, p 6, and Janeway, CA, Travers, P, Walport, M., Capra, J.D. (eds) Immunobiology, 4th ed. Current Biology Publications, London, and Garland Publishing, New York, 1999.

50. What are cytokines, where are they made, and what do they do?
Cytokines are proteins produced by many cells, not necessarily only cells of the immune system, that function as intracellular signaling molecules, usually within the radius of a few cell diameters. There are presently more than 38 cytokines (Table 12-4).

TABLE 12-4. ACTIONS OF CYTOKINES RELEVANT TO ALLERGIC AND IMMUNE RESPONSES

Cytokine	Effects
GM-CSF	Secreted by activated macrophages, T cells, mast cells, eosinophils, and other cells
	Promotes differentiation of neutrophils and macrophages
	Activates mature eosinophils
	Prolongs eosinophil survival
IFN-γ	Derived mainly from TH1 lymphocytes, cytotoxic T cells, NK cells, but also macrophages
	Represents the most important cytokine activator of macrophages
	Increases expression of class I and II MHC antigens
	Stimulates B cell proliferation and differentiation
	Inhibits IL-4–induced IgE synthesis
	Inhibits TH2 lymphocytes
	Induces ICAM-1 expression
IL-1	IL-1 family contains IL-1α, IL-1β, the IL-1 receptor antagonist (IL-Ira), and IL-18
	Produced mainly by monocytes and macrophages, but also by lymphocytes and other cells
	Induced by endotoxin, microorganisms, antigens, and cytokines
	Increases proliferation of B cells and antibody synthesis
	Promotes growth of Th cells in response to APCs
	Stimulates production of T cell cytokines and IL-2 receptors
	Without IL-1, tolerance develops or immune response is impaired
	Promotes formation of arachidonic acid metabolites, including PGE_2 and LTB_4
	Induces proliferation of fibroblasts and synthesis of fibronectin and collagen
	Increases ICAM-1, VCAM-1, E-selectin, and P-selectin expression
	IL-1 receptor antagonist (IL-1ra) antagonizes proinflammatory effects of IL-1
IL-2	Induces clonal T cell proliferation
	Enhances proliferation of cytotoxic T cells, B cells, NK cells, macrophages
IL-3	Derived primarily from TH cells, but also from mast cells and eosinophils
	Stimulates development of mast cells, lymphocytes, macrophages
	Activates eosinophils
	Prolongs eosinophil survival
IL-4	Preformed peptide in mast cells and eosinophils
	Also secreted by TH2 cells, cytotoxic T cells, and basophils
	Promotes growth of TH2 cells, cytotoxic T cells, mast cells, eosinophils, basophils

(continued)

TABLE 12-4. ACTIONS OF CYTOKINES RELEVANT TO ALLERGIC AND IMMUNE RESPONSES *(continued)*

Cytokine	Effects
IL-4	Initiates IgE isotype switching
	Upregulates expression of high- and low-affinity IgE receptors
	Increases expression of class I and II MHC antigens on macrophages
	Stimulates VCAM-1 expression
IL-5	Produced by TH2 cells and mast cells
	Attracts eosinophils
	Activates eosinophils
	Prolongs eosinophil survival
IL-6	Synthesized primarily by monocytes and macrophages, but also by T, B, and other cells
	Mediates T-cell activation, growth, differentiation
	Induces B-cell differentiation into plasma cells
	Inhibits TNF and IL-1 synthesis and stimulates IL-Ira synthesis
IL-7	Necessary for development of B and T cells
	Enhances growth of cytotoxic T and NK cells
	Increases tumor killing by monocytes and macrophages
IL-8	Produced mainly by monocytes, phagocytes, and endothelial cells
	Exerts potent chemoattraction for neutrophils
	Attracts activated eosinophils
	Induces neutrophil degranulation and activation
	Inhibits IL-4–mediated IgE synthesis
IL-9	Produced by Th2 cells
	Promotes mast cell and T-cell proliferation
	Stimulates IgE synthesis
	Produces eosinophilia
	Induces bronchial hyperreactivity
IL-10	Secreted primarily by monocytes and B cells
	Inhibits monocyte/macrophage function
	Stimulates growth of mast cells, B cells, and cytotoxic T cells
	Induces permanent tolerance in TH lymphocytes
	Decreases synthesis of IFN-γ and IL-2 by TH1 cells
	Inhibits IL-4–induced IgE synthesis and promotes IgG4 production
	Decreases eosinophil survival
IL-11	Produced in response to respiratory viral infections
	Promotes generation of mast cells and B cells
	Induces bronchial hyperreactivity
IL-12	Synthesized by monocytes/macrophages, dendritic cells, B cells, neutrophils, mast cells
	Induced by IFN-γ and microorganisms

TABLE 12-4. ACTIONS OF CYTOKINES RELEVANT TO ALLERGIC AND IMMUNE RESPONSES *(continued)*

Cytokine	Effects
IL-12	Promotes TH1 and inhibits TH2 cell development
	Inhibits IL-4 induced IgE synthesis
	Enhances activity of cytotoxic T cells and NK cells
IL-13	Produced by TH1 and TH2 cells, mast cells, and dendritic cells
	Exerts effects similar to IL-4 on B cells and macrophages but does not affect T cells
	Induces IgE isotype switching
	Increases VCAM-1 expression
	Promotes airway hyperreactivity and mucus hypersecretion
	Suppresses production of proinflammatory cytokines and chemokines
	Decreases synthesis of nitric oxide
IL-16	Secreted by $CD8^+$ T cells, eosinophils, mast cells, and epithelial cells
	Promotes growth of $CD4^+$ T cells
	Provides major source of $CD4^+$ T cell chemotactic activity after antigen challenge
	Induces IL-2 receptors and class II MHC expression on $CD4^+$ T cells
IL-18	Produced by lung, liver, and other tissues, but not by lymphocytes
	Stimulates secretion of IFN-γ and GM-CSF
	Enhances IgE synthesis
	Promotes TH1 responses and activates NK cells (similar to IL-12)
	Induces synthesis of TNF, IL-1, Fas ligand
	Decreases IL-10 synthesis
IL-23	Induces secretion of IFN-γ
TGF-α	Synthesized by macrophages and keratinocytes
	Stimulates proliferation of fibroblasts
	Promotes angiogenesis
TGF-β	Secreted by platelets, monocytes, some T cells (TH3), and fibroblasts
	Stimulates monocytes and fibroblasts, inducing fibrosis and extracellular matrix formation
	Attracts mast cells, macrophages, fibroblasts
	Inhibits B cells, T helper cells, cytotoxic T cells, NK cells, mast cells
	Induces IgA isotype switching and secretory IgA synthesis in gut lymphoid tissue
	Inhibits airway smooth muscle cell proliferation
TNF-α	Produced primarily by mononuclear phagocytes; stored preformed in mast cells
	Induced by endotoxin, GM-CSF, IFN-γ, IL-1, and IL-3
	Binds to cell surface receptors TNFR I and TNFR II
	Enhances class I and II MHC expression
	Activates neutrophils, modulating adherence, chemotaxis, degranulation, respiratory burst
	Increases cytokine production by monocytes and airway epithelial cells

(continued)

TABLE 12-4. ACTIONS OF CYTOKINES RELEVANT TO ALLERGIC AND IMMUNE RESPONSES *(continued)*

Cytokine	Effects
TNF-α	Promotes ICAM-1, VCAM-1, and E-selectin expression
	Stimulates COX-2 expression in airway smooth muscle
	Induces bronchial hyperreactivity
	Mediates toxic shock and sepsis
	Produces cachexia associated with chronic infection and cancer
TNF-β	Synthesized primarily by lymphocytes
	Binds to cell surface receptors TNFR I and TNFR II
	Mediates functions similar to TNF-α

From Hamilton ME: Immunology and pathophysiology of allergic disease. In Naguwa SM, Gershwin ME (eds): Allergy and Immunology Secrets. Philadelphia, Hanley & Belfus, 2001.

51. **What is anergy?**
Anergy is the lack of an immunologic response to an antigen under circumstances in which one would normally expect to see one. T-cell anergy, for example, is demonstrated by the lack of reaction to common delayed-type hypersensitivity recall antigens. Clinically this is seen frequently in patients with miliary tuberculosis, Hodgkin's disease, or HIV infection. B-cell anergy is failure to develop a specific antibody response in a person who has been immunized with antigens that are known to routinely stimulate antibody responses in other individuals of the same species. Anergy may be temporary, as occurs during measles infection, or of indeterminate duration, as in sarcoidosis, AIDS, and certain disseminated malignancies and overwhelming infectious diseases, including lepromatous leprosy.

52. **How is anergy established?**
To establish that someone is T-cell anergic, DTH skin testing is customarily used. Typically one employs four or five recall antigens to ensure a > 90% chance of using at least one antigen against which normal age-matched individuals would mount a delayed hypersensitivity response. Recall antigens are antigens that a person has already encountered before; thus, during the test the immune responses are asked to mount a secondary response.

53. **Which antigens are available for anergy testing?**
Readily available antigens include *Trichophyton* (1:30 dilution) from Hollister Stier Labs, tetanus toxoid used at 10 Lf/mL from Wyeth Labs, mumps antigen at 40 cfu/mL from Connaught Labs, *Candida* extract at 500 PNU/mL from Greer Labs, and purified protein derivative (PPD) at 50 TU/mL, also from Connaught Labs.

54. **How is the test performed?**
To perform the test, 0.1 mL of each antigen is injected intradermally at widely spaced sites, usually on the volar surface of the forearms. Mean diameter of induration is read at 48 h. There is disagreement as to whether a 5- or 10-mm diameter indurated lesion represents a positive result. To assess nonspecific reactions, one can use 0.1 mL of saline as a negative control, but most forego this procedure because there is nothing to show at 48 h unless the tester inadvertently triggers a capillary bleed at the site of the injection.

55. Summarize the clinical significance of anergy.
Anergic individuals have increased susceptibility to infections that require cell-mediated immune responses for adequate host defense.

56. What are antigen-presenting cells (APCs)? What is their role in the immune response?
APCs are cells that present antigen principally to T lymphocytes, as a result of which the T cells are activated and stimulated to perform one of their many functions. Classic APCs are dendritic cells, B cells, and monocyte/macrophages (including those specialized forms found in specific tissues such as microglial cells, Kupffer cells, etc). All three of these express MHC class II molecules so that they can display antigens to CD4 T cells. Like all somatic cells, they also express MHC class I molecules and can display antigen peptides to CD8 T cells.

57. How do APCs activate naive T cells?
To activate naive T cells, APCs must present costimulatory signals to the T cell along with antigen. These costimulatory molecules include CD80 and CD86 (also known as B7.1 and B7.2), which interact with CD28 on T cells. Dendritic cells are often considered to be the most effective APC because of their constitutive expression of costimulatory molecules. The other APCs tend to up-regulate their expression of costimulatory molecules after encounter with microbes or microbially induced molecules. Stimuli with cytokines such as IFN-δ can up-regulate MHC molecules on these cells.

58. What is major basic protein (MBP)?
MBP is the principal bioactive protein in the cytoplasmic granules of eosinophils. It is the only one localized to the crystalline core. It is also present in much smaller amounts in basophils. It should not be confused with myelin basic protein from Schwann cells, which is also abbreviated as *MBP*.

59. List the biologic effects of MBP.
- Highly toxic to many parasites (including *Schistosoma mansoni, Trichinella spiralis*, and *Trypanosoma cruzi*).
- Toxic to a wide variety of mammalian cells (including human cells).
- Stimulates histamine release from basophils and mast cells.
- Neutralizes heparin.
- Causes bronchospasm.

60. Describe the mechanism of immediate hypersensitivity reactions and give some clinical examples.
Type I, or immediate hypersensitivity, reactions are classic allergic reactions initiated by degranulation and activation of mast cells. There are several mechanisms by which mast cells can be induced to degranulate. One is by cross-linking of several IgE molecules bound in Fc receptors on the mast cell membrane. Cross-linking can also be achieved by autoantibodies that react with either IgE or with the mast cell receptor for the Fc of IgE.

Autoantibodies specific for these antigens have recently been recognized as the agents responsible for 20% or more of cases with chronic idiopathic urticaria/angioedema. Mast cells can also be degranulated by the anaphylatoxins C3a and C5a. Both are products of complement activation. Finally, mast cells can be degranulated by direct chemical and physical stimuli, such as those provided by iodinated radiocontrast dyes and opiods.

61. Distinguish between an anaphylactic reaction and an anaphylactoid reaction.
Degranulation resulting from cross-linking of cell-bound IgE is called an **anaphylactic reaction**; degranulation caused by activation of antigen nonspecific receptors like those for C3a or C5a, which does not involve the IgE receptors, is called an **anaphylactoid reaction**.

62. Explain the clinical significance of immediate hypersensitivity reactions.
Mast cells release granules containing preformed mediators, including histamine, heparin, and tryptase. They also mobilize arachidonic acid to generate prostaglandins and leukotrienes. Several hours later, the mast cell begins to release cytokines such as TNF-alpha. Immediate reactions resulting in release of preformed mediators like histamine become clinically evident within seconds to minutes. Clinical examples include anaphylaxis, allergic rhinitis (hay fever), food allergy, extrinsic (allergic) asthma, immediate drug allergy (such as to penicillin), and acute urticaria (hives).

63. What are the four types of hypersensitivity reactions?
The four classic types of hypersensitivity reactions referred to by Coombs and Gell in their attempt to classify immunologically mediated reactions are summarized in Table 12-5.

TABLE 12-5. FOUR TYPES OF HYPERSENSITIVITY REACTIONS

Type	Mechanism	Timing to Onset	Clinical Example
I	Mast cells and basophils, often involving IgE	1–15 min	Atopy, hay fever, urticaria
II	Antibody reacts with host cells leading to phagocytosis or lysis. Stimulatory or blocking antibodies may also cause disease	Hours	Autoimmune hemolytic anemia (lysis), diabetes (blocking antibodies), Graves' disease (stimulatory antibodies)
III	Immune complexes of any specificity deposit in tissues (typically the walls of small vessels, and the kidney) leading to frustrated phagocytosis and complement activation	Hours	Arthus reaction, polyarteritis nodosa, serum sickness, small vessel vasculitis
IV	T-cell mediated either by CD4 cells activating macrophages or by cytolytic CD8 cells	36–48 h	Granulomatous reactions in tuberculosis and sarcoidosis; PPD reaction

64. How do type IV, or delayed-type hypersensitivity (DTH), reactions differ from types I–III?
Type IV, or DTH, reactions are a reflection of cell-mediated immunity and initiated by T cells. Unlike reaction types I–III, DTH can be transferred by T cells, but not by serum.

65. Describe the mechanism of type IV reactions.
When antigen-sensitized T cells are re-exposed to the same antigen by antigen-presenting cells, T-cell activation occurs. Activated T cells secrete IFN-gamma, IL-2, and other cytokines,

causing monocytes to accumulate at the site of the reaction and differentiate into macrophages. Over 90% of the T cells that accumulate at the site of a DTH reaction are not antigen-specific; rather, they have been called to that site by the activity of the chemokines and cytokines produced by the infiltrating monocytes and few antigen-specific T cells that have localized in the vicinity of the antigen-presenting cells.

66. **Summarize the clinical effects of type IV reactions.**
Additional inflammatory mediators and cytokines are released that cause edema and sometimes necrosis of bystander cells. If the antigen persists or can be degraded only with difficulty, as is the case with the antigenic lipids of *M. tuberculosis*, lymphocyte and macrophage activation continues and may result in granuloma formation. Delayed hypersensitivity reactions differ in tempo, depending on the cells involved (Table 12-6).

TABLE 12-6. EXAMPLES OF DELAYED HYPERSENSITIVITY REACTIONS

Time to Type	Inducing Antigen	Peak	External Signs	Histologic Appearance
Tuberculin	Tuberculin	48 h	Indurated, painful skin swelling	Intradermal lymphocyte and monocyte infiltration
Jones-Mote	Foreign proteins such as ovalbumin	24 h	Slight skin thickening	Intradermal, lymphocyte and basophil infiltration
Contact	Urushiol, the antigen of poison ivy	48 h	Eczema	Same as tuberculin
Granulomatous	Talcum powder silica, and other substances that stimulate phagocytosis but cannot be metabolized	4 wk	Skin induration	Epithelioid cell granuloma formation, giant cells, macrophages, fibrosis, necrosis

Modified from Klein J: Immunology. Oxford, Blackwell Scientific Publications, 1990.

67. **Describe the mechanism of cytotoxic reactions.**
Type II, or cytotoxic, reactions occur when antibody binds to specific antigens on circulating cells or antigens fixed in tissues. Antibody binding activates complement. If the target site lacks decay-accelerating factor or other complement regulatory proteins, as is the case with red blood cells (RBCs), the complement cascade can go to completion, causing lysis of the target cell. Target cells coated with both antibody and bound complement fragments can be opsonized for phagocytosis by macrophages that reside within the reticuloendothelial system and by circulating phagocytes.

68. **Give a clinical example of a type II reaction.**
Rarely antigens localized in basement membranes can become a target of autoantibodies. In Goodpasture's syndrome, the antigen is localized in the basement membranes of the renal glomeruli and the lung. Deposition of antibody binds and activates complement and induces

leukocytes to localize at the sites of antigen-antibody and complement deposition with the result that the leukocyte proteases break down the basement membranes.

69. Describe the mechanism of immune complex reactions and give some clinical examples.
Type III, or immune complex–mediated, reactions are caused by the formation of soluble or not-so-soluble antigen and antibody complexes in the circulation. These deposit preferentially in (a) fenestrated endothelia, as are found in the choroid plexus and in the renal glomeruli and (b) bifurcations of postcapillary venules where eddy currents slow the flow of blood. Immune complexes usually activate complement in situ. This activation causes neutrophils to accumulate and these cause tissue damage.

70. Give clinical examples of type III reactions.
Examples include the Arthus reaction, such as happens in hyperimmunized people who receive a tetanus toxoid booster, and generalized serum sickness as occurs following the injection of foreign proteins into the circulation in people who have preformed antibodies to that protein.

71. What is an Arthus reaction?
Arthus reactions are caused by antigen-antibody complexes (immune complexes) and were first described by Nicolas-Maurice Arthus, a French physiologist, in 1903. The reaction is an acute inflammatory response at the site of deposition of antigen in tissue. The common site is skin near a site of subcutaneous injection of an antigen.

72. When does an Arthus reaction occur in the clinical setting?
Arthus reactions develop when there are high serum levels of complement-fixing antibodies. Immune complexes form in the blood vessel walls of the dermis and subcutaneous tissues causing a localized vasculitis. Arthus reactions depend on both neutrophil and complement function. In humans, localized Arthus reactions have been reported at the sites of injection of second and subsequent tetanus and diphtheria immunizations, and rarely at the site of injection of insulin in diabetics.

73. What is an allergen?
An allergen is a special type of antigen that commonly induces synthesis of IgE antibodies that sensitize mast cells and basophils. Whether the host makes IgE depends on multiple factors, but most particularly it depends on the type of cytokines that the T helper cells make following the injection of the antigen.

74. What are the major differences between mast cells and basophils?
See Table 12-7.

75. Are all mast cells alike?
No. Mast cell heterogeneity exists in both animals and humans. Differences have been most extensively studied in mice, which appear to have two major mast cell populations, labeled mucosal mast cells (MMCs) and connective tissue mast cells (CTMCs). MMCs are found principally at mucosal surfaces, whereas CTMCs are found within connective tissue, lining blood vessels, and at serosal surfaces. They differ with respect to histamine content, the extent to which they degranulate following non-IgE stimuli, arachidonic acid metabolite production, and histochemical-staining characteristics. MMCs respond to stimulation by the T-cell cytokine IL-3. In contrast, expression of the CTMC phenotype depends on stimulation by fibroblasts.

76. What are the types of mast cells in humans?
Humans also appear to have two major mast cell populations that are identified by differences in neutral protease content of their cytoplasmic granules. Both populations contain tryptase, but

TABLE 12-7. COMPARISON OF MAST CELLS AND BASOPHILS

Parameter	Mast Cells	Basophils
Life span	Weeks to years	Days
Origin	Probably bone marrow	Bone marrow
Location	Tissues, noncirculating	Normally circulating
Size	8–20 mm	5–7 mm
Nucleus	Round to oval, may be indented	Multilobulated
Cytoplasmic granules	Smaller, more numerous,	Larger, fewer granules
High-affinity IgE receptor	Present	Present
Histamine release	Yes	Yes
Major arachidonic acid metabolites	PGD2, LTC4, -D4, -E4	LTC4
Staining characteristics		
Toluidine blue	Yes	Yes
Tryptase	Yes	No
Chloroacetate esterase	Yes	No

PG = prostaglandin, LT = leukotriene.

only one contains both tryptase and chymase. The tryptase-only mast cells (MC^T) are located primarily at mucosal surfaces, whereas the tryptase- and chymase-positive mast cells (MC^{TC}) are located primarily in connective tissue, around blood vessels, and at serosal surfaces. The factors responsible for human mast cell growth remain to be clearly defined. Although human IL-3 appears to have some mast cell growth-promoting activity, its effects are less well defined. Of interest is that MC^T mast cells, but not MC^{TC} mast cells, appear to be T lymphocyte–dependent. This is suggested by a marked decrease in MC^T but not MC^{TC} mast cell numbers in the tissues of patients with severe T-cell immunodeficiency disorders.

77. **What is the reticuloendothelial system (RES)? What are its principal functions?**
The RES (mononuclear/phagocyte system) comprises a heterogeneous population of fixed-tissue phagocytic cells throughout the body. Components of the RES include Kupffer cells of the liver, microglial cells of the brain, pulmonary alveolar macrophages, and macrophages in endothelial lined channels in bone marrow, lymph nodes, lung, gut, and other tissues.

78. **Summarize the principal functions of the RES.**
Cells in the RES remove particulate and soluble substances from the circulation and tissues, especially if the substances are coated with antibody and complement. Substances removed include immune complexes, bacteria, toxins, and exogenous antigens. These may be internalized by nonspecific endocytosis, nonimmune but receptor-mediated phagocytosis, or immunologic phagocytosis mediated by binding to Fc or complement receptors.

79. **How is the RES relevant to idiopathic thrombocytopenic purpura (ITP)?**
Blockade of the RES is one postulated mechanism for prevention of platelet destruction by high-dose IV immunoglobulin (IVIG) in ITP. The binding of IgG-sensitized platelets to the IgG-Fc receptors on RES cells, particularly in the liver and spleen, leads to phagocytosis and platelet destruction in ITP. This IgG-Fc receptor mechanism may be “blocked” or overwhelmed by the

infusion of high dose IVIG. IgG-Fc receptors are lost during phagocytosis and may take as long as several days to be reexpressed.

80. **How can antibody measurements be used to indicate an active infection?**
IgG antibodies can persist for years after an infection has resolved and cannot be used to prove active infection. However, IgM antibodies are produced as new B cells are stimulated by the infection; their development indicates an active ongoing infection. The presence of a rising titer of antibodies also indicates an active response, regardless of antibody class. The first serum sample, typically called the acute sample, and a second sample, drawn one or more weeks later, typically called the convalescent sample, should be sent to the lab together for simultaneous testing. Many titrations, that is antibody measurements, are done using serial twofold dilutions of serum. Results are not considered significant until there is a fourfold or greater rise in titer.

81. **Name some of the characteristics of antibody deficiency disorders.**
Antibody deficiency disorders, whether acquired or congenital, have several general characteristics that are manifestations of the defect in antibody-mediated immune responses (Table 12-8).

TABLE 12-8. CHARACTERISTICS OF ANTIBODY DEFICIENCY DISORDERS

1. Recurrent infections with extracellular encapsulated pathogens.
2. Relatively few problems with fungal or viral (except enteroviral) infections.
3. Chronic sinusitis and pulmonary disease; some patients may develop bronchiectasis.
4. Growth retardation is not a striking feature.
5. Low antibody levels measured in serum and secretions. Low Ig levels by themselves are not sufficient evidence of an antibody deficiency syndrome, and titers of specific antibodies should be measured.
6. The hallmark of these deficiency syndromes is the inability to make antibodies to new antigens when challenged with vaccines or following infection with one or another microbe.
7. Patients may or may not lack B lymphocytes. If they have B lymphocytes these may lack surface immunoglobulins or complement receptors, indicating that they are arrested relatively early in ontogeny.
8. Absence of cortical follicles in lymph nodes and spleen are seen in X-linked agammaglobulinemia.
9. Scanty cervical lymph nodes and small or absent tonsils and adenoids are characteristic of X-linked agammaglobulinemia.
10. Replacement therapy with IV Ig has greatly increased lifespan and reduced morbidity.

From Wyngaarden JB, Smith LH: Cecil Textbook of Medicine, 18th ed. Philadelphia, W.B. Saunders, 1988, p 1943.

82. **What is the most common immunoglobulin deficiency disorder?**
Selective IgA deficiency has a frequency of approximately 1 in 500–700 persons.

83. **Describe the clinical significance of seletive IgA deficiency.**
Many patients are asymptomatic, but some have recurrent infections, particularly of the respiratory tract. IgG_2 deficiency sometimes accompanies IgA deficiency, and these patients are partic-

ularly prone to infectious complications with encapsulated bacteria (such as *Streptococcus pneumoniae*, or *Haemophilus influenzae*) because the principal IgG antibody response against bacterial polysaccharide is usually IgG_2. In selective IgA deficiency, the serum IgA level is less than 5 mg/dL (0.05 mg/cc). IgA in secretions is almost always depressed as well. IgG and IgM levels are normal. A few patients have autoimmune disorders (including SLE and rheumatoid arthritis).

84. **How is selective IgA deficiency treated?**
Treatment is supportive. Even if patients have an increased incidence of infections, IVIG therapy is unlikely to be effective since infused IgG will not be transported into secretions. Ig infusions also pose a risk because 50% of these patients may have the ability to develop antibodies to the small quantities of IgA present in most IVIG preparations. Life-threatening anaphylaxis can occur with the second and subsequent infusion of IVIG. A similar risk is associated with blood transfusions. IgA deficient patients can develop antibodies to IgA in the plasma that accompanies packed RBCs. Subsequent transfusions, if needed, should be performed with well-washed RBC to remove all traces of IgA.

85. **What is common variable immunodeficiency disease (CVID)?**
CVID is a heterogeneous group of disorders characterized by hypogammaglobulinemia (total IgG < 250 mg/dL and total Ig usually < 350 mg/dL), decreased ability to produce antibody following antigenic challenge, and recurrent infections. A significant fraction of patients whose serum IgG level is depressed, but still greater than 250 mg/dL. may have a similar clinical presentation. The most common serum Ig pattern, however, is panhypogammaglobulinemia—a deficiency of IgG, IgM, and IgA.

86. **How does CVID present?**
CVID usually presents in late childhood or early adulthood but may present at any age. Recurrent bacterial infections of the upper and lower respiratory tract with encapsulated bacteria (e.g. *Str. pneumoniae, H. influenzae*) are common pathogens, and bronchiectasis may develop. Patients may also have defective cell-mediated immunity and may have mycobacterial, fungal, and protozoal (i.e., *Giardia lamblia*) infections. Patients with CVID have an increased frequency of autoimmune disorders, including pernicious anemia, Coombs-positive hemolytic anemia, autoimmune thrombocytopenia, and thyroiditis. GI disorders are common, including diarrhea, malabsorption, and nodular lymphoid hyperplasia of the small intestine. Finally, there is an increased incidence of malignancy, particularly of the lymphoreticular system and the GI tract.

87. **Identify the principal immunologic defects in CVID.**
The most commonly appreciated defect appears to be a defect in B-cell maturation. The B cells cannot terminally differentiate into antibody-producing plasma cells. This subset of patients generally has normal numbers of circulating, surface Ig-positive B cells. Up to 20% of patients may have increased suppressor-cell activity, causing decreased antibody production. But a host of other immunologic defects are seen in some patients, including T-cell immunoregulatory defects. Depressed cell-mediated immunity, as demonstrated by cutaneous anergy, may be present in up to 30% of patients.

88. **Discuss treatment for CVID.**
The principal therapy for CVID is IVIG replacement and aggressive management of infections with appropriate antibiotics. IVIG is given every 3–4 weeks. The usual dose is 200 mg/kg, and the infusion is given slowly over several hours. Adverse reactions consisting of pruritus, headache, and nausea usually resolve with slowing or stopping of the infusion. IVIG often dramatically decreases the frequency and severity of infections and may also alleviate some of the symptoms, such as arthralgias, that sometimes accompany CVID.

89. What immunologic defects are heralded by recurrent bacterial infections?
Before the emergence of HIV-1, development of serial severe bacterial infections, defined as three or more episodes of bacterial sinusitis, pneumonia, or sepsis within the span of 1 year, was an indication to evaluate patients for a congenital or acquired antibody deficiency syndrome. Less commonly, recurrent bacterial infections may suggest complement deficiency or defective neutrophil function. Patients with antibody deficiency syndromes commonly experience repeated infections with encapsulated organisms (e.g., *H. influenzae, Str. pneumoniae*) that are common upper respiratory tract commensals.

90. How are patients screened for antibody deficiencies?
Screening for antibody deficiency first requires the measurement of serum Ig levels (IgG, IgM, and IgA) and IgG subclasses. Further evaluation may include measuring serum isohemagglutinin titers (IgM antibodies) and serum IgG antibody levels following immunization wth protein (tetanus toxoid) and carbohydrate antigen-containing vaccines. Ideally antibody levels found in pre-immunization and 3-week post-immunization sera are compared to accurately measure the antibody response to a specific antigen challenge.

91. How do complement deficiencies present?
Isolated C3 deficiency typically presents at a very early age, most often shortly after birth. Because C3 deficiency has such a profound negative effect on leukocyte phagocytic function, patients experience recurrent life-threatening pyogenic infections. Deficiencies of the terminal complement components, with the possible exception of C9 deficiency, increase susceptibility to bacteremia with neisserial species, typically *Neiserria gonorrhoeae.* Deficiency of properdin, an alternative complement pathway component, may also be accompanied by recurrent pyogenic and neisserial infections. Complement deficiency can be evaluated by obtaining a CH50 (or CH100) and by measuring levels of specific complement components thereafter as indicated.

92. How do defects of neutrophil function present?
Most defects of neutrophil function associated with recurrent infections occur in the pediatric age group. However, some adults may have a variant of chronic granulomatous disease of childhood (CGD) in which the defect in respiratory burst is qualitatively less than in typical CGD.

93. How is neutrophil function evaluated?
Specialty reference laboratories can provide diverse functional tests that identify defects in the ability of leukocytes to traverse endothelial barriers, phagocytose bacteria, and generate antimicrobial substances intracellularly. This testing can be usually arranged by community hospital laboratories by sending appropriately collected blood samples to experienced laboratories. For example, a nitroblue tetrazolium test can be performed to assess neutrophil respiratory burst in patients with a clinical history suggestive of CGD. Leukocyte adhesion deficiency syndrome can be assessed functionally and by flow cytometric analysis for defects in cell surface expression of CD18-dependent beta integrins. Patients with neutrophil functional defects are particularly susceptible to catalase-positive organisms.

94. Chronic or recurrent meningococcemia or gonococcemia are commonly associated with which host immune defects?
Deficiencies of the late components of complement (C6, C7, and C8) are the predominant defects associated with these disorders. Low C3, absent C5, or properdin deficiency have also been associated with such infections.

95. What gonococcal infection is of special concern in sexually active adults?
In sexually active adults, acute monoarticular arthritis may be a consequence of bacteremia with *N. gonorrhoeae.* Such patients must be evaluated for complement deficiency after treat-

ment of the septic joint. The intense neutrophilic infiltrate triggered by these infections is considered an orthopedic emergency requiring immediate drainage of the pus and irrigation of the joint to reduce the residence time of the inflammatory leukocytes in the joint space. The aim of this emergency treatment is to reduce the damage to the articular cartilage caused by leukocyte proteases and reactive oxygen products.

Ross S, et al: Complement deficiency and infection: Epidemiology, pathogenesis and consequences of neisserial and other infections in an immune deficiency. Medicine 63:243–273, 1984.

96. What clinical conditions are associated with deficiencies of the various components of the complement system?
See Table 12-9.

TABLE 12-9. DISEASES ASSOCIATED WITH INHERITED COMPLEMENT DEFICIENCIES

Deficient Component	Reported Cases	Associated Diseases
C1	31	Autoimmune diseases, SLE-like syndromes
C4	20	Autoimmune diseases, SLE-like syndromes
C2	109	Autoimmune diseases, SLE-like syndromes
C3	20	Bacterial infections, mild glomerulonephritis
C5	28	Gram-negative coccal infections
C6	76	Gram-negative coccal infections
C7	67	Gram-negative coccal infections
C8	68	Gram-negative coccal infections
C9	18	Gram-negative coccal infections
Properdin	70	Gram-negative coccal infections
Factor I	17	Bacterial infections
Factor H	13	Bacterial infections
Factor D	3	Bacterial infections
C4-binding protein	3	—
C1 Inhibitor	100	Hereditary angioedema

From David J: Immunology. In Dale DC, Federman DD (eds): Scientific American Medicine. New York, Scientific American, Inc., 1996, Section 6, Subsection VII, Table 12-9, p 26, with permission.

97. What are the clinical characteristics of disorders of cell-mediated immunity?
The manifestations of cellular immunodeficiency disorders, due to a partial or total defect in T-cell function, include:

- Recurrent infections with low-grade or opportunistic infectious agents, such as fungi, viruses, or protozoa (e.g., *Pneumocystis carinii*).
- T-cell anergy, defined as a general lack of T-cell–mediated immune responses.
- In children, one sees growth retardation, a dramatically shortened life span, wasting, and diarrhea.
- Graft-versus-host disease (GVHD) may occur if patients are given fresh blood or unmatched allogeneic bone marrow.

- Fatal infections after live virus vaccines and after vaccination with other attenuated microorganisms including bacille Calmette-Guérin (BCG).
- High incidence of malignancy.

Wyngaarden JB, Smith LH (eds): Cecil Textbook of Medicine, 18th ed. Philadelphia, W.B. Saunders, 1988, p 1945.

98. **Is skin testing useful for estimating T-cell–mediated responses to *Histoplasma capsulatum* as it is in evaluating immunologic responses to *M. tuberculosis*?**
Skin testing is rarely useful in the diagnosis of histoplasmosis and should be principally limited to epidemiologic surveys. As with a positive PPD, a positive skin test to *Histoplasma* indicates prior exposure and not necessarily active infection. But in contrast to a positive PPD, injection of the histoplasmin reagent often causes a significant rise in antibody titers, thereby complicating interpretation of subsequent serologic studies. A negative skin test is highly suggestive of the absence of disease (even during dissemination stages), unless the patient is anergic. So it is necessary to apply other skin test reagents at the same time that will estimate the ability of the subject to mount a delayed-type hypersensitivity reaction to recall antigens.

99. **List the common secondary causes of hypogammaglobulinemia and the mechanism by which they cause disease.**
See Table 12-10.

TABLE 12-10. SECONDARY CAUSES OF HYPOGAMMAGLOBULINEMIA

Cause	Mechanism
Drugs	Drugs
a. Anticonvulsants (especially with phenytoin)	a. Decreased B and T cells responses, often hypogammaglobulinemia
b. Cytotoxic agents as used in cancer chemotherapy	b. Decreased Ig production and T-cell activity
Multiple myeloma	Decreased Ig production
Chronic lymphocytic leukemia	Decreased Ig production and T-cell activity
Myotonic dystrophy	Selective hypercatabolism of IgG
Nephrotic syndrome	Ig loss in urine (particularly IgG)
Intestinal lymphangiectasia	Ig loss through GI tract, increased Ig catabolism
Radiation therapy	Decreased Ig production

100. **Why should RBCs be irradiated before transfusion into immunocompromised patients, such as those on immunosuppressive chemotherapy?**
Packed red cells in freshly acquired blood may include lymphocytes that can mount a graft-versus-host disease (GVHD) reaction if the patient's own immune system is unable to rapidly kill and inactivate these transfused allogeneic leukocytes. GVHD is mediated by mature donor T cells that recognize the recipient as nonself.

101. When is the radioallergosorbent test (RAST) useful?
The RAST is used for measurement of antigen-specific IgE antibody in serum. The test is only semiquantitative.

102. How is the RAST performed?
Purified allergen is coupled to a carrier (particles, paper discs, plastic wells) and incubated with the patient's serum. After washing, ^{125}I-labeled anti-IgE is added and radioactivity present on the immunoabsorbent material (carrier) is measured. The RAST is increasingly being converted to an enzyme-linked immunosorbent assay (ELISA) system that uses enzymatic color change rather than radioactivity. Recently, Pharmacia has produced quantitative antigen-specific tests of IgE to selected allergens that may be more useful than the RAST in the diagnosis of allergic diseases.

103. How does the RAST compare with skin testing in the diagnosis of allergy?
The RAST is less sensitive, and its correlation with the clinical history of allergy to specific agents is less clear cut than with skin testing. Furthermore, validity of the RAST is highly dependent on proper controls and interpretation of the results by the reporting laboratory. However, the RAST may be useful in patients in whom skin testing cannot be done for one reason or another, such as patients with extensive skin diseases or dermatographism, urticaria pigmentosa, or cutaneous mastocytosis. It may also be useful in patients receiving H_1 antihistamines and patients in whom skin testing is considered to carry a high risk of severe anaphylaxis.

104. Is a positive RAST result diagnostic of allergy?
No test of immediate hypersensitivity, whether skin testing or the RAST, is by itself diagnostic and cannot be taken as evidence of allergy to a specific agent unless the clinical history also suggests that the patient is highly reactive to the same substance. In practice while the specificity of the RAST (and skin testing, for that matter) is low, the sensitivity is relatively high and a negative RAST (or, for that matter, negative intradermal testing) is good evidence that the patient is *not* sensitive to a specific allergen.

105. Describe the advantages of ELISAs.
The ELISA has, to a great extent, replaced the radioimmunoassay (RIA) in diagnostic testing. The ELISA eliminates the radioactive hazards of RIA and has a sensitivity that is comparable or better (sensitivity of 1 ng or less, depending on test substance and components used in the assay).

106. How is the ELISA performed?
The ELISA is typically performed in plastic, flat-bottomed, 96-well, microtiter plates. The concentration of the substance to be measured is determined by comparing the optical density of the test samples against negative controls and a standard curve. The basic ELISA procedure used to test for antibody against specific antigen is outlined below:

1. Coat wells with antigen (by incubating appropriate concentration of antigen in the wells) and then wash.
2. Add test sample and incubate.
3. Wash.
4. Add enzyme-linked anti-species Ig and incubate.
5. Wash.
6. Add developing substrate and measure optical density.

107. Which principal components of house dust have been implicated in causing allergic disease?
House dust is a frequent cause of allergic rhinitis and asthma. House dust is a mixture of variable amounts of antigens from dust mites, cockroaches, cats, dogs, pollens, molds, and other environmental substances. Dust mites and cockroach-related antigens are often the most important sources of offending allergens in the home and are particularly prevalent in clothing, carpets, and mattresses. Both species of dust mite (*Dermatophagoides pteronyssinus* and

Dermatophagoides farinae) can be found in bedding, upholstered furniture, and carpets in offices and homes in the U.S. The allergens are released into the excretions of the mites. Dust mites thrive optimally at 25°C and 80% relative humidity. Human epidermal scales are a major substrate for dust mite growth.

108. Describe the approach to treatment of house dust allergy.
Efforts to minimize exposure to dust and to decrease favorable environments available for dust mite growth may be highly beneficial for allergic patients. Antiallergic medications and, when necessary, immunotherapy (allergy shots) are effective forms of therapy. In practice, symptoms of allergic rhinitis can be controlled in 90% of patients if the patients use prescribed medications regularly for prophylaxis as well as treatment, and if proper attention is given to eliminating sources of dust mite and other allergens from the home.

109. Which biologic functions are mediated via H_1, H_2, or a combination of H_1 and H_2 histamine receptors?
See Table 12-11.

TABLE 12-11. BIOLOGIC FUNCTIONS MEDIATED BY H_1, H_2, OR A COMBINATION OF H_1 AND H_2 RECEPTORS

H_1 Receptors	H_2 Receptors	H_1 and H_2 Receptors
Smooth muscle contraction	Gastric acid secretion	Hypotension
↑ Vascular permeability	↑ Cyclic AMP	Tachycardia
Pruritus	Mucous secretion	Flushing
Stimulation of prostaglandin synthesis	Inhibits basophil, but not mast cell histamine release	Headache
Tachycardia	Stimulates IL-5 production by	
↑ Cyclic GMP production	TH2 cells	

↑ = increased, ↓ = decreased.
Note that although the majority of histamine receptors in the skin are H_1, some H_2 receptors and recalcitrant cases of urticaria may require treatment with both H_1- and H_2-specific antihistamines.

110. List the modes of therapy for allergic rhinitis.

- Avoidance of the offending allergens
- Medical therapy
- Allergen-specific immunotherapy

111. List the options for medical therapy.

- H_1 antihistamines
- Topical corticosteroid nasal sprays: highly effective but must often be used for 1–2 weeks before there is evidence of efficacy, and they must be used continuously through the patients' allergy season. They are very safe even with continuous year-round use and can be used even during an upper respiratory infection.

- Cromolyn sodium: in patients who have ocular pruritus as part of their symptom complex, cromolyn sodium eyedrops or some other mast cell stabilizer are necessary to control the problem fully. Nasal sodium cromolyn is a useful adjuct to control nasal symptoms of allergic rhinitis.
- Parasympathetic blockers (ipratropium bromide) nasal spray: can be used to control troublesome rhinorrhea.
- Sympathomimetics: among the most effective is nasal inhalation of topical oxymetazoline, but it must only be used intermittently to avoid rhinitis medicamentosa.

112. Does systemic corticosteroid therapy have a role in the treatment of allergic rhinitis?

Systemic therapy with corticosteroids is indicated only rarely for severe acute exacerbations and for control of nasal polyps.

113. How does allergy immunotherapy work?

The mechanisms are not definitively known. Allergen-specific immunotherapy involves the subcutaneous injection of extracts of the specific allergens responsible for a patient's symptoms. Patients do produce more IgG specific for the allergen, which may have a blocking function. There is a decrease in IgE antibodies specific for the allergen, and there may be some induction of T-cell anergy. Recruitment of effector cells is reduced. There is also a shift of T-cell cytokine production from those produced by TH2 cells (i.e., IL-4, IL-5, and IL-13) to those produced by TH1 cells (IL-2 and IFN-δ). Immunotherapy with bacterial vaccines has no proven efficacy.

114. What immunologic changes occur in patients who undergo allergen-specific immunotherapy?

- Diminished seasonal increases of allergen-specific IgE
- Increased allergen-specific IgG
- Decreased basophil histamine release
- Development of allergen-specific suppressor T cells

115. Name common diseases associated with elevation of the total serum IgE level.

- **Atopic (allergic)** diseases (allergic rhinitis, allergic asthma, allergic bronchopulmonary aspergillosis)
- **Primary immunodeficiency disorders** (Wiskott-Aldrich syndrome, Nezelhof's syndrome [cellular immunodeficiency with IgE], selective IgA deficiency with concomitant atopic disease, Job's syndrome)
- **Infections** (parasitic; viral, including infectious mononucleosis and others; fungal, including candidiasis and others)
- **Malignancies** (Hodgkin's disease, bronchial carcinoma, IgE myeloma)
- **Dermatologic disorders** (atopic dermatitis, bullous pemphigoid, eczema, and others)
- **Acute GVHD**

116. How useful is measurement of total serum IgE in such diseases?

In many of these diseases, IgE levels may be normal, mildly elevated, or markedly elevated. The clinical usefulness of measurement of total serum IgE is usually limited to diagnosis and monitoring of exacerbations, remissions, and/or treatment of allergic bronchopulmonary aspergillosis, parasitic infections, and immunodeficiency disorders.

117. What causes rhinitis medicamentosa?

Rhinitis medicamentosa results in intense nasal congestion, often with complete obstruction of the nasal airway due to rebound vasodilation. It is caused by long-term use of inhaled topical vasoconstrictors to treat symptoms of allergic rhinitis that may have been complicated by recurrent episodes. The causative agents are typically over-the-counter medications such as oxymetazoline nasal spray (e.g., Afrin 12-h nasal spray) that patients have used to excess before seeking professional help.

118. How is rhinitis medicamentosa treated?

Treatment consists of discontinuation of the offending drug. For severe cases it may be necessary to use a short course of oral corticosteroids.

119. Should alpha-adrenergic topical vascoconstrictors be avoided in the treatment of allergic rhinitis?

The risk of rhinitis medicamentosa should not preclude the use of alpha-adrenergic topical vasoconstrictors such as oxymetazoline in treatment of allergic rhinitis. When used correctly, these agents help to open up the nasal passages and increase nasal airflow for 8–12 hours to ensure that inhaled topical corticosteroids can be effectively delivered throughout the nasal passages and as far as the posterior nasopharynx.

120. How can the risk of rhinitis medicamentosa be minimized with use of these agents?

To be certain that there are no complications from the use of these potent vasoconstrictors, treatment must be interrupted from time to time. This can be achieved by taking a drug holiday every 3 or 4 days. Some patients may be able to use these drugs daily if treatment is limited to once per day, preferably in the evening or at bedtime.

121. What is the triad of Kartagener's syndrome?

Originally described by Kartagener in 1904, the syndrome consists of the triad of recurrent sinopulmonary infections, bronchiectasis, and (sometimes) situs inversus. It must be considered in the differential diagnosis of chronic sinusitis and/or bronchitis that appears to be refractory to conventional treatment. Male patients may also have immotile spermatozoa and as a result are sterile.

122. What causes Kartagener's syndrome?

Kartagener's syndrome is an autosomal recessive disorder resulting in the defective functioning of the cilia, which lack dynein arms. As a result, patients do not move mucus secretions out of the respiratory tract except by coughing and blowing their noses.

Eliasson R, et al: The immotile cilia syndrome. N Engl J Med 297:1–6, 1977.

123. Describe the mechanism of action of cromolyn sodium.

Cromolyn sodium is available for use via inhalational, intranasal, and topical ophthalmic routes. Topical mucosal application inhibits the degranulation of mucosal mast cells, thereby preventing the release of the mediators of immediate hypersensitivity. The mechanism by which this occurs is unknown, although inhibition of calcium influx is one of several proposed explanations. This drug has no intrinsic antihistamine, bronchodilator, or anti-inflammatory activity.

124. When is cromolyn sodium particularly useful?

Cromolyn is used as a prophylactic agent in patients with sufficiently frequent symptoms to justify continuous therapy because it is most effective when administered prior to exposure to an allergen (i.e., prior to mast cell degranulation). Cromolyn inhibits both immediate hypersensitivity and late-phase reactions. It requires a run-in period of 3 weeks to reach maximum effectiveness.

125. How would 2 weeks of treatment with H_1 or H_2 antihistamines be expected to affect the results of allergy and DTH skin testing?

Allergy skin testing is used to evaluate a patient for immediate hypersensitivity reactivity (a type I reaction) against a specific allergen. Thus, if a patient's mast cells have been sensitized with

IgE antibody against the injected allergen, mast cell degranulation occurs, resulting in release of mediators such as histamine into the skin. The wheal-and-flare reaction of a positive skin test is primarily due to histamine stimulation of H_1 receptors in small blood vessels. Consequently, treatment with H_1 antihistamines markedly inhibits positive skin test reactivity and must be discontinued, usually 2 days, prior to skin testing.

H_2 antihistamines may occasionally depress skin test reactivity as well and should also be avoided prior to skin testing. To guard against the chance that the patient has forgotten to stop these drugs, a histamine standard should be used as a positive control in performing allergy skin testing.

126. How would 2 weeks of treatment with corticosteroids affect the results of allergy and DTH skin testing?

Corticosteroids do not affect mast cell degranulation, nor do they affect the biologic effects of histamine. Thus, corticosteroids do not alter allergy skin test results. In contrast, DTH skin testing is a type IV reaction and is a sensitive measurement of T-cell function. Histamine does not play a significant role in DTH, and antihistamines (both H_1 and H_2) do not affect DTH skin testing. However, corticosteroids may substantially depress cell-mediated responses, including the mobilization of T cells to specific antigen depots. Thus, DTH reactions (e.g., PPD skin tests) may be profoundly depressed by treatment with corticosteroids.

127. Which types of infections play a role in the exacerbation of asthma?

Strong evidence implicates upper respiratory infections caused by viruses and *Mycoplasma pneumoniae* as important exacerbating agents of asthma. The association is especially pronounced in the pediatric age group. Respiratory syncytial virus parainfluenza, influenza A, rhinovirus, and adenovirus have also been implicated.

128. What factors determine the severity of the exacerbation?

The severity of the exacerbation depends on multiple factors, including age, severity of the underlying asthma, concurrent medical problems, site and severity of the infection, and specific infectious agent.

129. Do bacterial infections play a role in the exacerbation of asthma?

Bacterial infections of the respiratory tract, except as causative agents for chronic sinusitis, have not been commonly associated with exacerbations of asthma, but they may be a significant cause of exacerbation in patients with COPD, in whom bronchospasm is triggered by allergenic stimuli. Considering these relationships, empirical antibiotic therapy, while frequently used during exacerbations of asthma in children and adults, frequently does not result in a remission of symptoms. More important in such cases is increased use of inhaled corticosteroids.

130. A 22-year-old patient complains of symptoms of asthma after playing basketball. What is a likely explanation?

The patient probably has exercise-induced asthma (EIA). Bronchoconstriction typically begins following cessation of exercise and is usually maximal 3–12 minutes later. The severity varies, but it is almost always short-lived.

131. How is the diagnosis of EIA confirmed?

The diagnosis of EIA is confirmed by a decrease in the forced respiratory volume following exercise or isocapnic hyperventilation, although the former is the preferred form of testing.

132. What causes EIA?

The cause of EIA is believed to be water loss from the bronchial mucosa, resulting in hyperosmolarity in the bronchial tissue. This mechanism has been demonstrated by prevention of EIA during exercise by means of air that is fully saturated with water vapor at body temperature.

Water content of the inspired air is probably the single most important factor affecting bronchospasm, but the level of ventilation achieved, the temperature of the inspired air, and the interval since the previous episode of EIA are also contributing factors. The severity of EIA cannot be predicted by baseline pulmonary function tests (PFTs).

133. Why is the interval since the previous episode of EIA an important factor?
The last factor is important because a refractory period usually occurs for as long as 2 hours following the previous episode. During this period, a second challenge invokes less than half of the initial airway response.

134. What treatment is available for prevention of EIA?
Inhaled beta agonists are the most effective treatment, giving 90% or greater response rates. Approximately 60–70% of patients respond to inhaled cromolyn alone. Some patients require combination therapy, and ipratropium bromide (an anticholinergic agent) may offer additional relief. Patients should inhale these medications from a hand-held nebulizer immediately before exercise. The protective effects of pharmacologic therapy may last for only 2 hours, even though in non–exercise-related bronchospasm benefits may continue for an additional 2–4 hours. Inhaled corticosteroids, when taken over several weeks, may decrease both the severity of EIA and the doses of the other medications required for control. Finally, nasal breathing may attenuate EIA but it is not practical in strenuous exercise.

135. What exercise should be recommended for asthmatics?
Whenever possible, asthmatics should be encouraged to swim for exercise.

136. What are the two major pathways of arachidonic acid metabolism?
Prostaglandin D_2 (PGD_2) and thromboxanes A_2 and B_2 are the major products of the **cyclooxygenase (COX) pathway** of arachidonic acid metabolism. Leukotrienes, especially LTC4, LTD4 and LTE4, are major products of the **lipoxygenase pathway**. These eicosanoids exhibit an array of potent inflammatory and immunoregulatory properties.

137. What effects do aspirin, NSAIDs, eicosapentaenoic acid (fish oil), and corticosteroids have on mediator production by these pathways?
Aspirin and NSAIDs inhibit COX; that is, they inhibit PG and thromboxane but not LT production. Eicosapentaenoic acid (fish oil) inhibits both PG/thromboxane and LT formation by preferential fatty acid substitution for arachidonic acid in the cell membranes of eicosanoid-producing cells. Corticosteroids also inhibit both PG/thromboxane and LT generation by stimulating production of the intracellular protein, lipocortin, which inhibits the activity of phospholipase A.

138. What is aspirin-exacerbated respiratory disease?
This condition is most dramatically evident in patients who in adult life have developed three manifestations of atopic disease sometimes known as Samter's triad: (1) rhinosinusitis, (2) nasal polyposis, and (3) asthma that is typically severe and exacerbated by aspirin and other nonsteroidal COX-1 inhibitors. In such people COX-1 inhibitor therapy is sometimes also associated with hives, flushing, and abdominal pain. Because selective inhibition of COX-2 does not provoke these responses, patients can be treated with COX-2 inhibitors with impunity.

139. What causes aspirin-exacerbated respiratory disease?
The underlying mechanism remains unknown, but there are several distinctive features of arachidonic acid metabolism in people who are aspirin sensitive. Their mast cells and eosinophils produce cysteinyl leukotrienes at a very high rate. Prostaglandin E_2 (PGE_2), a product of the COX pathway, inhibits 5-lipoxygenase, the enzyme that is responsible for the production of leukotrienes from arachidonic acid. One explanation is that aspirin-induced reduction in

synthesis of PGE_2 disinhibits synthesis of downstream bronchospastic metabolites in the 5-lipoxygenase pathway (Fig. 12-6). Indeed, during aspirin-induced asthma one can measure increased quantities of LTE4 in the urine and LTC4 in nasal and bronchial secretions. Recent studies indicate that patients also have increased numbers of receptors for cysteinyl leukotrienes in the nasal mucosa.

Sousa AR, Parikh A, Scadding G, et al: Leukotriene-receptor expression on nasal mucosal inflammatory cells in aspirin-sensitive rhinosinusitis. N Engl J Med 347:1493–1499, 2002.

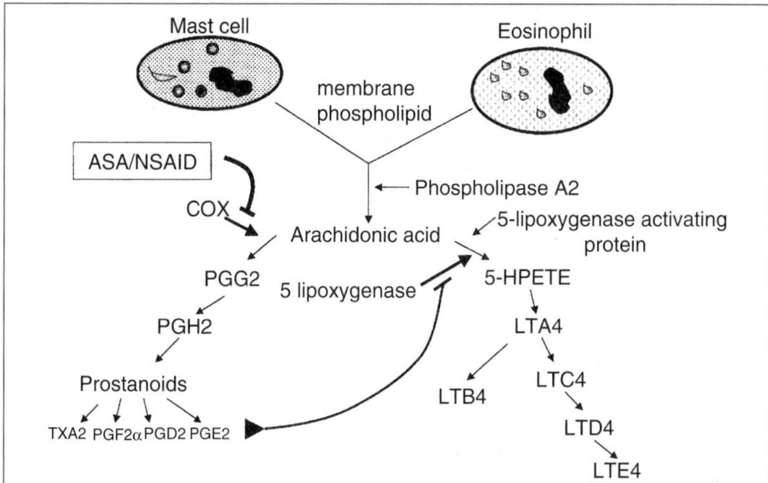

Figure 12-6. Effects of aspirin and NSAIDs on the two major pathways of arachidonic acid metabolism. (From Middleton E Jr, Reed Ce, Ellis EF, et al [eds]: Allergy: Principles and Practice, 5th ed, vol II. St Louis, Mosby, 1998, p 1229.)

140. How is aspirin-exacerbated respiratory disease treated?

Treatment options include strict avoidance of aspirin and other NSAIDs and desensitization therapy, which is typically attempted by treating patients with as much as 650 mg of aspirin twice daily on a continuous basis. While long-term desensitization therapy has been reported to reduce disease activity in many aspirin-sensitive patients, as shown by a reduced need for surgery for nasal polyps and reduced requirements for corticosteroids, in others the gastric irritation caused by aspirin has prevented them from continuing with the therapy.

141. Discuss the role of circadian rhythms in a patient who complains of nocturnal worsening of asthma.

Considerable attention has been directed toward the role of circadian rhythms in nocturnal exacerbations of asthma (usually between 3 AM and 7 AM). Cortisol levels decrease, plasma histamine levels increase, and epinephrine levels decrease during the night. The decrease in plasma cortisol is not thought to be a major factor since administration of corticosteroids in the evening is ineffective in preventing nocturnal exacerbations. Plasma histamine levels do not correlate with changes in PFTs. However, epinephrine levels do correlate, suggesting a possible important physiologic role. Circadian changes in the airways themselves are also important. Both airway caliber and reactivity change at night, with an overall 5–10% decrease in flow rates in normal individuals, but up to a 50% decrease in asthmatics. Increased vagal tone, impaired mucociliary clearance, and airway cooling and drying have also been reported as contributing factors in nocturnal asthma.

142. How does gastroesophageal reflux disease (GERD) affect nocturnal exacerbations of asthma?
GERD may also exacerbate asthma at night by microaspiration or reflex bronchoconstriction caused by stimulation of nerve endings by acid in the lower esophagus. GERD may be exacerbated by theophylline, which decreases lower esophageal sphincter tone.

143. Describe the treatment of symptoms due to GERD.
H_2 antihistamines and/or proton pump inhibitors may be helpful in patients with GERD. Possibly more important is a change in dietary habits to lengthen the interval between the last meal of the day and bedtime. A high content of fat or protein in food stimulates closure of the pylorus by a cholecystokinin-driven mechanism for 4 hours or more in some people, resulting in prolonged retention of food in the stomach. Some patients with GERD are helped by raising the head of the bed on blocks by as much as 4–6 inches in order that they may sleep with the head and thorax elevated.

144. How can adjustment in beta-agonist therapy improve nocturnal worsening of asthma?
The patient's pharmacologic regimen should be carefully reviewed and compliance assured. Use of longer-acting, inhaled beta agonists should be encouraged. The introduction of the long-acting form of albuterol, salmeterol, has a beneficial effect on nocturnal asthma in some patients. A recent randomized trial suggests that simultaneous administration of salmeterol and fluticasone by means of a Diskus inhaler significantly reduced nocturnal symptoms in patients with moderate-to-severe asthma. The comparison group received conventional therapy with corticosteroids and the long-acting beta agonist delivered by separate inhalers. Some patients also benefit from the use of leukotriene receptor antagonists.

Ringdal N, Chuchalin A, Chovan L, et al, for the PJ EDICT Investigators: Evaluation of Different Inhaled Combination Therapies (EDICT): A randomized, double-blind comparison of seretide (50/250 microg bd diskus versus formoterol (12 microg bd) and budesonide (800 microg bd) given concurrently (both via Turbuhaler) in patients with moderate-to-severe asthma. Respir Med 96:851–861, 2002.

145. How can adjustment of theophylline therapy improve nocturnal asthma?
Theophylline absorption may be decreased at night, leading to lower serum levels. If necessary, the evening dose should be adjusted so that peak levels occur approximately 6 hours later.

146. Do corticosteroids help in the treatment of nocturnal asthma?
Oral corticosteroids should not be given in the evening because the hypothalamic-pituitary-adrenal axis is more readily suppressed at that time of day by exogenous corticosteroids. There is also no evidence that differences in the time of administration either improve or reduce the benefits associated with the use of these drugs.

147. What other measures may improve the symptoms of nocturnal asthma?
Patients who have an allergic component to their asthma and who are on maximal pharmacologic therapy should be considered for immunotherapy. Potential environmental and dietary agents should be considered as exacerbating factors. For example, dust mites may cause immediate hypersensitivity reactions during the night. Allergen or irritant exposure several hours before going to sleep can also be important. The late-phase response that may occur following such exposure typically peaks 6–12 hours later and may cause severe, prolonged bronchospasm.

148. Which nonasthmatic factors may lead to nocturnal worsening of symptoms?
Nonasthmatic causes of wheezing such as cardiac diseases should be considered. Older patients who by other criteria are at risk for atherosclerotic cardiovascular disease should be

systematically evaluated to be certain that the nocturnal asthma is not an early or subtle manifestation of paroxysmal nocturnal dyspnea. One also should consider that what the patient perceives to be nocturnal asthma may actually be sleep apnea. Nocturnal asthma is not related to any particular stage of sleep. The patient's sleep partner should be interviewed to describe what type of sleep problems the patient is having and, if indicated, a formal sleep study should be performed.

149. Why is it critical that nocturnal asthma be treated aggressively?

The importance of the treatment of nocturnal asthma cannot be overemphasized, since the majority of fatalities due to asthma occur during the early morning hours.

150. What are Charcot-Leyden crystals, Creola bodies, and Curschmann's spirals?

- **Charcot-Leyden crystals** are composed of lysophospholipase, and their presence in tissue or secretions has been considered as specific for eosinophil activity. However, lysophospholipase is also found in basophils.
- **Creola bodies** are clumps of epithelial cells and suggest a desquamating disease process.
- **Curschmann's spirals** are mucus plugs composed of mucus, proteinaceous material, and inflammatory cells in a swirling, spiraling pattern. They usually conform to the configuration of the involved airways.

These three entities may be found alone or together as part of the clinical presentation of asthma. They are characteristically seen in patients who have died from status asthmaticus.

151. List the clinical manifestations of anaphylaxis.

- **General:** flushing, sense of foreboding
- **Skin:** urticaria/angioedema, flushing, pruritus
- **Eyes:** lacrimation, pruritus
- **Upper respiratory tract:** sneezing, nasal pruritus, discharge and congestion, hoarseness, laryngeal edema, stridor
- **Lower respiratory tract:** bronchospasm, tachypnea, intercostal retractions, use of accessory muscles of respiration
- **Cardiovascular:** hypotension, tachycardia, arrhythmia
- **GI:** nausea, vomiting, abdominal pain, diarrhea
- **Neurologic:** headache, syncope, seizure

152. A 20-year-old man presents with hypotension, wheezing, and urticaria 30 minutes after a beesting. What is the likely diagnosis?

This presentation suggests systemic anaphylaxis, an immediate hypersensitivity reaction, triggered by bee venom, that results in mast cell/basophil release of mediators like histamine, prostaglandins, and leukotrienes, into tissues and the circulation.

153. What is the first priority of treatment?

Prompt treatment is critical and should be directed toward maintaining cardiovascular and pulmonary function. Initial treatment should be epinephrine either by subcutaneous or intramuscular routes (0.3–0.5 cc of a 1:1000 dilution). With cardiovascular collapse, IV epinephrine may be indicated.

154. What other immediate steps should be taken?

Other immediate steps include applying a tourniquet proximal to the site of allergen inoculation (for example, a beesting or allergen injection in the forearm). If the anaphylaxis is due to oral intake of an allergen, a nasogastric (NG) tube may be inserted and residual gastric contents removed to prevent further antigen absorption. The patient's legs should be elevated, oxygen and airway support provided, and IV fluids (such as normal saline) given for blood pressure support.

155. Summarize the pharmacologic treatment of systemic anaphylaxis.
Parenteral H_1 and H_2 antihistamines may be administered. Inhaled beta-I agonists can be given prophylactically, especially when bronchospasm occurrs. Repeat doses of medication such as epinephrine should be given as needed, and vasopressor agents should be added when indicated. Although steroids do not alter the acute course of anaphylaxis, they may be given to attenuate a subsequent late-phase response. The aggressiveness of therapy depends on the severity of the anaphylaxis and the response to treatment.

156. When should a patient be desensitized to a needed drug (e.g., penicillin)?
Desensitization should only be considered in patients with life-threatening conditions for which the drug is so necessary for a favorable therapeutic result that this potential benefit outweighs the risks associated with desensitization therapy. The patient should be skin tested to verify presence of an IgE-mediated hypersensitivity to the drug. Desensitization should be done in a highly monitored situation, typically an intensive care unit, where cardiopulmonary resuscitation can be carried out under optimal conditions, if necessary.

157. How is desensitization performed?
Desensitization is achieved by starting treatment with a minute quantity of a drug that, if given in the full therapeutic dose, all at once, would cause anaphylaxis. After the initial test dose, serial, closely spaced injections of systematically increasing quantities of the drug are given at approximately 20-min intervals. The aim of this treatment is to slowly discharge the anaphylactogenic mediators of mast cells that display surface IgE antibodies to the drug. Essentially the treatment is designed to cause a controlled anaphylaxis. Patients should *not* be premedicated with antihistamines or glucocorticoids that mask the allergic reaction since it is necessary to titrate the rate of desensitization based on the patient's response. Once a patient has been desensitized, it is critical that there be no lapse in therapy since any significant interruption could allow the patient's mast cells to regenerate mast cell mediators like histamine that upon resumption of therapy would be discharged and induce anaphylaxis.

158. What are the major distinguishing factors between Churg-Strauss syndrome (allergic angiitis and granulomatosis) and classic polyarteritis nodosa (PAN)?
Both are systemic necrotizing vasculitides. Their distinctions are outlined in Table 12-12. Patients who have characteristics of both Churg-Strauss and PAN are classified as having polyangiitis overlap syndrome. Patients who fail corticosteroid therapy or who have fulminant disease should receive cytotoxic drug therapy.

159. What does palpable purpura indicate?
Palpable purpura indicates cutaneous vasculitis.

160. What is the classic triad of Wegener's granulomatosis (WG)? Describe the clinical presentation and laboratory findings.
WG is a systemic necrotizing vasculopathy of unknown etiology. The classic triad includes necrotizing granulomatous vasculitis of (1) the upper respiratory tract and (2) lungs as well as (3) glomerulonephritis. Vasculitis of many other organs, including the skin, ears, eyes, joints, and central nervous system (CNS), may also be present. Vasculitis typically involves *both* small arteries and veins. The glomerulonephritis is usually focal or crescentic without vasculitis or granulomas. Since the original description by Wegener in Germany in 1939, many more limited forms of the disease have been recognized.

161. Describe the clinical presentation of WG.
The clinical presentation may include fever, chronic sinusitis, serous otitis media (often unilateral), cough, chest pain, hemoptysis, and arthralgias. Upper airway infections are common,

TABLE 12-12. COMPARISON OF CHURG-STRAUSS SYNDROME AND PAN

	Churg-Strauss	PAN
Pulmonary involvement	Yes	No
Histology	Necrotizing vasculitis with granulomas	Necrotizing vasculitis
Vessel involvement	Small-to-medium arteries	Medium muscular arteries; veins, venules with aneurysmal dilation
Asthma/atopic disease	Yes*	No
Eosinophilia (blood and/or tissue)	Yes	No
Association with serum hepatitis B surface antigen (HBsAg)	No	Yes

*Often present for years before onset of vasculitis.

with *Staphylococcus aureus* the most common pathogen. Such infections may mimic exacerbation or recurrence of disease following remission. With the inflammatory process unchecked, nasal septal perforation may occur, leading to a saddle-nose deformity.

162. Which laboratory tests help in the diagnosis of WG?
Laboratory data are generally nonspecific, although recently an antibody to cytoplasmic components of the polymorphonuclear leukocyte (antineutrophil cytoplasmic antibody [ANCA], also known as antibody to proteinase 3) has been associated with active disease. The erythrocyte sedimentation rate (ESR) is markedly elevated (often > 100 mm/h) and is a sensitive indicator of disease activity. Mild anemia, leukocytosis, and an increase in serum IgG and IgA levels are commonly seen. Chest x-ray patterns include multiple nodules (which frequently cavitate), infiltrates, and solitary nodules. The mean age of onset is 40 years with a male predominance.

163. Describe the general approach to treatment for WG.
Before the use of cytotoxic drugs, specifically cyclophosphamide, WG was an almost uniformly fatal disease, with a mean survival of 5 months. Corticosteroid therapy did not significantly alter the disease's outcome. However, treatment with cyclophosphamide results in complete remission in over 90% of patients. Combination treatment with corticosteroids and cyclophosphamide should be given initially to gain benefits from the rapid anti-inflammatory effects of the steroid while the cytotoxic actions of the cyclophosphamide are taking effect.

164. How should cyclophosphamide and corticosteroid therapy be administered?
Prednisone may be started at 1 mg/kg daily, maintained for 1 month, tapered to alternate day therapy, and then gradually discontinued, depending on the patient's response. Cyclophosphamide should be started at 2 mg/kg orally and continued for at least a year. If, at the end of the year, clinical remission has been obtained, the cyclophosphamide may be tapered and discontinued. The patient's hematologic parameters should be closely monitored for cyclophosphamide toxicity. The patient's WBC count should be maintained above

3000/mm^3 with a neutrophil count above 1000/mm^3 to lessen the risk of infectious complications.

165. Are any other drugs helpful in the treatment of WG?
Other cytotoxic drugs, such as azathioprine, are less effective than cyclophosphamide in the treatment of WG. In a recent study of patients who had a partial or complete remission following cyclophosphamide/prednisolone induction therapy, leflunomide together with low-dose prednisone was used for maintenance therapy.

166. What are the major differences between WG and Goodpasture's syndrome?
See Table 12-13.

TABLE 12-13. WEGENER'S GRANULOMATOSIS VERSUS GOODPASTURE'S SYNDROME

	Wegener's	Goodpasture's
Etiology	Unknown	Unknown, but hydrocarbon exposure increases risk
Patients	Male > female Fifth decade	Male >> female Young adults
Histopathology	Necrotizing granulomatous vasculitis of upper/lower respiratory tract	Linear deposition of IgG along basement membrane of lung and kidney demonstrated by immunofluorescence, vasculitis absent
Target organs	Lung > kidney; may also affect: CNS, eyes, ears, joints, skin, heart, others	Kidney > lung
Primary symptoms	Chronic sinusitis/rhinitis, fever, weight loss, cough, chest pain, hemoptysis may occur	Hemoptysis, dyspnea, easy fatigability
Typical chest x-ray findings	Pulmonary nodule(s) with or without cavitation	Diffuse bilateral infiltrates
Diagnosis	Clinical picture with biopsy showing necrotizing vasculitis with granulomas of small arteries and veins	Demonstration of circulating or tissue-bound anti-basement membrane antibodies, pulmonary hemorrhage, glomerulonephritis
Treatment	Cyclophosphamide, corticosteroids	Vigorous plasmapheresis, corticosteroids, cyclophosphamide

167. What clinical and laboratory findings are most important in illuminating the cause of angioedema?
The majority of angioedema cases are idiopathic, and an extensive evaluation fails to reveal a specific cause or associated underlying disease. However, a careful history is of the utmost importance. For example, allergic angioedema may be suggested by a temporal relationship to exposure to specific allergens (such as food). Cold urticaria/angioedema is indicated by onset

following exposure to cold temperatures. A number of findings may indicate hereditary angioedema (HAE), including a positive family history, low C4 during and between attacks, and low antigenic or functional activity of C1 esterase inhibitor (C1INH). Because patients may have one gene producing functional C1INH and one gene producing a nonfunctional C1INH, it may be necessary to measure the quantity of functional or biologically active inhibitor as opposed to just the total quantity of C1INH protein.

168. What other diseases may be associated with angioedema?
The list of diseases reported to be associated with angioedema is exhaustive, but some of the most widely recognized are connective tissue diseases, malignancies, thyroid disease, and liver disease (such as hepatitis B). Not infrequently, angiotensin-converting enzyme (ACE) inhibitors may increase the risk of angioedema. Consider an alternative drug to control hypertension. Patients who have an episode of angioneurotic edema after use of one ACE inhibitor should not be treated with another ACE inhibitor.

169. What is the cause of angioedema in the HAE?
HAE is caused by deficiency of C1INH. Eighty-five percent of HAE patients have depressed serum levels of C1INH (by antigenic assay), whereas the remaining 15% have normal enzyme levels but lack functional activity. The clinical presentation and inheritance patterns are similar for both groups. Decreased C1INH leads to unchecked activation of the classical complement pathway and decreased inhibition of Hageman factor–dependent activation of the kinin and plasmin pathways. This results in increased generation of C2 kinin, bradykinin, and other molecules that can increase vascular permeability. C1INH is an inhibitor of multiple enzymes, including many in the clotting cascade. Tissue injury can lead to angioedema because consumption of C1INH during clotting leaves the conversion of bradykinin to kinin unchecked.

170. What are some of the most important clinical characteristics of HAE?
HAE is transmitted in an autosomal dominant pattern, although sporadic cases do occur. The age of onset is variable, and the diagnosis can be hindered by a predilection for nonlaryngeal sites, such as the abdominal viscera. Inciting causes are not usually identified, although trauma, even minor, can lead to attacks. Most patients have a high propensity for life-threatening laryngeal edema that is not characteristic of angioedema due to other causes. Abdominal pain may also be noted during attacks.

171. How is HAE distinguished from urticaria?
Urticaria, although commonly seen in association with other causes of angioedema, is not part of the HAE syndrome. Pain, not pruritus, is typical of HAE lesions. If pruritus is intense, it is likely that one is dealing with urticarial angioedema. Patients typically have depressed serum C4 levels even when they are asymptomatic between attacks.

172. Summarize the treatment of HAE.
Attenuated androgen (i.e., stanazolol) therapy dramatically decreases the severity and frequency of attacks. Androgens should be tapered to the lowest dose that adequately controls disease activity in order to minimize potential adverse effects such as virilization and hepatic toxicity.

173. What elements in the history are important in the evaluation of a previously healthy 26-year-old patient who presents with an 8-week history of daily urticaria?
Urticaria persisting for longer than 6 weeks is deemed chronic. A careful history should be obtained to determine whether the urticaria is related to the ingestion of a specific food or liquid, environmental exposure, animal exposure, physical condition (e.g., heat, cold, water, sunlight, pressure, exercise), or stress. The history should also seek to rule out symptoms suggestive of an underlying systemic disease. A careful medication history should also be obtained for the

ingestion of both prescription and over-the-counter medications (particularly aspirin and aspirin-containing compounds).

174. What elements of the physical examination are important in evaluating chronic urticaria?
A thorough physical examination should be performed to identify potential underlying illnesses, such as thyroid disease, malignancy, infection, and rheumatic diseases.

175. Summarize the role of imaging modalities in the evaluaton of chronic urticaria.
A chest x-ray usually should be obtained, particularly if the patient has not had one within the past 6 months. CT scanning may help to detect more difficult to diagnose and treat malignancies such as pancreatic cancer. If the patient has poor dental health or findings suggestive of a dental abscess, dental x-rays may reveal the source of an occult infection.

176. What laboratory tests may be useful in patients with chronic urticaria?
Screening laboratory tests should include a complete blood count with WBC count and differential, urinalysis, ESR, and liver function tests. In patients over the age of 40, a serum protein electrophoresis should be obtained to rule out paraproteinemia.

177. Which other tests may be helpful in specific cases?
Other tests that may rarely be helpful include cryoglobulins, screening for antinuclear antibodies, thyroid function studies, complement C3 and C4, and rheumatoid factor. In patients who have traveled abroad recently to third-world countries, testing stool for ova and parasites may be helpful; also to be considered is screening for hepatitis B and C. In patients from South or Central America, American trypanosomiasis (Chagas' disease) should also be considered. Whether these and other tests for the evaluation for systemic diseases are obtained depends on the degree of clinical suspicion based on the history, physical examination, and initial laboratory results. Tests for specific types of the physical urticarias can be performed as indicated. Some investigations attribute a significant fraction of chronic urticaria cases to the development of autoantibodies either to the mast cell receptor for IgE or to IgE itself.

178. Describe the first-line treatment for chronic urticaria.
Despite extensive evaluation, more than 90% of the cases of chronic urticaria are ultimately classified as idiopathic. If an underlying treatable cause for the chronic urticaria cannot be detected, it is appropriate to try empirical therapy with a combination of nonsedating H_1 antagonists and H_2 antagonists (e.g., 60 mg fexofenadine and 150 mg ranitidine every 12 h). In the great majority of cases, this treatment is sufficient to reduce the frequency and duration of the urticarial episodes to a tolerable level.

179. What other alternatives are available for treatment of chronic urticaria?
If combined H_1 and H_2 antagonist treatment is not sufficient, it may be necessary to add systemic corticosteroids at the lowest dose needed to control symptoms. Typical urticarial lesions do not usually require biopsy. However, in particularly severe, persistent cases, and especially when urticarial lesions are very painful (as opposed to pruritic), very erythematous, or persist longer than 24 hours, a skin biopsy may reveal urticarial vasculitis. Some of these cases are accompanied by hypocomplementemia and may require more aggressive medical therapy.

180. What is the usefulness of rheumatoid factors (RFs) in the diagnosis of rheumatoid arthritis (RA)?
RFs are autoantibodies (most commonly IgM) that react with the Fc portion of IgG. The presence of RF is not diagnostic of RA and may not be detected in approximately 20% of patients with this disease. When present, RF may be detected in blood, synovial fluid, and pleural fluid.

KEY POINTS: ALLERGY AND IMMUNOLOGY ✓

1. The biologic effects of glucocorticoids are not synchronized with blood levels of the drug; effects do not start until a minimum of 4–6 hours after administration.
2. The presence of specific IgM antibodies is indicative of an active infection.
3. The kinetics of a hypersensitivity response is an important diagnostic clue to the underlying mechanism.
4. Corticosteroids are anti-inflammatory, not immunosuppressive.
5. Chronic sinusitis may in fact represent allergic rhinitis.
6. Smoking cessation is critical for successful management of asthma, COPD, and allergic rhinitis.
7. Classification of collagen vascular diseases is based on clinical criteria, with laboratory testing playing a useful but subsidiary role.

Neither on the basis of specificity nor on the basis of sensitivity is RF warranted as a screening test for collagen vascular disease. In cases of RA documented by clinical criteria, it may be useful to follow RF titers because high titers of RF are found mainly in patients who have more aggressive joint and extra-articular manifestations of disease.

181. With what other disorders is RF associated?
RF is also found in a long list of other illnesses, including other systemic inflammatory diseases, malignancies, infectious diseases (such as tuberculosis, viral, subacute bacterial endocarditis), and sarcoidosis. Furthermore, RF can be detected in a small percentage of normal individuals, particularly in the elderly.

182. What is Sjögren's syndrome?
Sjögren's disease is a chronic inflammatory disease of the exocrine glands characterized by keratoconjunctivitis sicca and xerostomia. The inflammatory infiltrate is composed primarily of lymphocytes and plasma cells. Primary Sjögren's disease is exocrine gland disease alone, whereas secondary Sjögren's occurs with another connective tissue disease, most commonly RA.

183. What is the single best diagnostic test for Sjögren's syndrome?
Biopsy of the labial minor salivary glands is the most specific diagnostic procedure available.

184. How can eye involvement in Sjögren's disease be confirmed?
Eye involvement may be confirmed by the Schirmer test. This test measures tear production very simply. If the patient's tears wet only 10 mm of the filter paper in 5 minutes, tear production is poor and the test is considered positive. Other ophthalmologic tests include rose bengal staining of the conjunctivae, and/or the finding of keratitis on slit lamp examination.

185. What other tests are useful in Sjögren's disease?
Parotid salivary flow rates and salivary radionuclide scanning may be used to assess salivary gland function. Autoantibodies in sera may include Ro(SS-A), La(SS-B), RF, and Epstein-Barr–related nuclear antigen.

186. What do the direct and indirect Coombs' tests measure?

Once the presence of hemolytic anemia has been confirmed, additional testing should be performed to determine whether an immune mechanism causes the hemolysis. The **direct Coombs' test** (direct antiglobulin test) measures antibody or complement already deposited on the surface of the patient's RBC. Titrations are performed to determine the degree of RBC sensitization. The **indirect Coombs' test** (indirect antiglobulin test) measures the presence of antibody in the patient's serum. In the case of hemolytic anemia caused by penicillin-specific antibodies reacting with penicillin bound to the surface of RBCs, the direct Coombs' would be positive. However, the indirect Coombs' would be negative since normal RBCs do not have penicillin on their surface and would not bind the anti-penicillin antibodies in the patient's serum.

187. How is the direct Coombs' test performed?

Briefly, the test is performed by incubating the patient's RBCs with anti-Ig or anti-C3 reagent. If surface-bound Ig or complement is present, agglutination occurs with the appropriate antisera.

188. How is the indirect Coombs' test performed?

The patient's serum is added to normal RBCs, and after incubation and washing, an anti-Ig reagent is added. If the antibody from the patient's serum has bound to the RBCs, agglutination occurs.

189. What is the cold agglutinin syndrome? How is it diagnosed?

The cold agglutinin syndrome is characterized by hemolytic anemia secondary usually to IgM antibodies, although low-affinity IgG antibodies have also been implicated. The IgM antibodies can cause RBC lysis with decreasing temperature. IgG antibodies can, in addition, facilitate uptake of the antibody coated RBC by phagocytes. Agglutination of normal RBCs at 20°C occurs with serum from virtually all patients with the cold agglutinin syndrome.

190. How is the cold agglutinin syndrome diagnosed?

The direct Coombs' test is typically positive for complement and negative for Ig. This finding reflects the fact that the antibody involved has a high affinity for RBC only in the cold. Warming the antibody causes it to dissociate. Hence only RBCs in cold extremities (e.g., fingers, toes, tip of the nose) are likely to show a positive direct Coombs test.

191. What causes cold agglutinin syndrome?

The cold agglutinin syndrome is typically idiopathic, with the presentation of hemolytic anemia in the sixth or seventh decade of life. Despite the monoclonal nature of the antibody response, patients typically do not develop multiple myeloma or Waldenstrom's macroglobulinemia. Cold agglutinin syndrome may also occur in association with the lymphoproliferative disorders (i.e., non-Hodgkin's lymphoma), infections (*M. pneumoniae*, infectious mononucleosis), and rarely in connective tissue disorders such as SLE. The cold agglutinins in these disorders may be anti-I, or directed at other RBC antigens. Determination of antibody specificity is not necessary for either diagnosis or blood transfusion.

192. What is the "innocent bystander" mechanism of drug-induced hemolysis?

Some drugs can cause an immune hemolytic anemia even though they do not bind to RBCs. These drugs, bound to plasma proteins, stimulate the formation of complement-fixing antibodies that activate the classical complement pathway. The C3b generated by these reactions in the plasma binds covalently to nearby RBC. Occasionally this process leads to full assembly of the terminal components of the complement cascade, causing intravascular hemolysis of these "innocent bystanders."

193. When does a food allergy occur?
True food allergy occurs when ingested food antigens bind to IgE on the surface of intestinal mast cells, causing an immediate hypersensitivity reaction. Basophils may also participate if food antigens appear in the circulation. Foods that commonly cause true food allergies include peanuts, true nuts, shellfish, eggs, milk proteins, and wheat. Cooking may destroy allergenic substances in some foods.

194. Summarize the symptoms of food allergy.
Symptoms of food allergy localized to the GI tract result in nausea, vomiting, diarrhea, bloating, and pain. Systemic symptoms may include urticaria, angioedema, headache, wheezing, hypotension, and other manifestations of anaphylaxis.

195. What can mimic a food allergy?
The diagnosis is complicated by a bewildering array of other factors that may cause adverse reactions to food and that mimic allergic reactions. Examples include allergic as well as pharmacologic reactions to food additives, preservatives, dyes, and toxins. GI disorders such as eosinophilic gastroenteritis, malabsorption syndromes, enzyme deficiencies, gluten-sensitive enteropathy, gallbladder disease, peptic ulcer disease, and scrombroid poisoning are among a long list of important, nonimmunologic causes of adverse food reactions. Finally, the psychological aspect of food intolerance may be important, particularly in patients who are convinced that allergy is the cause of their GI symptoms.

196. How is a food allergy generally diagnosed?
A careful history and physical examination should be performed to rule out other potential causes of adverse reactions to food. In an allergic reaction, symptoms should occur after each ingestion of the specific food. This and the resolution of symptoms with elimination of the food from the diet support a diagnosis of food allergy. The onset of symptoms may be delayed for up to 2 hours. The longer time until onset of symptoms with some GI reactions compared to the typical 15–20 minutes for most immediate hypersensitivity reactions may be due to the need to transport the antigen into the GI tract or other processes related to digestion and absorption. In practice, the patient's own experience is frequently the best guide. If the symptoms have been truly dramatic, the patient will tell you straight out, "Doctor, I think I'm allergic to peanuts." If the history is that of an acute GI or systemic allergic response, further tests for all practical purposes are not necessary.

197. Which test is the gold standard for diagnosis of food allergy?
The gold standard for diagnosing food allergens is a double-blind, placebo-controlled ingestion of the suspected food. To disguise the food's appearance, it is often desirable to put the food in gelatin capsules.

Bock SA: Double-blind, placebo-controlled food challenge (DBPCFC) as an office procedure: A manual. J Allergy Clin Immunol 82:986, 1988.

198. Discuss the role of skin testing for food allergy.
Skin testing by means of a prick/puncture test with extracts of the suspected foods is also useful but mainly when the result is negative. Like skin testing for inhaled allergens, skin testing for food has a high sensitivity. If the result is negative it is unlikely that a particular food, at least in the form that was used for testing, is the offending agent. By itself, a positive skin test is not diagnostic of food allergy unless the history independently suggests that this particular food has caused allergic symptoms. Skin testing can be used to narrow the choices of foods to be used for a double-blind, placebo-controlled trial of ingestion.

199. Discuss the role of RAST in the diagnosis of food allergy.
The RAST and other more quantitative in vitro tests may also be used, but they should be reserved for patients in whom skin testing cannot be properly performed and interpreted

and patients thought to be at particular risk of a severe anaphylactic reaction to skin testing.

200. Is a direct food challenge safe?

Food challenge should be performed only in an appropriate medical setting, since life-threatening anaphylaxis may occur. In some patients, such as those with a low probability of a positive reaction, an open challenge may be useful. If positive, then a double-blinded, placebo-controlled challenge can be used to confirm the diagnosis.

201. Define Chinese restaurant syndrome.

It is a reaction to glutamate ingested as MSG (monosodium glutamate), a flavoring agent commonly used in Chinese cooking. It occurs within 15–30 minutes of ingestion and consists of a sensation of warmth and tightness on the face and anterior chest. It is occasionally confused with angina pectoris but is benign and requires no therapy except avoidance of foods cooked with MSG.

Kwok RHN: Chinese restaurant syndrome. N Engl J Med 278:1122, 1968.

202. What is the treatment for food allergy?

The treatment for food allergy is avoidance. Treatment with antiallergic medications, such as antihistamines or oral cromolyn, cannot be expected to decrease the risk of life-threatening reactions. Anaphylaxis caused by food ingestion should be treated like any other anaphylactic reaction, except that NG tube placement and lavage may be useful to remove residual food antigen. Immunotherapy has no place in the treatment of food allergy.

203. Compare drug allergy, drug intolerance, and idiosyncratic drug reaction.

All three are types of adverse drug reactions. A true **drug allergy** is an immunologically mediated adverse reaction to a drug. It can occur with very small doses of the offending agent and accounts for only 54% of all adverse drug reactions. **Drug intolerance**, which also can occur with very small doses, is the result of an undesirable pharmacologic effect of the drug. An **idiosyncratic drug reaction** is based on the individual patient's biochemical alterations of a drug's metabolism.

204. What confounding factors may complicate the diagnosis of adverse drug reactions?

Be aware that the listed drug is only one of many ingredients in a pill or capsule. Patients may develop allergic reactions to the dyes used as colorants, excipients, and other agents that either stabilize the medication, slow its absorption, or make it resistant to stomach acids. The tip-off to this type of problem is the patient who confidently states that he or she is allergic to a long list of pharmacologically unrelated oral medications. Further investigation reveals that what they all have in common is the same colorant. One can test this hypothesis by giving the patient the intravenous form of the offending drug by mouth in a gelatin capsule. If the reaction is to the additives, there will be no reaction to the pure drug.

205. What are the indications for skin testing for penicillin allergy?

Skin testing for penicillin allergy is indicated in patients with (1) a possible or definite past history consistent with immediate hypersensitivity to penicillin, (2) in whom penicillin therapy is indicated, and (3) for whom effective alternative antibiotic therapy is not available.

206. How does penicillin hypersensitivity develop?

Penicillin sensitization occurs by haptenation of host serum proteins or cell proteins. It may involve a number of structural components (or "determinants") of the penicillin molecule.

The penicilloyl determinant is referred to as the major determinant, and other degradation products of penicillin G, including penicilloate, are referred to as minor determinants. This "major" and "minor" nomenclature refers only to the abundance of the breakdown product and does not necessarily indicate relative clinical importance. Indeed, some reports suggest that the minor determinants may be responsible for the majority of life-threatening anaphylactic reactions.

207. How do you test for penicillin hypersensitivity?
One can purchase the major determinant antigens for immediate hypersensitivity skin testing purposes as penicilloyl-polylysine. The minor determinants are not available except in a research setting. The next best option is to prepare dilutions of the particular formulation of penicillin that you need to use to treat the patient and proceed to use serial dilutions for skin testing, if the test with penicilloyl-polylysine is negative.

208. Which class of medications should be used with particular caution in patients prone to develop anaphylaxis?
Beta blockers should be avoided whenever possible, because they may accentuate the severity of anaphylaxis, prolong its cardiovascular and pulmonary manifestations, and greatly decrease the effectiveness of epinephrine in reversing the life-threatening manifestations of anaphylaxis. For similar reasons, this class of drugs should be avoided in patients with asthma who require treatment with selective beta agonists.

209. What is the mechanism of action of cyclosporine? What are its principal adverse effects?
Cyclosporine inhibits calcineurin-dependent signal transduction. It binds to cytoplasmic immunophilins, and this interaction inhibits the phosphatase activity of calcineurin. The result is a reduction of IL-2 production and T-cell activation.

210. List the principal side effects of cyclosporine.
- Nephrotoxicity (25–75% of patients)
- Hypertension
- Hirsutism
- Hepatotoxicity
- Gingival hyperplasia
- Seizures (5% of patients)
- Tremor (> 50% of patients)

211. What are the limitations of using monoclonal antibodies as therapeutic agents?
Monoclonal antibodies are almost always made in mice, and the mouse Ig is sufficiently different from human immunoglobulin that it triggers production of human antibodies in recipients. Although serum sickness is a possibility, as was seen after infusion of horse antitoxins in the past, this problem is vanishingly rare. The main limitation is the shortened half-life of the mouse monoclonal after it complexes with human antimouse antibodies in the recipient.

212. How can monoclonal antibodies be "humanized"?
Monoclonal antibodies can be "humanized" using genetic engineering techniques so that almost all of the molecule, with the exception of the antigen-binding site, becomes a human IgG. Whereas unmodified murine monoclonal antibodies may have a half-life of less than 2 days, humanized antibodies can circulate with a half-life of 20 days, which is close to that of human IgG. Monoclonal antibodies are now used to help control allergic reactions, transplant rejection, and autoimmune responses, and as an adjunct to cancer chemotherapy.

213. Give the serum half-lives and relative potencies of the common glucocorticoids.
See Table 12-14.

TABLE 12-14. RELATIVE POTENCIES AND EFFECTS OF COMMON GLUCOCORTICOIDS

Preparation	Potency Relative to Hydrocortisone	Relative Sodium-Retaining Potency	Approximately Equivalent Dose of Action (mg)	Duration of Action
Hydrocortisone	1	1	20	Short
Cortisone	0.8	0.8	25	Short
Prednisolone	4	0.8	5	Intermediate
Prednisone	4	0.8	5	Intermediate
6α-Methylprednisolone	5	0.5	4	Intermediate
Triamcinolone	5	0	4	Intermediate
Dexamethasone	25	0	0.75	Long
Betamethasone	25	0	0.75	Long

From Schleimer RP: Glucocorticosteroids. In Middleton E, et al (eds): Allergy: Principles and Practice, 3rd ed. St. Louis, Mosby, 1988, p 742.

214. What are the effects of corticosteroids on circulating leukocytes?
The short answer is that neutrophil numbers increase, partly due to accelerated release from the bone marrow and partly due to the decreased ability of neutrophils to migrate out of the circulation during corticosteroid treatment. The numbers of circulating lymphocytes, monocytes, and particularly eosinophils decreases. Overall, the total white count is increased. Table 12-15 offers a more detailed answer.

215. What are the target organs of the common autoantibodies that characterize organ-specific autoimmune diseases?

- Myasthenia gravis: acetylcholine receptors
- Graves' disease: thyroid-stimulating hormone receptor
- Thyroiditis: thyroid (often involves T cells as well)
- Insulin-resistant diabetes with acanthosis nigricans: insulin receptor
- Insulin-resistant diabetes with ataxia telangiectasia: insulin receptor
- Allergic rhinitis, asthma, and autoimmune abnormalities: $beta_2$-adrenergic receptors
- Juvenile insulin-dependent diabetes: pancreative islet cells, insulin
- Pernicious anemia: gastric parietal cells, vitamin B_{12}–binding site of intrinsic factor
- Addison's disease: adrenal cells
- Idiopathic hypoparathyroidism: parathyroid cells
- Spontaneous infertility: sperm
- Premature ovarian failure: interstitial cells, corpus luteum cells
- Pemphigus: intercellular substance of skin and mucosa
- Bullous pemphigoid: basement membrane zone of skin and mucosa
- Primary biliary cirrhosis: mitochondria
- Autoimmune hemolytic anemia: erythrocytes
- Idiopathic thrombocytopenic purpura: platelets
- Idiopathic neutropenia: neutrophils
- Vitiligo: melanocytes
- Chronic active hepatitis: nuclei of hepatocytes

TABLE 12-15. EFFECTS OF CORTICOSTEROIDS ON THE NUMBERS OF LEUKOCYTES IN THE BLOOD

Cell Type	Effect on Numbers	Effect on Function	Comment
Neutrophil	Increase	Minimal effect on chemotaxis, phagocytosis, bactericidal activity; transendothelial migration in response to chemotactic stimuli is almost abolished	Decrease in numbers sequestered in marginating pools, increased production and release from bone marrow, increased half-life incirculation
Lymphocytes	Decrease	Decreased proliferative response, inhibition of mediator production and release, altered helper and suppressor function	Greater effect on T cells than on B cells; priming for antibody formation to new antigens is unaffected
Lymphocytes			
T cells	Decrease a. Helper/inducer (CD4)—decrease b. Cytotoxic/ suppressor (CD8)—no change		
B cells	Minimal decrease or no change		
Monocytes	Decrease	Depressed chemotaxis, suppression of cytotoxic activity, decreased transendothelial migration	Possible sequestration
Eosinophils	Decrease	Inhibition of mediator production and release	Possible sequestration
Basophils	Decrease	Inhibition of degranulation	Possible sequestration
NK cells	No effect	No effect	
Null cells	No effect	Unknown	

216. What are the targets of the common autoantibodies that characterize systemic autoimmune diseases?

- Goodpasture's syndrome: basement membranes of lung and kidney
- RA: IgG, Epstein-Barr virus–related antigens, types II and III collagen
- Sjögren's syndrome: IgG, SS-A (Ro), SS-B (La)
- SLE: nuclei, double-stranded DNA, single-stranded DNA, Sm, ribonucleoprotein, lymphocytes, erythrocytes, neurons, IgG, phospholipids such as cardiolipin, and other antigens.
- Scleroderma/CREST: nuclei, Scl-70 (topoisomerase I), fibrillin SS-A (Ro), SS-B (La), centromere

- Polymyositis: nuclei, Jo-1, (histadyl-tRNA synthetase), PL-7, (threonyl-tRNA synthetase), PM-1, Mi-2
- Rheumatic fever: myocardium, heart valves, collagen of joints, renal glomerulus, caudate nucleus of brain

217. What is Guillain-Barré syndrome (GBS)?
GBS is the name reserved for the acute form of the acquired demyelinating neuropathies. In patients who do not spontaneously remit within 4–6 weeks and develop chronic weakness, the condition is called chronic inflammatory demyelinating polyradiculopathy. The causes of these conditions remain obscure and the principal therapy is supportive, particularly with regard to decreased respiratory function. But there is a growing consensus that these conditions are immunologically mediated.

218. Summarize the recommended treatment for GBS.
Management involves a carefully orchestrated mix of anti-inflammatory and immunomodulatory therapy. Agents that have been used include azathioprine, cyclosporine, and cyclophosphamide as well as plasmapheresis or high-dose IVIG. Dramatic but often unsustained remissions have been observed with these treatments, particularly if instituted within 7 days of the onset of symptoms, when the disease process is still classified as acute GBS.

219. How is plasmapheresis used for treatment of GBS?
Since plasmapheresis is an inefficient procedure for reducing circulating Ig levels, typically six to ten plasmapheresis procedures or more are performed at the rate of two or three per week. Each procedure consists of the exchange of total plasma volume (usually 2–3 L in an adult) with an albumin/saline/electrolyte solution. The frequency of procedures varies with the overall medical condition of the patient and the availability of venous access.

220. Explain the role of IVIG in the treatment of GBS.
Plasmapheresis can theoretically be followed by IV infusions of Ig to prevent rebound synthesis of autoantibodies, but this strategy would add significantly to the expense. At present it is not clear that the added cost would be worth it. However, a recent report suggests that IVIG treatment may be superior for the subset of patients who have IgG autoantibodies to GM1 gangliosides.

Kuwabara S, et al: Intravenous immunoglobulin therapy for Guillain-Barré syndrome with IgG anti-GM1 antibody. Muscle Nerve 24:54–58, 2001.

221. A patient has a history of hypotension following an intravenous pyelogram (IVP). What is the likely explanation?
Systemic reactions to the older hyperosmolar radiocontrast media occur in 1% of patients with a fatality rate of about 0.0009%. The reaction may begin just after the onset of the infusion or up to 30 minutes after its completion. Cardiovascular collapse can result in death. The cause is unknown. It does not appear to be a true IgE-mediated immediate hypersensitivity reaction. It has been suggested that these anaphylactoid reactions result from the ability of the dyes to initiate acute degranulation of mast cells and basophils by activating the alternative complement pathway. A method for detecting patients at risk is not available. Specifically, skin testing with IV contrast material or iodine is of no value.

222. The same patient now requires a radiocontrast study. What procedure should be followed?
The considerable risk of a repeat reaction on reexposure can be minimized by use of the newer lower osmolar radiocontrast agents and by appropriate prophylaxis. Management of patients

who require the radiocontrast procedure includes careful evaluation and documentation of the essential nature of the procedure. Informed consent should be obtained from the patient and the family (especially with regard to the small but definite risk of a fatal outcome). Necessary personnel and supplies for emergency treatment, adequate patient hydration, and preprocedure medical prophylaxis are also necessary.

223. Summarize the usual prophylactic regimen.

The usual prophylactic regimen consists of steroids (usually methylprednisolone, 32 mg orally at 13, 7 and 1 hour before the procedure) and H_1 antihistamines (diphenhydramine, 50 mg parenterally or orally 1 hour before radiocontrast media administration). When not contraindicated, ephedrine, 25 mg orally, may offer additional benefit. The usefulness of H_2 antihistamines and/or ephedrine is controversial. Reactions after prophylactic therapy are usually mild. However, it is important that the procedure be started at the scheduled time or the efficacy of the prophylaxis may be decreased. It has been suggested that in patients with a history of radiocontrast media reactions, nonionic radiocontrast media do not seem to offer significant protective advantage over medical prophylaxis, but since the consequences of an adverse reaction are life-threatening, it is wise to error on the side of caution and use both prophylaxis and the newer low osmolar reagents.

Patterson R, et al: Drug allergy and protocols for the management of drug allergies. N Engl Reg Allergy Proc 7:325–342, 1989.

224. What percentage of patients with SLE lack detectable antinuclear antibodies?

Five percent or fewer patients with SLE have been reported to test negative for ANA. However, these patients have probably been tested using mouse kidney as the test substrate. This substrate does not readily detect antibodies against Ro/SSA, ssDNA, Jo, or centromere that are sometimes found in SLE patients. The majority (93–95%) of lupus patients show detectable ANA antibodies if the substrate contains either WIL-2 or HEP-2 cells. Antibodies specific for double-stranded DNA or anti-Sm antibodies are diagnostic for SLE. Other substrates for detection of antinuclear antibodies offer less assurance of a diagnosis.

225. Which drugs may cause drug-induced lupus?

Hydralazine and procainamide exemplify agents that cause drug-induced lupus. Up to 50–75% of patients receiving procainamide and a high but somewhat lower frequency of those receiving hydralazine may develop a positive ANA. A much smaller number develop lupus-like symptoms. Hydralazine-induced lupus is most commonly encountered when the total daily dose administered exceeds 400 mg; 10–20% of patients receiving this dose range develop a lupus-like syndrome. Other drugs that cause a syndrome resembling SLE, albeit rarely, are isoniazid, chlorpromazine, methyldopa, quinidine, IFN-alpha, and drugs that sequester or inhibit TNF-alpha.

226. Describe the presentation of drug-induced lupus.

Drug-induced lupus manifests many of the same symptoms as idiopathic SLE, although they are generally milder. However, lupus nephritis and cerebritis rarely, if ever, complicate the syndrome. Drug-induced lupus is more frequent in women than men and in people with HLA DR4 phenotype. Symptoms resolve shortly after discontinuation of the drug, although laboratory abnormalities may persist for months or years. The ANA pattern in drug-induced lupus is usually homogeneous or speckled and is caused by anti-histone antibodies. Antibodies to double-stranded DNA, as seen in SLE, are not found in drug-induced lupus.

227. A patient with SLE asks whether she should be vaccinated against measles. What is your recommendation?

The major live attenuated vaccines currently available are rubella (measles), poliomyelitis, BCG (bacille Calmette-Guérin), mumps, and yellow fever. Vaccinia (small pox) is no longer given, and attenuated poliomyelitis vaccine is only used in special circumstances. Live vaccines should not be administered to immunologically compromised patients, particularly those with depressed cell-mediated immunity, including SLE. Conditions in which live vaccination of patients should be avoided are listed in Table 12-16. In addition, household contacts of immunocompromised patients should not receive oral live polio vaccine because the live attenuated strain may revert to the wild type in the GI tract and spread by the fecal-oral route.

TABLE 12-16. PATIENTS IN WHOM USE OF LIVE VACCINES SHOULD BE AVOIDED

- Patients with primary immunodeficiency disorders (especially those with defective cell-mediated immunity such as SCID)
- Patients given immunosuppressive therapy (e.g., corticosteroids, cytotoxic drugs, radiation therapy)
- Patients with malignancies that cause immunosuppression (e.g., leukemia, lymphoma, Hodgkin's disease)
- Patients with systemic immunoregulatory, inflammatory, or infectious diseases associated with defective cell-mediated immunity (e.g., SLE, diabetes mellitus, sarcoidosis, HIV-1 infections, atopic dermatitis)
- Children less than 1 year of age
- Patients with severe malnutrition or burns
- Pregnant women (because of potential harm to fetus)*

*The exception is yellow fever vaccine when the mother must travel to an endemic area. The risks of infection and detrimental effects without the vaccine are greater than the risks of receiving immunization.

228. What is erythema multiforme (EM)?

EM is an immunologic reaction of the skin and mucous membranes to a variety of antigenic stimuli. The specific antigen cannot be identified in up to 50% of cases. The lesions may be localized or widespread and consist of bullae, erythematous plaques, and epidermal cell necrosis. The lesions are usually bilaterally and symmetrically distributed on the extensor surfaces of the limbs, on the dorsal and volar aspects of the hands and feet, and on the trunk. The lesions, which resemble "targets" or "bull's eyes," are diagnostic. They appear as a central vesicle or dark purple papule, surrounded by a round, pale zone that is in turn surrounded by a round area of erythema.

229. List the precipitating factors in EM.

- Viral diseases: herpes simplex, hepatitis, influenza A, vaccinia, mumps
- Fungal diseases: dermatophytoses, histoplasmosis, coccidioidomycosis
- Bacterial diseases: hemolytic streptococcal infections, tuberculosis, leprosy, typhoid
- Collagen vascular disease: RA, SLE, dermatomyositis, allergic vasculitis, polyarteritis nodosa

- Malignant tumors: carcinoma, lymphoma after radiation therapy
- Hormonal changes: pregnancy, menstruation
- Drugs: penicillins, sulfonamides, barbiturates, salicylates, halogens, phenolphthalein
- Miscellaneous: rhus dermatitis, dental extractions, *M. pneumoniae* infection

230. What is the Stevens-Johnson syndrome?
Stevens-Johnson syndrome is a severe form of EM with fulminant, disseminated, multisystem involvement. Patients appear toxic, with fever, chills, malaise, tachycardia, tachypnea, and prostration. Diffuse vesicular, bullous, and ulcerative lesions of the skin and mucous membranes develop and desquamate, leading to secondary infections, which in turn may lead to sepsis and even death. It is associated with all causes of EM.

231. Hepatitis B surface antigenemia is associated with which of the vasculitides?
Polyarteritis nodosa, which is seen in 40% of HBSAg-positive patients. The severity of the vasculitis and hepatitis is not correlated.

232. An 18-year-old male presents with abdominal pain, bloody diarrhea, peripheral neuropathy, and demonstration of IgA deposits on biopsy of the GI tract. What is the most likely diagnosis?
The clinical presentation is characteristic of Henoch-Schönlein purpura, although the age of onset is typically younger. The disease is almost always limited to males. This type of hypersensitivity vasculitis principally involves the skin, joints, intestine, and kidney. The disease is usually self-limited, although chronic renal failure may rarely occur. A history of recent infection, usually of the upper respiratory tract, is often reported. Circulating IgA immune complexes are common. Serum IgA levels may be elevated and IgA deposition can be demonstrated in the affected tissues.

233. How do anticentromere antibodies help differentiate between the CREST syndrome and scleroderma (progressive systemic sclerosis)?
The anticentromere antibody, which is found by ANA testing, is found in 60–80% of CREST patients but is often undetectable in patients with diffuse scleroderma.

234. Which other laboratory and clinical findings distinguish the CREST syndrome from diffuse scleroderma?
In CREST syndrome, skin involvement is principally limited to the extremities, and internal organ involvement generally develops more slowly and is less severe than in diffuse scleroderma. Particularly noteworthy of the CREST syndrome (but very rarely seen in diffuse scleroderma) is the development of pulmonary arterial hypertension in the absence of pulmonary fibrosis. This occurs in somewhat less than 10% of patients with limited systemic sclerosis or CREST. Intimal proliferation of the small and medium-sized pulmonary arteries is prominent. Pulmonary hypertension may be progressive and is almost uniformly fatal. Biliary cirrhosis also may occur in the CREST syndrome but is uncommon in systemic sclerosis.

235. In a patient who complains of fatigue with hair-combing and stair-climbing, what are the most likely diagnoses?
Diseases characterized by proximal muscle weakness, such as myasthenia gravis, Eaton-Lambert syndrome (myasthenic syndrome), polymyositis, dermatomyositis, and polymyalgia rheumatica.

236. Explain the importance of HLA typing in solid organ and bone marrow transplantation (BMT).
HLA compatibility of donor and recipient affects graft outcome in both solid organ transplantation (such as kidney, heart, lung, and liver) and BMT. For solid organs, matching for the HLA-D

or MHC type II antigens is more important than matching at HLA-A or HLA-B, the MHC type I antigens, because MHC class II molecules are involved in activating CD4 helper T cells that are needed for both humoral and cell-mediated effector functions that attack the graft. HLA incompatibility may lead to graft rejection of solid organ transplantation and to GVHD in BMT.

237. **Is HLA compatibility a major graft survival factor in corneal transplants?**
HLA compatibility is not a major graft survival factor for first-time, nonvascularized corneal transplants.

238. **Explain how the mechanism of graft rejection differs from the mechanism of GVHD in BMT.**
In graft rejection, the graft is attacked by the recipient's immune system. In contrast, in BMT with GVHD, the immunocompetent cells from the donor attack the recipient, whose own immune system has been ablated prior to the transplant.

239. **Explain the importance of ABO typing in solid organ transplantation and BMT.**
ABO blood typing is critical in solid organ transplants because ABO antigens are expressed on all tissue cells of the transplanted organ, and because type O, type A, or type B recipients almost always have preformed antibodies to these blood group antigens. Thus, transplantation of solid organ grafts at a minimum requires compatibility at ABO. However, ABO compatibility, oddly enough, is not a requirement for bone marrow grafting because the donor graft will thereafter supply all blood cells.

240. **List the four types of graft rejection and their immunologic mechanisms.**
See Table 12-17.

TABLE 12-17. TYPES OF SOLID ORGAN GRAFT REJECTION

Type	Onset	Major Effector Mechanisms
Hyperacute	Minutes to hours	Humoral: preformed cytotoxic antibody in the recipient against donor graft antigen(s) a. ABO system b. Anti-HLA class I
Accelerated	2–5 days	Cell-mediated: due to prior T-cell sensitization against donor antigen(s)
Acute	7–28 days	Principally cell-mediated immunity: allogeneic reactivity by recipient T cells against donor antigen(s) Humoral immunity to HLA antigens
Chronic	> 3 months	Principally cell-mediated immunity allogeneic reactivity by recipient T cells against donor antigen(s) Humoral immunity to HLA antigens

BIBLIOGRAPHY

1. Abbas AK, Lichtman AH: Cellular and Molecular Immunology, 5th ed. Philadelphia, W.B. Saunders, 2003.
2. Adkinson NF, Yunginger A, Busse W, et al (eds): Middleton's Allergy: Principles and Practice, 6th ed. St. Louis, Mosby, 2004.
3. Janeway CA, Travers P, Walport M, Shlomchik MJ: Immunobiology: The Immune System in Health and Disease, 6th ed. New York, Garland, 2004.
4. Klein J: Immunology, 2nd ed. Oxford, Blackwell Scientific Publications, 1997.
5. Paul WE (ed): Fundamental Immunology, 5th ed. Philadelphia, Lippincott Williams & Wilkins, 2003.
6. Rich RR, Fleisher TA, Shearer WT, et al: Clinical Immunology, Principles and Practice, 2nd ed. St. Louis, Mosby, 2001.

AIDS AND HIV INFECTION

Christopher J. Lahart, M.D.

CHAPTER 13

1. **How is HIV transmitted?**
   Sexual intercourse, both vaginal and anal, whether hetero-or homosexual, is the leading cause of HIV transmission. Other common means include percutaneous transmission as during injection drug use or as a result of occupational needle sticks, perinatal maternal-fetal transmission, and transmission via breast-feeding by an infected mother to her infant.

2. **List the symptoms of acute HIV infection along with their incidence.**

Fever (95%)	Headache (30%)
Fatigue (80%)	Nausea, vomiting, diarrhea (30%)
Lymphadenopathy (75%)	Weight loss (15%)
Pharyngitis (70%)	Thrush (15%)
Rash (70%)	Central/peripheripheral neurologic symptoms (10%)
Myalgias/arthralgias (55%)	

   Central/peripheral neurologic symptoms include aseptic meningitis, encephalitis, facial palsy, peripheral neuropathy, and Guillain-Barré syndrome.

   Department of Health and Human Services Guidelines. Ann Intern Med 137:381, 2002.

3. **How soon after acute HIV infection do symptoms develop? How long do the symptoms persist?**
   Symptoms develop 1–8 weeks after the initial infection. It is believed that symptoms are due to the development of specific immune responses to HIV. Patients presenting with these symptoms should have a specific risk history taken for possible recent exposure to HIV. The symptoms that develop are transient and generally are present for 1–3 weeks; however, cases have been reported with symptoms lasting up to 8 weeks.

4. **Do all persons newly infected by HIV exhibit symptoms? How many present for care?**
   It is estimated that fewer than 80% of newly infected people have any of these symptoms. The majority of them, however, do seek medical care. Unfortunately, only one quarter are correctly diagnosed with acute HIV infection. This represents a tragic lost opportunity not only to diagnose HIV infection at a very early stage but also to interrupt HIV transmission through early diagnosis and counseling. Undiagnosed or misdiagnosed people remain unaware of their infection and do not receive directed counseling to halt further HIV transmission.

5. **How can acute HIV infection be diagnosed?**
   HIV infection is typically diagnosed through the detection of HIV-specific antibodies. During acute infection these antibodies are not yet formed, and HIV antibody tests are negative. This demonstrates the absence of previously established HIV infection and is part of showing that the syndrome is acute in nature. Tests based on detection of HIV itself are positive. Blood donations are screened for acute infection with a test detecting the p24 antigen. This test also can be used clinically for making a diagnosis. HIV can also be detected by the tests for HIV RNA commonly used to assess the efficacy of HIV treatment. During acute infection, levels of HIV RNA are extremely elevated.

6. Should anti-HIV therapy be initiated when acute HIV infection is diagnosed?
If acute HIV infection is diagnosed, the patient should be referred to an HIV specialist. The best approach to acute HIV infection is not known. Although HIV infection cannot be eradicated by treatment at any stage of infection, early treatment during acute infection may assist in promoting and preserving HIV-specific immune function. This approach may beneficially alter the natural history of the infection. Additional consideration must be given to the source of the recently transmitted virus. Virus resistant to medication can be transmitted. For this reason, viral resistance testing should be performed in patients with acute infection while empirical therapy is begun.

7. Who should be tested for established HIV infection?
- Men who have had sex with other men
- Injecting drug users
- Anyone who has had sex for money or drugs
- Anyone diagnosed with another STD (including hepatitis B)
- Persons who received blood products prior to screening (before 1986)
- Anyone who has had sex with any of the above
- Patients with tuberculosis
- Pregnant women
- Anyone who requests it

8. Who else should be considered for testing?
A clinician should recommend HIV testing for any patient with a high index of suspicion for infection. Additionally, consider those who may have been unable to consent to sexual activity such as people in abusive relationships, those with psychiatric disability or a history of substance abuse (including alcohol), and those who have been or are incarcerated. The CDC recommends HIV testing for any man aged 15–54 admitted to the hospital if the hospital has an AIDS diagnosis rate > 1 per 1000 discharges or if it has an HIV prevalence rate > 1%.

9. Is HIV treatment effective in preventing perinatal HIV transmission?
Absolutely! Testing for HIV infection during pregnancy is recommended so that early treatment can be initiated. In the absence of treatment, perinatal transmission rates are 20–33%. With combination therapy, transmission rates have been lowered to less than 2%. In general, therapy recommendations are the same during pregnancy as in the nonpregnant patient. The major exception is the avoidance of efavirenz in the first trimester due to possible fetal toxicity with neural tube defects.

10. List a differential diagnosis for acute HIV infection.
- Epstein-Barr virus
- Cytomegalovirus
- Influenza
- Hepatitis
- Syphilis
- Rubella
- Toxoplasmosis

11. List common causes of false-positive HIV ELISA tests.
- Autoimmune diseases
- Other recent viral infections
- Recent viral vaccination, including influenza
- Hepatic disease
- Renal failure
- Lymphoma and other hematologic malignancies
- Positive rapid plasma reagin (RPR)

12. What is the risk of HIV transmission via needlestick?

The average risk of transmission in a large group of health care workers suffering percutaneous exposure to HIV is approximately 0.3%. However, each exposure needs to be evaluated individually. There is tremendous variation in the degree of exposure, which affects the likelihood of infection.

Tokars JI, et al: Surveillance of HIV infection and zidovudine use among health-care workers after occupational exposure to HIV-infected blood. Ann Intern Med 118:913–919, 1993.

13. What variables increase the risk of occupational exposure?

Exposure to a large volume of infectious material (or material with a high viral load), a deep injury, visible blood on the device causing the injury, prolonged contact with the infectious material, and the body area exposed (portal of entry) are important factors. Mucosal splashes and exposure on intact skin are not routes of transmission (no transmission in > 12,500 exposures followed prospectively). Associated with increased risk are intramuscular injection, exposures via hollow needles (as opposed to suture needles and pins), and exposure to material from a viremic HIV-infected patient.

14. Does postexposure antiretroviral therapy prevent occupational infection?

No controlled trial has been performed and, most likely, none ever will be. However, a retrospective case-control study involving 31 exposed and infected health care workers and 679 exposed, uninfected workers found that postexposure zidovudine reduced the risk of HIV infection by 79%. The study design is not the proper one for evaluating drug efficacy, but it does provide important information. Drug therapy must be part of a program that includes immediate availability of counseling as well as medication. Close follow-up should be provided and confidentiality guaranteed. Therapy recommendations include combination antiretroviral therapy based on the treatment status of the source patient. Consideration must be given to possible drug resistance.

Centers for Disease Control and Prevention: Case-control study of HIV seroconversion in health-care workers after percutaneous exposure to HIV-infected blood—France, United Kingdom, and United States, January 1988–August 1994. MMWR 44(50):929–933, 1995.

15. When should a health care worker be evaluated after a possible exposure? If needed, when should medication be started, and for how long should it be taken?

Once the immediate medical care situation is stable, the worker should seek attention immediately. The evaluation should take place as soon as possible and, if indicated, medication should be initiated as soon as possible. There may be benefit to medication begun 24–36 hours after exposure, but this is uncertain. The recommended course of therapy is 4 weeks.

CDC. Updated US Public Health Service Guidelines for the Management of Occupational Exposures to HBV, HCV, and HIV and Recommendations for Postexposure Prophylaxis. MMWR 50(No. RR-11):1–67, 2001.

16. Describe the difference between HIV infection and AIDS.

A diagnosis of HIV infection means only that antibodies to HIV have been detected and that HIV infection is established. A diagnosis of AIDS is made when a person with HIV infection is also diagnosed with a specific condition designated as an AIDS indicator. These conditions are associated with marked immunosuppression or are seen with markedly increased frequency in persons with HIV. Examples include opportunistic infections, malignancies, other symptomatic disease, or a $CD4^{+}$ lymphocyte count of less than 200. HIV infection can be thought of as a spectrum of illness with AIDS occupying the far advanced segment of the spectrum.

Centers for Disease Control and Prevention: 1993 revised classification system for HIV infection and expanded case surveillance definition for AIDS among adolescents and adults. MMWR 41(RR-17):1–19, 1992.

17. What are the AIDS indicator diseases?

See Table 13-1.

TABLE 13-1. AIDS INDICATOR DISEASES
Candidiasis of lungs, bronchi, trachea
Candidiasis of esophagus
Coccidioidomycosis, disseminated or extrapulmonary
Cryptococcus, extrapulmonary
Cryptospoidiosis, chronic intestinal
Cytomegalovirus, other than liver, spleen, nodes
Cytomegalovirus retinitis
Herpes simplex, chronic ulcers of bronchi, lungs, or esophagus
Histoplasmosis, disseminated or extrapulmonary
HIV encephalopathy
HIV wasting
Isosporiasis, chronic intestinal
Kaposi's sarcoma
Lymphoid interstitial pneumonia
Lymphoma, non-Hodgkin's
Lymphoma, primary central nervous system
Mycobacterium avium complex, disseminated or extrapulmonary
Mycobacterium kansasii, disseminated or extrapulmonary
Mycobacterium tuberculosis, any site
Pneumocystis carinii pneumonia
Pneumonia, recurrent bacterial
Progressive multifocal leukoencephalopathy
Salmonella bacteremia, recurrent
Strongyloides, non-gastrointestinal
Toxoplasmosis of central nervous system

18. **What is a T-cell count? What is its use?**
A T-cell count (CD4 count or $CD4^+$ lymphocyte count) is a laboratory measurement of the $CD4^+$ lymphocytes, or the helper-inducer cells in the peripheral blood. HIV targets these cells, and their progressive death accounts for the immunosuppression of HIV infection. By measuring these cells, a clinician can place a patient along the spectrum of HIV infection. A normal count is 800–1000. An AIDS diagnosis is made when the count is < 200. Since various opportunistic infections occur at or below certain counts, a count can be used to identify patients at high risk and initiate prophylaxis against specific infections. Thus, the CD4 count is of prognostic and therapeutic value.

19. **How much time elapses between infection with HIV and the diagnosis of AIDS?**
This period is not easily defined. Studies of large patient cohorts indicate that in the absence of treatment 50% of HIV-positive patients progress to AIDS in approximately 10 years. The rate of disease progression is not stable over this period, because few develop disease early after exposure and proportionally more develop AIDS with each passing year (Fig. 13-1). Several studies indicate that the average loss of $CD4^+$ lymphocytes is 80 cells per year. It is not certain at this time that 100% of HIV-infected individuals will develop AIDS, even without specific antiretroviral therapy.

Litson AR, et al: The natural history of human immunodeficiency virus infection. J Infect Dis 158:1360–1367, 1988.

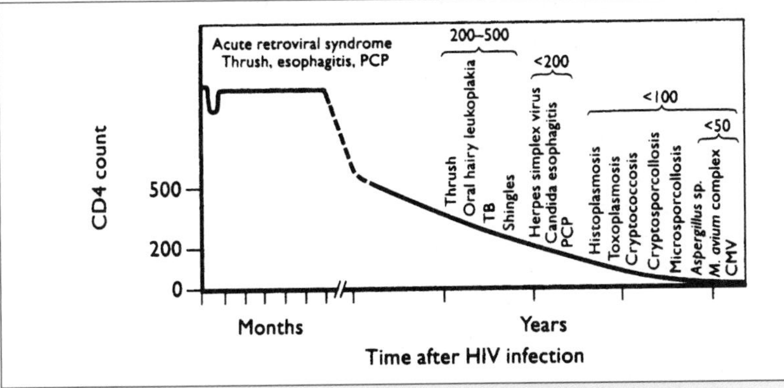

Figure 13-1. Onset of opportunistic infections with CD4+ count. (From Mildran D [ed]: Atlas of Infectious Diseases. I: AIDS. Philadelphia, Current Medicine, 1995, p 15.2, with permission.)

KEY POINTS: HIV INFECTION 

1. HIV infection is a lifelong condition. It is not curable. It is treatable.
2. A person with HIV infection should always be considered infectious.
3. Adherence to lifestyle changes (e.g., safer sex, no needle sharing) should be complete and lifelong.
4. HIV infection does not automatically carry a poor prognosis. Delayed diagnosis and poor adherence confer a poor prognosis upon HIV infection.
5. If you're thinking mononucleosis, think HIV.
6. Test for both HIV antibodies and HIV p24 antigen or HIV RNA.
7. Perform HIV resistance testing and initiate treatment.

20. What is a "viral load" test?

A viral load test measures the amount of HIV messenger RNA in the plasma as an indicator of viral replication. This test has been shown to be the single best prognostic indicator in HIV infection, with a higher level of mRNA indicative of a worse prognosis. The test is routinely performed as part of the initial assessment of newly diagnosed HIV infection. The viral load is also used to assess the efficacy of anti-HIV therapy. Once therapy has been initiated, the viral load should decrease rapidly. There should be at least a 1.0-log decrease in the viral load within 8 weeks of start of therapy. Within 24 weeks, the viral load should be below the limits of detection.

21. What is the meaning of an "undetectable" viral load?

Assays approved to measure HIV mRNA are approved with a certain range of accuracy. Results of testing are reported within this range. The lower limits of the approved ranges are currently between 50 and 500 copies of mRNA per milliliter, depending on the exact test performed. If a specimen has an amount of mRNA below this lower limit, it is said to be "undetectable" or, more accurately, "below the limits of detection." This is the goal of anti-HIV therapy: to lower the level of viral replication to below that detectable by any current assay.

22. Does "undetectable" mean "cured" or "not infectious"?
Neither, and never. An undetectable viral load means only that the current medical regimen has effectively halted viral replication at any level that can be detected by the assay being used. HIV infection is still present, and HIV infection is still transmissible. Evidence indicats that an undetectable viral load is associated with a decreased likelihood of transmission. This appears to be true for sexual transmission, transmission via needlesticks, and perinatal transmission.

23. What stages of the HIV life cycle are targets of currently available therapy?
- Fusion of viral and cell membrane
- Reverse transcription
- Protease activity

Current therapy can attack these steps in the HIV life cycle. The most common site of therapeutic attack is at reverse transcription with both nucleoside analog and nonnucleoside analog reverse transcriptase inhibitors. Protease inhibitors (PIs) also have a long clinical track record. Finally, fusion inhibitors are a recent addition to the list of therapeutic options.

24. Describe the mechanism of action of the reverse transcriptase inhibitors (RTIs).
The RTIs act during the initial infection of a new host cell. They inhibit viral reverse transcriptase during the transcription of viral RNA to host complementary DNA. The RTIs are nucleoside analogs (NRTIs) or nonnucleoside analogs (NNRTIs). The analogs become phosphorylated to a triphosphate form and competitively interfere with native nucleosides during transcription, causing viral DNA chain termination. The NNRTIs bind to reverse transcriptase, altering the active site and inactivating the enzyme.

25. How do PIs work?
In host cells with established infection, after the synthesis of mRNA and then HIV pro-proteins and polyproteins, HIV protease must cleave the polyproteins to result in the production of functional proteins. PIs act at this stage, preventing cleavage. Viral particles can still be formed and bud from the host cell, but they are nonfunctional and noninfective.

26. When should therapy against HIV be started?
This question has been debated since the first anti-HIV medication became available. In patients with advanced disease (AIDS diagnosis or $CD4^+$ count < $200/mm^3$), antiretroviral therapy has been shown to prolong life. The study of patients in less advanced stages has been complicated by the slowly progressive nature of the disease and the need for almost complete adherence to complicated medical regimens. Clinically significant benefit in patients with $CD4^+$ counts > $500/mm^3$ has been difficult to demonstrate. Newer findings of cumulative toxicities as well as evidence for immune reconstitution from even advanced disease have moved treatment guidelines into later stages of infection

TABLE 13-2. GUIDELINES FOR INITIATION OF ANTIRETROVIRAL TREATMENT

Clinical Stage	CD4 Count	Plasma Viral Load	Recommendation
Symptomatic disease, AIDS	Any value	Any value	Treat
Asymptomatic (AIDS diagnosis by CD4 count)	< 200	Any value	Treat
Asymptomatic	> 200 but < 300	Any value	Offer treatment
Asymptomatic	> 350	> 55,000	Consider treatment
Asymptomatic	> 350	< 55,000	Defer treatment

From U.S. Department of Health and Human Services Guidelines at www.AIDSinfo.nih.gov (March 23, 2000).

(Table 13-2). Several cohort studies have demonstrated poorer outcomes if treatment initiation is delayed until after the CD4 count is under 200.

27. What medications are available for use against HIV?
See Table 13-3.

TABLE 13-3. DRUGS FOR TREATMENT OF HIV INFECTION

Generic Name	Brand Name	Also Known As	FDA Approval
NRTIs (nucleoside analog reverse transcriptase inhibitors)			
Zidovudine	Retrovir	ZDV, AZT	1987
Didanosine	Videx	ddl	1991
zalcitabine	Hivid	ddC	1992
Stavudine	Zerit	d4T	1994
Lamivudine	Epivir	3TC	1995
Abacavir	Ziagen	ABC	1998
Tenofovir	Viread	TDF	2002
Emtricitabine	Emtriva	FTC	2003
	Combivir	CBV	Fixed dose ZDV/3TC
	Trizivir	TZV	Fixed dose ZDV/3TC/ABC
NNRTIs (nonnucleoside reverse transcriptase inhibitors)			
Nevirapine	Viramune	NVP	1996
Delavirdine	Rescriptor	DLV	1997
Efavirenz	Sustiva	EFV	1998
PIs (protease inhibitors)			
Saquinavir	Invirase	SQV-HGC	1995
Ritonavir	Norvir	RTV	1996
Indinavir	Crixivan	IDV	1996
Nelfinavir	Viracept	NLV	1997
Saquinavir	Fortovase	SQV-SGC	1997
Amprenavir	Agenerase	APV	1999
Lopinavir	Kaletra	LPV/r	2000
Atazanavir	Reyataz	ATV	2003
Fosamprenavir	Lexiva	FPV	2003
Fusion inhibitors			
Enfuvirtide	Fuzeon	T-20	2002

28. What is HAART?
HAART is an acronym for highly active antiretroviral therapy. The term grew out of the development of the use of a combination of at least three medications that could suppress HIV viral replication below the level of detection on the viral load test.

29. How are the guidelines for therapy against HIV infection developed?
Treatment guidelines for HIV infection change frequently and are developed by a panel established by the U.S. Department of Health and Human Services. This panel has typically updated the guidelines two to three times per year over the past several years. Since the adoption of HAART, therapy has traditionally been a combination of two nucleoside RTIs plus either a third nucleoside, a nonnucleoside RTI, or a PI.

Some recent studies have caused a downgrading of the three nucleoside RTI approach.

30. What are the most recent guidelines?
The most recent guidelines (March 2004) list the different regimens as either "preferred" or "alternative." The current preferred regimens are either NNRTI-based with efavirenz plus a dual NRTI backbone or PI-based with lopinavir/ritonavir with a dual NRTI backbone. In both cases, one of the NRTIs is suggested to be lamivudine. Triple nucleoside therapy is now listed as an alternative approach.

31. How do you assess the efficacy of anti-HIV therapy?
The goal of therapy against HIV is to inhibit HIV replication. The way to assess this goal is to perform a viral load test, an assay for HIV mRNA. A baseline viral load level should be obtained before initiating anti-HIV therapy. Within 6–8 weeks, a repeat viral load should be performed. This level should be at least 1.0 log less (down by 90%) than the baseline level. Within 24 weeks, the viral load level should be below the limit of detection of a test limit at 400 copies, and at 48 weeks the viral load should be below 50 copies.

32. List the predictors of long-term virologic success in HIV therapy.
- Low baseline viral load
- High baseline CD4 count
- Rapid reduction of viral load to undetectable levels
- Adherence to prescribed therapy

33. What level of adherence to therapy is necessary to sustain virologic success?
In general, the level of adherence required for successful therapy in HIV infection surpasses that required for almost any other condition (Table 13-4).

TABLE 13-4. LEVEL OF ADHERENCE IN RELATION TO SUCCESS OF THERAPY

Level of Adherence (%)	% Patients with Undetectable Viral Load at 48 wk
95–100	84
90–95	64
80–90	47
70–80	24
<70	12

KEY POINTS: HIV THERAPY

1. HIV therapy is complicated and potentially toxic.
2. The adherence necessary to secure durable viral control (95+%) is beyond many people's abilities.
3. Poor adherence creates and promotes viral resistance to anti-HIV medications.
4. The optimal time to initiate HIV therapy remains unknown.

34. How would you define treatment failure in anti-HIV therapy?
Treatment failure can be viewed from several perspectives: as virologic failure, immunologic failure, or clinical failure. **Virologic failure** is shown by an incomplete viral response with the viral load never becoming undetectable or by a viral rebound when a previously undetectable viral load again becomes detectable. Although CD4 count responses to therapy vary widely and are related to the nadir CD4 count, the mean CD4 count increase after a year of effective therapy is 150 cells. **Immunologic failure** can be termed the failure to increase the CD4 count by greater than 50 cells during the first year of treatment. **Clinical failure** is the development of HIV-related clinical events after at least 3 months of therapy.

35. Can HIV be resistant to medications?
Yes. The most common cause of virologic failure is the development of viral resistance to the medications being taken by the patient. This resistance may result from the selection of a preexisting resistant virus, as after transmission of a resistant virus to a new host, or as a result of inadequate therapy.

36. How can you test for HIV resistance?
Two types of resistance assays are available: genotypic resistance tests and phenotypic resistance tests. **Genotypic tests** are more readily available at this time. They involve sequencing HIV viral genes (i.e., reverse transcriptase, protease) and identifying mutations associated with drug resistance. **Phenotypic tests** assess the virus's ability to replicate in the presence of different concentrations of antiretroviral medications.

37. What vaccines are recommended in HIV-infected patients?
- Hepatitis A, one complete series
- Hepatitis B, one complete series
- Pneumococcal, every 5 years
- Influenza, annually
- Tetanus, every 10 years

38. What vaccines should be avoided in persons with HIV infection?
Live virus vaccines should not be administered to persons with HIV infection due to the risk for disseminated disease. MMR and varicella-zoster vaccinations should not be given. If bioterrorism concerns are heightened, smallpox vaccine should also be avoided.

39. How well do HIV-infected patients respond to the influenza vaccine?
Administration of the influenza vaccine has been recommended for all persons infected with HIV, although the antibody response to the vaccine is lower than in non–HIV-infected control subjects. A two-dose regimen is not superior in efficacy to the traditional single-dose regimen. $CD4^+$ counts < 100 are associated with poor antibody responses. Studies showing increased HIV viral load and decreased $CD4^+$ counts in study participants receiving influenza vaccine compared with placebo-injected controls have raised concerns, but no adverse clinical events have been demonstrated.

Tasker SA, et al: Effects of influenza vaccination in HIV-infected adults: A double-blind placebo-controlled trial. Vaccine 16:1039–1042, 1998.

40. Do HIV-infected patients respond to the pneumococcal polysaccharide vaccine?
The response is impaired compared with normal control subjects. HIV-infected patients mount an adequate antibody response to fewer of the serotypes contained in the 23-valent vaccine, and this response rate decreases with decreasing $CD4^+$ counts. As with influenza vaccination, there appears to be increased HIV viral activity after pneumococcal vaccination, but because morbidity due to pneumococcal disease is clearly and substantially increased in HIV-infected patients, the risk/benefit ratio supports vaccination.

Moore D, et al: Pneumococcal vaccination and HIV infection. Int J STD AIDS 9:1–7, 1999.

41. What is thrush?

Thrush is oropharyngeal pseudomembranous candidiasis, which often presages AIDS. It usually presents as white plaques (pseudomembranes), either scattered small plaques or large sheets, on any oral mucosal surface. Candidiasis also may present in an atrophic or erythematous appearance without plaques. Significant oral pain may be present along with altered taste. The diagnosis can be made clinically, with KOH smear, or by culture. A clinician should not confuse thrush with oral hairy leukoplakia, a whitish corrugated growth along the margins of the tongue.

42. Explain the significance of thrush.

Thrush often indicates significant immune suppression, and if it is found during an initial exam, evaluation should begin for other HIV-related medical interventions, such as PCP prophylaxis. Thrush seen in a person without previously diagnosed HIV infection absolutely deserves an evaluation for the presence of HIV infection.

43. Define HIV wasting syndrome.

This AIDS-defining diagnosis includes profound weight loss of > 10% of body weight, with either chronic diarrhea or weakness and fever for > 30 days. These clinical events should be evaluated for other HIV-related illnesses; in the absence of other causes, a diagnosis of wasting can be made.

44. How often does HIV infection result in anemia or thrombocytopenia?

Patients with AIDS are frequently pancytopenic. Anemia occurs in up to 80%, neutropenia in 85%, and thrombocytopenia in 65% of cases. HIV-infected but asymptomatic patients are much less frequently cytopenic. Clinically significant thrombocytopenia indistinguishable from that seen in idiopathic thrombocytopenic purpura (ITP) may be a presentation of HIV infection. Typically, bone marrow is normal with adequate numbers of megakaryocytes. The disorder behaves much like classic ITP in that patients respond to steroids and splenectomy. An HIV antibody test is recommended in patients presenting with ITP. Of interest is the recent recognition of thrombotic thrombocytopenic purpura in association with HIV infection.

45. Does thrombocytopenia improve with zidovudine therapy?

Thrombocytopenic patients have improved on zidovudine therapy, although AZT may cause anemia.

46. What rheumatic syndromes may occur in HIV-positive patients?

- Arthralgia
- Painful articular syndrome
- Psoriasis and psoriatic arthritis
- Spondyloarthropathy
- Septic arthritis
- Reactive arthritis (Reiter's)
- Avascular necrosis

47. How common is arthralgia in HIV-positive patients?

Arthralgia has been described in up to 35% of patients followed prospectively. Joint involvement is oligoarticular in 55%, monoarticular in 11%, and polyarticular in 34%. Knees, shoulders, and elbows are most commonly affected.

48. What are the major characteristics of painful articular syndrome and septic arthritis in HIV-positive patients?

Painful articular syndrome is of short duration and often requires narcotics or hospitalization for relief. Septic arthritis is similar in prevalence, presentation, and causation to HIV-negative patients.

49. What related abnormalities may be found in laboratory tests?

In addition to clinical syndromes, lab evaluations often reveal low titers of rheumatoid factors, antinuclear antibodies, and anticardiolipin antibodies. Generalized hypergammaglobulinemia is also seen, as are elevated CK levels of uncertain significance.

Mody GM, Parke FA, Reveille JD: Articular manifestations of human immunodeficiency virus infection. Best Prac Research Clin Rheum 17:580–591, 2003.

50. What is AIDS dementia complex?

Patients with AIDS may develop cognitive, behavioral, and motor dysfunction in the course of their illness. Although multiple opportunistic infections need to be ruled out (e.g., cryptococcosis, toxoplasmosis, tuberculosis), direct CNS infection by HIV seems to cause this complex of signs and symptoms. Early in its course, neuropsychologic testing may be needed to support a clinical suspicion of dementia, but the dementia can progress to a vegetative state. Patients may first complain of concentration difficulties, and family and friends may note personality changes. Thorough neurologic evaluation and investigation into other causes are needed. The exact cause of this dementia is not known.

51. What is PCP?

PCP stands for *P. carinii* pneumonia. Before routine prophylactic treatments, PCP was the presenting diagnosis in over 60% of patients with AIDS and eventually was seen in 80% of patients with AIDS at some time during their illness. With more proactive HIV testing and the initiation of effective primary PCP prophylaxis, the incidence of PCP should approach zero. Unfortunately, not enough patients receive early HIV testing, and a number progress asymptomatically to a point of immunosuppression at risk for PCP.

52. When is an HIV patient at risk for PCP?

Although some patients may present with PCP earlier in their progressive immunosuppression, PCP becomes a clinical concern in all HIV patients with a CD4 count of 200 or less, those with thrush, and those with constitutional symptoms such as weight loss or unexplained fever for 2 weeks. In addition, all patients with a history of prior PCP are at high risk for a second episode. In the absence of secondary prophylaxis and effective HIV therapy, the recurrence rate is 40% within 6 months.

53. Describe the typical symptoms of PCP.

Cough, fever, and dyspnea on exertion are the most common presenting symptoms. The cough is usually nonproductive or productive of only scant, whitish sputum. Patients also may relate a sensation of chest tightness or an inability to take a full, deep inspiration. Other less common complaints include nonspecific weight loss, night sweats, and malaise. Findings on physical examination include fever, tachypnea, persistent cough, and dry rales. Rarely, a patient may endure symptoms long enough to present with cyanosis. Oxygen saturation is decreased and further desaturates with exertion.

Moe AA, Hardy WD: *Pneumocystis carinii* infection in the HIV-seropositive patient. Infect Dis Clin North Am 8:331–364, 1994.

54. What laboratory findings are associated with PCP?

Laboratory findings include hypoxemia with an elevated A–aO_2 gradient. Elevated serum lactate dehydrogenase levels are seen.

55. How is PCP diagnosed?

By pathologic demonstration of the organism in lung specimens. Several centers have reported success with examination of induced sputum, but most centers rely on bronchoscopy with bronchoalveolar lavage (BAL). Lavage alone has a sensitivity of > 95%; thus, transbronchial biopsy is usually withheld except for cases not diagnosed by BAL. Open lung biopsy is rarely needed. An experienced HIV clinician may make an empiric diagnosis of PCP, but this approach should be reserved for patients known to be HIV-infected.

56. Describe the chest x-ray findings in PCP.

Typically seen is a diffuse, bilateral, interstitial infiltrate, often more pronounced in the hilar region (butterfly distribution). Areas of focal consolidation are less common, as are cystic and cavitary changes. Normal chest x-rays are also seen, especially in patients presenting early in the illness. Pleural effusion is rare and, if present, should raise the suspicion of another diagnosis. The same goes for hilar adenopathy: if present, consider alternative diagnoses.

57. How is PCP treated?
Conventional treatment comes down to a choice among three agents: trimethoprim-sulfamethoxazole (TMP-SMX), pentamidine isethionate, or atovaquone.

58. How do TMP-SMX and pentamidine compare in efficacy and administration?
They seem to be equally effective in clinical use but differ in routes of administration. Both are available for IV use, but TMP-SMX also can be administered orally, enabling outpatient therapy. The usual daily dose is 20 mg/kg of TMP and 100 mg/kg of SMX in divided doses, three to four times/day for 21 days. A lower dose (15/75 mg/kg) may be equally effective with fewer side effects. Pentamidine usually is given at a dose of 4 mg/kg/day. The 3-mg/kg, once-daily dose may be effective in mild pneumonias.

59. When is atovaquone used?
Atovaquone is an alternative oral therapy for mild-to-moderate PCP (PO_2 > 60 mmHg, A–a O_2 gradient < 45 mmHg) in patients who cannot tolerate TMP-SMX. In studies comparing it with TMP-SMX or pentamidine, atovaquone was less toxic and better tolerated. However, it is less effective than TMP-SMX, although equally as effective as pentamidine. The dosing regimen with the oral suspension is 750 mg twice daily, taken with a fatty meal, usually for 21 days. Because absorption depends on food intake, more acutely ill patients are not candidates.

60. When is secondary prophylaxis begun in all patients with PCP?
Secondary prophylaxis is begun as soon as primary treatment is completed.

61. What are the expected side effects of treatment of moderate-to-severe PCP?
TMP-SMX is very well tolerated in non-AIDS patients, but it produces side effects in 65–100% of patients with AIDS. Severe rash and neutropenia are often treatment-limiting but reversible with drug cessation. Progressive renal insufficiency and pancreatitis with dysglycemias are the most serious side effects of pentamidine infusion (Table 13-5). Atovaquone is associated with treatment-limiting rash in only 4% of patients and no other adverse reaction in more than 1%. However, as noted in the question above, it is not indicated in severe cases, only mild-to-moderate disease.

TABLE 13-5. DRUG-ASSOCIATED ADVERSE EFFECTS OF TMP-SMX VERSUS PENTAMIDINE

	TMP-SMX (%)	Pentamidine (%)
Fever (> 37°C)	78	82
Hypotension	0	27
Nausea, vomiting	25	24
Rash	44	15
Anemia	39	24
Leukopenia	72	47
Thrombocytopenia	3	18
Azotemia	14	64
Alanine aminotransferase	22	15
Alkaline aminotransferase	22	15
Alkaline phosphatase	11	18
Hypoglycemia	0	21
Hypocalcemia	0	3

62. **List the indications for PCP prophylaxis.**
- Prior episode of PCP (secondary prophylaxis)
- CD4⁺ count < 200/mm^3 (or CD4⁺ < 14% of total lymphocytes)
- Earlier initiation (CD4 > 200) warranted for patients with oral candidiasis, unexplained fever, or rapid fall in CD4⁺ count

63. **What agents and regimens are recommended for PCP prophylaxis?**
TMP-SMX appears virtually 100% effective in patients who can tolerate the side effects, whereas dapsone and pentamidine have a 5–10% failure rate per year. Failure means that PCP may be mild or atypical. In a practical, clinically pertinent study comparing the three agents, all had similar effectiveness when treatment-limiting toxicities were included. Table 13-6 summarizes typical prophylactic regimens.

TABLE 13-6. REGIMENS FOR PCP PROPHYLAXIS
TMP-SMX
■ TMP 160 mg, SMX 800 mg daily (one double-strength [DS] tablet)
■ Side effects similar to but less common than with primary PCP treatment
■ Decreasing dose by 50% (1 DS tablet 3 times/wk or single-strength daily) may limit side effects while preserving efficacy
■ Also provides prophylaxis against CNS toxoplasmosis
Dapsone (+ pyrimethamine)
■ 50 mg twice daily or 100 mg/day
■ Provides prophylaxis against toxoplasmosis with addition of pyrimethamine
Aerosolized pentamidine
■ 300 mg once monthly via nebulizer
■ Transient taste alterations and coughing or wheezing (can be minimized by pretreatment with inhaled bronchodilators)
■ Evaluate patients for active TB before starting therapy – administer in negative pressure room or booth
Atovaquone
■ 1500 mg/day
■ Gastrointestinal discomfort is main adverse event
■ Also covers toxoplasmosis

KEY POINTS: *PNEUMOCYSTIC CARINII* PNEUMONIA 

1. PCP is uniformly preventable.
2. A diagnosis of PCP usually represents a failed earlier opportunity to diagnose and treat HIV infection.
3. The onset of PCP is insidious but always progressive.
4. Specific PCP treatment is necessary. There is no "broad-spectrum" antibiotic coverage.

Bozzette SA, et al: A randomized trial of three antipneumocystis agents in patients with advanced human immunodeficiency virus infection. N Engl J Med 332:693–699, 1995.

64. How does aerosolized pentamidine prophylaxis change the presentation of breakthrough PCP?

Because aerosolized pentamidine is not 100% effective, new episodes of PCP may occur during prophylaxis. These episodes may present with an atypical radiographic appearance, with more upper-lobe infiltrates rather than the traditional diffuse interstitial infiltrates. The yield of BAL for pathologic diagnosis also is decreased.

Jules-Elysee KM, et al: Aerosolized pentamidine: Effect on diagnosis and presentation of Pneumocystis carinii pneumonia. Ann Intern Med 112:750–757, 1990.

65. When should adjunctive steroids be used in therapy for PCP?

- Indicated in patients with $PaO_2 < 70$ mmHg or $A–aO_2$ gradient > 35 mmHg on room air
- Corticosteroids are begun within 72 hours of initiating PCP treatment
- Improve clinical outcome and reduce mortality rate by 50%
- Avoid in presence of coincident pulmonary infection (TB, histoplasmosis) or process (KS)

66. Summarize the recommended regimen for adjunctive steroids.

Oral prednisone given as follows:

- 40 mg twice daily for 5 days, then
- 40 mg once daily for 5 days, then
- 20 mg once daily for 11 days (total duration 21 days)

67. What is extrapulmonary pneumocystosis?

Pneumocystis infection can involve anatomic sites literally from head (otitis) to foot (vasculitis). The use of nonsystemic (i.e., inhaled) pentamidine therapy for PCP prophylaxis appears to be involved in such cases, although current clinical practice prefers systemic therapy with TMP-SMX or dapsone.

68. Describe the relationship between HIV and tuberculosis (TB).

Until the mid-1980s there had been a steady and rapid decline in the morbidity and mortality attributed to TB. In 1986 the number of new TB cases increased for the first time since nationwide reporting was initiated in 1953. Cross-matching public health registers for TB and AIDS cases and found a high number of patients on both lists. HIV patients are highly susceptible to primary TB, and there is a high rate of progression from latent to active TB in HIV patients with preexisting latent TB.

69. How is this relationship explained?

The relationship is predictable from knowledge of the pathogenesis of each infection. Control of TB depends on cell-mediated immunity, precisely the most profound deficit in HIV infection. The incidence of TB in an HIV-infected population can be expected to mirror that population's previous exposure to *M. tuberculosis*. Immigrants, inner-city minorities, and IV drug users, groups with a high prevalence of both HIV infection and previous TB infection, will develop a high number of active TB cases unless prophylaxis is used. HIV is the strongest promoter of the development of active tuberculosis from latent infection. A person with latent TB is at a 5% lifetime risk of activation in the absence of HIV. With HIV infection, a person with latent TB is at a 5–9% risk per year of developing active disease.

Shafer RW, Edlin BR: Tuberculosis in patients infected with human immunodeficiency virus: Perspective on the past decade. Clin Infect Dis 22:683–704, 1996.

70. Does TB differ in presentation in HIV-infected patients?

TB in HIV-infected patients remains primarily a pulmonary disease, but the incidence of extrapulmonary disease is much higher in the HIV-infected population compared with the general population. Miliary and disseminated cases of TB are seen more often, and "typical" apical or cavitary disease is less common. Although the symptoms of chronic productive cough and hemoptysis are less common, TB in HIV infection remains a progressive, febrile, wasting disease. The more "typical" TB cases appear in HIV-infected patients with a better preserved immune status, whereas the more "atypical" presentations are seen in patients further along in HIV-related illness.

71. Is TB more contagious in patients with AIDS?

M. tuberculosis, a communicable pathogen in people with normal immunity, is the rare organism that may be transmitted from an HIV-infected person to a noninfected person. Patients with AIDS as a whole may be less contagious than non-AIDS patients since cavitary lung disease is less common, but the bottom line is that any patient capable of aerosolizing respiratory droplets containing *M. tuberculosis* is contagious. From the other perspective, patients with AIDS are much more susceptible to TB infection, and care should be taken to minimize new exposures.

72. Describe the treatment of TB in HIV infection.

TB is a curable infection in HIV patients. The recommended treatment is currently the same for both HIV-infected and non–HIV-infected patients—isoniazid, 300 mg/day, plus rifampin, 600 mg/day for 6 months, plus pyrazinamide, 20–30 mg/kg/day, during the first 2 months of therapy. Ethambutol, 25 mg/kg/day, is added initially to protect against the possibility of drug resistance. Directly observed therapy is the standard of care and treatment is continued for a minimum of 6 months. Therapy is extended to 9 months if cultures are still positive after the initial 2 months of therapy.

73. What precautions must be taken in treating TB in an HIV-infected patient?

Care must be taken when TB and HIV are treated simultaneously. The metabolism of the drugs that have revolutionized HIV treatment (nonnucleosides and PIs) is affected by the cytochrome p450 system. Rifampin is one of the strongest known inducers of this system. Combining rifampin with these agents may result in subtherapeutic levels of the antiretrovirals and subsequent HIV treatment failure with drug-resistant HIV. Rifabutin should be substituted for rifampin, decreasing the induction of cytochrome p450. This combined therapy must be supervised by physicians experienced with both diseases.

American Thoracic Society/Centers for Disease Control and Prevention/Infectious Diseases Society of America: Treatment of tuberculosis. Am J Respir Crit Care Med 167:603–662, 2003.

74. Is tuberculin skin testing (TST) with purified protein derivative (PPD) of any use in HIV-infected patients?

The benefits derived from PPD skin testing depend on the prevalence of underlying TB infection in the screened population and the degree of immunosuppression already present. TST is recommended in all patients after the diagnosis of HIV infection. Patients with a reaction > 5 mm should receive isoniazid prophylaxis for 9 months, regardless of age at the time of diagnosis. The risk of developing active TB is greater than the risk of treatment-related toxicity.

75. What about TB reporting and contact tracing?

TB remains a reportable disease in all states, and all cases should be reported. This reporting is wholly independent from reporting of HIV infection or cases of AIDS. Because many localities have protocols to protect the confidentiality of HIV-infected patients, often the report of a TB case may not include HIV status. In areas where these protocols are not present, it is a good idea to add this information, which assists the local health department in prioritizing its cases.

KEY POINTS: TUBERCULOSIS AND HIV

1. All TB patients need to be tested for HIV infection.
2. All patients with HIV need to have the tuberculin skin test.
3. Induration of 5 mm is a significant reaction, and treatment for latent TB should be strongly considered.
4. For reactions between 5 and 10 mm, you need to know HIV status to make a proper assessment.
5. The risk of TB reactivation from latent infection is almost always higher than the risk of significant toxicity from treatment of latent infection.

76. Should patients with TB be screened for HIV infection?

Absolutely. Because a larger number of TB cases are now related to HIV infection and because early diagnosis of HIV infection has many benefits, all patients with TB should be asked to consent to HIV testing. In many large cities, the rates of HIV infection in TB cases are as high as 30–40%.

77. What is a paradoxical reaction?

Paradoxical reactions during TB treatment are defined as transient worsening or appearance of new signs, symptoms, or radiographic manifestations of TB that occur after initiation of treatment and are not the result of treatment failure or a second process. Such reactions were seen prior to the HIV epidemic and are still seen in HIV-negative TB cases, although they are rare. Paradoxical reactions have been reported in up to 35% of HIV/TB cases. Most reactions are also associated with the initiation of antiretroviral therapy, usually within days or weeks. They are most common in patients with advanced (CD4 < 50) AIDS. Common manifestations include: fever, new or increased adenopathy, new or worsening pulmonary infiltrates, and serositis, such as pleural effusions.

Burman WJ, Jones BE: Treatment of HIV-related tuberculosis in the era of effective antiretroviral therapy. Am J Respir Crit Care Med 164:7–12, 2001.

78. What other mycobacterial infections are seen in HIV-infected patients?

Very early in the HIV epidemic, a large number of patients had disseminated *M. avium* complex (MAC) infection. Autopsy series have demonstrated a prevalence of up to 50% at the time of death from AIDS, and clinical studies have shown an annual risk of approximately 20% in patients with AIDS. Multiple other mycobacteria have been found to cause infection in patients with AIDS, but the only one seen in significant numbers is *M. kansasii.*

Nightingale SD, et al: Incidence of *M. avium–intracellulare* complex bacteremia in human immunodeficiency virus-positive patients. J Infect Dis 165:1082–1085, 1992.

79. How does infection with MAC present?

MAC infection usually is associated with advanced HIV disease (CD4 count < 50), and the patient often has concurrent conditions. Thus, the individual contribution of MAC infection to the patient's overall condition can be difficult to ascertain. Usually seen are systemic symptoms such as fever, night sweats, weight loss, fatigue, and malaise. Laboratory exam may reveal increasing anemia or mild hepatitis. Chronic diarrhea with abdominal pain and/or malabsorption is also seen. The frequency of GI symptoms and pathologic changes suggest that the GI tract may be the portal of entry.

80. How is MAC infection diagnosed?

Diagnosis of MAC infection is made by culture of blood. The yield from blood cultures is excellent, and there is often only a short delay before results are available. Positive results can be reported in as few as 5–10 days. Specimens from biopsies quickly reveal acid-fast organisms on stains, thus facilitating the diagnosis.

81. Describe the standard therapy for MAC in patients with AIDS.
Current recommendation is to include at least two drugs with good activity against MAC. One of these agents should be either azithromycin (500 mg/day) or clarithromycin (500 mg twice daily). The second drug is usually ethambutol (15 mg/kg/day). Other active agents include rifabutin (300 mg/day) and ciprofloxacin (750 mg twice daily). Rifabutin is often not used due to significant drug-drug interactions with anti-HIV medications.

82. Which drugs are used as prophylaxis against MAC?
Three drugs have been approved for prophylaxis against MAC: rifabutin, clarithromycin, and azithromycin. Due to ease of dosing and lack of drug interactions, most practitioners use azithromycin (1200 mg once per week). Rifabutin may cause cross-resistance to rifampin in a patient with TB who is inadequately evaluated and then treated with this single drug inadvertently. Rifabutin also has significant pharmacologic interactions with antiretroviral drugs. Many MAC breakthroughs on clarithromycin prophylaxis have been shown to be clarithromycin-resistant, thus negating the efficacy of the most active drug used in treatment.

83. In which HIV-infected patients should a serologic test for syphilis (STS) be obtained?
Every HIV-infected patient needs an STS as well as a detailed history for all STDs and past treatments. The body of literature in the pre-HAART era suggested the possibility of an accelerated course and unusual progression of syphilis in patients also infected with HIV. With this finding in mind, along with the fact that the routes of transmission for HIV and syphilis are similar, all patients with a positive serology for one infection should be tested for the other. In a patient presenting for primary syphilis, if the initial HIV test is negative, a second test should be done in 3 months. This is to evaluate for the possibility of early HIV infection with the absence of antibodies at the initial visit.

84. What if the STS is positive but the patient gives no history of syphilis?
Because of the concern about altered progression of syphilis in HIV infection, the discrimination between early syphilis, early latent syphilis, and late latent syphilis may be less important, because most practitioners aggressively treat early infection. A question does arise over the use of lumbar puncture (LP) to evaluate neurosyphilis. Currently, LP is not recommended in early syphilis but is recommended in late latent syphilis (> 1-year duration). With no patient history to guide treatment decisions, it may be best to err on the side of caution and proceed with LP in HIV-infected patients, especially those with any neurologic signs or symptoms or a serum antibody titer > 1:32. An inquiry to the local public health office may provide additional history that the patient has not recalled.

85. Which HIV-infected patients with syphilis need an LP?
Although a few authorities recommend an LP in all patients, most agree that patients with a clear episode of primary or secondary syphilis do not need an LP. Examination of the CSF should be done for all HIV-infected patients with syphilis of > 1 year's duration or any clinical signs or symptoms of CNS involvement. Patients with early syphilis whose serologic titers increase or fail to decrease appropriately (fourfold in 6 months) also should undergo an LP to evaluate CNS involvement before retreatment.

86. What is the treatment for neurosyphilis in HIV-infected patients?
It is the same whether or not the patient has HIV infection: aqueous crystalline penicillin G, 2.4 mU IV every 4 hours (12–24 mu/day) for 10–14 days. No non–penicillin-based therapy is considered wholly satisfactory. Patients with remote histories of unclear penicillin allergy may need skin testing.

87. If a chancre is present, is initial therapy for syphilis changed?
No. The recommended regimen remains one dose of benzathine penicillin G, 2.4 mU IM, but many authorities treat primary syphilis more aggressively in patients coinfected with HIV and administer a total of 7.2 mU given as 2.4 mU weekly for 3 consecutive weeks.

88. How should patients with HIV infection and primary syphilis be followed?
Patients should have repeat serologic testing at 1, 3, 6, and 12 months. If at any time there is a fourfold increase in titer, an LP should be done. If by 3 months there has not been a fourfold decrease in titer, an LP should be recommended so the CSF can be examined.

89. Should all patients with syphilis be tested for HIV?
Of course. HIV infection may alter the course of syphilis or the response to treatment. Obviously, there are common risk factors for both infections. In addition, any condition that causes open sores in the genital area can facilitate the transmission of HIV. As noted previously, if the initial HIV test is negative, it should be repeated in 3 months. This is to evaluate for the possibility of early HIV infection with the absence of antibodies at the initial visit.

90. What is the most common cause of meningitis in AIDS patients?
Cryptococcus neoformans. Depending on which series is examined, cryptococcus may cause 5–10% of AIDS-defining opportunistic infections. Because patients also develop cryptococcal infections after a previous AIDS diagnosis, the overall estimate is 8–15%. Studies suggested a decreasing incidence of cryptococcosis, even before the era of more effective HIV therapy, possibly related to the more general use of fluconazole for either prophylaxis or treatment for other fungal diseases, such as oral and esophageal candidiasis.

91. How does cryptococcal infection present?
Meningitis is the most common presentation in AIDS. Extraneural disease is frequently seen with meningitis but is much less common in its absence. Meningismus is present in only 25–30% of patients with meningitis, but fever and headache are seen in 80–90%. Focal neurologic symptoms or signs are seen in a small minority of patients (Table 13-7).

TABLE 13-7. FEATURES OF MENINGEAL CRYPTOCOCCOSIS

Symptoms			
Fever	58 (65%)	Altered mentation	25 (28%)
Malaise	68 (76%)	Focal deficits	5 (6%)
Headaches	65 (73%)	Seizures	4 (4%)
Stiff neck	20 (22%)	Cough/dyspnea	28 (31%)
Nausea/vomiting	37 (42%)	Diarrhea	19 (21%)
Photophobia	16 (18%)		
Signs			
Fever	50 (56%)	Altered mentation	15 (17%)
Meningeal signs	24 (27%)	Focal deficits	13 (15%)

From Chuck SL, Sande MA: Infections with *Cryptococcus neoformans* in AIDS. N Engl J Med 321:795, 1989, with permission.

92. Which patients with cryptococcosis need an LP?
All patients with a culture or a serum antigen titer positive for cryptococcus require an LP, regardless of which site originally yielded the positive specimen. In any HIV-infected patient with an undiagnosed fever and/or headache in a medically urgent situation, an LP should be considered to assess the possibility of cryptococcal disease. If the situation is less urgent, a serum antigen titer can be obtained, and if a negative LP is not needed from the standpoint of diagnosing cryptococcal disease.

93. Is an LP done only for diagnosis in cryptococcal disease?
An LP is performed at the time of diagnosis of cryptococcal infection. If the LP is indicative of meningitis and the patient responds to therapy, a repeat LP should be performed after 2 weeks of therapy to help evaluate microbial response and to decide on the appropriateness of continued IV or oral therapy. Subsequent LPs should be done as clinically indicated until adequate microbial response is documented. If the clinical response is poor or if the initial opening pressure was elevated (> 25 cmH_2O), frequent LPs, sometimes as often as daily, may be needed to relieve increased intracranial pressure and to guide therapy.

94. What CSF findings are seen in cryptococcal meningitis?
The CSF can appear remarkably normal. However, you should always perform an India ink test, which is usually positive and can yield an immediate diagnosis without waiting for other laboratory results (Table 13-8).

TABLE 13-8. CEREBROSPINAL FLUID FINDINGS IN CRYPTOCOCAL MENINGITIS

Finding	No. with Finding/No. Tested	%
WBC < 20 cells/mL	96/128	75
Glucose > 40 mg/dL	87/127	68
Protein < 45 mg/dL	53/127	42
Positive India ink	92/125	74
Positive CSF antigen	116/126	92

Adapted from Chuck SL, Sande MA: Infections with *Cryptococcus neoformans* in the acquired immunodeficiency syndrome. N Engl J Med 321:794–799, 1989, with permission.

95. What treatment is recommended for cryptococcosis in AIDS?
Amphotericin B, or its liposomal preparations, should be administered via IV therapy with oral flucytosine for the first 14 days. If the patient is stable, give oral fluconazole at a dose of 400 mg/day for 8 weeks. Maintenance fluconazole is then prescribed at 200 mg.

96. Are serum cryptococcal antigen levels good indicators of response to therapy?
No. Although the serum antigen test can be very helpful in the diagnosis of cryptococcal infection, it cannot be used to judge therapeutic response. In most cases of meningitis, the CSF antigen titer should be determined by repeat lumbar puncture. If after therapy the serum titer does revert to very low titer or negative, an increasing titer in the future should raise concern about a relapse.

97. Is primary prophylaxis indicated against cryptococcosis?
No. Some clinicians have adopted primary prophylaxis because of the frequency of other fungal diseases (such as oral and esophageal candidiasis) as well as cryptococcosis. A study

comparing fluconazole with clotrimazole troches found that fluconazole (200 mg/day) decreases the frequency of cryptococcosis and esophageal candidiasis, especially in persons at highest risk (i.e., CD4$^+$ count < 50/mm^3). However, no survival benefit was demonstrated, and it was estimated that > 11,000 doses of fluconazole were given to prevent one case of invasive fungal disease.

98. **Is there an interaction between HIV and hepatitis B virus (HBV) infection?**
Maybe. There is no clear HBV effect seen upon the course of HIV infection, unless the extent of hepatic disease prohibits the safe use of antiretroviral therapy. HIV may affect HBV infection if HIV infection is present at the time of HBV exposure. In the HIV-infected patient, there is an increased likelihood of HBV persistence. The actual course of disease, however, does not appear to be changed.

99. **How would you treat HIV and HBV simultaneously?**
Lamivudine, a nucleoside analog, is approved for both HIV and HBV treatment. While monotherapy for HBV is not uncommon, it is contraindicated for HIV. Tenofovir, while not FDA approved for HBV, does have good anti-HBV activity. A related drug, adefovir, is HBV approved, but did not obtain HIV approval. Thus, a good initial therapy for HIV that would also provide HBV therapy would be lamivudine 300 mg/day plus tenofovir 300 mg/day with the addition of either a non-nucleoside RTI or a PI. Care must be taken with the withdrawal of lamivudine from a course of HIV therapy when HBV is present. Such withdrawal can cause a clinically significant flare of hepatitis.

100. **Is there an interaction between HIV and hepatitis C virus (HCV) infection?**
Probably. Most studies have shown a more rapid course of HCV infection in the HIV-infected patient, but some studies have not. The positive studies have shown an increased percentage of patients developing cirrhosis and a shorter time from infection to cirrhosis. There has been demonstrated an increased risk of a liver-related death in HIV-infected HCV patients. The complication of administration of HIV treatment with potentially hepatotoxic medications makes it difficult to sort out true causation. Mother-to-infant transmission of HCV is in the range of 2–5%, but in HIV-infected mothers the rate is increased two to three times. There does not appear to be any effect of HCV infection on the course of HIV. Chronic and continued alcohol use is a major contributor to the progression of HCV disease.

101. **How common is HIV/HCV coinfection?**
Very common. Many HIV clinics have reported coinfection rates. They are generally in the range of 15–30%. That is, in large clinical populations followed at HIV clinics, up to 30% of the HIV-infected patients also have HCV infection.

102. **How effective is HCV treatment in the HIV patient?**
The most important determinant is the HCV genotype, just as in the HIV-negative population. Unfortunately, as in HIV negatives, in HIV/HCV coinfection genotype 1 is most common and least responsive to treatment. The response rate to the standard interferon-plus-ribavirin therapy is 25–30%.

103. **Can you treat HIV and HCV together?**
Yes. While not going into the specifics of each therapy, they are not exclusive from a pharmacologic standpoint. They are very complicated therapies and require extreme adherence levels. HCV therapy also adds important toxicities, especially depression, bone marrow suppression, and flulike symptoms that may impair the patient's ability to adhere to his or her HIV therapy. If HIV therapy is not immediately warranted, many experts recommend initial treatment of HCV with HIV treatment to follow. This may help minimize hepatic toxicity of HIV therapy and prevent flares of hepatitis due to immune reconstitution from HIV therapy.

104. What is the cause of blindness experienced by some patients with AIDS?
Chorioretinitis caused by cytomegalovirus (CMV) is a vision-threatening infection formerly experienced by 5–10% of patients with AIDS during the course of their illness. The incidence has declined dramatically during the era of more effective antiretroviral therapy. CMV is an AIDS-defining diagnosis if it occurs as the initial opportunistic infection; however, this infection appears later in the disease process, after a patient has already been diagnosed with AIDS.

105. How is CMV retinitis diagnosed?
Patients often present with nonspecific complaints of blurred vision, decreased visual acuity, or increasing "floaters," but occasionally CMV retinitis may present with a clear visual field cut. Ophthalmologic examination is essential and typically shows large white granular areas with hemorrhage. Diagnosis is based on this characteristic fundoscopic appearance because no tissue is obtained for pathologic examination. All patients with advanced HIV infection (CD4 counts < 100) should undergo routine retinal screening on a quarterly basis.

106. Should all HIV-infected patients have eye exams?
Because CMV retinitis usually presents later in HIV infection, patients with less-advanced disease do not need an immediate referral to an ophthalmologist. However, a baseline exam should be performed, with subsequent exams as clinical symptoms and signs dictate. Patients with $CD4^+$-lymphocyte counts chronically below $100/mm^3$ should be examined regardless of symptoms, with scheduled follow-up two to three times/year.

107. How else can CMV infection manifest in HIV infection besides chorioretinitis?
- Interstitial pneumonia
- Colitis
- Esophagitis
- Adrenal insufficiency
- Encephalitis

108. What does Kaposi's sarcoma (KS) look like?
KS in HIV-infected patients is most often seen as cutaneous or oropharyngeal nodules ranging in size from 0.5 to 2.0 cm, although multiple nodules may coalesce. The nodules usually are raised and readily palpable, painless, and nonpruritic, with no evidence of inflammation or exudate. Rarely, lesions may become friable or verrucous (warty) and weep or bleed with trauma. Their color is usually blue or violet-to-purple; in darker-skinned patients, they often appear black. Nodules are often multiple when first diagnosed, reflecting the relatively aggressive nature of this malignancy in HIV infection. Any area of the body may be involved, although the palms of the hands are rarely affected despite the more common involvement of the soles of the feet.

109. Does a lesion suspicious for KS need to be biopsied?
In general, yes. If a patient with HIV infection has no previous diagnosis of KS or any opportunistic infection, suspicious lesions should be uniformly biopsied to establish a diagnosis. In a patient who has had previously diagnosed opportunistic infections and is under regular supervision and care, the need for confirming a clinical diagnosis by biopsy is less clear. However, there are other causes of pigmented cutaneous lesions in HIV infection. Patients with previously diagnosed KS do not need biopsy of new lesions unless they have been in remission after therapy.

110. Does antiretroviral therapy treat KS?
In the era of highly active antiretroviral therapy, regression of otherwise untreated KS lesions has been widely described. It is now generally accepted practice, depending on the stage and severity of KS, to initiate effective antiretroviral therapy first and observe KS for any response. Suboptimal responses are then treated with specific anti-KS therapy in addition to HIV therapy.

111. Define immune reconstitution inflammatory syndrome.

This syndrome is analogous to paradoxical reactions in TB treatment. In the setting of effective antiretroviral therapy, there is a rapid control of HIV viral replication and subsequent improvements in CD4 cell count and function. This immune reconstitution may then lead to inflammatory responses to clinically known or subclinical opportunistic infections. Most commonly seen is lymphadenitis due to MAC, the paradoxical reactions in TB, and exacerbations of cryptococcal meningitis and CMV retinitis. The more severe reactions, such as meningitis and retinitis, may result in administration of steroidal therapy.

Shelburne SA, Hamill RJ: The immune reconstitution inflammatory syndrome. AIDS Rev 5:67–79, 2003.

112. What are the clinical benefits to this immune reconstitution?

It has been shown that as a result of this response, both primary and secondary prophylaxis against many pathogens may be discontinued. Most commonly, many patients are able to discontinue prophylaxis against PCP. Also common is cessation of MAC prophylaxis and even maintenance therapy. Chronic maintenance therapy against cryptococcal disease and histoplasmosis can also be stopped. Less is known about cerebral toxoplasmosis and its maintenance therapy.

113. What are the most common causes of CNS mass lesions in AIDS?

Cerebral toxoplasmosis and primary CNS lymphoma. Other causes include progressive multifocal leukoencephalopathy (PML), cryptococcoma, tuberculoma, bacterial and fungal abscesses, and metastatic neoplastic disease. The increasing use of TMP-SMX as prophylaxis for PCP may coincidentially decrease the proportion of CNS mass lesions attributable to toxoplasmosis. The advancing age of many patients has made lung cancer more common than in the past and the female prevalence of 30% has made breast cancer more common as a potential cause of metastatic CNS disease.

114. What are the characteristic CT scan findings in CNS toxoplasmosis as opposed to lymphoma?

Characteristic findings are summarized in Table 13-9. If a single lesion is seen on CT scan, a more sensitive test such as an MRI should be performed. If only a single lesion is still seen, an alternative diagnosis other than toxoplasmosis should be strongly considered. Centers with access to SPECT (single-photon emission computed tomography) scanning can increase the suspicion for lymphoma when an increased signal ratio is demonstrated.

TABLE 13-9. CT FINDINGS IN TOXOPLASMOSIS VERSUS LYMPHOMA

CT Finding	Toxoplasmosis	Lymphoma
Area involved	Deep gray matter and basal ganglia	White matter, periventricular areas
Mass effect	Yes	Yes
Enhancement	Ring enhancement	Weakly, not ring-shaped
Number of lesions	Multiple	1–2

115. How is the differentiation between CNS toxoplasmosis and lymphoma made?

Most clinicians recommend empirical treatment for toxoplasmosis (pyrimethamine, 100-mg loading dose, then 25 mg/day, and sulfadiazine, 4–6 gm/day in divided doses), using this treatment trial as an additional diagnostic tool. Response is judged clinically as well as on CT or MRI scanning. Response should be rapid (3–5 days). If it does not occur, an etiology other than toxoplasmosis is suggested.

116. Should primary toxoplasmosis prophylaxis be given?
Yes. Patients positive for toxoplasma antibodies who also have a $CD4^+$ count < 100 should receive primary prophylaxis. TMP/SMX 160/800 mg is the preferred daily regimen, providing protection against both PCP and toxoplasmosis. If this regimen is not tolerated, dapsone-pyrimethamine or atovaquone can be given. With immune reconstitution to a sustained CD4 count over 100, specific anti-toxoplasma prophylaxis may be stopped.

117. Besides KS and non-Hodgkin's lymphoma, what other malignancies are seen in HIV infection?
An additional AIDS-defining malignancy is invasive cervical cancer. Although not specific to HIV infection, it appears the clinical course is more aggressive in advanced HIV infection. All HIV-infected women need to receive routine screening for cervical cancer. Human papillomavirus (HPV) is involved in practically all cases of cervical cancer. Other non–AIDS-defining malignancies seen more frequently in HIV infection include Hodgkin's disease, anal cancer (also associated with HPV), lung cancer, and testicular cancer.

118. What metabolic complications have been associated with HIV treatments?
- Alterations in glucose metabolism: insulin resistance, glucose intolerance, diabetes mellitus
- Hyperlipidemia: hypercholesterolemia, hypertriglyceridemia
- Hyperlactatemia and lactic acidosis
- Fat redistribution: visceral fat accumulation, subcutaneous fat atrophy

119. Describe sensory neuropathy seen in HIV.
Many patients with HIV experience a distal sensory polyneuropathy. This may be due to HIV itself or treatment of HIV with certain neurotoxic nucleoside analogs, most commonly zalcitabine, didanosine, and stavudine. Patients present with paresthesias, numbness, or pain in the distal extremities. Symptoms are symmetrical and move proximally when advancing. The temporal relationship to medication is the only way to infer one cause over the other. HIV-related neuropathy often responds to effective anti-HIV therapy, but this response is not uniform and can be delayed.

120. What is PML?
Progressive multifocal leukoencephalopathy (PML) is a CNS demyelinating disease resulting from infection with Jakob-Creutzfeldt (JC) virus. Although spread throughout the population, JC virus requires profound immunosuppression to cause disease; in HIV the CD4 count is typically < 50. Any part of the CNS can be involved. As the name implies, lesions are multifocal and result in focal neurologic defects. Diagnosis is based on the typical presentation in late AIDS, abnormal CT or MRI imaging, positive PCR testing of CSF for JC virus, or a brain biopsy. Treatment is directed at anti-HIV therapy with immune reconstitution.

BIBLIOGRAPHY

1. Mandell GL, Bennett JE, Dolin R: Principles and Practice of Infectious Diseases, 6th ed. Philadelphia, Churchill Livingstone, 2005.
2. Sande MA, Volberding PA: The Medical Management of AIDS, 6th ed. Philadelphia, W.B. Saunders, 1999.

CHAPTER 14

NEUROLOGY

Loren A. Rolak, MD

This apoplexy, as I take it, is a kind of lethargy, an't please your lordship; a kind of sleeping in the blood, a whoreson tingling. . . . It hath it original from much grief, from study and perturbation of the brain. I have read the cause of his effects in Galen. It is a kind of deafness.

William Shakespeare (1564–1616)
Description of stroke, Henry IV, Part II

APPROACH TO THE PATIENT

1. What is the initial approach to evaluating patients complaining of neurologic symptoms?

The first step is to localize the lesion to a specific part of the nervous system. Only then should an etiology be sought, since defining the anatomy usually implies certain causes. Because each part of the brain, spinal cord, and peripheral nervous system has such specialized functions, lesions in these areas produce specific clinical deficits. Therefore, symptoms can often be localized, sometimes to the millimeter, to discrete parts of the nervous system.

2. What are the most important regions for anatomic localization?

For clinical purposes, the most important neuroanatomy is limited to a few large regions. The regions where lesions should be localized are (proceeding from distal to proximal):

1. Muscle
2. Neuromuscular junction
3. Peripheral nerve
4. Root
5. Spinal cord
6. Brain stem
7. Cerebellum
8. Subcortical brain
9. Cortical brain

3. How are symptoms localized to these neuroanatomic regions?

As in all aspects of medicine, the history guides the diagnosis. By asking the proper questions, a clinician can accurately localize most neurologic lesions. A useful system for diagnosis is to begin distally (with the muscle) and to ask the patient questions about each part of the neurologic anatomy, working backward (proximally) from the muscle, through the neuromuscular junction, peripheral nerve, root, spinal cord, cerebellum, brain stem, subcortex, and ending with the cortex of the brain. By sequentially asking about each of these areas, you can "examine" the patient thoroughly. Only after the lesion is localized by history-taking should the physical exam begin. If localization of the lesion is still unclear after a careful history, do not begin the physical exam—take a better history!

MYOPATHIES

4. Which tests and procedures are used in the diagnostic evaluation of a patient with a suspected myopathy?

The diagnostic evaluation of a myopathy generally entails a triad of tests:

- Serum creatine kinase (CK)
- Electromyography (EMG)
- Muscle biopsy

5. **Explain the significance of serum CK.**
Muscle destruction usually liberates CK, making elevation of this enzyme a good screening test for muscle disease. (The MM isoenzyme of CK is the most common.)

6. **What can you learn from the EMG?**
An EMG is done by inserting a fine-needle electrode into the muscle to record the electrical impulses related to contractions. Myopathies cause low-voltage, short-duration muscle contractions, and this test can thus confirm the presence of myopathy.

7. **Summarize the role of muscle biopsy.**
A muscle biopsy is often needed to define the cause of a myopathy, since most myopathies are clinically similar. The tissue may show inflammation (polymyositis), mitochondrial abnormalities, or other specific diseases.

8. **List the most important myopathies.**
   - Muscular dystrophies (e.g., Duchenne's muscular dystrophy)
   - Congenital myopathies (e.g., Kearns-Sayre syndrome, central cord syndrome)
   - Inflammatory myopathies (e.g., polymyositis, dermatomyositis)
   - Toxic myopathies (e.g., alcohol, zidovudine, clofibrate, steroids)
   - Endocrine myopathies (e.g., hypothyroidism, hypoadrenalism)
   - Infectious myopathies (e.g., trichinosis, AIDS)

9. **Which of the myopathies is most common on the medical ward?**
Polymyositis is the most common. It is an inflammatory, T cell–mediated autoimmune disease of the muscles, characterized by the subacute onset of proximal weakness of the arms and legs, often with dysphagia. It may accompany connective tissue disease (such as systemic lupus erythematosus) or vasculitis but usually appears alone. It runs a variable course but can be severe or even fatal.

10. **Which is the second most common myopathy?**
Dermatomyositis is a distinct clinical entity characterized by similar subacute proximal muscle weakness in association with a rash, often over the face and trunk. Dermatomyositis is a humeral-mediated microangiopathy. It has an increased incidence of concomitant malignancies.

11. **How are polymyositis and dermatomyositis treated?**
Treatment for polymyositis and dermatomyositis is the same and involves high-dose oral prednisone (at least 1 mg/kg body weight/day) as the mainstay of therapy. Azathioprine or methotrexate may be used in steroid-resistant cases or when complications develop from steroid use. IV immunoglobulin (IVIG) may also be safe and effective, especially during acute exacerbations.

Briember HR, Amato AA: Dermatomyositis and polymyositis. Curr Treat Opt Neurol 5: 349–356, 2003.

NEUROMUSCULAR JUNCTION

12. **Name the most common neuromuscular junction disease seen on the medical ward. Summarize its prevalence and distribution.**
Myasthenia gravis (MG). MG has a prevalence of 1 case/10,000 population and a bimodal age distribution, occurring in young women in their teens and 20s and older men aged 60 and above.

13. **What causes MG?**
MG is an autoimmune disease in which patients produce antibodies that destroy the acetylcholine receptors on muscle. Acetylcholine is the neurotransmitter that makes muscles contract.

14. How does MG present?

MG presents with proximal weakness, especially ptosis and diplopia, with fatigue on use and recovery with rest. Because MG can involve the respiratory muscles, pulmonary failure is the most feared complication.

15. How is MG treated?

Treatment consists of acetylcholinesterase inhibitors, which block the enzymatic breakdown of acetylcholine, thus allowing greater concentrations of acetylcholine at the receptor. **Pyridostigmine** (Mestinon) is the drug of choice, but immunosuppressive drugs, including prednisone, azathioprine, and cyclosporine, are often necessary to attack the underlying autoimmune process. Plasmapheresis and IVIG have also been shown to help. Surgical thymectomy is probably beneficial, but its role in treating MG remains controversial.

Gronseth GS, Barohn RJ: Practice Parameter: Thymectomy for autoimmune myasthenia gravis. Neurology 55: 7–15, 2000.

16. What other disease may cause neuromuscular junction problems?

Lambert-Eaton myasthenic syndrome (LEMS).

17. What causes LEMS?

Like MG, LEMS is an autoimmune condition, although its target is the presynaptic voltage-gated calcium channel involved in acetylcholine release, not the receptor. It is commonly seen in the association with occult carcinoma, especially small-cell carcinoma of the lung. LEMS clinically resembles MG because of fluctuating proximal weakness.

18. How is LEMS treated?

It is generally treated by therapy for the underlying neoplasm, sometimes accompanied by plasmapheresis and other immune suppressors, especially in cases where no occult cancer can be found. Guanidine may provide symptomatic relief.

Neusom-Davis J: A treatment algorithm for Lambert-Eaton myasthenic syndrome. Ann NY Acad Sci 841: 817–822, 1998.

19. Which drugs may worsen neuromuscular junction diseases?

1. Aminoglycosides
2. Tetracycline antibiotics
3. Corticosteroids (acutely)
4. Thyroid hormone
5. Phenothiazines (e.g., chlorpromazine)
6. Quinidine
7. Lidocaine
8. Propranolol
9. Lithium
10. Dilantin

PERIPHERAL NEUROPATHIES

20. Which peripheral neuropathies are seen most commonly on the medical ward?

Peripheral neuropathies are probably the most frequent neurologic problems seen on a medical ward, unlike myopathies and neuromuscular junction diseases, which are rare. The most common peripheral neuropathies can be remembered by the mnemonic **DANG THE RAPIST**:

D = **D**iabetes
A = **A**lcohol
N = **N**utritional (e.g., vitamin deficiencies)
G = **G**uillain-Barré syndrome
T = **T**rauma (e.g., carpal tunnel)
H = **H**ereditary
E = **E**nvironmental (toxins, drugs)
R = **R**emote effects of cancer
A = **A**myloid
P = **P**orphyria
I = **I**nflammation (e.g., collagen vascular disease)
S = **S**yphilis
T = **T**umors

21. The evaluation of a patient with a peripheral neuropathy usually begins with which study?

An electromyogram and nerve conduction velocity (EMG/NCV) study. This test applies electrical current directly over the nerves and uses an electrode to record the speed with which the nerves conduct the current. It thus documents the extent and degree of impairment of nerve conduction. The EMG uses a needle electrode within the muscles to record muscle contractions and thus show denervation of the muscles.

22. Describe the management of a patient with a neuropathy.

Once a neuropathy has been confirmed, work-up for the etiology focuses on the conditions listed in question 21, requiring evaluation for diabetes, alcoholism, vitamin B_{12} deficiency, metabolic abnormalities such as thyroid disease or uremia, familial illnesses, toxic exposure, and collagen vascular disease. A spinal tap is seldom needed to detect inflammatory neuropathies. Only rarely is a nerve biopsy required. Many neuropathies improve with treatment of the underlying etiology.

Zochodne DW: Diabetic neuropathies. Curr Treat Options Neurol 2: 23–29, 2000.

23. What is the most common entrapment neuropathy?

Carpal tunnel syndrome (CTS), caused by compression of the median nerve at the wrist.

24. Describe the presentation of CTS.

Most commonly the result of mechanical overuse, CTS usually presents with symptoms of pain and tingling in the hand (especially at night), weakness, and/or numbness. Pain in the hand at night is considered CTS until proved otherwise.

25. How is CTS diagnosed?

There may be no objective neurologic findings in CTS. As with other peripheral neuropathies, EMG/NCV studies are helpful in making the diagnosis.

26. How is CTS treated?

Treatment is usually surgical, involving open or endoscopic release at the wrist, although conservative measures (such as wrist splinting) may be sufficient for mild cases.

27. What is Guillain-Barré syndrome (GBS)?

GBS is an acute inflammatory polyradiculopathy with inflammation of the nerve roots and peripheral nerves. It is presumably autoimmune and often follows viral infections, surgery, pregnancies, and other immune-altering events. It runs a monophasic course, with weakness progressing for several days to weeks, reaching a plateau, and then recovering over a period of several weeks to months.

28. What are the symptoms of GBS?

GBS causes weakness, often but not always in an ascending pattern (from legs up the trunk to the arms and face). The weakness is hyporeflexive, but there is no significant sensory loss. *Rapidly progressive weakness with absent reflexes and no sensory change is almost always GBS. The diagnosis is supported by high CSF protein and slowed nerve conduction velocities on EMG.*

29. Treatment of GBS is based on which of its abnormalities?

Although GBS is presumably autoimmune, no specific antigen or well-defined immune abnormality has been confirmed. Nevertheless, treatment is directed toward an immunologic cause, employing IVIG or plasmapheresis. If done early in the disease, these treatments shorten the overall course. Because autonomic dysfunction frequently complicates the syndrome and because respiration is often impaired by the weakness, patients usually require management in the intensive care unit. Therapy thus focuses on the day-to-day concerns of respirators, vital signs, nutrition, and other aspects of critical care.

Plasma Exchange/Sandoglobulin Guillain-Barré Syndrome Trial Group: Randomized trial of plasma exchange, intravenous immunoglobulin, and combined treatments on Guillain-Barré syndrome. Lancet 349: 225–230, 1997.

RADICULOPATHIES

30. What is the most common cause of radiculopathies on the medical ward?
Mechanical compression, as from spondylosis or a herniated disk. The common manifestations are neck or low back pain radiating into a limb.

31. How should the patient with a radiculopathy be evaluated?
The diagnostic evaluation generally begins with an MRI of the area where the root emerges from the spinal cord, since this is the most common site of disorders causing radiculopathies. If imaging studies are negative, showing no root compression, then nonmechanical causes such as inflammation or infection should be considered.

32. Discuss the treatment for radiculopathies.
For most mechanical radiculopathies, the recommended treatment consists simply of analgesics, such as aspirin or other NSAIDs. Avoid muscle relaxants and chronic opioid use. There are surprisingly few careful, controlled studies analyzing the value of bed rest, traction, spinal manipulation, or invasive procedures such as acupuncture or trigger point injection. At this time, these methods have no proven benefit in the treatment of radiculopathy.

Bigus S, et al: Acute Low Back Problems in Adults [Clinical Practice Guideline 14.] Rockville, MD, Agency for Health Care Policy and Research, 1994. [AHCPR publ no. 95–0643.]

33. What is the main indication for surgery in the treatment of a radiculopathy?
Many experts believe that the presence of focal neurologic findings—such as weakness, atrophy, or fasciculations in the muscles affected, an absent reflex, or dermatome sensory loss (Fig. 14-1)—is a strong indication for surgery. Such hard findings are unlikely to improve spontaneously and may well progress unless pressure on the nerve is relieved.

34. Is surgery ever appropriate for patients without focal neurologic findings?
This issue is much more controversial. Even in well-chosen patients with clear lesions and no overlying complications (such as litigation or secondary gain), surgery to alleviate pain is effective in only about half the cases. It is therefore often reserved for patients who have "failed medical management," which is a clinical decision and generally implies persistent, severe pain after an adequate trial of analgesics.

35. What are the most common causes of back pain?
Only about 20% of back pain is caused by a slipped disk or root compression. There are many other causes, such as arthritis of the facet joints, but most back pain is thought to be musculoskeletal, due to strain placed on the tendons, ligaments, and muscles of the back. Many experts feel that this pain is largely mechanical, secondary to the inherent instability of the lordotic spine required for the human upright posture and aggravated by the problems of obesity, lack of exercise, and other precipitating factors in the modern lifestyle. For most such pain, conservative therapy and patience are indicated.

Van Tulder MW, Koes BW, Bouter LM: Conservative treatment of acute and chronic nonspecific low back pain: A systematic review of randomized controlled trials of the most common interventions. Spine 22: 228–256, 1997.

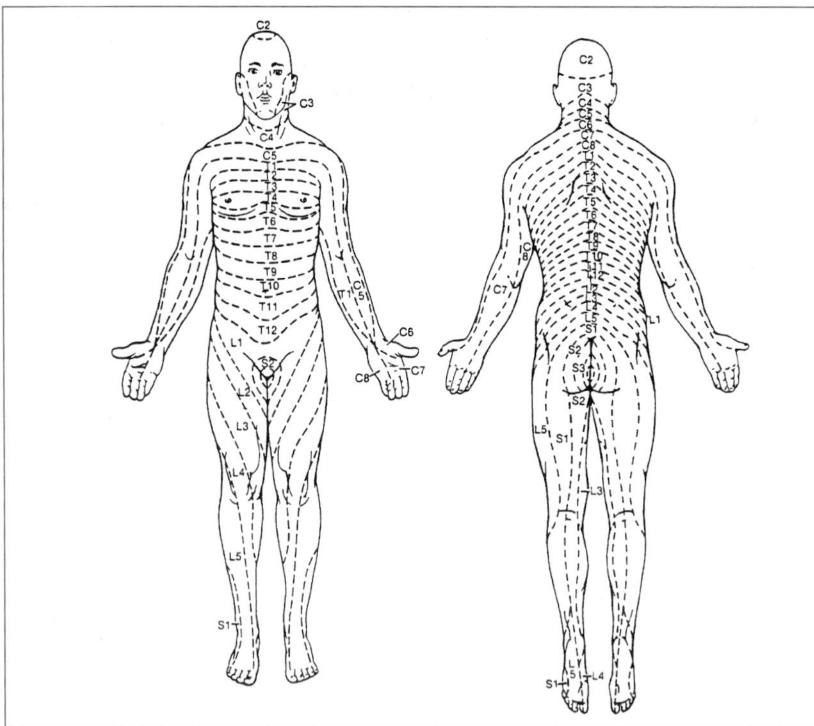

Figure 14-1. Map of the sensory dermtomes in the anterior and posterior aspects.

MYELOPATHIES

36. What are the most common causes of spinal cord disease?

The most common cause of chronic spinal cord compression is cervical spondylosis. If there is no history of trauma, the acute syndrome is often due to compression by a neoplasm, usually metastatic. Such compression may develop almost instantaneously and may or may not cause back pain. Besides compression, other causes include cord infarction, vitamin B_{12} deficiency, HIV infection, and inflammation such as multiple sclerosis or transverse myelins.

37. How does spinal cord compression present clinically?

Spinal cord compression causes the classic cord syndrome of a sensory level, bowel and bladder changes, and upper motor neuron weakness with spasticity, hyperreflexia, and a positive Babinski sign. Superficial reflexes, such as abdominal reflexes and the anal wink, may be diminished.

38. How is spinal cord compression best diagnosed?

The first step is to localize the site of the lesion. Plain x-rays of the spine have a high yield for showing metastatic disease, as evidenced by lytic lesions and erosion of pedicles. Bone scans lack specificity and are generally of low yield. MRI has largely replaced myelography for the definitive documentation of compression.

39. Summarize the treatment for spinal cord compression.

Surgical intervention is indicated for compression due to cervical spondylosis or mechanical deformation, such as spondylolisthesis. For neoplastic compression, radiation therapy is increasingly favored over surgical decompression, since results are equally good in many studies. Otherwise, surgery may be needed for diagnosis as well as treatment. In either case, high-dose IV steroids, such as 100 mg of dexamethasone daily, may provide additional relief.

Armstrong R: Myelopathies. In Rolak LA (ed): Neurology Secrets. Philadelphia, Hanley & Belfus, 1998, pp 103–111.

KEY POINTS: NEUROLOGY I

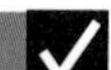

1. Myopathies cause proximal symmetric weakness without sensory loss and with little change in tone or reflexes.
2. Neuromuscular junction diseases cause proximal symmetric weakness that fluctuates (fatigues), without pain or sensory loss.
3. Neuropathies usually cause distal weakness, often asymmetric, with atrophy, sensory loss, and pain.
4. Most back pain is not caused by a radiculopathy.
5. Myelopathies cause a sensory level.

VESTIBULAR DISEASE

40. What is the first step in evaluating a patient with dizziness?
The first question should be whether the problem is true vestibular dizziness or "dizziness" because of near-syncope, ataxia, or another etiology. Patients with true vestibular dizziness complain of **vertigo**, which is a feeling of spinning.

41. What is the second step in evaluation of dizziness?
The next step is to determine whether the vertigo is central (due to a brain-stem lesion) or peripheral (due to an ear lesion).

42. How do you distinguish between central and peripheral vertigo?
Although many accompanying signs and symptoms have been promulgated to differentiate central from peripheral vertigo, none has great sensitivity or specificity. The most useful way to diagnose vertigo is by the company it keeps. **Central vertigo** is almost always accompanied by other signs of brain-stem dysfunction, such as double vision, weakness or numbness of the face, dysarthria, or dysphagia. **Peripheral vertigo** may be accompanied by tinnitus or hearing loss, but no other neurologic abnormalities.

43. Name the common causes of peripheral vertigo and central vertigo.

Peripheral	**Central**
Ménière's disease	Stroke
Vestibular neuronitis	Multiple sclerosis
Local trauma	Tumors
Drugs (antibiotics, diuretics)	
Acoustic neuroma	
Benign positional vertigo	

44. How is dizziness best treated?
Nonvertigo dizziness (including near-syncope, anxiety, and ataxia) should be treated by addressing the underlying cause. True vertigo can be treated symptomatically, almost regardless of the cause. **Scopolamine** has proved to be the best available treatment in comparative trials against other drugs and placebos. Benzodiazepines and antihistamines are of some value, including meclizine (Antivert) and diazepam. Canalith repositioning maneuvers (epley maneuvers) effectively treat benign paroxysmal positional vertigo.

CEREBELLAR DISEASE

45. What is the most common cause of cerebellar disease?
Alcoholism. Alcohol causes an anterior, midline (vermal) atrophy that leads to leg and truncal instability and thus to ataxic gait. Other metabolic causes of cerebellar disease include hypothyroidism and drugs such as 5-fluorouracil and phenytoin. Structural lesions, such as cerebellar infarcts, hemorrhages, and neoplasms (both primary and metastatic) are another cause.

46. Is there any treatment for cerebellar dysfunction?
Cerebellar tremor, dysmetria, and ataxia are among the most difficult symptoms to mask or treat effectively. Some studies have shown that high doses of isoniazid, 900–1200 mg/day, are superior to placebo for minimizing cerebellar dysfunction. However, the toxic effects on peripheral nerves, requiring pyridoxine supplementation, and on the liver, requiring constant blood monitoring, complicate use of this drug at these high doses. Other medications, such as propranolol, primidone, and trihexyphenidyl, have provided occasional success.

STROKE

47. What is a stroke?
A stroke is focal brain dysfunction due to ischemia. The ischemia may arise from atherosclerotic narrowing of a blood vessel, an embolus, hemorrhage, or other causes.

48. Distinguish among the four main kinds of stroke.
See Table 14-1.

49. What are the clinical features of a thrombotic stroke?
Thrombotic strokes are the most common type and account for approximately 40% of all strokes. They may have a gradual, stuttering, or stepwise onset rather than an abrupt deficit. The cause is generally atherosclerosis affecting large intracranial vessels. The large-vessel involvement explains why these strokes tend to cause considerable neurologic deficit. About one-third to one-half of thrombotic strokes are preceded by transient ischemic attacks (TIAs), which are focal but totally reversible deficits that last a few minutes.

50. Describe the major clinical features of an embolic stroke.
Embolic strokes generally arise from the heart with an underlying cardiac disease, such as atrial arrhythmias, valvular disease, or mural thrombus. They tend to be abrupt in onset, with more rapid resolution, and tend to cause smaller neurologic deficits than a thrombotic stroke. Because the embolus travels in the arterial stream until it reaches a blood vessel of sufficiently small caliber to occlude it, it often travels distally all the way to the cortex. Cortical deficits, such as aphasia, are thus characteristic of embolic strokes.

TABLE 14-1. TYPES OF STROKES

Type	% of All Strokes	Onset	Preceding TIAs (%)	Altered Mental Status (%)	MRI or CT Scan	Other Features
Thrombotic	40	May be gradual	Up to 50	5	Ischemic infarction	Carotid bruit Stroke during sleep
Embolic	30	Sudden	10	1	Superficial (cortical) infarction	Underlying heart disease, peripheral emboli, or strokes in different vascular territories.
Lacunar	20	May be gradual	30	0	Small, deep infarction	Pure motor or pure sensory stroke
Hemorrhagic	10	Sudden	5	25	Hyperdense mass	Nausea and vomiting, decreased mental status

51. Explain the mechanisms of a lacunar stroke.

Lacunar strokes are very small, discrete infarcts, < 1 cm^3 in size, occurring deep within the brain or brain stem (*lacune* means little lake or pond). These strokes are due to occlusion of tiny penetrating arterioles that supply the deep brain substance, usually in the region of the basal ganglia, thalamus, and internal capsule, as well as the brain stem. These small strokes may cause discrete clinical symptoms, such as a pure motor stroke (hemiparesis without sensory loss) or pure sensory stroke.

52. How do hemorrhagic strokes differ from the other three types?

An intracerebral hemorrhage is classified as a stroke because of its abrupt onset with focal neurologic deficits, but it is due to rupture of a blood vessel, with subsequent bleeding and intracerebral mass, rather than to ischemia directly. Intracerebral bleeds have an abrupt onset and are usually accompanied by a significant headache and other signs of increased intracranial pressure, such as nausea, vomiting, and a diminished mental status. These are often devastating events with a poor prognosis. Bleeds tend to occur in the same deep locations as lacunae (i.e., the basal ganglia and brain stem).

53. What are the leading causes of death shortly after a stroke?

The three leading causes of death in the first 30 days after a stroke are not related primarily to the stroke itself or to neurologic deficits:

- Pneumonia
- Pulmonary embolus
- Ischemic heart disease

54. Discuss the medical management of the patient with acute stroke.

Medical management of the stroke patient should focus on the complications that develop after the stroke. Since the leading cause of death is **pneumonia**, care should be taken that the patient does not aspirate—keep the patient NPO until it is clear that swallowing is not impaired by neurologic damage. Fever should always be presumed to be pneumonia until proved otherwise. Measures to prevent **pulmonary embolus** should be instituted, including early mobilization. **Ischemic heart disease** commonly causes death, since atherosclerosis affecting the cerebral vasculature probably also involves the coronary arteries. Cardiac assessment should be individualized.

55. When should thrombolysis be used to treat acute ischemic strokes?

Recombined tissue plasminogen activator (TPA) is approved for the acute treatment of ischemic stroke, but only in certain settings. It must be given as soon as possible after the stroke and certainly within the first 3 hours. A CT scan of the head must not show any evidence of infarction (i.e., tissue damage must not be severe or hemorrhage). The patient must have significant deficits (the drug should not be used if the patient will recover well without it), and there should be no other contraindications, such as active bleeding or severe hypertension. Few patients, in fact, meet all these requirements and are candidates for TPA.

56. How is thrombolytic therapy given?

Patients are treated with 0.9 mg/kg TPA given over 1 hour after an initial 10% bolus. Studies suggest that such patients show approximately 30% more recovery of function than untreated patients. The risk of intracranial hemorrhage is approximately 6%; patients should be carefully monitored.

Halley EC: Thrombolysis in the treatment of acute ischemic stroke. Curr Treat Opt Neurol 5: 377–380, 2003.

57. When is anticoagulation indicated in cerebrovascular disease?

The role of anticoagulation in cerebrovascular disease is highly controversial. The consensus among neurologists is that anticoagulation is mainly of benefit to prevent embolic stroke from the heart. Following an initial brain embolus from a cardiac source, the risk of subsequent emboli is high, especially within the first few days and weeks, and evidence suggests that immediate anticoagulation reduces the risk. Although there is a chance that anticoagulation will worsen a stroke by converting the ischemia into hemorrhage, data suggest that this worsening is more than outweighed by the benefits in preventing further emboli.

Brott T, Bogousslavsky J: Treatment of acute ischemic stroke. N Engl J Med 343:710–722, 2000.

58. Discuss the role of aspirin in the management of cerebrovascular diseases.

Aspirin, given at the time of a stroke, may have some protective effects. Patients with TIA or minor stroke are often treated with aspirin, usually 1 tablet (325 mg) per day, to prevent further episodes of cerebrovascular ischemia. There may be additional benefits to combining aspirin with dipyridamole.

59. What is the role of ticlopidine and clopidogrel in the management of cerebrovascular disease?

Ticlopidine, like aspirin, acts as a platelet inhibitor and similarly decreases the risk of further cerebrovascular ischemia. Unlike aspirin, it does not affect the cyclo-oxygenase pathway and instead acts by interfering with platelet membrane interactions. **Clopidogrel** is another antiplatelet agent with similar properties. Their current role is primarily for the prevention of stroke in patients with cerebral ischemia for whom aspirin therapy has failed, has caused intolerable side effects, or is otherwise contraindicated.

60. What is the main indication for carotid endarterectomy in cerebrovascular disease?
For patients with symptomatic atherosclerotic stenosis of > 70% in the carotid artery, carotid endarterectomy is clearly beneficial, significantly decreasing the risk of ipsilateral stroke.

61. Discuss the role of carotid endarterectomy in asymptomatic patients.
In asymptomatic patients with atherosclerotic stenosis of the carotids, the role of carotid endarterectomy is less clear. Three large randomized trials done in the early 1990s detected no benefit of endarterectomy in these patients. However, the Asymptomatic Carotid Atherosclerosis Study (ACAS) demonstrated a reduction in cerebral infarction in asymptomatic patients with as little as 60% stenosis, provided perioperative morbidity was kept to a minimum. The benefits were sufficiently modest that not all experts were convinced of the utility of surgery, and considerable individual variation remains among physicians managing such patients. Clearly, any surgical intervention in the treatment of carotid artery stenosis must be used in addition to, not in lieu of, aggressive control of modifiable risk factors.

North American Symptomatic Carotid Endarterectomy Trial Collaborators: Benefit of carotid endarterectomy in patients with symptomatic moderate or severe stenosis. N Engl J Med 339: 1415–1425, 1998.

APHASIA

62. Define aphasia.
Aphasia is an acquired disturbance in language functions (i.e., the ability to manipulate sounds and symbols into concepts, words, and phrases). It must not be confused with dysarthria or slurred speech, which is strictly a problem with the motor control of talking. Aphasics not only have difficulty with talking but also with writing, reading, and all other forms of language production.

63. What is the most common cause of aphasia in adults?
The most common cause of aphasia in adults is cerebrovascular disease.

64. Define fluent aphasias.
Fluent aphasias are due to lesions in the cortex in the posterior part of the dominant hemisphere, around the posterior temporal lobe. Such aphasias—also known as **Wernicke's**, sensory, receptive, or posterior aphasia—result in speech that is fluent and even loquacious, but senseless. These patients can talk but make no sense. They have many neologisms and paraphasic errors, inventing words and sounds as they go along and stringing words together in nongrammatical, meaningless fashions. Patients usually have impaired naming, repetition, and severely impaired comprehension as well.

65. How do nonfluent aphasias differ from fluent aphasias?
Nonfluent aphasias are generally produced by lesions in the cortex, in the anterior part of the dominant hemisphere around the sylvian fissure, and are often referred to by other expressions such as **Broca's**, motor, expressive, or anterior aphasia. Such patients have difficulty producing language and either cannot speak or do so only in monosyllables and short telegraphic phrases. Naming and repetition are also impaired, but comprehension is relatively preserved.

66. Compare the two main types of aphasia.
See Table 14-2.

TABLE 14-2. COMPARISON OF THE TWO MAIN TYPES OF APHASIA				
Type	Fluent	Names	Repeats	Comprehends
Broca's	No	No	No	Yes
Wernicke's	Yes	No	No	No

SEIZURES

67. What is an epileptic seizure?
An epileptic seizure is the abnormal discharge of a neuron or group of neurons that leads to excessive electrical activity in the brain, causing disruption of brain function sufficient to produce clinical symptoms such as staring spells or jerking of muscles.

68. What are the main kinds of epileptic seizures?

Generalized seizures	Partial seizures
Generalized tonic-clonic (grand mal)	Partial simple (focal)
Generalized absence (petit mal)	Partial complex (psychomotor)

69. Describe the clinical features of partial simple seizures.
Most partial simple seizures encountered in a medical setting consist of the focal jerking or twitching of an arm or leg on one side of the body. This is usually due to a structural lesion in the brain (such as a stroke, abscess, or tumor) that leads to local irritation and an epileptic discharge. If this discharge spreads, the focal seizure also spreads, sometimes involving the other side of the brain and causing twitching or jerking of both arms and legs (generalized tonic-clonic or grand mal seizure). Occasionally, metabolic lesions, especially hyperglycemia and hyperosmolar states, can cause focal lesions and focal partial seizures.

70. Describe the clinical features of partial complex seizures.
Partial complex seizures may be preceded by an aura of abnormal smells or tastes, visual sensations, or mental phenomena, such as *deja-vu.* The seizure itself may consist of an episode of staring, lip smacking, and automatic, semipurposeful movements, such as picking at clothes. Often there is no jerking of muscles, no loss of tone, and no falling down. Patients, however, are in a state of significantly altered mental status and often completely unresponsive. After a minute or two, the seizure passes, leaving a postictal state of confusion and lethargy.

71. Which group is most likely to develop generalized absence seizures?
Generalized absence seizures, sometimes referred to as petit mal, are seen almost exclusively in children. These seizures usually do not have a significant aura or postictal state but may consist of just a few seconds of staring and altered mental status. This may be so brief as to escape detection by untrained observers. At other times, children are thought to be daydreaming rather than experiencing a seizure.

72. How do generalized tonic-clonic seizures present?
Generalized tonic-clonic seizures, the so-called grand mal seizures, consist of the sudden onset, often without any preceding aura, of jerking tonic and clonic activity of both arms and both legs, with a generalized increase in muscle tone and loss of consciousness. There may be tongue biting or incontinence. Seizures usually last a minute or two and then resolve, often with a period of postictal lethargy and confusion.

73. How do the identifiable causes of seizures vary by age?
See Table 14-3.

TABLE 14-3. COMMON CAUSES OF SEIZURES BY AGE

Neonate to 3 Yr	3–20 Years	20–60 Years	> 60 Years
Prenatal injury	Genetic predisposition	Brain tumors	Vascular disease
Perinatal injury	Infections	Trauma	Brain tumors, esp. metastatic tumors
Metabolic defects	Trauma	Vascular disease	
Congenital malformations	Congenital malformations	Infections	Trauma
CNS infections	Metabolic defects		Systemic metabolic derangements
Postnatal trauma			Infections

74. What are the most common causes of seizures seen in the emergency department or on the medical ward?
Anticonvulsant withdrawal. Most patients seen here are known epileptics who have been taking medicine and, for one reason or another, are noncompliant with their drugs. Alcohol withdrawal, drug overdose, and metabolic derangements such as hyponatremia are other common causes. Structural brain disease, including stroke and meningitis, is a less common cause of seizures.

75. How do alcohol withdrawal seizures present?
Such seizures generally occur 12–48 hours after cessation or abrupt reduction in the intake of alcohol. These seizures are always generalized tonic-clonic seizures, without focality. They are often single, isolated seizures, but sometimes patients may have two or more over a span < 6 hours. Status epilepticus is rare after alcohol withdrawal but does occasionally occur. Alcohol withdrawal seizures seldom persist and are self-limited.

76. What are the most important principles of seizure management?
Most seizures can be controlled completely, or nearly so, by following three basic principles:

- Pick the most appropriate anticonvulsant for the type of seizure that the patient is experiencing.
- Steadily increase the dose of that drug, guided by serum anticonvulsant levels, until seizures are controlled. If drug toxicity develops before the seizures stop, the drug is not the appropriate one; try a different one. Obviously, increase the new anticonvulsant to therapeutic levels before tapering of the old drug.
- Monotherapy is preferable. Good therapeutic levels of one drug are preferable to subtherapeutic levels of multiple drugs.

77. Which drugs are the most useful anticonvulsants for the different types of seizures?
See Table 14-4.

78. How is status epilepticus treated?

1. Rapid history and physical examination, including airway, breathing, circulation.
2. Start IV and draw blood for complete blood count (CBC), electrolytes, anticonvulsant levels. Administer thiamine and glucose.

TABLE 14-4. USEFUL ANTICONVULSANTS FOR THE DIFFERENT TYPES OF SEIZURES

	Pheny-toin	Carba-mazepine	Phenobar-bital	Etheo-suximide	Valproate	Gaba-pentin	Lamo-trigine
Partial simple	+	+	+		+	+	
Partial complex	+	+	+			+	+
Generalized absence			+	+			
Generalized tonic-clonic	+	+	+		+		

Adapted from Brodie MJ, French, JA: Management of epilepsy in adolescents and adults. Lancet 356:323–329, 2000.

3. Infuse fosphenytoin by slow IV push at 50 mg/min to a dose of ~20 mg/kg (1500 mg). To break a continuous seizure, give diazepam up to 20 mg or lorazepam up to 8 mg.
4. Infuse IV phenobarbital, 100 mg/min up to 600 mg.
5. Institute general anesthesia.

79. When should you intubate a patients with status epilepticus?
Experts disagree about when to intubate that patient. Some do it in step 2; others wait until step 4. You should always be prepared to immediately intubate any patient in status epilepticus.

Treiman DM: Convulsive status epilepticus. Curr Treat Options Neurol 1:359–369, 1999.

MOVEMENT DISORDERS

80. What is Parkinson's disease?
Parkinson's disease is a gradual, progressive, degenerative disease of the basal ganglia (extrapyramidal) motor system.

81. List the four cardinal features of Parkinson's disease.
- Tremor
- Rigidity
- Bradykinesia (slowness of movement)
- Postural instability

82. Describe the tremor of Parkinson's disease.
The tremor is usually a to-and-fro, pronation-supination, resting tremor that diminishes with voluntary movement. It is coarse and slow and most prominent in the hands and head.

83. Describe the rigidity of Parkinson's disease.
The rigidity is associated with a diffuse increase in muscular tone and sometimes a "cog-wheeling" property to the joints when passively moved.

84. How does bradykinesia manifest in Parkinson's disease?
Patients exhibit a paucity or lack of movement and tend to show minimal axial expression. They often sit quite immobile, almost like statues.

85. What is the differential diagnosis of Parkinson's disease?
A few conditions can cause parkinsonism, a symptom complex that mimics idiopathic Parkinson's disease. The most common examples are the neuroleptic drugs. Similar symptoms also can be mimicked by multiple strokes, hydrocephalus, and degenerative conditions such as Alzheimer's disease.

86. How is Parkinson's disease treated?
The best treatment is a combination of levodopa plus carbidopa (Sinemet). The main cause for the symptoms of Parkinson's disease is a deficiency of dopamine within the pathway running from the substantia nigra to the basal ganglia. Since dopamine cannot be given directly (because it does not cross the blood-brain barrier), it is given as levodopa. Other dopamine agonists are sometimes used to supplement Sinemet. Anticholinergic agents, which suppress the overactive cholinergic system and bring it into balance with the diminished dopamine system, can also alleviate symptoms.

87. What are the important types of tremors other than the resting tremor of Parkinson's disease?
- **Essential tremor.** This rapid, fine tremor involving the head and arms becomes more noticeable with sustained postures or intentional movement. A family history, with an autosomal dominant inheritance, is seen in about half the cases. Treatment may include a beta blocker (propranolol, 80 mg/day) or primidone (starting at 50 mg/day).
- **Cerebellar tremor.** Damage to the cerebellum disturbs motor control by causing a tremor. The tremor is absent at rest and appears only with intentional or voluntary movements. It is a slow, coarse, dyssynergic tremor. Other evidence of cerebellar dysfunction may be present. Pharmacologic treatment is generally unsatisfactory.

Lambert D, Waters CH: Essential tremor. Curr Treat Options Neurol 1: 6–13, 1999.

88. What are dystonias?
Dystonias, as the name suggests, are disorders of muscle tone that result in involuntary, sustained muscle contractions. They can lead to abnormal posturing or unique repetitive movements. Examples include spasmodic torticollis, blepharospasm, and oromandibular dystonia.

89. How are dystonias treated?
Relief can often be obtained by injecting the muscles with botulinum toxin (Botox).

HEADACHE

90. What are the three key principles in evaluating headache?
- The brain is anesthetic. This means that most causes of head pain do not arise from the brain itself but rather from surrounding structures, such as blood vessels or periosteum. Since most headaches are not caused by brain disease, most are benign.
- The more severe the headache, the more benign the disease. The exception to this rule is intracranial hemorrhage, but, in general, most severe headaches are due to self-limited causes.
- Eye problems and sinus disease seldom cause headaches. Patients tend to blame their headaches on eye strain or sinusitis, but, in fact, these are rare causes.

91. List the common types of headache.
- Common migraine (without aura)
- Classic migraine (with aura)
- Tension headaches

92. What are the less common types of headaches?
Other less common or rare types of headaches include cluster headaches and headaches from brain tumor, meningeal irritation, and temporal arteritis.

93. Which serious diseases capable of causing permanent neurologic dysfunction can present as headaches?
Most processes causing headache are benign, but some are serious. Examples include:

1. Primary brain tumor
2. Metastatic brain tumor
3. Abscess
4. Subdural hematoma
5. Intracerebral hemorrhage
6. Subarachnoid hemorrhage
7. Meningitis
8. Temporal artery disease
9. Hypertension
10. Hydrocephalus
11. Glaucoma

94. What clinical features are seen with increased intracranial pressure (ICP)?
Because the brain is completely surrounded by the hard bony skull, any increase in ICP can impair brain function. The most sensitive indicator of increased ICP is an altered mental status, and it is usually the first symptom to change as the pressure rises. With increased pressure, the brain can herniate downward through the foramen magnum, compressing and destroying the brain stem. Herniation can be recognized by the development of brain-stem signs as the top of the brain stem (midbrain) becomes impaired. In addition to altered mental status, these signs include dilatation of one or both pupils ("blown pupil"), hyperventilation, and focal neurologic signs such as hemiparesis. Herniation can progress to coma and death.

95. What basic principle underlies all techniques of lowering ICP?
Lowering ICP requires reduction of the intracranial contents to make room for the mass lesion and increased pressure. The intracranial contents consist essentially of the brain, CSF filling the ventricles, and blood within the blood vessels.

96. List four specific techniques for lowering ICP.

- **Lowering blood pressure** lowers the ICP and can be accomplished with a diuretic such as furosemide.
- **Incubation and hyperventilation** cause vasospasm that reduces the blood volume intracranially.
- **Steroids** can reduce swelling secondary to vasogenic edema. They may take hours or days to work and have little value acutely.
- **Shunting** can be used in emergency situations to remove CSF and to lower ICP.

97. How does intracranial hemorrhage present?
Intracranial hemorrhage causes the abrupt onset of an extremely severe headache. Patients report that it is "the worst headache in my life." Approximately half of these patients die at the time of the bleed. The remainder usually present to an emergency department with an altered mental status but may not have significant focal neurologic findings.

98. What causes intracranial hemorrhage?
The bleeding may result from the rupture of a vessel outside the brain (subarachnoid hemorrhage) or inside the brain (intracerebral hematoma). **Subarachnoid hemorrhage** is usually due to the rupture of a small intracranial aneurysm, called a berry aneurysm, often located on the anterior communicating artery, middle cerebral artery, or their branches.

99. What is temporal arteritis?
Temporal arteritis is a **giant cell arteritis,** which is a systemic illness with generalized symptoms such as fevers, myalgias, arthralgias (polymyalgia rheumatica), anemia, and elevated liver function tests. The headache is a mild-to-moderate diffuse pain, not necessarily confined to the

temples or frontal region of the head. The disease should be suspected in elderly people, over age 55, who develop new headaches.

100. How is temporal arteritis diagnosed?
The erythrocyte sedimentation rate (ESR) is usually very elevated, >100 mm/min, and is a good screening test. The confirmatory test is a temporal artery biopsy showing granulomatous arteries.

101. How is temporal arteritis treated?
High-dose steroids for a period of 1–2 years are often required, sometimes in doses of 60 mg/day of prednisone equivalent or more. Approximately 15% of patients, if left untreated, develop significant visual loss.

102. What are migraine headaches?
Migraine headaches are paroxysmal, intermittent headaches occurring on an average of once a month and lasting from 4–12 hours or more. Migraines typically begin in the teenage years, sometimes even in childhood, and diminish in both frequency and intensity of attacks in later adulthood. About half of all patients with migraine have a family history of the problem.

103. What are the common symptoms of migraines?

- About one third of patients have hemicranial pain, but in two thirds of patients the headache is diffuse over the entire head.
- Some patients have a preceding aura for 20–40 minutes before the headache. This often consists of visual changes, such as flashing lights.
- Gastrointestinal disturbances are very common, including nausea, vomiting, and anorexia. If the patient can eat during the headache, it is probably not migraine!
- Photophobia and phonophobia.
- Mood changes.
- Visual or sensory loss.

104. What causes migraine headaches?
The cause is not entirely understood. Probably low serotonin levels in the brain trigger certain brainstem neurons to fire, which alters cerebral function and blood flow. The nausea, neurologic deficits, and head pain result from low brain serotonin levels, aggravated by concomitant vascular changes.

105. What is the best treatment for a migraine headache?
For symptomatic relief from mild to moderate migraines, simple analgesics or NSAIDs such as aspirin or naproxen may be sufficient. For more severe attacks, triptans are the drugs of choice. Sumatriptan, a 5-hydroxytryptamine receptor agonist, was the first triptan to be used, but multiple other triptans are now available in various routes of administration. Patients should be warned of the flushing, sweating, and chest tightness that can occur as side effects.

106. When is prophylactic therapy indicated for migraine headaches?
For patients having frequent headaches (2–3/month or more) or for the occasional patient whose headache is complicated by persistent neurologic deficits, prophylactic treatment may be indicated.

107. Which drugs may be used for prophylaxis of migraine headaches?

- **Amitriptyline**, a tricyclic compound. Doses of 100 mg/day or more may be necessary. Many other tricyclics are not effective.
- **Propranolol**, a beta-adrenergic blocking agent. Again, doses of 100 mg/day or more may be needed. Most other beta-adrenergic blockers are not effective.
- **Calcium channel blockers**. Both nifedipine and verapamil are useful.
- **Anticonvulsants**, especially valproic acid, are sometimes effective.

Ferrari MD: Migraine. Lancet 351:1051–1093, 1998.

108. Describe the clinical features of tension headaches.
Tension headaches are diffuse headaches, often described as a band around the head, usually bifrontal but sometimes occipital. Unlike migraine, these headaches are usually not paroxysmal but are constant and chronic. Like migraine, they are more common in women and generally begin early in life. About half of the patients have a family history. Usually, there are no associated neurologic symptoms (such as visual changes) or nausea and vomiting.

109. What causes tension headaches?
The cause is not known. There is no convincing evidence that they are due to psychological factors or emotional stress, nor do sound data show that they are related to muscle contraction. Some of them may be transformed migraines.

110. How should tension headaches be treated?
Amitriptyline, up to 75–150 mg/day, works independently of its antidepressant effects. NSAIDs are useful for common headaches but are seldom successful in chronic persistent tension headache. Muscle relaxants are not effective.

DEMENTIA

111. Define dementia.
Dementia is a progressive decline in cognitive and intellectual functions in the presence of a clear sensorium. Dementia implies that the person has lost intellectual function from a baseline state—i.e., he or she was not born mentally retarded (the process is acquired) and is not delirious, lethargic, or otherwise suffering from an impaired level of consciousness.

112. List the major causes of dementia along with their incidence.
- Senile dementia of Alzheimer's type (50–60%)
- Multi-infarct dementia (MID) (10–20%)
- Combination Alzheimer's and MID (10–20%)
- Other disorders (5–10%)
- Reversible or partially reversible causes (20–30%)

113. What are the other possible causes of dementia?
Other causes of dementia include neurosyphilis, hypothyroidism, HIV infection, neoplasm, subdural hematoma, and head trauma. The old belief that generalized atherosclerosis and global reduction in blood flow can cause dementia has proved correct in only rare cases.

Cerebrovascular disease essentially does not cause dementia except by actual destruction (infarction) of brain tissue, as in MID.

Small GW, et al: Diagnoses and treatment of Alzheimer's disease and related disorders. JAMA 278:1363–1371, 1997.

114. Summarize the general approach to the patient with dementia.
Most dementias, such as Alzheimer's disease, have no effective treatment, so the evaluation of any patient presenting with dementia generally focuses on finding the treatable causes, even though these are uncommon.

115. List the reversible causes of dementia.
The reversible causes can be remembered with the aid of the mnemonic **DEMENTIA:**

D = Drugs
E = Emotional disorders (pseudodementia or depression)
M = Metabolic and endocrine disorders (hepatic encephalopathy, hypothyroidism, chronic renal failure)

E = Eye and ear dysfunction
N = Nutritional deficiencies, normal pressure hydrocephalus (NPH)
T = Tumor, trauma (including chronic subdural hematoma)
I = Infections (neurosyphilis, chronic meningitis)
A = Alcohol, arterosclerotic complications

116. After the history and physical exam, what tests are used to screen for reversible diagnosis?
A work-up includes CT scan or MRI to image the brain, an electroencephalogram (EEG) to show metabolic encephalopathies (diffuse slowing) or some specific dementias (e.g., periodic sharp waves seen in Creutzfeldt-Jakob disease), and sometimes lumbar puncture to rule out neurosyphilis, cryptococcal meningitis, or other chronic infections. CSF analysis may reveal normal pressure hydrocephalus. Blood studies detect most other causes of dementia, such as hypothyroidism, vitamin B_{12} deficiency, and vasculitis.

117. What is Alzheimer's disease?
Alzheimer's disease is a degenerative dementing process of unknown etiology. Most elderly patients who were once termed "senile" probably had Alzheimer's disease, which is now thought to be a specific, distinct disease entity rather than the mere loss of intellectual function with normal aging. Pathologically, Alzheimer's disease is characterized by degenerative changes in the brain, especially senile plaques, neurofibrillary tangles, and granulovacuolar degeneration.

118. How is Alzheimer's disease diagnosed?
There is no biologic marker or specific test for Alzheimer's disease. The clinical diagnosis is largely one of exclusion. Clinical criteria for the diagnosis of Alzheimer's disease include:
- Proof of dementia by neuropsychological testing
- Deficits in two or more areas of cognition (i.e., not just memory loss)
- Progressive worsening
- No disturbance of consciousness
- Onset between ages 40 and 90 (usually after age 65)
- Absence of other causes of dementia

119. Is there any treatment for Alzheimer's disease?
Because levels of the neurotransmitter acetylcholine are low in Alzheimer's disease, treatment aims to increase concentrations by inhibiting cholinesterase. The drugs donepezil and rivastigmine are among the most commonly used. Memantine, an NMDA receptor antagonist, may also have some modest benefits. However, no treatment alters the underlying degenerative process.

MULTIPLE SCLEROSIS

120. What is multiple sclerosis (MS)?
MS is the most common disabling neurologic disease of young people under age 40, affecting approximately 250,000 Americans. It is probably an autoimmune disease, characterized by relapsing and remitting episodes of inflammation in the brain and spinal cord. This inflammation destroys the myelin, which is the insulating sheath around nerve cells, and hence destroys the ability of the nerves to conduct electrical impulses (action potentials).

121. Describe the clinical symptoms of MS.
Clinically, MS may affect almost any part of the brain or spinal cord (Table 14-5). Generally, symptoms come on fairly abruptly, over a period of hours to days, persist for several weeks, and then resolve over a period of several more weeks, often returning completely to normal. On average, patients have one attack per year, although about 20% of patients have a chronic

progressive course with steady worsening deficits, without abrupt attacks. The highly variable presentation of MS reflects the fact that it may involve the optic nerves, spinal cord, pyramidal tracts, spinothalamic tracts, brain stem, or cerebellum.

TABLE 14-5. MOST COMMON SYMPTOMS OF MULTIPLE SCLEROSIS

Focal weakness	45%	Cerebellar ataxia	30%
Optic neuritis	40%	Diplopia and nystagmus	25%
Focal numbness	35%	Bowel and bladder changes	20%

122. **Can any treatments alter the natural course of MS?**
While a cure for MS remains elusive, some therapies may actually alter the natural course of MS. Beta interferon-1a (Rebif or Avonex), beta interferon-1b (Betaseron), and glatiramer acetate (Copaxone) decrease the number of yearly relapses in patients with MS, as demonstrated in large clinical trials. The drugs seem equally effective, cutting attacks by approximately one third. Major side effects of beta interferon include flulike symptoms and leukopenia. Copaxone has relatively few side effects; mild injection site inflammation is the only one of note. Despite their apparent benefit in decreasing relapses of MS, none of the drugs has shown much benefit in patients with chronic progressive MC, nor is it clear how well they prevent ultimate disability.

Rolak LA: Multiple sclerosis. Clin Med Res 1:57–60, 2003.

123. **How long do patients survive the onset of MS?**
MS may be disabling but is seldom fatal. Most patients experience intermittent relapses for 5–15 years, followed by a more chronic progressive phase of variable duration. The life expectancy is almost normal and about one third of patients never experience significant disability.

COMA

124. **What are the most common causes of coma?**
- Drugs (e.g., alcohol, illicit drugs, accidental or intentional overdose)
- Hypoxia
- Hypoglycemia
- Other metabolic derangements (e.g., sepsis, uremia, hepatic failure)
- Structural brain disease (e.g., stroke, intracranial hemorrhage)

125. **Outline the approach to the patient in coma.**
- ABCs—protect the airway, breathing, and circulation.
- Draw blood to check for metabolic derangements, infections, and drugs.
- Infuse glucose, thiamine, and naloxone.
- History and physical exam for clues to the cause of coma. Focus on pupils and extraocular movements for evidence of brain-stem dysfunction.
- Definitive diagnosis (and therapy) may require CT scanning, lumbar puncture, EEG, and other studies, depending on the situation.

KEY POINTS: NEUROLOGY II

1. The most common cause of dizziness is benign paroxysmal positional vertigo.
2. The leading causes of death after a stroke are medical complications, not the stroke itself.
3. Although heparin may prevent some future strokes, it has no value in the acute treatment of strokes.
4. The sudden onset of a severe headache may be an intracranial hemorrhage.
5. Despite a long differential, it is rare to find a treatable cause of dementia.
6. Most etiologies of coma are medical problems, not primary neurologic diseases.

126. What is the prognosis of coma?

Almost 70% of patients admitted to a hospital in a coma die. Brain-stem abnormalities—absent extraocular movements, gag reflex, or spontaneous respirations, or unreactive pupils—carry an especially grim prognosis.

Hamel MB et al: Identification of comatose patients at high risk for death or severe disability. JAMA 273:1742–1484, 1995.

OTHER MEDICAL CONDITIONS

127. How does alcohol affect the nervous system?

Alcohol can affect virtually any part of the nervous system:

- Alcoholic myopathy: occurs in heavy drinkers in a fashion analogous to alcoholic cardiomyopathy.
- Acute rhabdomyolysis: rare, associated with heavy alcohol consumption.
- Peripheral neuropathy: usually a distal, symmetric, stocking-and-glove sensory and motor polyneuropathy.
- Nerve compression: increased susceptibility in alcoholics (e.g., "Saturday night" palsy).
- Fulminant necrotic myelopathy: rare, associated with heavy alcohol intake.
- Wernicke's encephalopathy: due to thiamine deficiency secondary to alcoholism.
- Cerebellar ataxia: alcohol leads to degeneration of the anterior (dermis) region of the cerebellum, causing an ataxic gait.
- Alcoholic dementia: amnesia (Korsakoff's syndrome) and generalized dementia.

Charness ME: Alcohol. In Noseworthy JH (ed): Neurological Therapeutics. London, Martin-Dunitz, 2003, pp 1502–1503.

128. What triad of findings is seen in Wernicke's encephalopathy?

Alcohol can affect the brain stem in the classic Wernicke's encephalopathy, which causes a triad of:

- Nystagmus with extraocular abnormalities
- Cerebellar ataxia
- Confusion

129. How is Wernicke's encephalopathy treated?

Wernicke's is really due to a thiamine deficiency rather than to alcohol ingestion itself. The brain-stem signs reverse readily with parenteral thiamine infusion, but the confusion resolves more slowly.

130. How does HIV affect the nervous system?

HIV can cause widespread damage in the nervous system, probably entering through macrophages that cross the blood-brain barrier. Approximately 10% of all AIDS patients present initially with neurologic symptoms, and up to 50% develop neurologic complications at some point during their illness.

131. What are the most common neurologic complications of HIV infection?

- Inflammatory myopathy: similar to polymyositis, with symptoms of slowing progressive proximal weakness. Zidovudine may also cause a similar reversible myopathy.
- Peripheral neuropathy: distal symmetric (glove-and-stocking) pattern, with distal burning and other dysesthesias, seen in approximately 30% of patients.
- Acute inflammatory demyelinating polyneuropathy: like Guillain-Barré syndrome but with CSF pleocytosis.
- AIDS myelopathy: vacuolar degeneration resembling vitamin B_{12} deficiency, a chronic progressive spinal cord syndrome.
- HIV encephalopathy: progressive dementia manifested by apathy, personality change, and/or loss of higher cognitive functions.
- Aseptic meningitis: due to HIV itself.

Klepser ME, Klepser TB: Drug treatment of HIV-related opportunistic infections. Drugs 53: 40–73, 1997.

132. What two conditions should be suspected when a CT scan reveals CNS mass lesions in a patient with AIDS?

Cerebral toxoplasmosis and primary CNS lymphoma.

133. What are the effects of diabetes mellitus (DM) on the peripheral nervous system?

The primary effect of DM on the nervous system is on the peripheral nerves. The most frequent problem is a distal, symmetric, stocking-and-glove sensory and motor **polyneuropathy**.

134. Discuss the mononeuropathy associated with DM.

Mononeuropathy can occur because the small vessel disease that accompanies DM frequently leads to infarction of nerves by occlusion of the vasa nervorum. Femoral neuropathies and cranial nerve palsies are particularly common. Another type of neuropathy is thoracoabdominal neuropathy, in which a thoracic root is damaged leading to severe chest or abdominal pin that is often mistaken for a visceral crisis.

135. How does DM affect the autonomic nervous system?

Effects on the autonomic nervous system may lead to impotence, bowel and bladder dysfunction, gastroparesis, orthostatic hypotension, or arrhythmias.

136. In what ways does diabetes affect the CNS?

Involvement of the CNS by diabetes is more indirect than its effects on the peripheral nerves. Because diabetes is a risk factor for atherosclerosis, there is an increased incidence of stroke. **Hypoglycemia** from overmedication can lead to focal neurologic findings, such as hemiparesis or aphasia, or, if severe, altered mental status including coma. **Hyperglycemia**, from diabetic ketoacidosis or from nonketotic hyperosmolar states, also causes altered mental status, sometimes accompanied by seizures.

137. How does renal failure affect the nervous system?

- Uremia is one of he most common metabolic abnormalities affecting the nervous system, especially the peripheral nerves, where there is a stocking-and-glove distal, symmetric, sensorimotor neuropathy.

- Patients with renal failure are prone to metabolic encepahalopathies causing confusion, lethargy, and even coma.
- Because of the anticoagulation necessary for dialysis, there is an increased incidence of intracerebral hemorrhage, such as subdural hematomas.

138. What is dialysis encephalopathy?
A special type of mental status change is the syndrome of dialysis encephalopathy, which is a progressive deterioration in mental status, with hyperreflexia and dysarthria, usually accompanied by myoclonus and seizures. This syndrome is often irreversible and progressive until death.

139. How does metastatic cancer present in the brain?
Cancer affects the nervous system primarily by direct invasion. Metastases to the brain occur in 10–30% of patients with primary neoplasms, most commonly in lung and colon cancer in males and breast cancer in females. Metastatic cancer usually presents as a focal neurologic deficit, such as hemiparesis, but may also cause seizures.

140. How does metastatic cancer present in the spinal cord?
Cancer may metastasize or spread locally to the spinal cord, leading to acute spinal cord compression. Usually, this is accompanied by back pain from vertebral body destruction. The onset of symptoms may be sudden with paraparesis, sensory level disturbances, and bowel and bladder disturbances.

141. What other effects of cancer may be seen?
Carcinomatous meningitis is most common in lymphomas and leukemias but can be seen with solid tumors as well. Usually it presents as altered mental status, sometimes with fever and sometimes with focal neurologic deficits as the cancer invades cranial nerves and roots as they emerge from the CNS. Involvement of the peripheral nervous system by direct extension is sometimes seen, such as when a Pancoast's tumor invades the brachial plexus. Peripheral neuropathies are uncommon.

142. How common are paraneoplastic syndromes?
Paraneoplastic syndromes (remote effects of cancer) are quite rare. They may include myopathy (polymyositis), neuromuscular junction deficit (LEMS), and a peripheral neuropathy, predominantly sensory.

WEB SITES

1. www.neuroguide.com
2. www.aan.com (American Academy of Neurology)
3. www.medmatrix.org
4. www.internets.com/mednets/sneurolo.htm
5. www.medwebplus.com/subject/Neurology.html

BIBLIOGRAPHY

1. Aminoff M: Neurology and General Medicine, 3rd ed. Philadelphia, Churchill-Livingstone, 2001.
2. Noseworthy JH (ed): Neurologic Therapeutics. London, Martin Dunitz, 2003.

3. Bradley WG, Daroff RB, Fenichel GM, Jankovic J: Neurology in Clinical Practice, 4th ed. Philadelphia, Butterworth-Heinemann, 2004.
4. Caplan LR: Stroke: A Clinical Approach, 3rd ed. New York, Butterworth-Heinemann, 2000.
5. Samuels MA, Feske S (eds): Office Practice of Neurology, 2nd ed. Boston, Churchill-Livingstone, 2003.
6. Johnson RT, Griffin JW: Current Therapy in Neurologic Disease, 6th ed. St. Louis, Mosby, 2002.
7. Rolak LA (ed): Neurology Secrets, 4th ed. Philadelphia, Hanley & Belfus, 2005.
8. Victor M, Ropper AH: Prinicples of Neurology, 7th ed. New York, McGraw-Hill, 2001.
9. Wyllie E: The Treatment of Epilepsy: Principles and Practice, 3rd ed. Philadelphia, Lea & Febiger, 2002.

CHAPTER 15

MEDICAL CONSULTATION

Jane M. Geraci, M.D., M.P.H.

Physicians who meet in consultation must never quarrel or jeer at one another.

Hippocrates
Precepts VIII

Whenever he [Thomas Jefferson] saw three physicians together, he looked up to discover whether there was not a turkey buzzard in the neighborhood.

Quoted by Dr. Everett,
private secretary to James Monroe

1. **List the characteristics of the best consultations.**
   - Specific question is asked of and answered by the consultant.
   - A conversation between the referring and consulting physician confirms mutual understanding of the recommendations.
   - Recommendations are highly specific (drug dosages, routes and duration of treatment for example) so there is no doubt as to how the plan will be carried out.
   - A follow-up plan is specified in the consult note.

PREOPERATIVE RISK ASSESSMENT

2. **What are the four essential "dos" of preoperative risk assessment?**
   - **Do** interview and examine the patient with respect to major organ-system disease, and describe the extent, severity, and stability of each disease in your assessment.
   - **Do** explain to the patient your estimate of his or her risk of complications of anesthesia and surgery, and document the explanation in your consultation note.
   - **Do** specify how the patient's current medications should be handled in the perioperative period (see also questions 90–106).
   - **Do** make recommendations for venous thromboembolism prophylaxis in patients who may benefit (see also questions 78-83).

3. **List the three essential "don'ts" of preoperative risk assessment.**
   - **Don't** tell the anesthesiologist which type of anesthesia and anesthetic agent to use; this determination is the anesthesiologist's job. The anesthesiologist relies on you for adequate characterization of the patient's burden of medical disease.
   - **Don't** "clear" the patient for surgery—such a step implies complete freedom from risk of adverse events, and we can never guarantee that a patient will not suffer an adverse outcome.
   - **Don't** directly try to change a patient's mind about proceeding with surgery—you are interfering in a patient-doctor relationship! Encourage patients to ask the surgeon questions about the proposed procedure. If you have serious concerns about surgery for a particular patient, call the referring surgeon and speak with him or her in a confidential manner and setting.

4. **Describe general anesthesia (GA).**
   GA provides a loss of sensation with the loss of consciousness. Patients under GA may receive inhaled agents, inhaled plus IV drugs, or IV drugs alone. Ventilation may be managed through a

mask, with or without an oropharyngeal or laryngopharyngeal airway, or through an endotracheal tube.

KEY POINTS: PURPOSE OF THE PREOPERATIVE RISK ASSESSMENT 

1. Describe the patient's current chronic diseases, their management, the patient's level of symptomatology, and whether the diseases are stable.
2. Make an estimate of the patient's risk of postoperative cardiac and noncardiac complications.

5. **How is regional anesthesia (RA) different from GA?**
   RA uses local anesthesia to produce loss of sensation to part of the body. Examples include epidural, spinal, axillary, and other regional blocks. Patients receiving RA also may receive some sedation. A patient undergoing RA may need to receive GA if the block is not adequate.

6. **Explain monitored anesthesia care (MAC).**
   MAC involves an anesthesiologist's management of the patient during a procedure and may include provision of IV sedation, antiemetics or narcotics, and other pharmacologic treatments. MAC sometimes resembles GA in the amount of sedation produced in the patient.

7. **List the three phases of GA.**
   Induction, maintenance, and reversal.

8. **Define induction, and list some of the potential problems.**
   Induction of anesthesia consists of administering medication to the conscious, perceiving patient to produce a state of unconsciousness and lack of perception. Although inhalational agents can be used to induce anesthesia, in current practice induction usually is accomplished by the IV route. Although it is advisable to intubate some patients before induction, endotracheal intubation usually is carried out immediately after induction. Potential problems include retching, vomiting, aspiration, cough, laryngospasm, hypotension, and cardiac dysrhythmias.

9. **Which anesthetic technique is safer for patients—spinal/epidural or general?**
   This is a trick question. The few available well-designed studies that have compared RA with GA found no difference in cardiac outcomes. GA with inhalational agents directly suppresses myocardial contractility and reduces functional residual capacity in the lungs, with increased mismatch of ventilation and perfusion. Hence, inhalational GA may not be optimal for patients with severe cardiac or pulmonary insufficiency. Although spinal and epidural blocks do not have these effects, patients receiving RA can develop hypotension and bradycardia. In addition, the patient's airway is not as easily protected with RA. The higher the level of the spinal/epidural block, the more prominent the hypotension. Spinal and epidural blocks can be administered somewhat more quickly than GA.

10. **What hemodynamic changes occur with spinal anesthesia?**
    Spinal anesthesia (the injection of local anesthetic into the subarachnoid space) blocks transmission of impulses from the sympathetic nervous system as well as impulses mediating motor and sensory functions. The sympathetic nervous system controls the caliber of the blood vessels. At basal levels of sympathetic tone, the vessels are maintained at about half their maximal

diameter. Sympathetic stimulation causes vasoconstriction, whereas sympathetic enervation, as in spinal anesthesia, causes vasodilatation. Vasodilatation causes a drop in systemic vascular resistance and consequent pooling of blood in the lower extremities. Arterial blood pressure usually decreases with administration of spinal anesthesia, and the drop is more severe in patients who are volume-depleted before the anesthetic is given. Patients with hypertension (controlled or not) also tend to have exaggerated hypotensive responses to spinal anesthesia.

11. List the major clinical predictors of perioperative adverse cardiovascular events after noncardiac surgery.

- Unstable coronary syndromes
- Decompensated congestive heart failure (CHF)
- Significant arrhythmias
- Severe valvular disease
- Acute or recent myocardial infarction (MI)

12. What are the intermediate clinical predictors of perioperative adverse cardiovascular events after noncardiac surgery?

Mild angina pectoris, prior MI, compensated/prior CHF, diabetes mellitus, and renal insufficiency.

13. List the minor clinical predictors of perioperative adverse cardiovascular events after noncardiac surgery.

Advanced age, abnormal electrocardiogram, rhythm other than sinus, low functional capacity, history of stroke, uncontrolled hypertension.

Eagle KA et al: ACC/AHA guideline update for perioperative cardiovascular evaluation for noncardiac surgery-executive summary. J Am Coll Cardiol 39:542–53, 2002.

14. Which surgical procedures place the patient at low risk (< 1%) of cardiac complications?

Endoscopic procedures, superficial procedures, cataract surgery, breast surgery.

15. Which surgical procedures place the patient at intermediate risk (< 5%) of cardiac complications?

Carotid endarterectomy, head and neck surgery, intraperitoneal and intrathoracic surgery, orthopedic surgery, prostate surgery.

16. List surgical procedures that place the patient at high risk (> 5%) of cardiac complications.

- Emergent, major surgery, especially in elderly patients
- Major vascular surgery, including aortic surgery
- Peripheral vascular surgery
- Prolonged surgery, with expected large fluid shifts and/or blood loss

Eagle KA et al: ACC/AHA guideline update for perioperative cardiovascular evaluation for noncardiac surgery-executive summary. J Am Coll Cardiol 39:542–53, 2002.

17. Summarize the relationship of patient functional status to postoperative complications.

Poor functional status increases a patient's risk of both cardiac and noncardiac complications of surgery. Assessment of functional status is an essential part of the American College of Cardiology/American Heart Association (ACC/AHA) perioperative assessment guideline.

18. How is functional status assessed?

Cardiologists express functional status in terms of metabolic equivalent (MET) levels. One MET is equal to the oxygen consumption (3.5 mL/kg/min) of a 70-kg, 40-year-old man in a resting state. With this benchmark, functional capacity is excellent in patients who can perform at a level of > 7 METs; moderate at 4–7 METs; and poor if patients cannot meet a 4-MET demand during most daily activities. The 4-MET cut point is used in the ACC/AHA guideline.

19. **Which specific activitites indicate that a patient's functional status is acceptable?**
   - Brisk walks of at least several blocks
   - Climb at least one flight of stairs
   - Heavy housework such as scrubbing tiles and floors and moving furniture
   - Golfing (without a cart) and participation in team sports such as doubles tennis or pitching in baseball
   - More strenuous activities (which approach 10 METs or more in energy consumption), including swimming, singles tennis, basketball, and skiing.

   Eagle KA et al: ACC/AHA guideline update for perioperative cardiovascular evaluation for noncardiac surgery-executive summary. J Am Coll Cardiol 39:542–553, 2002.

20. **Summarize the ACC/AHA approach to patients with major clinical predictors of cardiac risk.**
   Patients with major clinical predictors of cardiac risk (see question 11) should be evaluated and stabilized before elective surgery.

21. **What are the ACC/AHA guidelines for patients with intermediate clinical predictors of cardiac risk?**
   Patients with intermediate clinical predictors of cardiac risk (see question 12) who have poor functional status (< 4 METs) or moderate or excellent (> 4 METs) functional status but who are undergoing high surgical risk procedures (see question 16) should undergo noninvasive cardiac testing to refine risk assessment. Patients with intermediate clinical predictors who are undergoing low surgical risk procedures (see question 14) and patients with moderate to excellent functional status who are undergoing procedures of no more than intermediate risk (see question 15) may go to the operating room without further cardiac evaluation.

22. **Summarize the ACC/AHA guidelines for patients with low clinical predictors of cardiac risk.**
   Patients with minor or no clinical predictors (see question 13) should undergo noninvasive testing only if they have both poor functional status (< 4 METs) and are scheduled to undergo a high surgical risk procedure. All other patients with minor or no clinical predictors may go directly to the operating room.

KEY POINTS: INDICATIONS FOR PREOPERATIVE NONINVASIVE CARDIAC TESTING

1. Patients with intermediate clinical predictors who cannot exert to above 4 METs and need moderate- or high-risk surgery.
2. Patients with intermediate clinical predictors who can exercise to 7 METs but need high-risk elective surgery.
3. Patients with minor or no clinical predictors who cannot exercise to 4 METs and need high-risk elective surgery.
4. Patients who would be candidates for interventions were they not having surgery.

Eagle KA et al: ACC/AHA guideline update for perioperative cardiovascular evaluation for non-cardiac surgery-executive summary. J Am Coll Cardiol 39:542–53, 2002.

23. What is the prevalence of underlying coronary artery disease (CAD) among patients with peripheral vascular disease?

Patients with peripheral vascular disease are highly likely to have CAD. Among 1000 consecutive patients with vascular disease but *no* clinical evidence of CAD who underwent coronary angiography, 37% had at least one coronary artery stenosis > 70%. This can be considered the minimal pretest probability of CAD in a population of patients under consideration for peripheral vascular surgery. However, many patients with vascular disease may have some clinical evidence of CAD, and in such patients the prevalence is far higher. Thus, for the patient population as a group, the incidence is approximately 60%.

Gersh JB, et al: Evaluation and management of patients with both peripheral vascular and coronary artery disease. J Am Coll Cardiol 18:203–214, 1991.

Hertzer NR, et al: Coronary artery disease in peripheral vascular patients: A classification of 1000 coronary angiograms and results of surgical management. Ann Surg 199:223–233, 1984.

24. Discuss the major complication of the cross-clamping procedure and related maneuvers in repair of an abdominal aortic aneurysm.

Ischemia can result in the territories that are served by the clamped arteries. Decreased blood flow during the cross-clamping can result in a number of complications caused by ischemia, including acute renal failure, bowel infarction, and spinal cord damage that may result in paraplegia.

25. What is the risk of embolization of cholesterol fragments into the peripheral circulation?

Embolization of cholesterol and atheromatous fragments from the diseased aorta into the peripheral circulation is a rare complication. Although embolization can result from any angiographic procedure in which an atheromatous blood vessel is cannulated, a study obtained through a femoral artery seems to pose the highest risk.

26. What types of damage may result from embolization?

A shower of cholesterol emboli causes ischemic damage to the skin, extremities, and visceral organs (e.g., intestines and kidneys). Small emboli to the kidneys can cause progressive renal failure; large emboli can obstruct the main renal arteries and cause fulminant acute renal failure.

27. What factors are associated with a higher risk of cholesterol emboli syndrome?

Clues to the diagnosis of cholesterol emboli syndrome include a predisposing procedure in a patient with extensive vascular disease; the presence of leukocytosis, and especially eosinophilia, in the peripheral blood film; and cholesterol crystals in tissue specimens and retinal arteries.

28. Why do general anesthesia and surgery carry a higher risk for perioperative cardiac complications in patients with asymptomatic but significant aortic stenosis (AS)?

AS presents a fixed obstruction to the outflow of blood from the left ventricle (LV). In other words, the stenotic orifice limits maximal cardiac output (CO). In patients with moderately severe AS, arterial dilatation has little ability to increase the CO, because the stenotic valve remains the major obstruction to outflow. Because such patients do not have the normal response to peripheral dilatation, they are prone to hypotension with exercise or other situations in which peripheral dilatation is induced (e.g., anesthesia). Furthermore, because of LV hypertrophy such patients have stiff ventricles so that, for any given intracavitary volume, the pressure is higher than normal. When cardiac return is increased in an effort to augment CO, there is the potential for rapid rises in filling pressures with resultant pulmonary edema.

29. **What specific complications may develop in patients with AS?**
At the time of surgery, patients with AS are at risk for hypotension, pulmonary edema, and MI. Ischemia can develop in patients with AS for several reasons. First, atherosclerotic coronary disease frequently coexists with AS. In addition, the pathophysiologic features of AS also affect myocardial oxygen balance unfavorably. Myocardial hypertrophy is associated with an increase in myocardial oxygen demand, and decreases in aortic pressure, especially during diastole, lead to decreases in myocardial oxygen delivery.

30. **What are the risk factors for perioperative MI with noncardiac surgery?**
In theory, anything that increases myocardial oxygen demand or decreases oxygen supply to the myocardium so that irreversible cell injury occurs is a risk factor for perioperative MI. In practice, however, because of the remarkable range of the autoregulation of perfusion across the coronary bed in people with normal coronary arteries and myocardium, the most important risk factor is heart disease (e.g., stenotic coronary arteries, hypertrophied muscle, dilated chambers). These conditions make the heart less able to compensate for the perturbations of myocardial oxygen demand and supply that may occur with anesthesia and surgery. Sustained hypotension intraoperatively seems to be the most important extraneous risk factor. Sustained intraoperative hypertension does not seem to be as important.

Ashton CM: Perioperative myocardial infarction with noncardiac surgery. Am J Med Sci 308:41–48, 1994.

31. **Which surgical patients should undergo surveillance testing for perioperative MI?**
Patients with known or suspected CAD who undergo high-risk procedures (see question 16) should be considered candidates for electrocardiograms performed at baseline, immediately after surgery, and on postoperative day 2. Biomarkers such as creatine kinase and troponin levels may also be performed in these patients or only in those with electrocardiographic or clinical evidence of cardiovascular dysfunction.

Eagle KA et al: ACC/AHA guideline update for perioperative cardiovascular evaluation for noncardiac surgery-executive summary. J Am Coll Cardiol 39:542–53, 2002.

32. **Summarize the principles of evaluation and management of patients with CHF who must undergo noncardiac surgery.**
Whether CHF results from systolic impairment or diastolic dysfunction, determining the state of compensation is the most important component of the preoperative evaluation—even more important than the ejection fraction. The ejection fraction tells nothing about the state of compensation, and no consistent relationship has been found between ejection fraction and exercise tolerance as determined on a treadmill. It is important to have the patient as well compensated as possible before surgery. CHF is an independent risk factor for perioperative cardiac complications.

33. **What are the symptoms and signs of decompensation?**
New or recent declines in exercise tolerance, increasing fatigue, orthopnea, and paroxysmal nocturnal dyspnea are the symptoms of decompensation. The signs of decompensation are weight increase, jugular venous distention, S_3 gallop, hepatomegaly, and edema.

34. **Explain the significance of postoperative atrial fibrillation (AF).**
AF is common after intrathoracic or cardiac procedures, which may directly irritate the atria and precipitate fibrillation. Patients with chronic pulmonary or cardiac disease also may develop atrial fibrillation because of the combination of the disease and the high catecholamine state that exists after surgery.

35. How are patients with postoperative AF treated?

The evaluation and management of patients with postoperative AF are similar to those for nonsurgical patients. One difference is that, wherever possible, beta blockers or calcium channel blockers are preferred over digoxin for ventricular rate control. These drugs counter the excessive postoperative catecholamines and have anti-ischemic effects, which also may be beneficial. AF often resolves relatively quickly, but if it persists, the patient should be anticoagulated, if possible, to prevent development of atrial thrombus and embolic stroke.

Bach DS: Management of specific medical conditions in the perioperative period. Prog Cardiovasc Dis 40:469–476, 1998.

36. What are the clinically significant pulmonary complications of surgery?

Any pulmonary abnormality that affects the clinical course of the surgical patient is considered clinically significant. Examples include:

- Atelectasis
- Infection, including bronchitis and pneumonia
- Prolonged mechanical ventilation and respiratory failure
- Exacerbation of chronic obstructive pulmonary disease (COPD)
- Bronchospasm

37. What are the definite risk factors for postoperative pulmonary complications?

- Upper abdominal or thoracic surgery
- Surgery lasting more than 3 hours
- Poor general health status, as defined by high ASA class
- COPD
- Smoking history within the past 8 weeks
- Use of pancuronium as a neuromuscular blocker

38. List the probable risk factors for postoperative pulmonary complications.

General anesthesia (versus spinal or epidural anesthesia), obesity, and $PaCO_2 > 45$ mmHg.

39. List the possible risk factors for postoperative pulmonary complications.

Current upper respiratory tract infection, abnormal chest radiograph, and age.

Smetana GW: Evaluation of preoperative pulmonary risk. In UpToDate, vol. 11.3, 2003, with permission.

40. Which surgical patients should undergo preoperative spirometry?

The only group for whom preoperative pulmonary function tests (PFTs) are mandatory is the group under consideration for lung resection. For all other types of surgery, there is no absolute minimal lung function, as assessed by PFTs, for avoidance of postoperative pulmonary complications. In other words, even patients with severe COPD can be managed perioperatively with a satisfactory outcome. Patients with unexplained pulmonary symptoms may benefit from preoperative PFTs, as well as those whose symptoms due to known COPD or asthma may not be optimally controlled.

Smetana GW: Evaluation of preoperative pulmonary risk. In UpToDate, vol. 11.3, 2003, with permission.

41. Which surgical patients should undergo preoperative arterial blood gas (ABG) analysis?

Patients with a $PaCO_2 > 45$ mmHg are at increased risk for postoperative complications. Such patients usually have underlying severe COPD. The ACP recommends preoperative ABG testing for patients undergoing coronary bypass surgery or upper abdominal surgery who have a history of smoking or dyspnea and for patients undergoing lung resection.

Smetana GW: Evaluation of preoperative pulmonary risk. In UpToDate, vol. 11.3, 2003.

42. Which preoperative strategies help to reduce the risk of postoperative pulmonary complications in patients with chronic pulmonary disease?

- Smoking cessation 8 or more weeks before surgery
- Inhaled ipratropium for all patients with clinically significant COPD
- Inhaled beta agonists for patients who wheeze or are dyspneic
- Preoperative systemic corticosteroids for patients who are not optimized to baseline at the time of surgery
- Antibiotics for definite pulmonary infection
- Teaching lung expansion maneuvers to patients before the surgery

43. List intraoperative strategies that help to reduce the risk of postoperative pulmonary complications in patients with chronic pulmonary disease.

- Limit the surgical procedure and anesthesia to less than 3–4 hours in duration
- Surgery other than upper abdominal or thoracic, when possible
- Laparoscopic rather than open abdominal surgery, when possible
- RA for very high-risk patients
- Epidural/spinal anesthesia rather than GA for high-risk patients
- Avoid use of pancuronium in high-risk patients

44. Which postoperative strategies help to reduce the risk of postoperative pulmonary complications in patients with chronic pulmonary disease?

- Lung expansion maneuvers (deep breathing or incentive spirometry) in high-risk patients
- Epidural anesthesia rather than parenteral narcotics

Smetana GW: Evaluation of preoperative pulmonary risk. In UpToDate, vol. 11.3, 2003.

45. Describe the principles of management for asthmatic patients who must undergo nonpulmonary surgery.

The two major principles of managing asthmatic patients are control of bronchospasm and control of secretions. Tracheal intubation can exacerbate bronchospasm and also is associated with increased sputum production. This problem is minimized by ensuring that bronchospasm is under optimal control before the patient goes to the operating room. Inhaled bronchodilators should be administered on a regular schedule, and if the patient is receiving theophylline, the serum level should be kept in the therapeutic range. Secretions can be managed by a pulmonary toilet program perioperatively. Such a program includes incentive spirometry in addition to inhaled bronchodilators. Steroid-dependent asthmatics, in whom adrenal function is often suppressed, should receive IV corticosteroids in the perioperative period to cover the stress of anesthesia and surgery.

46. Are patients with obstructive sleep apnea (OSA) at increased risk for postoperative complications?

When patients undergo surgery, such as uvulopalatopharyngoplasty, to correct OSA, the most common complications are airway-related, but the complication rate is still low. There are no data about outcomes of other noncardiac surgical procedures in patients with OSA. In evaluating a patient with known OSA who is treated with continuous positive airway pressure (CPAP), the consulting physician should determine whether the patient is compliant. Noncompliance with CPAP is quite common. The physician should assess the patient for signs and symptoms of right heart failure. Room-air ABG and electrolyte analyses reveal CO_2 retention consistent with inadequately treated OSA.

Gupta RM, Gay PC: Perioperative cardiopulmonary evaluation and management: Are we ignoring obstructive sleep apnea syndrome? Chest 116:1843, 1999.

47. How can the risk of general medical complications be assessed in patients with chronic liver disease?

Patients with chronic liver disease are at increased risk for medical complications of surgery and anesthesia. The medical consultant should identify the nature of the liver disease (acute or chronic hepatitis and whether cirrhosis is present) and describe its severity. Most studies examining surgical outcomes have evaluated patients with cirrhosis. The Child-Pugh classification of cirrhotic severity has been shown to predict morbidity and mortality (Table 15-1). Patients with acute alcoholic or viral hepatitis, fulminant hepatic failure, or severe and uncorrectable hypoprothrombinemia are not candidates for elective surgery.

Friedman LS: Assessing surgical risk in patients with liver disease. In UpToDate, vol. 11.3, 2003.

TABLE 15-1. CHILD-PUGH CLASSIFICATION OF CIRRHOTIC SEVERITY

	Points Assigned		
Risk Factor	1	2	3
Ascites	Absent	Slight	Moderate
Bilirubin (mg/dL)	< 2	2–3	> 3
Albumin (gm/dL)	> 3.5	2.8–3.5	< 2.8
Prothrombin time			
Seconds over control	1–3	4–6	> 6
INR	< 1.7	1.8–2.3	> 2.3
Encephalopathy	None	Grade 1–2	Grade 3–4
Score interpretations:	5–6 points = grade A (well-compensated disease)		
	7–9 points = grade B (significant functional compromise)		
	10–15 points = grade C (decompensated disease)		
Predicted mortality rate:	Grade A ≅ 10%		
	Grade B ≅ 30%		
	Grade C ≅ 80%		

48. What measures should be undertaken to prepare patients with chronic liver disease for surgery?

- Treatment of hypoprothrombinemia with vitamin K or fresh frozen plasma to achieve a prothrombin time within 3 seconds of normal
- Platelet transfusion to maintain a count of at least 100,000/mL
- Cessation of all alcohol intake
- Treatment and control of ascites with diuretics to reduce the risk of wound dehiscence in the abdomen
- Correction of electrolyte abnormalities, such as hypokalemia
- Consideration of perioperative nutritional support for malnourished patients who must undergo major surgery (e.g., hepatic resection/transplant)

49. Why is cessation of alcohol intake particularly important for patients with alcoholic hepatitis?

For patients with alcoholic hepatitis, cessation of alcohol intake may improve liver function indices. Some experts recommend serum gamma glutamyl transferase (GGT) as a useful marker of hepatic inflammation due to alcohol. GGT levels should return to normal 3–5 weeks after cessation of alcohol intake.

50. What tests should be performed before cataract surgery?

Schein and colleagues randomized over 18,000 patients at nine medical centers to undergo or not to undergo a standard set of preoperative tests (EKG, serum electrolytes, renal function, complete blood count) in addition to the history and physical examination. They found no difference in complication rates between the two groups overall, nor did specific subgroups based on characteristics such as age or medical history benefit from preoperative tests. Based on these results, it appears reasonable to forego routine blood work and EKG for patients whose history and physical examinations reveal no need for such evaluation.

Schein OD, Katz J, Bass EB et al: The value of routine preoperative medical testing before cataract surgery. N Engl J Med 342:168–175, 2000.

51. What is the most useful screening tool for asymptomatic patients who may be at risk for perioperative bleeding due to hereditary hemorrhagic or coagulation disorders?

Patient history is the most useful screening tool for disorders that may cause perioperative hemorrhage, such as von Willebrand's disease or hemophilia. All patients should be questioned about a personal or family history of excessive bleeding after prior surgeries, procedures, or childbirth; history of transfusions; and medication use that may be associated with acquired coagulation defects.

52. What lab tests are used to assess hemostasis?

A prothrombin time, activated partial thromboplastin time, and platelet count should be performed in patients undergoing procedures that have a low risk of hemorrhage (lymph node biopsies, herniorrhaphy, dental extractions), if their history suggests a possible bleeding disorder. Patients undergoing most other procedures have a higher risk of possible hemorrhage, and these tests should be considered independently of the history and physical examination. Additional tests will probably be necessary if one of these parameters is abnormal.

Coutre S: Preoperative assessment of hemostasis. In UpToDate, vol 11.3, 2003, with permission.

53. How should you determine the cause of new-onset renal insufficiency in postoperative patients?

In postoperative patients, as in other populations, it is useful to classify new-onset renal insufficiency as prerenal, renal, or postrenal.

54. What causes prerenal azotemia?

Prerenal azotemia results from decreased renal perfusion. Its causes include intravascular volume depletion due to hemorrhage, GI losses (as with nasogastric suction or ileostomy), or third-spacing of fluids (as with peritonitis); decreased cardiac function due to pump failure, valvular abnormalities, dysrhythmias, or pericardial tamponade; excessive peripheral vasodilatation as seen in sepsis or with afterload-reducing agents; and obstruction of blood flow through renal arteries or veins.

55. What causes postrenal azotemia?

Obstruction to urine flow causes postrenal azotemia. In the work-up of postoperative renal insufficiency, obstruction at or below the bladder neck should be ruled out by the insertion of a catheter. For obstruction above the bladder to cause renal failure, it must be bilateral. Inadvertent ligation of the ureters during abdominopelvic surgery occasionally occurs. The presence of hydronephrosis/hydroureter can be ascertained by renal ultrasonography.

56. List the causes of renal azotemia.

Causes of postoperative renal azotemia include ischemia, as may occur with abdominal aortic aneurysm surgeries, and exposure to nephrotoxins, such as contrast agents and aminoglycosides.

57. Which class of acute renal failure (ARF) causes is most common in surgical patients?

Prerenal causes account for 90% of postoperative ARF.

Carmichael P, Carmichael AR: Acute renal failure in the surgical setting. Aust N Z J Surg:73:144–153, 2003.

58. What is the incidence of perioperative ARF?

Perioperative ARF occurs in 1.2% of all surgical patients.

59. What patient- and surgery-specific characteristics are associated with perioperative ARF?

Elderly patients and patients with jaundice, chronic renal failure, CHF, or diabetes are at increased risk. Cardiac and aortic surgical procedures are associated with higher rates of perioperative renal failure.

60. Explain the mechanism of perioperative ARF.

The mechanism of the renal failure is most commonly ischemic injury to the kidney, which can be caused by intraoperative hypotension and cardiopulmonary bypass and aortic cross-clamping procedures related to cardiac and aortic surgeries. Another important cause of ARF in patients undergoing aortic surgery is renal artery cholesterol embolism after clamping and unclamping of the atherosclerotic aorta during repair of aortic aneurysm. In the most severe cases, patients develop sudden, complete anuria during the release of the cross-clamp, as a manifestation of bilateral renal artery embolism. A careful skin and ophthalmologic exam may reveal cholesterol emboli, which provide essential evidence for the diagnosis.

Kellerman PS: Perioperative care of the renal patient. Arch Intern Med 154:1674–1688, 1994.

61. Are dialysis patients who undergo surgery at increased risk for adverse outcomes?

Yes. Dialysis patients appear to have an increased likelihood of postoperative complications compared with surgical patients with normal renal function and to require longer hospital stays, pressor support, and intensive care.

62. What causes postoperative complications in dialysis patients?

- High incidence of underlying coronary artery disease and myocardial dysfunction
- Lack of physiologic maintenance of volume and electrolyte status, leading to perioperative volume overload or sodium or potassium disturbances
- Underlying bleeding diathesis, leading to perioperative hemorrhage
- Poor blood pressure control
- Retarded excretion/metabolism of some anesthetics and analgesics

Kellerman PS: Perioperative care of the renal patient. Arch Intern Med 154:1674–1688, 1994.

Soundararajan R, Golper TA: Medical management of the dialysis patient undergoing surgery. In UpToDate, vol. 11.3, 2003.

63. When should dialysis be performed in relation to elective surgery?
Most nephrologists recommend that patients with end-stage renal disease (ESRD) undergo dialysis immediately before surgery to optimize volume status and electrolyte levels.

64. Many patients with ESRD have a bleeding tendency. Should bleeding time be assessed before surgery?
No. Experts do not recommend using the bleeding time to screen patients because (1) a normal bleeding time does not predict the safety of surgery, and (2) a prolonged bleeding time does not predict hemorrhage. This finding may be due in part to the effect of technical factors in test performance. However, nephrologists do recommend assessment of the bleeding time before renal biopsy.

65. What causes platelet dysfunction in uremia?
Platelet dysfunction in uremia is probably multifactorial; causative factors include uremic toxins (hence performance of dialysis immediately before surgery is advisable), anemia, excessive parathyroid hormone, and aspirin use. Some patients with chronic renal disease are hypercoagulable; therefore, one should not assume that all dialysis patients are safe from acute venous thromboembolism.

66. How does perioperative bleeding due to uremia typically present?
Uremic bleeding usually develops as hemorrhage in the skin or oozing at sites of trauma or surgery. Therefore, bleeding from an organ should be evaluated with the appropriate diagnostic tests to identify a cause, such as peptic ulcer disease.

67. Summarize the treatment options for perioperative bleeding due to uremia.
- Transfusion to increase the hematocrit to 25–30%
- Desmopressin (DDAVP) at a dose of 0.30 μg/kg either intravenously or intranasally (onset of action = 1 hour, duration = 4–24 hours)
- Cryoprecipitate, 10 units IV every 12–24 hours (duration of effect = 8–24 hours)
- Conjugated estrogens, 0.6 mg/kg/day IV for 5 days; Premarin, 2.5–5.0 mg/day orally, or 50–100 μg transdermal estradiol twice weekly (onset at 1 day after initiation, peak effect 5–7 days later, duration of effect up to 1 week or more after cessation of therapy)
- Dialysis

Rose BD: Platelet dysfunction in uremia. In UpToDate, vol. 11.3, 2003.
Soundararajan R, Golper TA: Medical management of the dialysis patient undergoing surgery. In UpToDate, vol. 11.3, 2003.

68. What is the first step in the diagnostic approach to patients with postoperative hyponatremia?
The first step in the approach to patients with postoperative hyponatremia (serum sodium of 127 mEq/L) is to assess volume status by performing a physical examination. Three possibilities exist, each with its own differential diagnosis: volume depletion, edema, and euvolemia.

69. What causes volume depletion?
The volume-depleted patient is salt- and water-depleted, with the salt deficit exceeding the water deficit. The deficits result from either renal losses (e.g., diuretic excess) or extrarenal losses (e.g., GI losses).

70. Discuss the possible causes of edema.
The edematous patient has an excess of total body water and salt, with the water excess greater than the salt excess. The excesses result from the kidneys' retention of salt and water in conditions such as cardiac failure and cirrhosis, in which the kidneys perceive a decrease in the

"effective arterial blood volume." Salt and water excesses also are seen in nephrosis and advanced renal failure, although the inciting causes are different.

71. **Explain hyponatremia in the euvolemic patient.**
The hyponatremic patient who appears to be euvolemic is usually modestly volume-expanded and has an excess of total body water, although this excess is not detectable on examination. The most likely explanation for "euvolemic" hyponatremia is prolonged release of antidiuretic hormone (ADH) in the face of persistent water intake. Postoperative pain is one stimulus for ADH release.

72. **Summarize the role of measuring urinary sodum concentration in patients with hyponatremia.**
Measurement of urinary sodium concentration is a useful adjunct in distinguishing among the diagnostic possibilities in the three categories. Hyponatremia is quite common in postoperative patients. Usually it results from a combination of hypotonic fluid administration and release of ADH.

Berl T, Schrier RW: Disorders of water metabolism. In Schrier RW (ed): Renal and Electrolyte Disorders, 5th ed. Philadelphhia, Lippincott-Raven, 1997, pp 32–72.

73. **Should postoperative adrenal insufficiency be a major concern?**
Adrenal insufficiency in the perioperative period is rare. Although it is an eminently treatable condition, clinicians often omit it from the differential diagnosis of intra- or postoperative deterioration. Surgery is a physiologically stressful situation that may unmask chronic adrenal insufficiency.

74. **What are signs and symptoms of adrenal insufficiency?**
The first sign may be persistent intraoperative hypotension. Postoperatively, the patient may be febrile (to 103°F) with nausea, vomiting, and severe abdominal pain—findings that often are misdiagnosed as an intra-abdominal catastrophe. Hypotension and shock can develop. Whenever the diagnosis is entertained, a serum cortisol level should be drawn, and corticosteroids should be administered without waiting for the result.

75. **What is the incidence of postoperative delirium?**
In a prospective cohort study, Marcantonio and colleagues identified postoperative delirium in 9% of patients undergoing general, orthopedic, or gynecologic surgery at a single institution.

76. **What risk factors may lead to postoperative dementia?**
Multivariate analysis revealed the following independent predictors of delirium:

- Age > 70 years
- Alcohol abuse
- Poor cognitive status, as measured by the Telephone Interview for Cognitive Status (a score of 30 correlates with a score of 24 on the Mini-Mental Status Exam)
- Poor physical functional status, as measured by a class IV assessment according to the Specific Activity Scale (patients are unable to walk 4 km/hr for one block, make their bed, or dress themselves without stopping to rest)
- Preoperative electrolyte abnormalities: serum sodium < 130 or > 150 mmol/L, serum potassium < 3.0 or > 6.0 mmol/L, or serum glucose < 60 or > 300 mg/dL
- Aortic aneurysm surgery
- Noncardiac thoracic surgery

77. How can these risk factors be used to score the patient's risk for postoperative dementia?

Each item in question 76 is scored with 1 point with the exception of aortic aneurysm surgery, which is scored with 2 points. In the validation study set, no patients with scores of 0 developed delirium, whereas 11% of patients with scores of 1 or 2 and 50% of patients with scores > 3 developed postoperative delirium.

Marcantonio ER, et al: A clinical prediction rule for delirium after elective noncardiac surgery. JAMA 271:134–139, 1994.

78. How can the risk of perioperative venous thromboembolism (VTE) be assessed?

The numerous risk factors for VTE may occur in combination in a single patient, in which case their effect is cumulative. The risk assessment for each surgical patient must be comprehensive, taking into account medical history, current illness, and planned surgical procedure. The VTE risk factors can be grouped as negligible risk, increased risk, and moderate-to-high risk to facilitate the choice of prophylactic treatment.

79. Which factors indicate negligible risk of VTE?

Age under 40 years and absence of chronic medical illness.

80. Which factors lead to an increased risk of VTE?

Age over 40 years
General surgery
Acute MI admission
General surgery
CHF
Hyperhomocysteinemia
Antithrombin III deficiency
Use of oral contraceptives
Obesity
Protein C deficiency
Protein S deficiency
Factor V Leiden
Acute cerebrovascular accident with lower extremity paralysis
Pneumonia admission
Pregnancy
Malignancy
Prior VTE

81. Which surgical procedures involve a moderate-to-high risk of VTE?

- Knee or hip replacement
- Hip fracture
- Pelvic/lower extremity trauma
- Spinal cord injury

82. In which patients is VTE prophylaxis recommended?

In general, patients with negligible risk who are not undergoing a moderate-to-high risk (question 81) surgical procedure do not need VTE prophylaxis. Patients at highest risk for VTE are those who are undergoing major orthopedic procedures or have suffered pelvic or lower extremity trauma. Such patients warrant aggressive VTE prophylaxis with low-molecular-weight heparin or warfarin compounds, as do patients with multiple risk factors (see question 80). Patients who combine high-risk surgery with at least several other risk factors should be considered for combined-modality prophylaxis (i.e., intermittent pneumatic compression plus low-molecular-weight heparin).

Pineo GF: Prevention of venous thromboembolic disease. In UpToDate, vol 11.3, 2003.

83. What is the optimal duration of VTE prophylaxis for patients undergoing total hip or knee replacement? For patients who have had repair of a hip fracture?

This is an area of ongoing inquiry. Such patients continue to be at risk for postoperative VTE after discharge from the hospital. In 2001, the Sixth American College of Chest Physicians

Consensus Conference recommended that patients who have had total knee or hip replacement should receive 7–10 days of postoperative warfarin or LMW heparin but noted that optimal prophylaxis may actually be longer in duration. Newly published data suggest a benefit to extending prophylaxis with LMW heparin in hip replacement patients to 35 days postoperatively. Warfarin is stopped with discharge. Unfortunately, no such data exist for patients who have undergone surgery for hip fracture. The best course is to treat such patients with VTE prophylaxis until they are fully ambulatory.

Greets WH, et al: Prevention of venous thromboembolism. Chest 119:132S–175S, 2001.

Hull RD, et al: Low-molecular-weight heparin prophylaxis using dalteparin extended out-of-hospital versus in-hospital warfarin/out-of-hospital placebo in hip arthroplasty patients. Arch Intern Med 160:2208–2215, 2000.

84. Two days after repair of a hip fracture, an elderly patient develops sudden dyspnea and tachypnea. He has been receiving LMW heparin for VTE prophylaxis. What diagnosis must be ruled out first?

Despite VTE prophylaxis, there is a good possibility that the patient has sustained a pulmonary embolism. In randomized, controlled trials of interventions to prevent VTE in patients with hip fracture, the groups that received prophylaxis (low-dose or LMW heparin or low-intensity warfarin) had a DVT prevalence of 24–27% by venogram (compared with 48% for the control/placebo groups). Thus, some patients who have received prophylaxis develop VTE, and the medical consultant and orthopedist must maintain a high index of suspicion.

Greets WH, et al: Prevention of venous thromboembolism. Chest 119:132S–175S, 2001.

85. What is malignant hyperthermia?

Malignant hyperthermia is a rare genetic disorder that develops in response to treatment with certain anesthetic agents, most commonly succinylcholine and halothane. The onset is within a few hours of anesthetic administration.

86. What clinical findings are associated with malignant hyperthermia?

Clinical findings include muscle rigidity, sinus tachycardia, cyanosis, and mottling of the skin, closely followed by marked hyperthermia with temperatures possibly as high as 45°C. Hypotension, arrhythmias, rhabdomyolysis, electrolyte disorders, and disseminated intravascular coagulation may ensue rapidly. The full syndrome can develop without hyperthermia, although this occurrence is rare.

87. How is malignant hyperthermia treated?

Dantrolene is the treatment of choice and should be administered as quickly as possible to ensure survival. Dantrolene is a nonspecific skeletal muscle relaxant that acts by blocking release of calcium from the sarcoplasmic reticulum. It should be given as a 2-mg/kg IV bolus and then repeated every 5 minutes until the symptoms resolve to a maximal dose of 10 mg/kg. This protocol may be repeated every 10–15 hours. Once the patient has responded, oral therapy may be initiated at 4–8 mg/kg/day in four divided doses for 3 days.

MANAGEMENT OF CHRONIC MEDICAL AND OTHER DISEASES IN THE PERIOPERATIVE PERIOD

88. What are the important issues in the preoperative care of patients with a permanent cardiac pacemaker?

Pacemakers and implantable cardioverter/defibrillators (ICDs) should be evaluated before any operation in which electrocautery is used. Two issues must be addressed: the cardiac status of the patient, including assessment of adequacy of pacemaker function, and safety in the operating room. In general, the adequately functioning pacemaker (1) senses the patient's own intracardiac signals and (2) delivers an electric stimulus to depolarize the myocardium at a time when it is excitable and at an appropriate rate. Pacemaker function should be assessed during the month before elective surgery at the usual source of pacemaker care.

89. How do you manage the problem of electromagnetic interference in the operating room?

In the operating room, electromagnetic interference (usually from electrocautery) may cause failure of the demand pacemaker. This problem can be solved by converting the pacemaker from a demand mode to a fixed-rate mode by placing a high-powered magnet over the generator. The possibility of electromagnetic interference can be minimized by placing the ground plate as far from the generator as possible and by using electrocautery in short bursts. In patients with a temporary pacemaker, the pacemaker leads provide a direct pathway by which extraneous external electrical impulses can go directly to the heart. The contact points between the leads and the generator should be covered with a surgical glove, and gloves should be worn when the unit is handled. The pacemaker/ICD should be evaluated again after the procedure. Similar precautions should be taken for patients with these devices who receive radiotherapy or lithotripsy.

Goldschlager N, Epstein A, Friedman P, et al: Environmental and drug effects on patients with pacemakers and implantable cardioverter/defibrillators: A practical guide to patient treatment. Arch Intern Med 161: 649–655, 2001.

90. Which patients undergoing noncardiac surgery are candidates for perioperative beta blockade to prevent adverse postoperative cardiac outcomes?

Two studies have demonstrated that perioperative beta blockade reduces adverse cardiac outcomes, including cardiac death, in high-risk patients undergoing noncardiac surgery. Thus, indications for such treatment include the following:

- Established CAD
- Peripheral vascular disease
- Multiple cardiac disease risk factors: tobacco use, hypertension, diabetes mellitus, hyperlipidemia, age > 65 years

For best results, patients should start beta-blocker therapy before their surgery, and the dose should be titrated to produce a heart rate of 50–60.

Mangano DT, Layug EL, Wallace A, et al: Effect of atenolol on mortality and cardiovascular morbidity after noncardiac surgery. N Engl J Med 335:1713–1720, 1996.

Poldermans D, Boersma E, Bax JJ, et al: The effect of bisoprolol on perioperative mortality and myocardial infarction in high-risk patients undergoing vascular surgery. N Engl J Med 341:1789–1794, 1999.

Eagle KA et al: ACC/AHA guideline update for perioperative cardiovascular evaluation for noncardiac surgery-executive summary. J Am Coll Cardiol 39:542–53, 2002, with permission.

91. In which patients on chronic or life-long warfarin therapy may warfarin be withheld before surgery without use of preoperative IV heparin?

Ambulatory patients taking warfarin for prevention of stroke due to chronic atrial fibrillation may stop the drug 4–5 days before surgery (to achieve an international normalized ratio [INR] ≥ 1.5). This practice has been inspired in large part by an analysis published by Kearon and Hirsh, who noted that most patients have partial protection against thromboembolism for several more days after the cessation of warfarin because of the slow decline in the anticoagulation effect. The argument against preoperative heparin also includes the fact that patients receiving heparin have a risk of hemorrhage that more than offsets the decrement in thromboembolism risk. Warfarin also may be withheld without preoperative heparin treatment in patients who suffered an acute arterial or VTE longer than 1 month before.

92. Should warfarin be withheld in patients with more recent thromboembolic events?
For patients with more recent thromboembolic events, Kearon and Hirsh recommend avoiding elective surgery if possible; if avoidance is not possible, patients should receive IV heparin and/or a vena caval filter.

93. Is it advisable to withhold warfarin from patients with mechanical heart valves?
Kearon and Hirsh suggest that patients with mechanical heart valves do not warrant either preoperative or postoperative IV heparin while off warfarin for surgery. However, the physicians providing longitudinal or primary care for such patients often are averse to leaving them unprotected against thromboembolic events. In patients with mechanical valves and patients on lifelong warfarin therapy with multiple prior arterial or VTEs, the author defers the decision about perioperative heparin to the patients and their primary care physicians.

Kearon C, et al: Management of anticoagulation before and after elective surgery. N Engl J Med 336:1506–1511, 1997.

KEY POINTS: PATIENTS IN WHOM CHRONIC WARFARIN THERAPY MAY BE WITHHELD WITHOUT PERIOPERATIVE IV HEPARIN

1. Patients taking warfarin for stroke prophylaxis related to atrial fibrillation
2. Patients at least 3 months from an episode of venous thromboembolism
3. Patients at least 1 month out from an episode of arterial thromboembolism

94. Which patients who have stopped warfarin before surgery should have postoperative IV heparin while awaiting therapeutic oral anticoagulation?
The risk of thromboembolism in the postoperative period is the combination of the patient's baseline risk plus risks associated with the surgery. An additional consideration is the risk of bleeding due to heparin therapy. Kearon and Hirsh recommend that patients within 3 months of an acute venous or 1 month of an acute arterial thromboembolic event receive postoperative heparin to prevent another such event while they are awaiting full oral anticoagulation. The risk of venous or arterial thromboembolism in untreated patients outweighs the risk of bleeding associated with postoperative IV heparin. Other patients should receive the appropriate therapy to prevent postoperative venous thromboembolism while resuming warfarin.

Kearon C, et al: Management of anticoagulation before and after elective surgery. N Engl J Med 336:1506–1511, 1997.

95. What are the adverse consequences of postoperative hyperglycemia in diabetics?
A number of uncontrolled studies in cardiac bypass surgery patients indicate that diabetics with poorly controlled blood sugar in the perioperative period have worse outcomes. The mechanism is not well defined, but most physicians believe that wound healing is impaired in patients with poorly controlled diabetes. A second adverse effect may be a predisposition to infection. Although the clinical ramifications are not yet known, several defects in host

defense mechanisms have been shown in poorly controlled diabetes, including impaired leukocyte chemotaxis, decreased intracellular bactericidal activity, and impaired cell-mediated immune response.

Furnary AP, Gao G, Grunkemeier GL, et al: Continuous insulin infusion reduces mortality in patients with diabetes undergoing coronary artery bypass grafting. J Thorac Cardiovasc Surg 125:1007–1021, 2003.

McAlister FA, Man J, Bistritz L, et al. Diabetes and coronary artery bypass surgery. An examination of perioperative glycemic control and outcomes. Diabetes Care 26:1518–1524, 2003.

96. What management principle applies to all diabetics undergoing surgery?
All diabetics should have preoperative and postoperative glucose checks, and hyperglycemia can be treated with sliding-scale insulin.

97. Why is proper management of the blood sugar of type 1 diabetics so crucial in the perioperative period?
Type 1 diabetics, who account for 10% of all diabetics, have an absolute deficiency of insulin and therefore require regular administration for survival. The physiologic stress induced by induction of anesthesia and surgery leads to increased blood glucose concentrations. Surgery induces release of catecholamines, adrenocorticotropic hormone, glucagon, and growth hormone, all of which cause gluconeogenesis. Without insulin to counteract this process, diabetic ketoacidosis may result.

98. Describe an appropriate protocol for blood sugar management.
One approach is to give the patient one half to two thirds of the usual morning dose of intermediate-acting (NPH) insulin, monitor blood sugar levels throughout the early postoperative period, administer sliding-scale regular insulin as needed, and then resume the patient's usual regimen when he or she is able to eat. Alternatively, a patient may be treated with a continuous insulin infusion with concomitant IV dextrose.

99. How should the insulin regimens of type 2 diabetics be managed perioperatively?
Type 2 diabetics who are treated with insulin may be managed as described in question 98, particularly if time in the operating room is expected to be long. For surgical procedures of minor or intermediate complexity, and especially for day surgery, patients may withhold the morning dose of insulin, have periodic checks of blood glucose during recovery, and resume their usual regimen the same evening when they are able to eat.

100. Describe the management of type 2 diabetics taking medications other than insulin.
Type 2 diabetics are currently treated with a variety of oral medications that remedy one or more of the specific defects associated with type 2 diabetes: target-tissue resistance to insulin, low insulin secretion by islet cells, and increased hepatic gluconeogenesis. These agents should be withheld before surgery.

101. What is the specific recommendation for metformin?
The manufacturer of metformin recommends that it be held 48 hours before a contrast-dye procedure is performed because of concerns that lactic acidosis may occur in a patient who develops ARF.

102. Summarize the recommendations for sulfonylureas.
The longer-acting, older sulfonylureas (chlorpropamide and tolbutamide) should be discontinued at least 3 days before surgery because of their long half-lives. The second-generation

sulfonylureas, as well as the newer agents, including alpha glucosidase inhibitors, biguanides and thazolidinediones, may be stopped on the day of surgery. Patients with chronic liver or renal disease should stop sulfonylureas at an earlier point because of their prolonged activity in such disease states.

103. When may oral antidiabetic drugs be resumed?

Oral antidiabetic drugs can be resumed with resumption of oral intake.

Khan NA, Ghali WA: Perioperative management of diabetes mellitus. In UpToDate, vol 11.2, 2003.

104. What are the two reasons for strict continuation of medications for comorbid diseases during the perioperative period?

1. Continued administration of medications minimizes the chance that patients will develop an acute exacerbation of chronic disease in the perioperative period. Patients with serious chronic disease should receive medications on the day of surgery and throughout the perioperative period. Such conditions include but are not limited to CAD, CHF, hypertension, seizure disorders (particularly if the seizure is generalized tonic-clonic), Parkinson's disease, and COPD.
2. Continued administration of medications avoids the development of a withdrawal syndrome with abrupt cessation (Table 15-2).

TABLE 15-2. WITHDRAWAL SYNDROMES ASSOCIATED WITH COMMON MEDICATIONS

Medication	Withdrawal Syndrome
Alpha blockers (clonidine)	Rebound hypertension
Benzodiazepines	Rebound anxiety and insomnia
Beta blockers	Rebound hypertension
Short-acting SSRI antidepressants (sertraline, venlafaxine)	Headache, nausea, dizziness

105. How should patients on chronic corticosteroid therapy be managed in the perioperative period?

Although it is possible to assess the reserve of the hypothalamic-pituitary-adrenal (HPA) axis in response to stress, this assessment is rarely done in clinical practice. Instead, it is assumed that most patients on chronic corticosteroid therapy are at risk for developing secondary adrenal insufficiency due to the stress of surgery and therefore should receive stress doses of steroids. Included are patients taking daily prednisone for more than 3 weeks and patients with Cushing's syndrome. In patients taking < 10 mg each morning, the HPA axis is unlikely to be suppressed, but many experts nevertheless recommend that they receive stress doses of steroids for surgery.

106. Suggest steroid regimens for moderate and severe illness.

- For **moderate illness**: hydrocortisone, 50 mg twice daily orally or intravenously; taper rapidly to maintenance dose.
- For **severe illness**: hydrocortisone, 100 mg IV every 8 hours; decrease dose by half each day, keeping in mind the course of the illness.

107. Suggest steroid regimens for minor, moderately stressful, and major procedures.

- For **minor procedures** under local anesthesia and most radiologic studies: no corticosteroid supplementation is needed.
- For **moderately stressful procedures** (e.g., barium enema, endoscopy, arteriography): single 100-mg dose of hydrocortisone IV just before the procedure.
- For **major surgery**: hydrocortisone, 100 mg IV just before induction of anesthesia and every 8 hours for the first 24 hours; then taper rapidly by decreasing the dose by half each day to maintenance level.

  Note: If IV access cannot be obtained, hydrocortisone can be administered rectally.

Nieman LK, Orth DN, Kovacs WJ: Pharmacologic use of glucocorticoids, and Nieman LK, Orth DN : Treatment of adrenal insufficiency. In UpToDate, vol. 11.3, 2003.

108. When should antiplatelet agents be discontinued before surgery?
See Table 15-3.

TABLE 15-3. TIMETABLE FOR DISCONTINUATION OF ANTIPLATELET AGENTS BEFORE SURGERY

Agent	Effect	Discontinuation Date
Aspirin	Irreversible defect	5–10 days
Cilostazol	Reversible inhibition of platelet aggregation	3 days
Clopidogrel	Irreversible defect	7–10 days
Dipyridamole	Inhibits platelet aggregation	2 days
NSAIDs	Reversible defect	4–5 half-lives before surgery
Ticlopidine	Irreversible defect	7–10 days

CARE OF THE PSYCHIATRIC PATIENT

109. Define somatization disorder.
According to the DSM-IV, it is a psychiatric condition characterized by multiple, recurrent physical complaints for which no organic basis can be found. The disorder begins before age 30 and is more common in females. Common physical complaints include vomiting, pain in the extremities, shortness of breath, amnesia, pain in the sexual organs or rectum, and dysmenorrhea. The patient makes frequent visits to physicians because of the physical symptoms, and internists often see and evaluate these patients.

110. How should the internist approach the patient with somatization disorder?
Because the cycle in somatization disorder (or any somatoform disorder) often is physical complaint → unrevealing work-up → empiric therapy → unsatisfying outcome → return to doctor, the danger of iatrogenic disease is quite real. The physician who can establish a long-lasting relationship with the patient is occasionally able to break the cycle with good history-taking and examination skills and diagnostic and therapeutic restraint. Even more important is that the patient trusts the physician—often patients develop substantial mistrust of health care providers after repeated

encounters are fruitless and they are labeled "crocks." A dedicated primary care physician may be able to identify underlying emotional or mental health issues (e.g., sexual abuse) that may be amenable to psychiatric consultation and treatment. The treating physician should express empathy for the patient, acknowledging the patient's difficulties and challenges, and a commitment to helping the patient cope with his or her symptoms.

111. What is a personality disorder?
A personality disorder is an enduring pattern of maladaptive behavior that interferes with a person's ability to achieve success and satisfaction in interpersonal and work relationships. Patients with personality disorders meeting DSM-IV criteria more frequently sustain injuries, attempt suicide, abuse substances, and have poorer outcomes for depression treatment than the general population.

112. Define the three groups of personality disorders.
The DSM-IV divides 10 personality disorders into three groups:
Cluster A: "odd or eccentric" (paranoid, schizoid, schizotypal)
Cluster B: "dramatic" (histrionic, narcissistic, borderline, antisocial)
Cluster C: "anxious" (avoidant, dependent, obsessive-compulsive)

American Psychiatric Association: Diagnostic and Statistical Manual of Mental Disorders, 4th ed., Primary Care Version (DSM-IV-PC). Washington, DC, American Psychiatric Association, 1995.

113. When should a clinician suspect that a patient has a personality disorder?
Such patients often pose severe challenges to a physician's professionalism and empathy. They often do not see a connection between their behavior and its outcomes, and pointing out such relationships can lead to considerable anger. It may be impossible to establish a mutually satisfying patient-physician relationship; the patient alternates between glowing approval and open distrust of the physician. A physician's own discomfort within a particular patient-physician relationship may signal the presence of a personality disorder. Patients with severe behavioral difficulties should be referred to mental health professionals for treatment. In addition, patients presenting with depression or anxiety disorders who also have symptoms suggestive of a coexistent personality disorder should be referred to mental health professionals, because the personality disorder frequently complicates the treatment of the mood disorder.

114. What is a panic attack?
A panic attack is a sudden feeling of extreme fear or terror. The DSM-IV criteria stipulate that the panic attack and the associated physical symptoms start abruptly and reach a peak within 10 minutes. Furthermore, sufferers should manifest at least four of the following symptoms:

- Cardiopulmonary: chest pain/discomfort, shortness of breath, palpitations
- Neurologic: trembling/shaking, paresthesias, dizziness, lightheadedness
- Autonomic: sweating, chills, hot flashes
- Gastrointestinal: nausea, abdominal pain, feeling of choking
- Psychiatric: feelings of unreality or of being detached from oneself, fear of losing control, fear of dying

American Psychiatric Association: Diagnostic and Statistical Manual of Mental Disorders, 4th ed., Primary Care Version (DSM-IV-PC). Washington, DC, American Psychiatric Association, 1995, with permission.

115. When is panic disorder diagnosed?
Panic disorder is diagnosed when a person has recurrent panic attacks and, after at least one of the attacks, one month or more of worry about the attack or a change in behavior related to the attack (e.g., avoidance of the place of occurrence).

116. List the differential diagnoses for panic attack.

Alcohol withdrawal
Amphetamine abuse
Asthma
Caffeinism
Cardiac dysrhythmias
Cardiomyopathies
Cocaine abuse
Complex partial seizures
CAD
Cushing's syndrome
Drug withdrawal
Electrolyte abnormalities
Hyperparathyroidism
Hyperthyroidism
Hypoglycemia
Hypothyroidism
Marijuana-induced palpitations
Menopausal symptoms
Mitral valve prolapse
Pheochromocytoma
Pulmonary embolism
Vertigo

Katon W: DHHS Pub. No (ADM) 89–1629, Washington, DC, U.S. Government Printing Office,1989.

117. How do you differentiate between delirium and dementia?

Both are associated with impairment of the three main aspects of cognition: thinking, perception, and memory. In dementia, however, the cognitive impairment develops insidiously and is enduring, whereas in delirium the impairment has an abrupt onset and is short-lived. Moreover, delirious patients are frequently not completely alert, whereas patients with dementia maintain alertness until the disease is quite advanced (Table 15-4).

TABLE 15-4. DELIRIUM VERSUS DEMENTIA

Characteristic	Delirium	Dementia
Onset	Sudden	Insidious
Course over 24 hours	Fluctuating, worse at night	Stable
Consciousness	Reduced	Clear
Attention	Disordered	Normal except in severe cases
Cognition	Disordered	Disordered
Hallucinations	Visual or auditory	Not common
Delusions	Poorly systematized	Not common
Orientation	Usually impaired	Often impaired
Psychomotor activity	Variable	Often normal
Speech	Often incoherent	Difficulty in word-finding, perseveration
Involuntary movements	Asterixis/coarse tremor	Often absent
Physical illness or drug toxicity	One or both present	Often absent

Adapted from Lipowski ZJ: Delirium in the elderly patient. N Engl J Med 320:578–582, 1989.

118. What is "steroid psychosis"?

Corticosteroid use is frequently associated with changes in mood (euphoria, dysphoria, or emotional lability), sleep pattern (insomnia, weird dreams, nightmares), and appetite (usually increased). Corticosteroids also can have important effects on behavior and thought processes, inducing frank psychosis in persons without a history of psychiatric disturbance or decompensation in known psychotics.

119. How should the diagnosis and treatment of hypertension be handled in patients with a major psychiatric disorder?
In patients with major depression, schizophrenia, or bipolar disorder, elevated blood pressure should be evaluated in the same way as for patients without these disorders. Diuretics must be used with caution in patients treated with lithium because they may cause volume depletion, lithium toxicity, coma, and even death. Beta blockers and central alpha agonists may not be advisable for patients with depression, and reserpine is contraindicated in depressed patients.

120. List reasonable medications for treatment of hypertension in patients with a major psychiatric disorder.

- Thiazide diuretics (for patients not on lithium therapy)
- Beta blockers
- Long-acting calcium channel blockers (e.g., verapamil, felodipine)
- Angiotensin-converting enzyme (ACE) inhibitors (monitor serum creatinine in patients taking lithium)

Beta blockers and central alpha agonists are best avoided if compliance is a problem, because sudden cessation of these medications is associated with rebound hypertension.

National Institutes of Health: The Sixth Report of the Joint National Committee on Prevention, Detection, Evaluation, and Treatment of High Blood Pressure. Washington, DC, NIH, 1997, NIH Publication No. 98-4080.

121. What renal lesions may be caused by chronic lithium treatment?
Up to 20% of patients on chronic lithium therapy develop resistance to antidiuretic hormone (ADH), resulting in polyuria and polydipsia. Lithium accumulates in the collecting tubule cells and interferes with the ability of ADH to increase water permeability. Nocturia not accompanied by fluid ingestion before sleep suggests a urinary concentrating defect. However, polyuria in a patient on lithium therapy cannot be automatically ascribed to the lithium. Psychiatric patients also may have primary polydipsia or central diabetes insipidus. Other renal complications of chronic lithium treatment are type I (distal) renal tubular acidosis and nephrotic syndrome due to minimal change disease or glomerulosclerosis.

122. What conditions and drugs can cause lithium retention and hence toxicity?

- Any condition that causes or predisposes a patient to volume depletion or renal ischemia can cause decreased lithium excretion and hence toxicity: GI losses, CHF, and cirrhosis.
- Certain types of drugs, if not monitored carefully, can disturb lithium excretion: diuretics, NSAIDs, and ACE inhibitors.

123. What are the symptoms of lithium toxicity?
Symptoms include coarse tremors, muscle weakness, ataxia, delirium, nausea, vomiting, diarrhea, leukocytosis, sinus bradycardia, hypotension, seizures, and, in the most severe cases, coma.

124. How is severity of lithium toxicity graded?

- Mild: lithium level of 1.5–2.5 mEq/L
- Moderate: lithium level of 2.5–3.5 mEq/L
- Severe: lithium level > 3.5 mEq/L

125. How is lithium toxicity treated?

- Volume repletion if the patient is hypovolemic
- Oral charcoal in cases of acute overdose (to adsorb other ingested drugs)
- Hemodialysis (treatment of choice in severe cases)

126. When should hemodialysis be initiated to treat lithium toxicity?

Hemodilaysis should be initiated if the serum lithium level is > 4 mEq/L, regardless of symptoms. With lower lithium levels, hemodialysis should be initiated if patients have severe symptoms or concomitant conditions (e.g., CHF, cirrhosis) that limit urinary excretion. Effective dialysis is likely to require several sessions or a long session of 8–12 hours, because the movement of lithium from within to outside cells is slow. In addition, there may be a rebound in the serum lithium level after cessation of a short hemodialysis session.

127. Define serotonin syndrome. What are the symptoms?

Serotonin syndrome can result when a patient takes two or more serotonergic agents with different mechanisms of action, either concurrently or in close succession. Symptoms include altered mental status, altered muscle tone (hyperreflexia, myoclonus, tremor, ataxia), autonomic instability with wide fluctuations in vital signs, hyperthermia, and diarrhea.

128. Which drugs may cause serotonin syndrome?

Any two agents from the list below may cause the syndrome. Of note, because some agents have very long half-lives, great caution must be used in starting a second agent in patients who have just stopped another serotonergic agent.

- Serotonin precursor: tryptophan.
- Serotonin release at the synapse: some amphetamines, selective serotonin-reuptake inhibitors (SSRIs: citalopram, fluoxetine, paroxetine, sertraline) and other newer antidepressants (e.g., venlaxafine), tricyclic antidepressants, trazodone, dextromethorphan, meperidine, tramadol.
- Decreased serotonin metabolism: monoamine oxidase (MAO) inhibitors; St. John's wort (has MAO inhibitor activity in vitro).
- Other serotonergic activity: buspirone, lithium, sumatriptan, dihydroergotamine.

129. What combination has caused most cases of serotonin syndrome?

To date, most reported cases appear to have resulted from the combination of SSRIs and MAO inhibitors. If a patient is to begin therapy with an MAO inhibitor after treatment with an SSRI, at least 2 weeks should be allowed for washout of the SSRIs. The exception is fluoxetine, which may require up to 5 weeks.

130. How is serotonin syndrome treated?

Treatment of serotonin syndrome chiefly involves withdrawal of the inciting drug(s). There are some reports of rapid resolution of symptoms with cyproheptadine.

131. Define neuroleptic malignant syndrome (NMS).

NMS is a clinical state of high fever, muscle rigidity, altered mental status, and dysautonomias that is thought to arise from depletion of dopamine in the central nervous system. The chief causative agents are the major tranquilizers (e.g., haloperidol), which are antidopaminergic in nature. Some patients develop the syndrome suddenly, after years of treatment with major tranquilizers; it also has been reported after sudden cessation of treatment with dopaminergic agents. Although NMS seems to resemble the serotonin syndrome in some of its features, experts currently believe that they are two distinct entities.

132. How is NMS treated?

Treatment of NMS consists of cooling, bromocriptine for mild or dantrolene for severe cases, and, most importantly, withdrawal of the offending agent.

133. Describe the diagnosis of anorexia nervosa.

Anorexia nervosa is a psychiatric disorder that predominantly affects young women. Because of disordered body image, patients labor to stay extremely thin by eating little; purging with induced vomiting, laxatives, or enemas; and sometimes exercising excessively. In addition to abnormal body image, the DSM-IV requires the following three findings for a diagnosis of anorexia nervosa: (1) refusal to maintain a body weight within 15% of the ideal for age and sex, (2) amenorrhea, and (3) fear of weight gain.

134. What medical complications may result from anorexia nervosa?

Anorectic patients develop numerous laboratory abnormalities and medical complications. Low electrolyte levels may lead to sinus bradycardia or arrhythmias. Amenorrhea is common and may persist after the weight gain that is a sign of successful treatment. Relative hypothyroidism may occur, with low serum T_3 but normal serum T_4 levels. Dry skin and hair and cold intolerance may be seen. The left ventricle may become thin, and anorectic patients may develop CHF with aggressive refeeding. Thus increased oral intake must be monitored carefully. Anorectics are prone to the development of osteoporosis because of estrogen deficiency and poor intake of calcium and vitamin D.

BIBLIOGRAPHY

1. Carey CF, Lee HH, Woeltjke KF (eds): The Washington Manual of Medical Therapeutics, 30th ed. Philadelphia, Lippincott Williams & Wilkins, 2003.
2. Desai SP, Isa-Pratt S (eds): Clinician's Guide to Laboratory Medicine: A Practical Approach. Cleveland, OH, Lexi-Comp, 2000.
3. Gross RJ, Caputo GM (eds): Kammerer and Gross' Medical Consultation, 4th ed. Philadelphia, Lippincott Williams & Wilkins, 2003.

AMBULATORY CARE

Mary P. Harward, M.D.

CHAPTER 16

The practice of medicine is an art, based on science.

Sir William Osler (1849–1919)

The sooner patients can be removed from the depressing influence of general hospital life, the more rapid their convalescence.

Charles H. Mayo (1865–1939)
Lancet, 1916

It's the humdrum, day-in, day-out everyday work that is the real satisfaction of the practice of medicine; . . . the actual calling on people, at all times and under all conditions, the coming to grips with the intimate conditions of their lives, when they were being born, when they were dying, watching them die, watching them get well when they were ill, has always absorbed me.

William Carlos Williams (1883–1963)
"The Practice" from
The Autobiography of William Carlos Williams, 1951

1. **What are the most common reasons for visits to an ambulatory care clinic or office?**

Reasons named by patients	Reasons named by physicians
General medical examination	Essential hypertension
Hypertension	Diabetes mellitus
Progress visit, no symptom	Chronic ischemic heart disease
Chest pain and related symptoms	Acute upper respiratory tract infection
Cough	General medical examination
Blood pressure test	Osteoarthritis and related diseases
Diabetes mellitus	General symptoms
Symptoms referable to throat	Chronic airway obstruction
Abdominal pain, cramps, spasms	Asthma
Headache, pain in head	Bronchitis
Upper respiratory tract infection (head cold)	Neurotic disorders
Back symptoms	Chronic sinusitis
Vertigo, dizziness	Acute pharyngitis
Tiredness, exhaustion	Miscellaneous (diagnosis missing or illegible)
Leg symptoms	Other disorders of soft tissue
Shoulder symptoms	Other respiratory symptoms
Neck symptoms	Congestive heart failure
Ischemic heart disease	Peripheral enthesopathies

Barker LR: Curriculum for ambulatory care training in medical residency: Rationale, attitudes, and generic proficiencies. J Gen Intern Med 5(Suppl 1):S13–S14, 1990.

CARDIOLOGY

2. **You see a new patient who is a 47-year-old African-American man with an initial blood pressure (BP) reading in his right arm of 150/90 mmHg. What is the first thing you should do?**
   The BP should be measured again in the right arm several minutes after the first reading and repeated until the BP readings are similar. Record the average of the readings. The BP should also be checked in the left arm. A difference between the two arms > 10 mmHg suggests arterial occlusion in the arm with the lower BP. The arm with the higher reading should be used for future measurements.

3. **What elements in a patient's history may suggest secondary hypertension (HTN) due to substance use?**
   - Drug-induced (over the counter): decongestants, stimulants, appetite suppressants, non-steroidal anti-inflamatory agents (NSAIDs)
   - Drug-induced (prescription): NSAIDs, corticosteroids, antidepressants (Effexor), cyclosporine
   - Drug use (illicit): cocaine, stimulants
   - Alcoholism: alcohol history, CAGE questionnaire (see question 103), family history of alcoholism

4. **What elements in a patient's history may suggest secondary HTN due to an endocrine disorder?**
   - Cushing's syndrome: weight gain, central obesity, easy bruising, "moon" facies, abdominal striae
   - Hyperthyrodism: weight loss, tachycardia, nervousness
   - Hypothyroidism: weight gain, fatigue, constipation, dry skin
   - Pheochromocytoma: labile HTN, sweating, headache, palpitations
   - Hyperaldosteronism: fatigue, muscle weakness due to low potassium

5. **List two elements in the history that may suggest secondary HTN due to sleep apnea.**
   Snoring and daytime sleepiness.

KEY POINTS: RISK FACTORS FOR CORONARY ARTERY DISEASE (CAD) IN PATIENTS WITH HYPERLIPIDEMIA

1. Cigarette smoking
2. Hypertension
3. Low HDL (< 40 mg /dL)
4. Family history of premature CAD (father or brother < 55 years; mother or sister < 65 years)
5. Diabetes mellitus

6. **List two elements in the history that may suggest secondary HTN due to renovascular disease.**
   Sudden onset of pulmonary edema and history of atherosclerotic disease

7. **What causes of secondary HTN can be detected by physical examination?**
   - Aortic insufficiency: diastolic murmur
   - Aotic coarctation: diminished femoral pulses, bruit best heard over the back
   - Renovascular disease: periumbilical bruit
   - Subclavian stenosis: BP difference > 10 mmHg between right and left arms
   - Cushing's syndrome: abdominal striae, "buffalo hump," "moon" facies
   - Hyperthyroidism: thyroid nodularity or tenderness
   - Sleep apnea: obesity, particularly of neck
   - Alcoholism: spider angiomata, hepatomegaly, gynecomastia

8. **Can licorice ingestion elevate the BP?**
   Yes, although glycrrhizic acid is found only in confectioner's black licorice. Most commercially sold licorice in the U.S. does not contain significant amounts, although glcyrrhizic acid may be found in chewing tobacco.

9. **How often should you check the BP in a patient with an initial systolic reading between 120 and 139 systolic and/or diastolic reading between 80 and 89?**
   Yearly.

10. **Should systolic BP between 120 and 139 and/or diastolic BP between 80 and 89 be treated?**
    Blood pressure readings such as these are called "prehypertension" and are associated with increased risk of cardiovascular events. Lifestyle modification (weight loss, salt restriction, limited alcohol use, stress reduction, smoking cessation, regular exercise, and low saturated-fat diet rich in fruits and vegetables) should be recommended. Pharmocologic therapy should be initiated if the BP increases to the hypertensive range (systolic ≥ 140 or diastolic ≥ 90).
    Chobanian AV, Bakris GL, Black HR, et al: The Seventh Report of the Joint National Committee on Prevention, Detection, Evaluation, and Treatment of High Blood Pressure: The JNC 7 Report. JAMA 289:2560, 2003.

11. **Which lipids can be measured without fasting?**
    Total cholesterol and HDL cholesterol. LDL cholesterol is calculated from the fasting triglyceride level and total and HDL cholesterol levels are calculated by the following formula:

    LDL cholesterol = Total cholesterol − HDL cholesterol + (Triglycerides/5)

12. **What are the characteristics of an innocent heart murmur? Mitral valve prolapse (MVP) murmur?**
    See Table 16-1.

TABLE 16-1. INNOCENT HEART MURMUR VERSUS MURMUR DUE TO MITRAL VALVE PROLAPSE

Characteristic	Innocent Murmur	MVP Murmur
Location	Base	Apex
Intensity	< 3/6	> 2/6
Timing in cardiac cycle	Early systole	Mid-to-late systole
Response to standing	Decreased	Begins earlier in systole
Response to Valsalva	Decreases	May increase
Associated findings	None	Midsystolic click

13. List the cardiac conditions that require prophylactic antibiotics when a patient has a dental procedure, gastrointestinal, genitourinary, or respiratory procedure.

- Congenital heart disease (except uncomplicated secundum atrial septal defects and surgically repaired atrial septal defect, ventricular defect, and patent ductus arteriosus)
- Rheumatic valvular heart disease
- Acquired valvular heart disease
- Hypertrophic cardiomyopathy
- MVP with mitral insufficiency (evidenced by systolic murmur in addition to click) or valve thickening
- Prosthetic heart valve
- History of infective endocarditis

14. For which of these conditions is the patient considered at high risk?

- Prosthetic valve
- Previous bacterial endocarditis
- Complex cyanotic congenital heart disease
- Surgically constructed systemic pulmonic shunts or conduits

15. For which of these conditions is the patient considered at moderate risk?

- Most other congenital heart disease
- Hypertrophic cardiomyopathy
- MVP with regurgitatioin

16. Which dental procedures require endocarditis prophylaxis?

- Extraction
- Periodontal procedures (surgery, planing, scaling, and probing)
- Dental implant
- Reimplantation of teeth
- Endodontic procedures
- Subgingival antibiotic fiber or strip placement
- Initial orthodontic band placement
- Local anesthetic injections
- Teeth cleaning with likely bleeding

17. Which nondental procedures require endocarditis prophylaxis?

- Tonsillectomy and/or adenoidectomy
- Rigid bronchoscopy
- Respiratory mucosa surgery
- Esophageal variceal sclerotherapy
- Esophageal stricture dilatation
- Endoscopic retrograde cholangiopancreatography
- Biliary tract surgery
- Intestinal mucosa surgery
- Prostatic surgery
- Cystoscopy
- Urethral dilation

18. What antibiotics are used for prophylaxis for endocarditis?

Depending on the procedure and underlying cardiac condition, patients should receive oral or intravenous/intramuscular antibiotics (Table 16-2).

TABLE 16-2. ANTIMICROBIAL PROPHYLAXIS FOR THE PREVENTION OF BACTERIAL ENDOCARDITIS IN PATIENTS WITH UNDERLYING CARDIAC CONDITIONS

Situation	Agent	Regimen
Dental, oral, respiratory tract, or esophageal procedures		
Standard general prophylaxis	Amoxicillin	2 gm PO 1 hr before procedure
Unable to take oral medications	Ampicillin	2 gm IM or IV within 30 min of procedure
Allergic to penicillin	Clindamycin *or* cephalexin[1] *or* cefadroxil[1]	600 mg PO 1 h before procedure 2 gm PO 1 h before procedure
	Azithromycin *or* clarithromycin	500 mg 1 h before procedure
Allergic to penicillin and unable to take oral medications	Clindamycin *or* cefazolin[1]	600 mg within 30 min of procedure 1 gm IM or IV within 30 min of procedure
For genitourinary/gastrointestinal (excluding esophageal) procedures		
High-risk (HR) patients[2]	Ampicillin + gentamicin	Ampicillin 2 gm IM or IV + gentamicin 1.5 mg/kg (not to exceed 120 mg) within 30 min of procedure; 6 h later, ampicillin 1 gm IM/IV or amoxicillin 1 gm PO
HR patient allergic to ampicillin/amoxicillin	Vancomycin + gentamicin	Vancomycin 1 gm IV over 1–2 h + gentamicin as above
Moderate-risk (MR) patients[3]	Amoxicillin or ampicillin	2 gm PO 1 h before procedure or ampicillin 2 gm IM/IV within 30 min of procedure
MR patients allergic to ampicillin/amoxicillin	Vancomycin	1 gm IV over 1–2 h; complete infusion within 30 min of procedure

[1]Cephalosporins should not be used in patients with immediate-type hypersensitivity reaction (urticaria, angioedema, or anaphylaxis) to penicillins.
[2]Defined in question 14.
[3]Defined in question 15.
Adapted from Gilbert DN, Moellering RC Jr, Sande MA: The Sandford Guide to Antimicrobial Therapy, 32nd ed. Hyde Park, VT, Antimicrobial Therapy, Inc., 2002, pp 122–123.

19. **What are the common causes of atrial fibrillation?**
Alcohol use (especially binge drinking), thyrotoxicosis, congestive heart failure, myocardial ischemia or infarction, pulmonary embolism, illicit or over-the-counter stimulant use, mitral valve disease, Wolff-Parkinson-White (WPW) syndrome, hypertensive cardiomyopathy, digoxin toxicity

20. **What range of the International Normalized Ratio (INR) is the target treatment for most patients receiving anticoagulation for atrial fibrillation?**
2.0 – 3.0

21. **Should a postmenopausal woman with known cardiovascular disease take hormone replacement therapy (estrogen and progesterone)?**
No. The American Heart Association recommends that women with known cardiac disease avoid hormone replacement therapy.
American Heart Association: www.aha.org

22. **If medications are taken with grapefruit juice, the absorption and blood level of the medication may be increased, resulting in toxicity. Which medications show this effect?**

Amiodarone	Felodipine	Nimodipine
Benzodiazepines	Fexofenadine	Nisoldipine
Buspirone	Fluoxetine	Quinidine
Carbamazepine	HMG-CoA reductase inhibitors ("statins")	Sertraline
Cyclosporine	Itraconazole	Sildenafil
Dextromethorphan	Methylprednisone	Theophylline
Diltiazem	Nicardipine	Verapamil
Erythromycin	Nifedipine	Warfarin
Estrogens		

23. **How much grapefruit juice can be consumed by patients on these medications?**
One cup of juice or ½ grapefruit is probably safe if taken at a different time from the medication.
Drug interactions with grapefruit juice. Med Let 46:2–3, 2004.

24. **Which is a greater risk factor for cardiovascular disease: cigarette smoking or obesity?**
Cigarette smoking.

DERMATOLOGY

25. **List your treatment recommendations to an adolescent with stage I acne (comedones or "blackheads" with small pustules but no scarring).**
    - Avoid oily cosmetics.
    - Do not rub your face.
    - Use mild cleansing soap.
    - Apply topical retinoic acid cream (or gel) or benzoyl peroxide at bedtime.
    - Use sunscreen.
    - For women, consider prescribing an oral contraceptive containing norgestimate.

26. **Define hidradenitis suppurativea and erythrasma.**
Hidradenitis suppurativa: an apocrine sweat gland infection of the axilla, groin, breasts, or buttocks that can cause inflammation and scarring.
Erythrasma: a skin infection caused by *Corynebacterium minutissimum* that occurs in the axilla or groin or sometimes between the toes.

27. **How do you treat hidradenitis suppurativa?**
Hidradenitis suppurative sometimes responds to dicloxacillin or erythromycin, although surgical excision is sometimes required.

28. **How do you treat erythrasma?**
Erythrasma responds to topical benzoyl peroxide or systemic erythromycin.

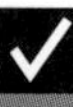

KEY POINTS: ABCDE CHARACTERISTICS OF SKIN LESIONS LIKELY TO BE MALIGNANT MELANOMA

1. **A**symmetric
2. **B**order that is irregular
3. **C**olors that vary within the lesion
4. **D**iameter > 6 mm
5. **E**nlarging lesion

29. How do you recognize tinea versicolor (pityriasis)?
Tinea versicolor is a macular lesion of various colors such as red, pink, or brown. Slight scale may be present. Involved areas do not tan and are hypopigmented.

30. How do you treat pityriasis?
Treatment consists of 2.5% selenium sulfide suspension or pyrithione zinc shampoo applied with a rough washcloth to the entire body, then allowed to remain for 10 minutes before rinsing. A topical antifungal agent such as clotrimazole or miconazole can be used for small areas, or systemic antifungal agents (fluconazole) can be used for severe cases or in immunocompromised patients.

ENDOCRINOLOGY

31. Describe the typical follow-up examination for a patient with non–insulin-dependent diabetes mellitus.

- **History:** Ask about the frequency, cause, and severity of hypoglycemic or hyperglycemic episodes. Review home glucose monitoring records. Update medication list. Ask about any recent illnesses. Review diet and life stressors.
- **Physical examination:** Weight, BP, foot exam, fundoscopic exam (in addition to annual dilated exam by ophthalmologist), peripheral pulse exam.

32. What laboratory testing should be ordered during follow-up visits?

- Glycohemoglobin ($HgbA_1C$) quarterly
- Lipids, including triglycerides, total cholesterol, HDL cholesterol, LDL cholesterol
- Liver function tests if taking statin drugs
- Urinalysis with annual testing for protein or microalbumin if proteinuria is absent

33. What immunizations do diabetics need?

- Pneumococcal vaccine every 5 years
- Annual influenza vaccination
- Tetanus-diphtheria (Td) vaccine every 10 years

34. Name the two most frequent causes of mild, asymptomatic hypercalcemia in ambulatory patients.
Thiazide diuretics and hyperparathyroidism.

KEY POINTS: COUNSELING FOR PATIENTS WITH DIABETES

1. Exercise
2. Diet
3. Foot care
4. Medication adjustment when ill
5. Regular ophthalmologic follow-up
6. Regular dental follow-up
7. Up-to-date immunizations
8. Smoking cessation
9. Management of hypoglycemic and hyperglycemic episodes

35. What is the BMI?

Body mass index. The BMI gives an estimate of risk of complications of obesity as it relates weight to height. It can be obtained from tables or normograms. Ideal BMI is < 25.

36. List the complications of morbid obesity.

- Hypertension
- Coronary artery disease
- Impaired glucose tolerance (metabolic syndrome)
- Diabetes mellitus
- Increased mortality from all causes, including cancer
- Sleep apnea
- Osteoarthritis
- Depression
- Recurrent skin infections (particularly intertriginous areas)

37. What is the target level of $HgbA_1c$ for diabetics?

Although there may be some variation among laboratories, in general an $HgbA_1c < 7.0$ suggests good control. If the level is > 8.0, a therapeutic change is warranted.

38. What test is most useful for monitoring thyroid replacement therapy?

Thyroid-stimulating hormone (TSH).

KEY POINTS: SYMPTOMS OF IRRITABLE BOWEL SYNDROME DISEASE (IBSD)

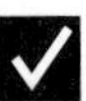

1. Abdominal pain
2. Altered bowel habits (diarrhea or constipation)
3. Abdominal bloating
4. Excessive belching or flatulence
5. Dyspepsia
6. Early satiety
7. Nausea
8. Heartburn
9. Noncardiac pain

GASTROENTEROLOGY

39. What medications can cause chronic constipation?

Calcium channel blockers
Antihistamines
Opiates
Iron
Tricyclic antidepressants
Anticholinergics
Aluminum- and calcium-based antacids
Calcium supplements
Sucralfate
Disopyramide
Laxatives (if abused)

40. Define proctalgia fugax.

A fleeting, deep pain in the rectum, possibly caused by muscle spasm. Tenderness is found on digital rectal examination.

GYNECOLOGY

41. What topics should you cover in the history of a 20-year-old, sexually active woman with the complaint of acute dysuria?

Hematuria, vaginal discharge; flank pain; fever; chills; last menses; sexual activity; use of barrier contraception; use of oral contraceptives; previous pregnancies, miscarriages, or abortions; illness or symptoms in sexual partner; recent new sexual partner; previous sexually transmitted diseases, human immunodeficiency virus (HIV) test results, if done.

42. What should the physical examination include in the same patient?

Temperature, pulse, BP, abdominal exam, evaluation for flank tenderness, and bimanual examination if cervicitis and/or vaginitis likely by history.

43. What laboratory tests should you order for this patient?

Wet mount of any vaginal discharge and testing for *Chlamydia* spp. and *Neisseria gonorrhoeae* if cervical or adnexal tenderness is present. If the history and exam suggest acute cystitis without complications, empirical treatment can be started with a fluoroquinolone without urinalysis or urine culture. If the symptoms continue after treatment, urinalysis and urine culture should be done.

44. List the common causes of abnormal vaginal bleeding in premenopausal women.

Theatened or complete abortion
Ectopic pregnancy
Hypothyrodism
Hypercortisolism
Polycystic ovary syndrome
Thrombocytopenia
Bleeding diathesis
Vulvar infection, laceration, or tumor
Vaginal laceration, tumor, or foreign body
Cervical infection, erosion, polyp, or carcinoma
Uterine infection, polyp, fibroids, or carcinoma
Ovarian infection
Intrauterine device
Idiopathic

45. How do you manage a woman with postmenopausal vaginal bleeding?

Refer her to a gynecologist for consideration of diagnostic studies to detect endometrial carcinoma.

46. List the characteristic vaginal discharges caused by *Candida albicans, N. gonorrhoeae, Gardnerella vaginalis,* overgrowth of lactobacilli (cytolytic vaginosis), and *Trichomonas vaginalis.*

See Table 16-3.

TABLE 16-3. CHARACTERISTIC VAGINAL DISEASES OF COMMON INFECTIONS

Organism	Discharge Characteristics
C. albicans	Thick, white, curdlike, adherent to vaginal wall with satellite lesions and erythema on perineum
N. gonorrhoeae	Mucopurulent with cervicitis
G. vaginalis	Foul-smelling ("fishy" with KOH), thin, scanty, adherent to vaginal wall
Lactobacilli	White, frothy with pH > 3.5 and < 4.5
T. vaginalis	Copious, yellow-green, frothy

47. What are clue cells?
Epithelial cells covered with cocobacilli or curved rods. Clue cells are found in the vaginal discharge of patients infected with *G. vaginalis.*

48. What are the absolute contraindications to the use of oral contraceptives (OCPs)?
- Pregnancy
- Lactation
- Thrombophlebitis
- History of stroke
- History of thromboembolic event
- History of hypercoaguable state (antiphospholipid syndrome, nephritic syndrome, factor V Leiden mutation)
- History of estrogen-dependent tumor (breast, endometrium)
- Liver disease
- Uterine bleeding of unknown cause
- Hypertriglyceridemia
- Heavy smoking (20 cigarettes/day) in women > 35 years old

49. What conditions are associated with an increased risk of complications from OCPs?
- Uncontrolled hypertension
- Diabetes mellitus (may require adjustment of insulin dose)
- Migraine headaches
- Use of anticonvulsants (may reduce effectiveness of OCPs)

50. Describe the evaluation of a new breast nodule discovered in a 50-year-old woman during routine exam.
- **History:** personal history of breast disorders and biopsies; family history of breast, ovarian, or colon cancer; use of hormone replacement therapy; use of OCPs.
- **Physical exam:** location, size, mobility, and consistency of nodule; presence or absence of nipple discharge; presence or absence of axillary adenopathy; complete exam of contralateral breast and axilla.
- **X-ray:** mammogram with appropriate needle aspiration or biopsy of suspicious lesions.

Most importantly, a new solitary nodule should always be biopsied even if a mammogram is normal.

51. What is the role of genetic testing in the risk assessment for breast cancer?
The gene mutations associated with an increased risk of beast and ovarian cancer (*BRAC1* and *BRAC2*) have been identified and can be commercially tested. The results may be difficult to interpret and women may be unduly concerned or relieved about their breast cancer risk if

improperly interpreted. If a woman requests genetic testing because of a perceived increased family risk, she should be referred to a genetic counseling center or specialists where a thorough family history can be obtained and appropriate counseling and testing provided.

52. What is premenstrual syndrome (PMS)?
PMS is a group of physical and psychological symptoms that occur consistently during approximately 5 days prior to menses consistently during a woman's menstrual cycle and lead to significant social and occupational functioning. Physical symptoms include abdominal bloating, fatigue, breast tenderness, and headaches. Emotional symptoms include depression, irritability, confusion, and isolation.

53. What are the treatments for PMS?
If a woman is only mildly impaired by her symptoms, calcium, vitamin B_6, and magnesium supplements may be useful. For a woman with significant depression, the selective seritonin reuptake inhibitors (SSRIs) such as fluoxetine, sertraline, paroxetine, and citalopram have the most clinical efficacy when taken daily. Other possibly effective medications include venlaxafine, nefazodone, clomimpramine, danazol, alprazalom, and GnRh agonists.

54. What are the risk factors for osteoporosis?
Women $\geq$ 65 years old, men $\geq$ 70 years old, postmenopausal state, medication use (glucocorticoids, chronic heparin, vitamin A, cyclosporine, methotrexate, anticonvulsants, thyroid replacement, and anxiolytics), chronic illnesses (systemic lupus erythematosus, rheumatoid arthritis, psoriatic arthritis, cancer treatment, cystic fibrosis, inflammatory bowel disease, celiac disease, hyperthyroidism, hypogonadism, vitamin D deficiency, and chronic liver disease), positive family history, cigarette smoking, excessive caffeine, low body weight, above average height, and lack of exercise.

55. List the available treatments for osteoporosis.
- Weight-bearing exercise (including walking)
- Calcium (1500 mg/day for postmenopausal women and older men, 1000 mg/day for premenopausal women) + vitamin D (400–800 IU/day)
- Biphosphonates (alendronate and risedronate)
- Raloxifene (tissue-selective estrogen receptor modifier)
- Salmon calcitonin (less effective but can be used intranasally)
- Calciferol (rarely used)

56. What is the role of estrogen-progesterone therapy in prevention and treatment of osteoporosis?
Although estrogen-progesterone therapy has been shown to reduce fracture risk in postmenopausal women, recent data from the Women's Health Initiative (WHI) suggest that the risks of cardiac events, breast cancer, and stroke are increased in treated women and outweigh potential benefit.

57. How should you instruct patients to take a biphosphonate?
- Take weekly preparation.
- Take the pill first in the morning with a full glass of water.
- Do not take with other pills or food.
- Do not eat, drink, or swallow any other pills for 30 minutes.
- Maintain upright posture (either sitting or standing) for 30 minutes.

58. Why should a patient follow the regimen in question 57 when taking biphosphonates?
The biphosphonates can cause esophageal ulceration, which can be prevented by following the directions in question 57.

INFECTIOUS DISEASES

59. List the high-risk factors that indicate the need for the pneumococcal vaccine.

- Age ≥ 65 years
- Chronic cardiovascular disease such as congestive heart failure and cardiomyopathies
- Chronic pulmonary disease (not including asthma)
- Diabetes mellitus
- Alcoholism
- Chronic liver failure
- CSF leaks
- Asplenia, either functional or anatomic
- Immunosuppression including hematologic malignancy, multiple myeloma, renal failure, organ transplants, chronic cortocosteroid use, and HIV infection
- Residence in long-term care facilities

60. List the symptoms of influenza.

Sudden onset of high fever*	Malaise
Myalgia	Coryza
Headache	Sore throat

* Although influenza infection may present with mild upper respiratory tract symptoms without fever

61. What are the complications of influenza?

- Pneumonia (either primary influenza pneumonia or secondary bacterial pneumonia)
- Encephalitis, myelitis
- Hepatitis, pancreatitis
- Myositis, rhabdomyolysis
- Asthenia, prolonged fatigue
- Reye's syndrome (in children and adolescents)

62. How do you diagnose influenza?

Influenza is a clinical diagnosis supported by community epidemiological data and confirmed by laboratory testing. Influenza A or B is very likely when a patient presents with the symptoms described in question 50 during the time when influenza is known to circulate in your community. The Centers for Disease Control and Prevention publishes influenza updates October through May on its website (http://www.cdc.gov/ncidod/diseases/flu/weekly.htm). Updates are also available through the CDC Voice Information System (888–232–3228) and by fax (888–232–3229). Local health departments also publish data from the local community. The suspicion of influenza can be confirmed through rapid tests done in the office from nasal or throat swabs. Most commercially available kits provide results within 45 minutes.

63. What are the treatments for influenza?

Antiviral agents are available that reduce the duration and severity of influenza. Amantadine and rimantadine were the first agents available to treat influenza but are only effective against influenza A and have CNS side effects, particularly in the elderly. Newer neuroaminadase inhibitors (zanamivir and oseltamivir) are effective against both influenza A and B. Zanamivir is given as an inhaled powder. All of these drugs should be given within the first 48 hours from the onset of symptoms and reduce the symptomatic phase by about a day. These treatments may not be effective in severe influenza. The symptoms may be relieved by cough suppressants and acetaminophen. Aspirin should not be used during influenza epidemics.

64. How do you prevent influenza?

Influenza virus vaccine is the most effective preventive agent for influenza and should be given in the fall. Influenza virus vaccine can be given in physicians' offices, at the time of hospital discharge, and in local health departments. Many community groups, churches, pharmacies, and groceries also sponsor opportunities to receive vaccine. The vaccine is reformulated each year and should be given annually to ensure protection against the current year's circulating virus. An intranasal preparation was first available for the 2003–2004 influenza season but is only recommended at this time for adults < 50 years old, children, and patients who are not at high risk for influenza complications. Amantadine, rimantadine, and zanamivir may also be used for prevention in those exposed to influenza before receiving the vaccine or those unable to receive the vaccine.

65. Which groups at high risk for complications of influenza should receive the vaccine?
- Patients with chronic pulmonary disease (including asthma)
- Patients with chronic cardiovascular disease
- Residents of nursing homes or long-term care facilities
- Those 50 years old or older
- Chronic medical conditions such as diabetes mellitus, renal dysfunction, hemoglobinopathies, and immunosuppression (including medication-induced)
- Adolescents on long-term aspirin therapy
- Women who will be in the second or third trimester of pregnancy during influenza season (usually late November to early March)

66. Who should receive the influenza vaccine because of high likelihood of transmitting the virus to high-risk groups?
- Physicians and allied health professionals, nurses, health professions students with patient contacts, and office and hospital staff with direct patient contact
- Emergency medical personnel
- Home care givers
- Employees of nursing homes and long-term care facilities
- Household contacts (including children)

67. What other groups should receive the influenza vaccine?
- Travelers to countries where influenza will likely circulate during the time of travel (southern hemisphere during April–September)
- Travelers to the tropics
- Travelers in organized tourist groups
- Essential community service providers (police, firefighters)
- Anyone interested in reducing personal risk of influenza

68. Who should not receive influenza virus vaccine?
- People with documented severe reaction to egg (i.e., anaphylaxis)
- People with a history of Guillain-Barré syndrome after previous influenza virus vaccination

69. Which patients with wounds should receive tetanus immune globulin (TIG) in addition to tetanus/diphtheria toxoid (Td)?
- Those who have received fewer than 3 previous doses of Td
- Those with wounds contaminated with dirt, feces, or saliva
- Those with injuries caused by puncture, sharp object penetration, frostbite, or burns

70. Who should receive the measles-mumps-rubella (MMR) vaccine?
- Women of child-bearing age
- College students
- Health care workers who may transmit infection to women of child-bearing age
- International travelers

At least two doses of MMR are required to obtain full immunity.

71. Who should receive meningococcal vaccine?

- College students
- New entrants to institutions with residential living (e.g., dormitories, military barracks)

72. Who should receive hepatitis A vaccine?

- Frequent travelers to Mexico, the Caribbean, Asia (excluding Japan), Eastern Europe, South America, and Africa
- Patients with chronic liver disease
- Residents of U.S. states with high prevalence (e.g., California)
- Illegal drug users
- Men who have sex with other men
- Day care center staff
- Adults who receive clotting factor replacement
- Food handlers

73. Which immunizations should a person who has had a splenectomy or functional asplenia (i.e., sickle cell disease) receive?

- Pneumococcal
- Meningococcal
- *Haemophilus influenza*

74. What organisms commonly cause nongonoccal urethritis (NGU) in men?

- *Chlamydia trachomatis*
- *Mycoplasma enitalium*
- *Trichomonas vaginalis*
- *Ureaplasma urealyticum*

75. What organisms commonly cause epididymitis?

- *C. trachomatic*
- *Neisseria gonorrhoeae*
- *U. urealyticum*
- Gram-negative organisms (older men)

76. List the bacterial causes of community-acquired pneumonia.

Streptococcus pneumoniae
Group A streptococci
Moraxella catarrhalis
Staphylococcus aureus
Klebsiella pneumoniae
Bordetella pertussis

77. List the nonbacterial cause of community-acquired pneumonia.

Mycoplasma pneumoniae
Influenza A and B viruses
Legionella pneumoniae
Chlamyida psittaci, C. pneumoniae
Coxiella burnetti
Pneumocystis carinii
Other viruses
Fungi

NEUROLOGY

78. What are the prodromal symptoms of herpes zoster (shingles)?

Headache, malaise, pain, and paresthesias (in the involved dermatome)

79. What is meralgia paresthetica?

Meralgia paresthetica is the entrapment of the lateral femoral cutaneous nerve producing pain and numbness over the anterolateral thigh.

80. **What causes meralgia paresthetica?**
- Diabetes mellitus
- Pregnancy
- Obesity
- Sudden weight loss
- Girdles, guns, belts, and other tight-fitting accessories

81. **List the typical symptoms of migraine, tension, and cluster headaches.**
See Table 16-4.

TABLE 16-4. SYMPTOMS OF MIGRAINE, TENSION, AND CLUSTER HEADACHES

Symptom	Migraine	Tension	Cluster
Location	Hemicranial	Entire head or bitemporal	Unilateral
Pain quality	Throbbing	Aching	Burning
Duration	2–6 h	Days	1–2 h
Frequency	Episodic	Daily	Flurry of attacks for several weeks
Associated Symptoms	Prodrome	Neck and shoulder aching	Ipsilateral sweating, flushing, lacrimation and rhinorrhea

82. **What are the prodromal symptoms of migraine headache?**
Scotoma, paresthesias, confusion, and behavioral changes.

83. **Compare the symptoms of a transient ischemic attack in the anterior (carotid) distribution and posterior (vertebrobasilar) distribution.**

Anterior	**Posterior**
Transient paresis of face and/or arm	Transient global amnesia
Paresthesia	Ataxia
Aphasia	Dysarthria
Amaurosis fugax	Weakness, dizziness
Homonymous hemianopia	Hearing loss

84. **What is amaurosis fugax?**
Sudden loss of vision in one eye associated with TIA. It may be described as a "shade" coming down over the eye.

85. **List the symptom triad of Ménière's syndrome.**
Paroxysmal vertigo, hearing loss, and tinnitus.

86. **What are the frequent causes of acute loss of or impairment of smell?**
Head trauma and viral infection.

87. **What is Phalen's maneuver?**
Forced flexion (hyperextension) of the wrist. If carpal tunnel syndrome is present, the symptoms of pain and paresthesia are reproduced.

88. What is Tinel's sign?
If carpal tunnel syndrome is present, tapping on the median nerve over the wrist reproduces the symptoms.

89. Compare the neurologic findings in a patient with the following nerve root compressions: L4, L5, and S1.
See Table 16-5.

TABLE 16-5. FINDINGS IN NERVE ROOT COMPRESSIONS AT L4, L5, AND S1

Root	Disk	Muscle Weakness	Sensory Loss	Absent Reflex
L4	L3–L4	Leg extensors (quadriceps)	Anterolateral thigh, medial lower leg	Patellar
L5	L4–L5	First toe dorsiflexion (extensor hallicus longus), heel walking (tibialis anterior)	Dorsum of foot	None
S1	L5–S1	Toe walking (gastrocnemius)	Lateral foot and fifth toe	Ankle

ORTHOPEDICS

90. How do you treat a coccygeal fracture?
A coccygeal fracture is treated conservatively with analgesics and seating cushions. Inflatable "donut" cushions should not be used because they can lead to pressure ulcers. Coccygeal fractures usually result from a fall.

91. Can hip pads prevent hip fractures?
Yes. Commercially available, small, light-weight pads can be easily worn daily and prevent hip fractures after falls.

92. Which toe fracture should be referred to an orthopedist?
Fractures of the proximal phalanx of the first toe. A fracture that involves the distal phalanx and extends into the interphalangeal joint also should be referred.

93. How do you manage a patient with acute low back pain?
If a patient has no signs of nerve root compression and mild-to-moderate pain, usual activity should be encouraged. Ice to the area of pain may be useful for the first 24 hours, but moist or dry heat is helpful later if used for 20 minutes 3–4 times/day. Pain can usually be controlled with regularly scheduled doses of acetaminophen, aspirin, or NSAIDs. Tramadol can be given by prescription. Muscle relaxants such as diazepam and cyclobenzaprine are needed only for patients with severe muscle spasm.

94. What should be done if the patient has severe pain or signs of nerve root compression?
If a patient has severe pain or signs of nerve root compression, bed rest may be needed but should be limited to only 2 days. Once a patient can sit comfortably, increasing exercise levels is

warranted. Patients with occupations that require prolonged sitting or standing, bending, or lifting will need evaluation and counseling to prevent future back injury.

95. **What is Tietze's syndrome?**
Mild inflammation of the costochondral junction that produces localized warmth, swelling, erythema, and pain. The symptoms are reproduced by palpation of the involved area.

PSYCHIATRY

96. **What are the diagnostic criteria for major depression?**
At least five of the following symptoms must have been present nearly every day for 2 weeks:
- Depressed mood most of the day
- Diminished interest or pleasure in nearly all activities (anhedonia)
- Weight loss or gain or decrease or increase in appetite
- Insomnia or hypersomnia
- Psychomotor agitation or retardation
- Feelings of worthlessness or inappropriate guilt
- Decreased ability to think or concentrate
- Recurrent thoughts of death, suicidal ideation, or suicide attempt

American Psychiatric Association. Diagnostic and Statistical Manual of Mental Disorders, 4th ed, Primary Care Version (DSM-IV-PC). Washington, DC, American Psychiatric Association Press, 1995.

97. **Which medical illnesses can also present with symptoms of depression?**
- **Endocrine disorders:** hyperthyroidism, hypothyroidism, Cushing's syndrome, Addison's disease, hypercalcemia, hyperparathyroidism
- **Rheumatic disorders:** rheumatoid arthritis, systemic lupus erythematosus, fibromyalgia.
- **Neurologic disorders:** temporal lobe epilepsy, chronic intracranial hematoma, cerebrovascular accident, multiple sclerosis, frontal lobe tumor, Alzheimer's disease, vascular dementia
- **Infections:** hepatitis, infectious mononucleosis, Lyme disease, HIV infection, tuberculosis, syphilis, influenza, viral illnesses
- **Nutritional deficiency:** vitamin B_{12}

98. **Which antidepressant causes priapism?**
Trazodone (Desyrel)

99. **List the risk factors for suicide.**
- Male sex
- Single or widowed status
- Unemployment
- Social isolation
- Urban residence
- Recent loss of health
- Recent surgery
- History of impulsive behaviors
- History of suicide attempts
- History of chronic illness such as chronic pain, depression, organic brain syndromes, or psychosis
- History of alcoholism or substance abuse
- Family history of suicide

100. What is an anniversary reaction?

As the anniversary of the death of a spouse, relative, or close friend approaches, the survivor may experience depressed mood or undefined somatic symptoms. An anniversary reaction may also occur after any significant loss such as that of a job, limb, or health or divorce.

101. What is agoraphobia?

Agoraphobia is the fear of being in public places. People with agoraphobia may live a reclusive life. Women are most often affected, and symptoms may present in adolescence or the early 20s. If panic attacks accompany agoraphobia, the patient has at least four of the following symptoms when in a public place:

Dyspnea	Dizziness, faintness	Sweating
Palpitations	Feelings of unreality	Trembling
Chest discomfort	Paresthesias	Feeling of doom or fear of death
Choking sensation	Hot and cold flashes	

102. What are some of the early signs and symptoms of anorexia nervosa?

- Amenorrhea
- Weight loss
- Distorted body image (feeling "fat" even though clearly emaciated)

103. What is the CAGE test?

The CAGE test is a rapid, simple, and reliable screening test for alcoholism that asks four questions. A positive answer to at least two of the questions warrants further evaluation for possible alcoholism.

C = Have you every felt the need to **c**ut down on drinking?
A = Have you ever felt **a**nnoyed by criticism of your drinking
G = Have you ever felt **g**uilty about your drinking?
E = Have you ever taken a morning **e**ye-opener?

Johnson B, Clark W: Alcoholism: A challenging physician-patient encounter. J Gen Intern Med 4:445–452, 1989.

VASCULAR DISEASE

104. What are the physical findings of deep venous thrombosis (DVT)?

Physical finding may be present in as few as 50% of patients with acute DVT. If present, unilateral leg swelling, warmth, pitting edema, or engorged superficial veins may be seen. Physical exam should not be relied upon to confirm or refute the suspected diagnosis. Any patient with suspected DVT should undergo immediate venous duplex scanning.

105. What are the complications of DVT?

Patients with DVT may have pulmonary emboli, which have a high mortality. Untreated DVT can also lead to chronic venous insufficiency with resultant swelling and predisposition to leg ulcerations.

106. What are the characteristics of a venous insufficiency ulcer?

Located on the medial leg with surrounding pigmentation with hemosiderin. The involved leg is usually swollen.

107. How is a venous insufficiency ulcer treated?

The ulcer should be surgically or chemically debrided and any underlying infection should be treated. Moist wound dressings are used. Compression wraps are absolutely necessary to reduce swelling and promote healing.

MISCELLANEOUS

108. Compare the characteristics of bacterial, viral, and allergic conjunctivitis.
See Table 16-6.

TABLE 16-6. CHARACTERISTICS OF BACTERIAL, VIRAL, AND ALLERGIC CONJUNCTIVITIS

Characteristic	Bacterial	Viral	Allergic
Foreign body sensation	–	+/–	–
Itching	+/–	+/–	++
Tearing	+	++	+
Discharge	Mucopurulent	Mucoid	–
Preauricular adenopathy	–	+	–

Adapted from Goroll AH, Mulley HG: Primary Care Medicine: Office Evaluation and Management of the Adult Patient, 4th ed. Philadelphia, Lippincott Williams & Wilkins, 2000, p 1079, with permission.

109. List the characteristics of a person capable of making medical decisions.
- Able to understand the medical information presented
- Able to understand the consequences of a medical decision
- Able to deliberate about the medical decision and its consequences
- Able to communicate decision

110. What is an advanced directive?
An advanced directive is a personal written or oral statement indicating preferences for end-of-life therapies. A living will is an example of an advanced directive. Living wills typically state that a person does not want life-sustaining treatments such as artificial ventilation or resuscitation started or continued if he or she has a terminal illness without the hope of effective treatment. A durable power of health care (DPAHC) designates the medical decision maker for a person who is unable to make his or her own treatment decisions because of incapacity or severe medical illness.

BIBLIOGRAPHY

1. Barker LR, Burton JR, Zieve PD: Principles of Ambulatory Medicine, 6th ed. Philadelphia, Williams & Wilkins, 2002.
2. Dale DC, Federman DD: Scientific American Medicine. New York, Scientific American, 2002.
3. Goroll AH, Mulley AC (eds): Primary Care Medicine: Office Evaluation and Management of the Adult Patient, 4th ed. Philadelphia, J. B. Lippincott, 2000.
4. Noble J, Greene HL, Levinson W, et al: Textbook of Primary Care Medicine, 3rd ed. St. Louis, Mosby, 2001.
5. www.UpToDate.com

CHAPTER 17

GERIATRIC SECRETS

Sarah E. Selleck, M.D.

1. **Why is geriatrics an increasingly important area of research and clinical practice?**
   Although some clinicians may choose practices that inherently limit contact with older adults, it is a rare clinician who entirely avoids elderly patients, younger patients with aging parents, or younger patients whose lives are touched by issues of aging family members. As the American population in 2030 is expected to increase by 32% from the population in 1995, the elderly are expected to more than double to 69 million by 2030. Despite public and personal efforts to remain healthy as we age, this trend will unavoidably be associated with increasing numbers of elderly people deserving specialized medical care for prevention, acute disease, and chronic conditions.

2. **Define "functional assessment."**
   A functional assessment evaluates how people are able to meet needs for self-care (activities of daily living [ADL]) and how they interact with their environment (instrumental activities of daily living [IADL] and gait and balance assessment). These are valuable screening tools, but some patients may not report accurately. They may be polite or tell the clinician only what they think the clinician wants to hear, or they may simply not have the memory or insight to report accurately. Therefore, it is imperative that clinicians probe and seek the corroboration of available informants, because a change in function is often the first sign of physical or mental illness.

3. **Summarize the three major theories of aging.**
   - **Cellular theory:** Proposes that genetic instability (such as accumulated errors in DNA replication) and progressive cellular damage (from both internal and environmental factors such as oxidative stress) cause the aging process.
   - **Autoimmune theory:** Proposes that aging is the result of progressive "self-destruction" through autoimmune mechanisms. This process may be mediated by genetic, environmental, endocrine, or other factors.
   - **Neuroendocrine theory:** Proposes that changes in the neural and endocrine systems cause aging. These changes may lead to the development of diseases that limit life span (e.g., cancers, atherosclerotic cardiovascular diseases).

4. **List the major organ-specific changes in human morphology and function associated with aging.**
   See Table 17-1.

5. **What percentage of persons over age 65 is fully independent in ADLs?**
   Despite the image of dependent, frail elders often seen in our society, 90% of people over age 65 do not require any assistance in performing ADL—bathing, toileting, dressing, walking, and eating.

6. **What is known about sexuality as people age?**
   The frequency of intercourse decreases for most men and women as they age but not to zero! For many people, interest in the expression of intimacy remains high and should be considered in terms of the quality of life of community-dwelling and institutionalized elders. Physiologically

TABLE 17-1. ORGAN-SPECIFIC CHANGES ASSOCIATED WITH AGING

System	Morphology	Function
Skin	↑wrinkling Atrophy of sweat glands	—
Cardiovascular	Elongation and tortuosity of arteries ↓maximum cardiac output ↑intimal thickening of arteries ↑fibrosis of media of arteries ↓rate of cardiac hypertrophy Sclerosis of heart valves	↓maximum cardiac output ↓heart rate response to stress ↓compliance of peripheral blood vessels
Kidney	↑number of abnormal glomeruli	↓creatinine clearance ↓renal blood flow ↓maximum urine osmolarity
Lung	↓elasticity ↓cilia activity	↓vital capacity ↓maximal oxygen uptake ↓cough reflex
GI tract	↓hydrochloric acid ↓saliva flow ↓number of taste buds	—
Bones	Osteoarthritis Loss of bone substance	—
Eyes	Arcus senilis ↓pupil size Growth of lens	↓accommodation Hyperopia ↓visual acuity ↓color perception ↓depth perception
Hearing	Degenerative changes of ossicles ↑obstruction of eustachian tube Atrophy of external auditory meatus Atrophy of cochlear hair cells Loss of auditory neurons	↓high-frequency perception ↓pitch discrimination
Immune	—	↓T-cell function
Nervous	↓brain weight ↓cortical cell count	↑motor response time Slower psychomotor performance ↓complex learning ↓hours of sleep ↓hours of REM sleep

TABLE 17-1. ORGAN-SPECIFIC CHANGES ASSOCIATED WITH AGING *(continued)*

System	Morphology	Function
Endocrine	↓free testosterone ↑insulin ↑norepinephrine ↑parathyroid hormone ↑vasopressin	—

From Kane RL, et al: Essentials of Clinical Geriatrics, 2nd ed. New York, McGraw-Hill, 1989, p 7, with permission.

KEY POINTS: COMPREHENSIVE GERIATRIC ASSESSMENT (CGA) 

1. A medical, psychosocial, and functional evaluation of an older adult.
2. Often employs a multidisciplinary team that may consist of physicians, nurses, social workers, pharmacists, and therapists.
3. Most effective in terms of time and money when used with patients for whom screening raises concerns of frailty, memory loss, depression, falls, anorexia or weight loss, or functional decline.
4. Commonly used tools include the Mini Mental Status Exam (MMSE), Geriatric Depression Scale (GDS), ADL, IADL, and Assessment of stability and mobility, such as the Tinnetti or "Get Up and Go" tests.

all four main phases of the sexual response—arousal, plateau, orgasm, and resolution—change with aging in both men and women, and these changes often combine with physical conditions, such as cardiac disease or arthritis, and with medications affecting libido to affect sexual enjoyment. Clinicians need to be comfortable taking a sexual history with all patients, starting first with open-ended questions and asking about symptoms such as dyspareunia, depression secondary to loss of a partner (be it because of death or illness), and homosexuality.

7. **Why are older people more prone to hypothermia?**
The "thermostat" within the hypothalamus is less responsive to changes in both skin temperature and core temperature and therefore signals shivering to begin at a lower temperature. Shivering in the elderly does generate normal amounts of heat, but the loss of subcutaneous tissue with aging results in a loss of insulation, leading to more rapid loss or gain of heat. Additionally, the basal metabolic rate of the older person is lower, resulting in less heat to conserve. Finally, some older people may have a reduced drive to microacclimatize (put on warm clothing) when the surroundings are cold. All of these small changes (especially in the presence of impaired cognition or sedative medications) can add up to a large risk of accidental hypothermia.

8. **Why are older people also prone to hyperthermia?**
Hyperthermia is increasingly common due to a higher threshold to initiate sweating combined with a lower maximum sweating rate due to both a decrease in the number of sweat glands

and a decrease in the maximum production of sweat by both eccrine and apocrine sweat glands.

9. **Why do so many older people become dehydrated?**
Water and salt homeostasis are well maintained in the healthy elderly in the absence of stress. With stress they are more vulnerable for several reasons. First, the elderly have a decreased thirst drive, and it takes a larger change in plasma osmolarity to stimulate water intake. Even then, the amount of water ingested is often less than necessary. Even the stress of ischemia or an early infection may be enough to cause an elder to drink or eat less, initiating a cycle that can lead to confusion and even less intake—a cycle that quickly escalates to serious dehydration.

10. **How do the age-associated changes in body composition affect drug pharmacokinetics?**
A marked increase in fat mass corresponds to a decrease in lean body mass during normal aging. These changes are less dramatic for women, who have significantly more fat mass throughout life. The results are more fat and less muscle (water volume) in which the drug can distribute. Therefore, water-soluble drugs may have higher concentrations due to decreased volume of distribution, and highly fat-soluble drugs may have lower concentrations at effector sites in the elderly. Furthermore, these drugs are stored in body fat, which then acts as a depot once therapy is discontinued, prolonging the time for drugs to "wash out."

11. **How are the three components of hepatic metabolism affected by aging?**
   - Blood flow decreases in both the arterial and portal systems, contributing to increases in the half-life of certain agents and narrowing the oral dose/parenteral dose discrepancies for drugs that are heavily metabolized during the "first pass" through the liver
   - Phase I reactions, oxidations and reductions, decrease
   - Phase II reactions, acetylations and glucuronidations, are generally unchanged

12. **What is the strongest risk factor for adverse drug reactions?**
Polypharmacy, the number of drugs to which the patient is exposed. Other contributing factors are female gender, small body size, hepatic or renal insufficiency, and previous drug reactions. The presence of multiple chronic medical conditions, altered compliance, and decreased homeostatic mechanisms may also predispose the older person to adverse drug reactions.

13. **Is anemia a normal part of aging?**
No. There is no age-associated decrease in hemoglobin in healthy men and women.

14. **Is there any benefit to smoking cessation for smokers after age 65?**
Yes. The most immediate benefit is to the heart and circulation. Furthermore, the FEV_1 decreases at a much faster rate in smokers than in nonsmokers. Thus, although the absolute level of FEV_1 does not improve with cessation of smoking, the rate of decline does. The elderly smoker is difficult to change; nevertheless, the smoker has much to gain by stopping and should be counseled about the behavioral and pharmaceutical aids available.

15. **Many old people complain about difficulties with sleeping. How many hours of sleep does the average 75-year-old person require?**
Controversy continues, but it is now thought that the number of hours of sleep per 24-hour period changes very little throughout adult life. Because older persons seem to increase daytime sleeping (naps) and decrease nocturnal sleeping, the number of hours of sleep at night decreases. There is a large change in the amount of sleep time spent in the various stages of sleep. Older persons spend more time in stage I (light sleep/sleep-awake transition) and less time in stage IV sleep.

16. **Sjögren's syndrome is more common than previously thought in older patients. What findings are seen in this syndrome?**
Sjögren's affects approximately 2% of older adults and is a chronic inflammatory disease of unknown etiology primarily involving the lacrimal, salivary, and excretory glands. Symptoms may include dry mouth, dry eyes, recurrent salivary pain or swelling, dyspareunia, cough, and dysphagia. In most patients, the ESR is elevated but nondiagnostic. A positive Shirmer test (< 5 mm of wetting of a paper strip placed inside the eye), biopsy, anti-Ro (SS-A), or anti-La (SS-B) is diagnostic. Treatment is symptomatic, and patients with Sjögren's have an increased risk of non-Hodgkin's lymphoma.

17. **How much money is spent annually on health care costs for each person over 65?**
Data from 1996, looking at per capita health care cost by age group (including hospital, home care, and prescription drugs) ranged from approximately $6000 per capita for those 65–69 up to more that $16,000 per capita for those over 85. Much of this expense is "out of pocket" for patients and their families.

18. **An older person under your care appears unable to live independently at home. What resources might you offer before suggesting that the person needs to move from his or her home?**
Many communities have programs offering home-delivered meals and friendly visitor programs. Day programs and home health aides may help an elder stay at home longer. Finally, never underestimate the informal network of family and friends that might offer assistance.

19. **What is required for Medicare to provide care at home?**
A patient must be certified by a physician as meeting criteria for being "homebound" and have a need for skilled care that is expected to be of limited duration. For example, Medicare may provide wound care or monitoring for urinary catheter function for a limited period. Medicare will not provide for custodial care or ongoing nursing care. Medicaid and private sources generally have similar criteria.

20. **What is elder abuse? How significant is the problem?**
Elder abuse refers to any mistreatment of an elder, by omission or commission, that results in actual harm or even threatened harm to the health or welfare of an older adult. This definition encompasses not only situations of direct physical and financial abuse but also neglect, abandonment, failure to provide adequate housing and medical care, and even self-neglect. Although extremely difficult to measure, there are reports that 3% of community-based elders in the United States acknowledge being victimized.

Lachs MS, Pillemer K: Abuse and neglect of elderly persons. N Engl J Med 332(7):437–443, 1995.

21. **What are some of risk factors for abuse? What are some of the signs?**
Poor health, cognitive decline, substance abuse by the elder or caregivers, shared living arrangements, external stresses, social isolation, and a history of violence in the home should be "red flags" prompting further investigation by the clinician. Behavioral withdrawal, agitation or depression, poor hygiene, signs of dehydration or trauma, and missed appointments are a few other signs of possible abuse.

Lachs MS, Pillemer K: Abuse and neglect of elderly persons. N Engl J Med 332(7):437–443, 1995.

22. **What is the Diogenes syndrome?**
The Diogenes syndrome is a condition of self-neglect, independent of depression and cognitive impairment, that may represent the evolution of a personality disorder. Individuals are unkempt

and may often exhibit hoarding behavior. As they retreat socially, their behavior may preclude proper nutrition so that malnutrition is common. The 1-year mortality rate may be as high as 50%.

Cooney C, Hamid W: Review: Diogenes syndrome. Age Ageing 24:451–453, 1995.

23. **At what age must a person give up driving?**
Driving is without a doubt fundamental to our sense of independence and a very difficult issue for older adults, families, and clinicians. There is no specific age at which one must stop, and statutes vary from state to state with regard to driver retesting. Furthermore, published studies have failed to settle the controversy of safety. Some studies even suggest that a diagnosis of early dementia may not preclude safe driving when a copilot is present. What is certain is that all older drivers need to be asked about their driving habits and accident history and need to be examined for sensory, cognitive, and neuromuscular function. In many areas, occupational therapists and private agencies can assist in referral for assessment and training.

24. **What are some of the risk factors of physical restraints?**
In addition to being dehumanizing, even soft restraints to the wrist, vest, or pelvis carry a risk of physical injury and even death. Restraints may increase agitation and lead to lacerations, fractures, decubiti, thrombosis, or even strangulation.

25. **What are some of the "restraint-free" options for a patient at risk for delirium, wandering, or falls?**
The individual at risk for delirium should first be offered behavioral interventions such as gentle reorientation. A wanderer should have supervision and be allowed to be as active as physically able. And the person at risk for falls should, where appropriate, have therapy to improve strength and balance and be offered assistive devices. Low beds should be used, and mattresses or other absorbent pads can be placed on the floor next to the bed. For those without the insight or physical ability to safely arise unassisted, bean-bag chairs can provide a minimally restrictive "restraint."

CARDIOVASCULAR DISORDERS

26. **Why is it important to identify diastolic dysfunction as distinct from systolic dysfunction?**
Diastolic dysfunction results from impaired relaxation in heart failure with preserved ejection fracture and may account for half of all cases of heart failure in people over 80. Clinically, the symptoms may be similar to those of systolic dysfunction, but the traditional therapy for systolic dysfunction can actually worsen ventricular filling and increase the risk of orthostasis and syncope. Treatment for diastolic dysfunction may include calcium channel blockers or beta blockers.

27. **How and why would you take postural blood pressure measurements?**
Blood pressure is measured 1–2 minutes after arising. A measurement that is least 20 mm (systolic) or 10 mm (diastolic) lower than the seated readings defines othostatic hypotension (OH). The etiology is often multifactorial, resulting from irreversible anatomic or neurovascular changes. It is important to identify OH because it can be caused by or exacerbated by many of the medications commonly used in the elderly, leading to falls, presyncope, or syncope.

28. **What is Osler's maneuver? How does it affect the diagnosis of hypertension?**
If the blood pressure cuff is pumped above the systolic blood pressure and the brachial or radial arteries are still palpable, this is a positive Osler's maneuver, resulting from the rigid, heavily calcified arteries commonly encountered in the elderly. The result is an overestimation of blood pressure with a lower, actual intra-arterial pressure.

29. **What does a fourth heart sound (S_4) signify?**
An S_4 likely results from the decreased compliance of the ventricular septum and is very common in older persons and usually of limited clinical significance. The presence of an S_3 gallop, however, is never normal in an older person and is characteristic of CHF.

30. **How common is atherosclerotic heart disease?**
Approximately 30% of people older than 75 have symptomatic heart disease. The prevalence increases with age, and autopsy findings suggest that nearly everyone has atherosclerosis, to some degree, at the time of death. However, many people remain completely asymptomatic throughout their lives or have atypical presentations of atherosclerotic heart disease.

KEY POINTS: FEATURES OF RENOVASCULAR HYPERTENSION AS A CAUSE OF SECONDARY HYPERTENSION 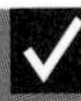

1. Sudden onset of hypertension
2. Sudden exacerbation of previously well-controlled hypertension
3. Hypertension with acute renal failure especially associated with an ACE inhibitor
4. Hypertension with an abdominal or flank bruit

31. **What is the difference between aortic sclerosis and aortic stenosis?**
Aortic sclerosis is the source of many benign murmurs in the elderly, resulting from hardening and fibrosis of the aortic cusps, and is not hemodynamically significant. **Aortic stenosis** is not uncommon in the elderly and is usually due to calcification of a bicuspid valve in the younger elderly patient or degenerative calcification in those over 75. By definition, impedance to flow accompanies aortic stenosis.

32. **How do you distinguish between aortic sclerosis and aortic stenosis?**
It is difficult to distinguish these two conditions by examination alone in all but the most severe cases of aortic stenosis. Therefore, an echocardiogram with Doppler is usually required for definitive diagnosis.

33. **Should one worry about frequent premature ventricular contractions in an asymptomatic, otherwise healthy man over 65?**
No. The key is that the patient is not believed to have any significant ischemic disease. However, once someone has experienced a myocardial infarction, age by itself is a risk factor for increased arrhythmias, and in the Cardiac Arrhythmia Suppression studies, subjects with ischemia and a low EF had decreased deaths when treated with antiarrhythmic agents.

34. **How common is atrial fibrillation?**
The prevalence in the elderly may be as high as 15% and increases with advancing age. The increased inability of the elderly to tolerate atrial fibrillation is due to the older heart's dependence on atrial systole for left ventricular filling.

35. **What does apple-green birefringence under polarized microscopy signify?**
Amyloid protein fibrils stained with Congo red stain appear bright, apple green. Amyloid is an extracellular, proteinaceous substance that exists in several forms. In its most innocent presentation, it is clinically silent and common at autopsy. In other forms, tissue infiltration can lead to amyloid angiopathy, arthropathy, restrictive cardiopathy, neuropathy, and nephropathy, and infiltrative liver disease—all of which are associatied with a high mortality.

36. What important points should be conveyed to an elder starting an exercise program?

Exercise programs carry tremendous therapeutic benefits in terms of prevention of illness and the treatment of chronic conditions, at any age. Even the oldest old derive real, measurable benefits from regular aerobic and strengthening programs. A target heart rate should be 70–80% of the calculated maximum heart rate. More simply, this is usually 15–20 bpm above the resting heart rate. Simpler still is to aim for a rate of exercise that still allows comfortable conversation.

NEUROLOGIC/PSYCHIATRIC DISORDERS

37. Why is it important to distinguish patients with cardiovascular syncope from those with syncope of other causes?

Patients with a cardiovascular etiology (anatomic, myocardial, or electrical) for syncopal episodes have a much higher 1-year mortality (20%) than those with a defined non-cardiovascular etiology or those whose etiology is uncertain after work-up. This is thought to be due to the underlying cardiovascular diseases for which syncope serves as a marker (especially aortic stenosis).

38. Does jaw pain with chewing have any significance? How about a headache with scalp tenderness?

Both of these unusual complaints may be the symptoms of temporal arteritis. Both problems are most common in (but not exclusive to) elderly, white women. Temporal arteritis may rapidly produce monocular or binocular blindness and needs to be addressed urgently when suspected, because corticosteroids can prevent blindness. The ESR is usually elevated, but the definitive diagnosis requires a temporal artery biopsy. Scheduling the procedure should not delay the initiation of steroid therapy with prednisone at 1 mg/kg per day.

KEY POINTS: CLASSIC FEATURES OF NORMAL PRESSURE HYDROCEPHALUS

1. Dementia
2. Urinary incontinence
3. Gait abnormalities
4. May be a reversible dementia when treated early
5. May be treated by ventriculoatrial shunting

39. Define dementia.

Dementia is not a single disease but a general term encompassing many neurologic conditions that lead to a cognitive decline that impedes normal functioning. This term includes impairments most commonly resulting from Alzheimer's disease as well as memory loss associated with Lewy body disease, cerebral vascular disease, Parkinson's disease, and Pick's disease. The clinical presentation, progression, and even post-mortem findings of the many etiologies may overlap, and an individual may suffer from more that just one type of dementia.

40. What is meant by "reversible dementia"?

A condition that is otherwise considered reversible but leads to a similar picture of cognitive decline and altered function is called a reversible dementia. Therefore the work-up for dementia, as guided by history and physical exam, should evaluate for delirium, depression, CNS processes, anemia, malignancy, and infection as well as any renal, metabolic, hepatic, and endocrinologic dysfunction.

41. How can you differentiate depression and dementia?

Apparent dementia by history, examination, or screening tools that actually results from depression is termed **pseudodementia**. On the mental status examination, the depressed patient may answer "I don't know," whereas a demented patient may try to answer even though the answer is incorrect. Depressed patients may have complaints about memory impairments that are out of proportion to the severity of findings on exam. A screening tool for depression, such as the Hamilton Depression Scale, is often helpful, as is neuropsychologic testing. If the uncertainty in the diagnosis persists, a diagnostic/therapeutic trial of an antidepressant followed by continued surveillance and retesting, is justifiable before making a diagnosis of dementia. Keep in mind that these two conditions commonly coexist; therefore, a patient with dementia may improve functionally when the depression is treated, even though the underlying dementia is not affected by the treatment.

42. How common is dementia? What is its cost?

In 2000, an estimated 4.5 million Americans suffered from Alzheimer's disease, and this number is rising. Cases of dementia do occur early in life, although they are rare before age 60. For those aged 65 and older, the prevalence of all forms dementia is 6–8%, while for those over 85 the prevalence soars to 30%. It is estimated that the cost in terms of direct care to the individual and lost wages by caregivers reaches $100 billion dollars annually. The emotional and personal costs cannot be estimated.

43. What percentage of dementia is caused by Alzheimer's disease (AD)?

At least 50–60% of patients with dementia have AD or have a component of AD coexisting with another dementing illness, commonly vascular dementia.

44. What are the two ways to make a definitive diagnosis of Alzheimer's disease?

Autopsy and the impractical option of a brain biopsy remain the only ways to make a definitive diagnosis. The diagnostic requirements are a clinical history consistent with AD and histopathologic confirmation. However, a thorough evaluation of the clinical history, physical examination, and diagnostic tests, as indicated to rule out other forms of dementia, allows most astute practitioners to be accurate in diagnosing AD in more than 90% of the cases.

45. What are the currently available treatment options for Alzheimer's disease?

For the treatment of memory symptoms, four acetylcholine esterase inhibitors are currently on the market in the U.S. The first to be approved by the FDA was tacrine, which requires monitoring for hepatoxicity and is less frequently used. The other three—donezepil, rivastigmine, and galantamine—work in a similar manner, and there is no convincing evidence that any one is more efficacious in slowing cognitive and functional decline. A fifth agent, memantine, targets acetylbuterase and also appears to slow the progression of the disease. To treat the behavioral or psychotic symptoms of AD, behavioral approaches are used as well as the typical and atypical antipsychotics and antidepressants, when indicated. Finally, any treatment plan should include education about the disease as well as resources for support for all of those involved.

46. Are any neurologic signs present in patients with dementia?

On initial evaluation, focal neurologic findings may provide a clue that the etiology of the dementia may be vascular and not purely AD. Furthermore, cranial nerve findings should suggest the presence of an intercranial lesion or chronic meningitis and prompt further imaging and lumbar puncture. Several findings can be seen in advanced dementia, perhaps because of the loss of inhibitory influences. Examples include the snout reflex, suck reflex, and glabellar blink; however, the sensitivity and specificity of these "soft" neurologic signs in identifying patients with dementia are poor relative to those of a mental status exam.

47. **Why is depression common after a stroke?**
Depression may affect up to 60% of stroke victims. The exact reason is unclear but appears to relate to the physical limitations produced by the stroke as well as the location of the stroke. Patients with left frontal infarctions have the highest risk of depression. This area of the brain may play a key role in maintenance of mood. Commonly used antidepressants are effective and may improve not only affect but also performance in rehabilitation.

KEY POINTS: COMMON FEATURES OF DELIRIUM

1. Sudden onset of impaired thinking
2. Fluctuating course
3. Inattention
4. High risk of mortality, morbidity, and increased cost of hospital stays

48. **What neurologic findings would be abnormal in a young patient but possibly normal in a healthy older adult?**
The passage of time has many effects on the nervous system. On cranial nerve exam, a marked limitation of upward gaze is seen in most elderly as well as relatively constricted pupils. There is a slowing of rapid alternation of movements, termed dysdiadochokinesia. In the distal extremities, there may be sensory impairments, and ankle jerks and abdominal reflexes may be diminished or absent in an otherwise neurologically intact older person.

49. **How can handwriting help with the differential diagnosis of tremor? What can a glass of wine do in this regard?**
An essential tremor worsens with intention or movement such as writing and usually diminishes with an alcoholic beverage; however, the resting tremor of parkinsonism is not significantly altered.

50. **Who gets tardive dyskinesia? How is it treated?**
Tardive dyskinesia usually follows prolonged use of neuroleptic agents. Although older patients seem to be more likely to develop tardive dyskinesia, it is not clear that the duration of use, the specific agent, or the total cumulative dose has any direct relation to the appearance of these involuntary movements. There is little evidence that tardive dyskinesia can be treated with drugs, and it is usually treated with discontinuation of the offending medication, although in a certain percentage of patients, the movements may disappear with time, even with continuation of the neuroleptic agent.

51. **Does an asymptomatic carotid bruit imply impending stroke?**
No. The risk of a cerebrovascular accident (CVA) without warning transient ischemic attacks (TIAs) is only about 1% in the year following the discovery of a bruit. However, the bruit is a marker of widespread atherosclerosis, and the risk of CVA is elevated. The scenario becomes quite different once the bruit becomes symptomatic with ipsilateral TIAs. At this point, therapy may be indicated.

DISORDERS OF THE SENSES

52. **Other than cataracts, which changes in the eye occur with normal aging?**
Other than the changes in the aging eye leading to cataract formation, the periorbital tissues atrophy, the upper lid may droop, and the lower lid can turn inward or outward. The pupil

becomes smaller, and adaptation of the eye to changes in lighting is much slower. The lens loses elasticity, leading to an inability to focus on near items (presbyopia) and to distinguish objects from the background.

53. **How common are macular degeneration and cataracts in older people?**
The prevalence of these two eye problems is very high. The Framingham study reported macular degeneration in about 6% of patients aged 65–74 and in 18% of those 75 or older. Cataracts were noted in 13% of those 65–74 and in approximately 40% of those 75 and older.

54. **What are the two types of senile macular degeneration?**
Nonexudative (dry) and exudative (wet).

55. **Characterize the nonexudative type.**
The nonexudative type is more common and is characterized by drusen (hyaline excrescences in Bruch's membrane). The underlying changes in the pigmented epithelia can produce geographic atrophy. This disorder produces a slowly progressive central visual loss, though only 10% of patients progress to legal blindness. There is no adequate therapy.

56. **How is the exudative form different from the nonexudative form?**
The exudative form of senile macular degeneration is accompanied by neovascularization that weeps and bleeds. Laser photocoagulation and nutritional therapies aim to slow the progression of visual loss in the exudative type, and vigorous research continues.

57. **Are changes in hearing part of normal aging?**
The most common loss of auditory function that occurs with aging is in the high-frequency range, and the minimum sound appreciated by the older ear is increased (louder). This sensorineural hearing loss usually begins in middle age but may not become problematic until later life.

58. **What other loss may complicate hearing loss?**
Complicating hearing loss is the decrease in speech discrimination. When the patient is given words to both ears simultaneously and then asked about information given to one ear, older people seem to have a large age-related loss in discriminant function. Because this test is performed with sounds above the individual's auditory threshold, it is thought to be due to a central processing deficit, independent of the sensorineural loss.

59. **Are there any types of hearing loss that do not respond to hearing aids?**
Although some elderly do not believe that sensorineural hearing loss responds to amplification, it appears that in most cases both of the common types of age-associated hearing loss, conductive and sensorineural, respond to amplification provided by hearing aids. The third type of communication defect, a central processing problem in which the words are heard but not properly understood, may be made worse by a hearing aid that also amplifies the background sound. Such patients need to have extraneous sound reduced for optimal function.

SKIN DISORDERS

60. **What are some of the major risk factors for developing pressure sores or decubitus ulcers?**
Intrinsic factors include chronic disease, immobility, impaired nutrition, vascular compromise, and any condition that impairs a person's ability to sense and respond to discomfort. Extrinsic risk factors include friction, shear, moisture, and urinary and fecal incontinence.

61. **How are pressure sores classified?**
All of the popular classification systems to grade pressure sores use maximum depth of penetration to measure the severity of the lesion.
- Stage 1: Non-blanching erythema limited to intact epidermis
- Stage 2: Penetrates the dermis
- Stage 3: Extends into the subcutaneous fat, limited by the fascia
- Stage 4: Extends beyond the fascia or without apparent boundaries

62. **Define seborrheic keratoses.**
Seborrheic keratoses are hyperpigmented, hyperkeratotic lesions that have distinct borders and an irregular, scaly surface. They are common, benign epidermal lesions in the elderly. They may be light or dark brown, wart-like papules of varying size, generally described as having a "stuck-on" or "greasy" appearance. They are usually multiple and are most commonly found on the trunk. They have no malignant potential, but because of their dark color they can sometimes be confused with malignant melanoma.

63. **Define actinic keratoses.**
Actinic keratoses (also called solar keratoses) are often irregular, scaly silver, or erythematous lesions generally in sun-exposed areas. While many may regress without treatment, many have malignant potential and progress to squamous cell carcinoma. Therefore, removal is recommended.

INFECTIONS AND IMMUNITY

64. **How frequently do elderly persons with active tuberculosis (TB) have a nonreactive skin test?**
As many as 30% of patients with active TB have a negative skin test. The frequency of this scenario appears to increase with increasing age. The booster effect (a more powerful reaction seen after a second PPD applied 7–10 days after the first) reveals that many of the patients who are initially negative have active disease. This approach is worthwhile when TB is suspected and may be an appropriate protocol for screening institutionalized elders.

65. **What is the most common infectious cause of death in the elderly?**
Pneumonia. Many of the changes that occur with aging make the older person more likely to develop pneumonia. Among them are an increased risk for aspiration of oral microflora and a reduced cough reflex. The organisms that inhabit the oropharynx are generally nonpathogenic in the younger person, while gram-negative organisms are increasingly prevalent in the oral flora of community-dwelling elderly individuals and present in almost all nursing home residents. In addition, age-associated alterations in T-cell and antibody affinity contribute to an increased risk for developing pneumonia.

66. **Summarize the treatment options for uncomplicated herpes zoster and postherpetic neuralgia (PHN).**
Antiviral therapy with acyclovir or pencyclovir may reduce acute pain and possibly decrease the risk of PHN, but corticosteroids have not been shown to be effective adjunctive therapy. PHN is more likely to occur in people with advanced age and in those who had extremely painful or sizable rashes. Opiates, tricyclic antidepressants, neurontin, capsaicin and lidoderm patches are also options for treating PHN.

67. **Which vaccinations are useful in preventing illness in the elderly?**
Influenza, pneumococcal, and tetanus-diphtheria (Td) vaccinations are recommended for older patients.

68. **How effective is the flu vaccine? When should it be given?**
The flu vaccine is about 70% effective in the elderly and should be given yearly, in the fall, to all people over 65 as well as to their close contacts who do not have a contraindication.

69. **How often should the pneumococcal vaccine be given?**
The pneumococcal vaccine includes antigen from 23 serotypes that cause more than 90% of cases of pneumococcal pneumonia. Antibody levels tend to decline over time so attention to the latest consensus regarding repeat immunization is important.

70. **How important is the tetanus vaccine? How often should it be given?**
Tetanus remains a fairly uncommon disease, but the percentage of patients over age 50 has been increasing and the mortality and morbidity rates are high. Booster immunizations with adult Td vaccine should be done every 10 years.

71. **Explain the significance of a positive antinuclear antibody test (ANA) in an older patient.**
The frequency rate of a positive ANA test in normal older people is 15%. ANA titers are usually low (1:16 or less) and, in isolation, are of little clinical significance.

UROLOGIC DISORDERS

72. **How common is urinary incontinence?**
The frequency of insignificant loss of urine is quite common in women of all ages. However, the frequency of urine loss of a sufficient magnitude to produce social compromise or health problems is found in 10–30% of community-dwelling elderly, with a lower frequency in men. Surveys of elderly nursing home residents have reported urinary incontinence in 50% of inhabitants. The very high frequency found in institutionalized populations is primarily due to other chronic conditions, but it sometimes results from the use of physical restraints or medications.

73. **What are the main causes of acute and reversible urinary incontinence?**
Because of the severe physical, psychological, social, and economic costs of urinary incontinence, it is important to identify reversible cases and render the needed treatment. The causes of acute and reversible forms of urinary incontinence can be remembered by the **DRIP** mnemonic:

D = **D**elirium
R = **R**estricted mobility, retention
I = **I**nfection, inflammation, impaction (fecal)
P = **P**olyuria, pharmaceuticals

Infection and inflammation refer to acute symptomatic urinary tract infection (UTI), atrophic vaginitis, and urethritis. Polyuria may be due to hyperglycemia or volume-expanded states causing excessive nocturia (e.g., CHF, venous insufficiency).

74. **What are the four different types of urinary incontinence?**
Urinary incontinence is not a part of normal aging, nor does aging cause it. However, many of the physiologic consequences of aging can contribute to urinary incontinence. The four types are stress incontinence, urge incontinence, overflow incontinence, and functional incontinence.

75. **Define stress incontinence. What causes it?**
Stress incontinence is the involuntary loss of small volumes of urine related to events that cause increased intra-abdominal pressure (coughing, laughing, and exercise). It is more common in

females (present with laughing in 50% of young females) and increases with aging. Its causes include weakness or laxity of pelvic floor muscles, bladder outlet, or urethral sphincter.

76. **Define urge incontinence. What causes it?**
Urge incontinence is the involuntary loss of larger volumes of urine due to the inability to delay voiding when the sensation of bladder fullness (urge) is perceived. Causes include detrusor motor and/or sensory instability, either alone or in combination with one of the following:
- Local GU conditions such as cystitis, urethritis, tumors, stones, diverticula, and outflow obstruction
- CNS disorders such as stroke, dementia, parkinsonism, and suprasacral spinal cord injury or disease

77. **Define overflow incontinence. What causes it?**
Overflow incontinence is the involuntary loss of small amounts of urine resulting from mechanical forces on an overdistended bladder or from other effects of urinary retention on bladder and sphincter function. Causes are anatomic obstruction by the prostate, stricture, or cystocele; acontractile bladder associated with diabetes mellitus or spinal cord injury; and neurogenic (detrusor-sphincter dyssynergy) associated with multiple sclerosis and other suprasacral spinal cord injury.

78. **Define functional incontinence. What causes it?**
Functional incontinene is leakage of urine associated with inability to toilet because of impairment of cognitive and/or physical functioning, psychological unwillingness, or environmental barriers. It is seen in severe dementia and other neurologic disorders as well as psychological conditions such as depression, regression, anger, and hostility.

79. **How are the four types of urinary incontinence treated?**
- **Stress incontinence:** pelvic floor (Kegel) exercises, alpha-adrenergic agonists, estrogen, biofeedback, behavioral training, periurethral injections, surgical bladder neck suspension.
- **Urge incontinence:** bladder relaxants, estrogen (if vaginal atrophy is present), training procedures (e.g., biofeedback, behavioral therapy), surgical removal of obstructing or other irritating pathologic lesions.
- **Overflow incontinence:** surgical removal of obstruction, intermittent catheterization (if practical), bladder retraining, indwelling catheterization.
- **Functional incontinence:** behavioral therapies (e.g., habit training, scheduled toileting), environmental manipulations, incontinence undergarments and pads, external collection devices, bladder relaxants (selected patients), indwelling catheters (selected patients).

80. **List the indications for a chronic indwelling Foley catheter.**
There are only a few indications for a chronic indwelling Foley catheter.
- Urinary retention should be treated with chronic catheterization if it produces renal dysfunction, infections, or overflow incontinence and if it is not treatable with surgery, medications, and intermittent catheterization.
- Decubitus ulcers, or skin irritations, whose healing is complicated by incontinence, may justify a catheter while wounds are healing.
- Severe disability in a patient with a terminal illnesses or a condition such as severe rheumatoid arthritis in whom any movement is very painful may benefit form a catheter. Rarely, such as at the end of life, a catheter may be acceptable when used for patient or caregiver convenience.

81. **What are the risks of a chronic indwelling Foley catheter?**
Risks of long-term catheter use include UTIs, pyelonephritis, stones, periurethral abscesses, urosepsis, and colonization with virulent or resistent bacteria and yeast.

GASTRIC DISORDERS

82. List the main causes of fecal incontinence.

- Fecal impaction with overflow diarrhea
- Laxative overuse or abuse
- Neurologic disorders (dementia, stroke, spinal cord injury)
- Colorectal disorders (diarrheal illnesses, rectal sphincter damage, neoplastic or inflammatory processes)

83. Does an enterostomal feeding tube eliminate aspiration in a chronically ill or demented patient?

The risks of aspiration and attendant complications of pneumonia are not eliminated by a feeding tube. Placement of such a tube should be done only after careful consideration of all issues surrounding the patient's functional status, potential for improvement, and previously expressed wishes regarding health care. Such an intervention in cases of an irreversible, progressive disorder such as dementia, may only extend life at the cost of increasing the likelihood of contractures, decubiti, and infection.

84. What are the common causes of lower GI bleeding in an elderly person?

Bleeding from diverticula is the most common cause, followed by bleeding due to angiodysplasia. These two causes explain 75% of the cases of lower GI bleeds. Colonic polyps, colon carcinoma, ischemic colitis, and inflammatory bowel disease are other causes of blood loss in the elderly.

CANCER

85. What differences are seen between breast cancers in younger women and older women?

Elderly women are much more likely to have estrogen receptor–positive breast cancer, implying a malignancy that will be more responsive to hormonal manipulation and possibly slower-growing.

86. What percentage of prostate cancers is confined to the prostate or local pelvis at time of diagnosis?

Only about 30% of prostate cancers are local at time of diagnosis. Two thirds are widespread and incurable at diagnosis. Fortunately, the malignancy is usually responsive to hormonal manipulation, which controls the disease and alleviates symptoms.

87. When an older person is found to a have a monoclonal gammopathy of undetermined significance (MGUS), what are the chances of developing a related malignancy in the next 10 years?

A monoclonal gammopathy is a condition in which a monoclonal protein (M spike) is identified on serum protein electrophoresis of IgG < 3.5 g/dl or IgA < 2 gm/dL without associated signs or symptoms of a hematologic abnormality. At 10 years of follow-up, 40% of elderly patients diagnosed with MGUS are stable, 40% have died from other causes, and 10–20% have myeloma, macroglobulinemia, amyloidosis, or non-Hodgkin's lymphoma.

88. What treatments are used for early chronic lymphocytic leukemia (CLL)?

CLL is the most common leukemia in the United States, and the incidence increases with age. Observation is generally chosen for patients in the early stages; alkylating agents and combination chemotherapy are offered to other selected patients.

MUSCULOSKELETAL DISORDERS

89. How is Paget's disease of the bone most often diagnosed in the elderly?
This disease of increased bone resorption with disordered formation is generally diagnosed following the work-up for an increased alkaline phosphatase found on routine blood work. Other serum markers of increased turnover suppport the diagnosis, which is confimed by classic radiographic findings.

90. What are the clinical manifestations of Paget's disease of bone?
About 10–20% of patients are asymptomatic, while others may have a combination of symptoms. Bone pain, deformities, and pathologic fractures are the most common. Other symptoms include more rare cardiovascular and neurologic manifestations, hypercalcemia, and osteogenic sarcoma.

91. How is Paget's disease treated?
Treatment goals are to minimize pain and to decrease the risk of orthopedic, neurologic, renal, and cardiac complications. NSAIDs or COX-2 inhibitors, bisphosphonates (chosen with respect to side effects), and calcium supplements (to decrease the risk of disordered bone formation) are commonly used. In some instances, surgery may be appropriate to increase joint mobility as well as to relieve nerve compression syndromes.

92. What are premonitory falls? With which diseases are they associated?
About 5% of falls are premonitory, signaling the presence of a serious systemic illness. These underlying illnesses are typically pneumonia, UTIs, or CHF exacerbations. A fall can even be the presenting complaint in an acute myocardial infarction or neoplastic process.

93. What types of falls are commonly seen in patients with parkinsonism?
Falls are very common in patients with parkinsonism, due to bradykinesia, rigidity, gait disturbance, and postural instability The typical festinating gait, in which patients appear to be accelerating as if to catch up with their center of gravity, may lead to forward falls. At the time of arising, postural instability may lead to falling backwards. Short steps that do not clear the ground adequately increase the likelihood of tripping over objects.

94. List common the risk factors for hip fracture.

Female sex	Increasing age
White race	Psychotropic drugs
Thin body habitus	Ethanol use
Hemiplegia	Previous hip fracture
Cigarette smoking	Surgical bilateral oophorectomy
Chronic corticosteroid use	(before natural menopause)
History of falls	

Many of these risk factors lead to osteopenia, thus increasing the risk for fracture.

95. How frequently do patients with hip fractures report prior falls?
Hip fractures are very common and one of the most dread sequelae of falling. About 15% of patients with hip fracture report previous falls. Therefore, early intervention in a patient who falls may prevent recurrent falls and significantly decrease the number of hip fractures that can ultimately lead to death, disability, or institutionalization.

96. When might you order a bone mineral density scan?
Bone densitometry, commonly of the spine and hip, should be done for any male or female with risk factors for osteoporosis, fractures, hyperthyroidism, hyperparathyroidism, Cushing's disease, height loss, or low testosterone.

97. What are the Z and T scores on a bone mineral density (BMD) test?

BMD is calculated in gm/cm^2 and then compared with standard values for the patient's age and standard values for a young adult. The number of standard deviations (SDs) above or below the standard for the person's age is the **Z value**, and the number of SD above or below the values for the young adult (supposedly replete bone) is called the **T value**. The World Health Organization defines a T value of less than 2.5 as osteoporosis and a T value of 1–2.5 as osteopenia. Fracture risk is considered to double for each SD below the mean.

98. Discuss major considerations in choosing to treat osteoporosis.

The goal of treatment is to stop any further bone loss and to increase BMD to a level that reduces fracture risk. Individual treatment is based on functional status, other medical conditions, and any possible adverse side effects of therapy. In addition to weight-bearing exercise, calcium, and vitamin D, the most commonly used agents now include bisphophonates, calcitonin, and raloxifene.

99. What are contractures? How do they develop?

Contractures are the result of fibrosis of periarticular structures and shortening of muscles and tendons. The process can occur within just 7 days if regular, full motion of the joint is not maintained for whatever reason. Contractures are difficult to treat once they are present; therefore, preventative measures, such as bedside passive range-of-motion exercises, should be used in all immobilized or ill patients. However, if they occur and are addressed early, contractures can be reversed.

BIBLIOGRAPHY

1. Cassel, CK, et al (eds): Geriatric Medicine: An Evidence-based Approach, 4th ed. New York, Springer, 2003.
2. Cobbs EL, Duthie EH, Murphy JB: Geriatrics Review Syllabus: A Core Curriculum in Geriatric Medicine. New York, American Geriatrics Society, 2002.
3. Forciea MA, Schwab EP, Raziano DB, Lavizzo-Mourey RJ: Geriatric Secrets, 3rd ed. Philadelphia, Hanley & Belfus, 2004.
4. Gallo JJ, et al (eds): Reichel's Care of the Elderly, 5th ed. Philadelphia, Lippincott Williams & Wilkins, 1999.
5. Hazzard WR, et al (eds): Principles of Geriatric Medicine and Gerontology, 5th ed. New York, McGraw-Hill, 2003.
6. Kane RL, et al: Essentials of Clinical Geriatrics, 5th ed. New York, McGraw-Hill, 2004.

INDEX

Page numbers in **boldface type** indicate complete chapters.

J

K

L

Q

R

S